MW00489512

Cardiac Surgery Essentials

for Critical Care Nursing

Sonya R. Hardin, PhD, RN, CCRN, NP-C
Roberta Kaplow, PhD, APRN-CCNS, AOCNS, CCRN

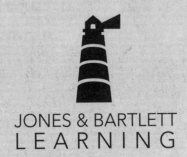

JONES & BARTLETT
LEARNING

World Headquarters
Jones & Bartlett Learning
5 Wall Street
Burlington, MA 01803
978-443-5000
info@jblearning.com
www.jblearning.com

Jones & Bartlett Learning books and products are available through most bookstores and online booksellers. To contact Jones & Bartlett Learning directly, call 800-832-0034, fax 978-443-8000, or visit our website, www.jblearning.com.

Substantial discounts on bulk quantities of Jones & Bartlett Learning publications are available to corporations, professional associations, and other qualified organizations. For details and specific discount information, contact the special sales department at Jones & Bartlett Learning via the above contact information or send an email to specialsales@jblearning.com.

Copyright © 2016 by Jones & Bartlett Learning, LLC, an Ascend Learning Company

All rights reserved. No part of the material protected by this copyright may be reproduced or utilized in any form, electronic or mechanical, including photocopying, recording, or by any information storage and retrieval system, without written permission from the copyright owner.

The content, statements, views, and opinions herein are the sole expression of the respective authors and not that of Jones & Bartlett Learning, LLC. Reference herein to any specific commercial product, process, or service by trade name, trademark, manufacturer, or otherwise does not constitute or imply its endorsement or recommendation by Jones & Bartlett Learning, LLC and such reference shall not be used for advertising or product endorsement purposes. All trademarks displayed are the trademarks of the parties noted herein. *Cardiac Surgery Essentials for Critical Care Nursing, Second Edition* is an independent publication and has not been authorized, sponsored, or otherwise approved by the owners of the trademarks or service marks referenced in this product.

There may be images in this book that feature models; these models do not necessarily endorse, represent, or participate in the activities represented in the images. Any screenshots in this product are for educational and instructive purposes only. Any individuals and scenarios featured in the case studies throughout this product may be real or fictitious, but are used for instructional purposes only.

The authors, editor, and publisher have made every effort to provide accurate information. However, they are not responsible for errors, omissions, or for any outcomes related to the use of the contents of this book and take no responsibility for the use of the products and procedures described. Treatments and side effects described in this book may not be applicable to all people; likewise, some people may require a dose or experience a side effect that is not described herein. Drugs and medical devices are discussed that may have limited availability controlled by the Food and Drug Administration (FDA) for use only in a research study or clinical trial. Research, clinical practice, and government regulations often change the accepted standard in this field. When consideration is being given to use of any drug in the clinical setting, the health care provider or reader is responsible for determining FDA status of the drug, reading the package insert, and reviewing prescribing information for the most up-to-date recommendations on dose, precautions, and contraindications, and determining the appropriate usage for the product. This is especially important in the case of drugs that are new or seldom used.

07901-2

Production Credits

VP, Executive Publisher: David D. Cella
Executive Editor: Amanda Martin
Acquisitions Editor: Teresa Reilly
Associate Acquisitions Editor: Rebecca Myrick
Editorial Assistant: Lauren Vaughn
Production Manager: Carolyn Rogers Pershouse
Production Editor: Sarah Bayle
Marketing Communications Manager: Katie Hennessy

VP, Manufacturing and Inventory Control: Therese Connell
Composition: Cenveo Publisher Services
Cover Design: Michael O'Donnell
Rights and Media Research Coordinator: Ashley Dos Santos
Media Development Assistant: Shannon Sheehan
Cover Image: green light blur image © Leah Groisberg/
    ShutterStock, Inc.
Printing and Binding: Edwards Brothers Malloy
Cover Printing: Edwards Brothers Malloy

Library of Congress Cataloging-in-Publication Data
Cardiac surgery essentials for critical care nursing / [edited by] Sonya R. Hardin, Roberta Kaplow. — Second edition.
    p. ; cm.
Includes bibliographical references and index.
ISBN 978-1-284-06832-0
I. Hardin, Sonya R., editor. II. Kaplow, Roberta, editor.
[DNLM: 1. Heart Diseases—nursing. 2. Cardiac Surgical Procedures—nursing. 3. Critical Care—methods. WY 152.5]
RC674
616.1'20231--dc23
                        2015005277
6048

Printed in the United States of America
19 18 17   10 9 8 7 6 5 4 3

Dedication

This book is dedicated to Susan, Grace, Jessie, James, and Bria. We are grateful for your love, support, patience, and encouragement as we worked on the production of this book.

A special thanks to James R. Perron, PE, our medical illustrator, who was responsive to all of our late-hour requests and showed great patience with our attention to detail. He was a true asset to the development of this book.

Contents

Contributors

Tracy D. Andrews, DNP, ACNP, APRN-BC
Program Director
Adult Gerontology Acute Care Nurse
 Practitioner Program
Columbia University School of Nursing
New York, New York

Mary Jane Bowles, DNP, RN, CCRN, CNS-BC
Mary Washington Healthcare
Clinical Nurse Specialist
Fredericksburg, Virginia

Susan K. Chase, EdD, RN, FNP-BC, FNAP
Associate Dean for Graduate Affairs and Professor
College of Nursing, University of Central Florida
Orlando, Florida

Becky Dean, MSN, APRN, ACNS-BS, CCRN
Clinical Nurse Specialist in Cardiology
Emory University Hospital
Atlanta, Georgia

Myra F. Ellis, MSN, RN, CCRN-CSC
Clinical Nurse IV
Duke Medical Pavilion 7 West (CTICU)
Duke University Hospital
Durham, North Carolina

Brianna Gee, FNP-C
Valve Clinic Coordinator/Nurse Practitioner
Department of Cardiac Surgery
East Carolina Heart Institute
Greenville, North Carolina

Tamara S. Goda, DNP, ANP-BC
Manager, Advanced Clinical Practice, Division
 of Cardiovascular Sciences
Nurse Practitioner, Cardiac Surgery
East Carolina Heart Institute
Greenville, North Carolina

Barbara Hutton-Borghardt, MSN, RN, CCRN, CMC
Clinical Nursing Supervisor
Memorial Sloan Kettering Cancer Center
New York, New York

Toni Patrice Johnson, DNP, MSN, APRN, CNS-BC, CPAN
Clinical Nurse Specialist, Cardiovascular
 Surgery
Emory University Hospital Midtown
Atlanta, Georgia

Julie Miller, BSN, RN, CCRN
Staff Development Educator
Critical Care
Trinity Mother Frances Hospitals and Clinics
Tyler, Texas

Vicki Morelock, MN, APRN-CNS, ACCNS-AG, CCRN
Clinical Nurse Specialist, Cardiothoracic
 Surgery ICU
Emory University Hospital Midtown
Atlanta, Georgia

Kristine J. Peterson, MS, RN, CCRN, CCNS-CMC
Cardiac Clinical Nurse Specialist
Aspirus Wausau Hospital
Wausau, Wisconsin

Noreen O. Peyatt, MSN Ed, RN-BC
Clinical Nurse
Emory University Hospital
Atlanta, Georgia

April Miller Quidley, PharmD, BCPS, FCCM
Cardiovascular ICU Pharmacist
Critical Care Pharmacy Residency Program
    Director
Department of Pharmacy
Vidant Medical Center
Greenville, North Carolina

Shelley K. Welch, MSN, RN, CCRN-CSC
Staff Development Educator—Cardiology
Trinity Mother Frances Hospitals and Clinics
Tyler, Texas

Mary Zellinger, MN, APRN-CCNS, ANP-BC, CCRN-CSC
Clinical Nurse Specialist in CVICU
Emory University Hospital
Atlanta, Georgia

Preface

Postoperative care of the cardiac surgery patient is both challenging and dynamic. Changes in technology, new research findings, the advent of minimally invasive procedures, and the development of off-pump procedures now afford patients of advanced age and with higher levels of acuity the opportunity to undergo procedures for which they were deemed unsuitable candidates not so long ago. Hence, patients with more—and more significant—comorbidities are receiving care in the immediate postoperative period in the intensive care unit (ICU).

Patients who undergo cardiac surgery are at risk for several adverse events not only related to their preoperative condition, but also as a result of effects of the surgical procedure and anesthesia. This requires ICU nurses to demonstrate high levels of clinical judgment, clinical inquiry, and caring practices to effectively manage patients and help optimize outcomes. High-level competency as a facilitator of learning is also required as nurses prepare their patients to undergo cardiac surgery. Clearly, ICU nurses, as members of a multidisciplinary team, play a pivotal role in promoting 10-year survival and high quality of life for patients who undergo cardiac surgery.

This book is designed to address the needs of both new and experienced nurses who care for patients in the ICU immediately following cardiac surgery. The purpose of this book is twofold. First, it is designed to prepare the nurse who is first learning to care for patients undergoing cardiac surgery. It addresses significant changes in cardiac surgery and the nursing responsibilities required to meet the needs of these acutely ill patients. Second, the book provides advanced knowledge and a scientific basis for care for nurses who have mastered the essential knowledge and skills necessary to care for this patient population, but who now seek to develop a more in-depth knowledge base about advances in this dynamic field and strategies to optimize patient outcomes. The emphasis throughout the book is providing an evidence-based foundation for care of patients during the vulnerable period immediately following cardiac surgery. A number of chapters in the book will also prove useful to nurses who work in other areas in which there are acute and critically ill patients, as many of the concepts discussed here can be translated into care of patients other than those who have undergone cardiac surgery.

Because this book uses a comprehensive approach to address the needs of patients in the immediate postoperative period following cardiac surgery, it can also be used to help prepare nurses who plan to take the Cardiac Surgery Certification (CSC®) subspecialty exam offered by the American Association of Critical-Care Nurses.

In addition to updating the text based on the changes in cardiac surgery that have occurred in the past few years, two new chapters have been added based on needs of patients, families, and readers. Chapters addressing needs of patients with obesity who are undergoing cardiac surgery and genetics implications complement the book. We sincerely hope the readers find this information helpful and that it augments patient outcomes.

Throughout the book, Clinical Inquiry Boxes highlight research findings that have implications for nursing practice. Other features that promote critical thinking and provide application of content are the Case Studies and Critical Thinking Questions that follow the respective chapter content. To further enhance critical thinking and for nurses preparing for the CSC exam, the Self-Assessment Questions found at the end of each chapter can be used as practice questions.

Chapter 1

Clinical Judgment in Critical Care

Susan K. Chase

INTRODUCTION

The critical care unit provides a location for continuous monitoring of unstable patients as well as a context for the use of invasive technology that supports basic life processes for acute and critically ill patients. Learning about technology and mastering its safe use are often the foci of basic critical care education and orientation. Aside from its technology, the more basic value of a critical care unit is the level of clinical judgment that occurs there. The thinking processes of clinicians from a variety of disciplines are essential to safe and effective care. The potential for optimal outcomes is enhanced when clinical judgments occur with the nurse synthesizing and interpreting multiple, often conflicting sources of data (Hardin & Kaplow, 2005).

Working in a critical care area is both exciting and rewarding, but it is also demanding and challenging. Nurses in critical care are central for rapid response to potentially life-threatening conditions and key in humanizing technological care. Since critical care units were first developed, the monitoring of, and early response to changes in, patients' conditions by nurses have revolutionized care. Nurses in critical care areas must make rapid and accurate decisions about diagnostic and treatment approaches in an independent way, which may include the use of protocols or standard orders. The nurse must constantly judge whether the standard protocols or orders are appropriate for a specific patient. This chapter describes the processes used by critical care nurses (CCNs) as they make these decisions. It will be useful to new CCNs as they learn to provide safe care and to experienced CCNs who wish to improve their processes of thinking and communicating.

The thinking processes used by CCNs differ quite dramatically from the schoolbook description of the "nursing process." The linear process of collecting information, forming a decision, choosing an action, and evaluating that action is rarely used in real-world practice. In critical care, multiple conditions are assessed simultaneously, a variety of actions and interventions are carried out concurrently, and the condition of the patient changes constantly. There is never just one single diagnosis or condition that is "resolved." Patients' conditions are constantly changing, and continual monitoring is required. Because the thinking work of CCNs is not a linear process, this chapter is likewise not linear. It deals in general terms with phases of the "thinking work" of nursing, but acknowledges that thinking and acting often overlap in real life.

Clinical judgment is one of the eight nurse competencies of the AACN Synergy Model for Patient Care adopted by the American

Association of Critical-Care Nurses (AACN) (Reed, Cline, & Kerfoot, 2007). Clinical judgment is defined as the use of clinical reasoning, which includes decision making, critical thinking, and achieving a global grasp of a situation, coupled with nursing skills acquired through a process of integrating education, experimental knowledge, and evidence-based guidelines (AACN, 2002).

CLINICAL JUDGMENT PROCESSES

Research has provided a window into how humans think and make decisions. Several models can help clinicians understand their decision-making processes and help them to become more efficient and to reduce errors in judgment. The three models that are useful in critical care are information processing, intuition, and decision analysis (Chase, 2004). Each model contributes a unique perspective to decision making, and clinicians can choose which model to apply based on matters of individual style. The nature of specific problems may also determine which model is useful in a particular situation.

Information Processing

The information processing model uses the analogy of the human brain working like a computer as it processes new information that becomes available. It also relies on the assumption that an "optimal" diagnosis can be made by taking into account the data that are available in the problem situation. The possible diagnoses or problems that might be present for a patient are called "hypotheses" before they are confirmed. There are usually multiple competing hypotheses to explain a particular pattern of data. For example, a nurse may notice that a diabetic patient has a serum glucose level above baseline. This finding might be a result of several causes—a faster

than expected glucose infusion, a new infection, or a missed insulin dose, among other possibilities. Each of these possibilities is a hypothesis. Further data collection can help to narrow the options by ruling out certain problems or increasing the likelihood of another explanation. In the example just given, if the nurse notes cloudiness in urine and an elevation of body temperature, then the probability that the hypothesis of infection is correct is increased. This, in turn, directs further action by the nurse. More data can be collected, such as a urinalysis and urine culture, to rule in (confirm) a urinary tract infection.

The information processing model focuses on reevaluating competing hypotheses based on new data (Thompson & Dowding, 2002). In critical care areas, nurses frequently work independently in choosing further data to be collected to support a hypothesis. Units may have protocols that authorize the nurse to proceed with further data collection without obtaining orders from a provider. This relative autonomy increases the necessity for CCNs to exercise appropriate judgment. It would not be appropriate judgment for the nurse to run expensive tests if the data do not warrant it. Judgment includes the decision to do things or not to do them. An economy of practice occurs when all appropriate actions—but only appropriate actions—are taken. To make the choice of further diagnostic testing, all information present must be considered.

In real life, nurses frequently need to act before all information necessary to confirm a diagnosis is available. If a condition that is suspected is particularly critical, such as impending respiratory failure, actions to support the patient must be taken even before a full understanding of the reason for such failure is obtained. To wait to offer support until the patient is in full respiratory failure is to miss the opportunity to offer timely interventions that support the patient's function. At times, by taking the most appropriate actions for the most likely problem and then noting the patient's response to those measures, the diagnosis is either confirmed or refuted. If the treatment approach does not work, additional reasons for the patient's problems must be investigated. New data must be considered to help develop a picture that answers the question, "What's going on with this patient?"

In any clinical situation, certain diagnoses or problems are possible, and some are more likely than others. Critical care units are places where monitoring equipment allows for the collection of a wider range of data than in less acute settings. Critical care nurses are the constant collectors and evaluators of clinical data. Early in their careers, nurses new to critical care may focus on the compilation of data through the use of new or unfamiliar equipment such as electrocardiography, monitoring systems that reflect and record hemodynamic parameters through the use of a pulmonary artery catheter, or continuous blood pressure through intra-arterial lines. It is appropriate that new nurses focus on perfecting their skills in managing and interpreting data from these systems. The assembly of information is just one small aspect of critical care nursing, however. The data obtained from monitoring systems represent key components to be utilized in understanding the full clinical picture presented by the patient.

Nurses collect and evaluate data to arrive at a diagnosis. Even after an initial medical diagnosis of acute myocardial infarction (AMI) is made, for example, the CCN has many diagnostic options to consider. Acute MI patients may develop dysrhythmias, cardiogenic shock, pulmonary edema, or anxiety. Early detection of these conditions can lead to early and more effective treatment and better outcomes. As more data are collected, they change the likelihood of recognizing each of the possible complications

that might occur. A normal respiratory rate and arterial blood gas values within normal limits for the patient's age, for instance, indicate that respiratory failure is not imminent. Even simple data, such as vital signs, offer a view of the wholeness of the patient and change the diagnostic possibilities. A normal respiratory rate might indicate that the patient is not in impending respiratory failure or experiencing anxiety. Standard support and monitoring will likely be sufficient to detect any changes in patient status. A rapid respiratory rate or restlessness in the patient should cause the nurse to set up different levels of support and to collect additional data.

Managing Data

In real life, multiple conditions may occur concurrently, and one finding (e.g., vital sign, hemodynamic parameter, lab value, assessment finding) may provide evidence for a variety of conditions. Because so much information is collected and used to form judgments in acute and critical care settings, flowsheets—either written on paper or assembled electronically—are used to organize and present the many pieces of information. Recognition of any condition depends on seeing patterns in the wide range of data available. Additionally, flowsheets enable healthcare providers to see how data points change over time. Individual values in isolation are not reflective of the whole person, nor are they reflective of the direction that a particular patient's condition is taking. Is the patient becoming more stable or less stable? Is mechanical ventilation providing adequate support of physiologic function, or is the patient so agitated or distressed by being unable to speak that expenditure of unnecessary energy is occurring? Is the patient failing to respond to any treatment approach such that multiple organ dysfunction syndrome is occurring? Experienced CCNs develop routine approaches to data collection and recognize patterns in the data. Seeing the whole of a situation comes with experience. It can lead to intuition, the topic of the next subsection.

Intuition

Once the nurse is oriented to critical care, the patterns of human response to challenges faced in critical situations become more evident and easily recognizable. Eventually, the nurse is able to see the wholeness of a situation. The pieces of data are not seen discretely, but rather as patterns indicative of the whole. The nurse may simply look at the patient and recognize impending loss of stability or the loss of the will to live. At times, experienced nurses will see a pattern or feel a "gut" response to a clinical situation that allows them to "know" the situation of the patient without spending time processing individual pieces of data. Of course, to provide the data that an interdisciplinary team needs to set up a treatment plan, nurses must generate data and check on those "gut" feelings they have about the patient. What is interesting is that the intuition precedes the action. Nurses can develop their intuitive skills by discussing their "hunches" about patients, by analyzing which indicators led them to their intuitive sense, and by checking their own accuracy. Experienced nurses can do this in unit nursing rounds or in clinical case discussions.

The AACN Synergy Model for Patient Care recognizes that as nurses gain expertise, they move from Level 1, which focuses on data collection, following decision trees, and using standard protocols, to Level 3, where nurses are able to see the wholeness of situations quickly. A sense of understanding of the direction of processes is part of the competency of these nurses. At Level 5, nurses

synthesize large amounts of data and help the entire team to recognize the "big picture" of what is happening with the patient (Reed et al., 2007).

Decision Analysis

Decision analysis is an approach to decision making based on mathematical models that take into consideration the likelihood of specific responses given action options. What is the likelihood that a patient who is intubated will develop pneumonia? What is the likelihood that the same intubation will allow for physiologic support during response from trauma or surgery? On a larger scale, if a new closed system suction device is used, what will be the reduced cost of care if the rate of a ventilator-associated condition is reduced? Decision analysis uses frequency and cost data to weigh options in care. It can be used for either individuals or groups of patients. Many current guidelines for practice are based on this kind of mathematical analysis. Electronic records and large dataset analytic techniques will support improved decision analysis in the near future. Nurses can participate in the use of decision analysis and can remind the team of the "whole person" view.

RELATIONSHIP-CENTERED CARING IN CRITICAL CARE

All nursing is carried out in the setting of relationships. Despite the fact that many critically ill patients are intubated and unable to speak, nurses form relationships with their patients and their families. Such relationships are not just "being nice"; rather, they are central to coming to know patients and how they respond to the challenges of illness. Critical care nurses learn to recognize the patterns of patient responses. How one patient responds to the physical challenge of weaning from mechanical ventilation is different from how another patient does. For example, one patient may become tachypneic in response to the increased work of breathing during weaning, whereas another patient may experience an increased heart rate. Recognizing and communicating patient response patterns are important to excellence in critical care nursing. Recognizing the patterns of how patients respond to challenges can help the nurse decide when in the day is best to provide physical care or to attempt a weaning trial. If a patient did not sleep the previous night, for example, then rest before weaning may result in a better response.

The relationships formed by nurses also extend to patients' families. Family members can provide needed comfort and a quiet presence, or they can spread their own anxiety to the patient. Supporting the family and managing their responses and connection to the patient are important interventions for optimal outcomes. Additionally, family members can assist CCNs in coming to know their patients, thereby helping ensure that the nurses can understand what matters most to the patients.

Now that we have explored the various ways of thinking that can be used in clinical judgment situations, we will see how CCNs can use these models in day-to-day practice.

DAY-TO-DAY PRACTICE

The use of specialized equipment to allow for the continuous collection of data related to a patient's status was discussed in the previous section. The quality of the data being collected and recorded is a central issue in its use. If an intra-arterial line is improperly calibrated, the readings will be consistent—but they will be consistently inaccurate, which can lead to improper treatment plans being established. Critical care nurses learn during orientation how to set up monitoring systems in anticipation of patient admission to the unit, and they learn routines of validating systems as they assume responsibility. In many units, technicians are available to set up lines and equipment, but verifying the accuracy of readings is the responsibility of the nurse. In addition, over time, readings can drift for various reasons such as lines moving, patient position changes, or mechanical equipment problems. Experienced nurses learn to constantly assess the reliability of the data they collect. If the data pattern does not match the apparent condition of the patient, the nurse rechecks the source of the data for accuracy. The adage, "Treat the patient, not the numbers," is good to remember regardless of whether the numbers are accurate. Other data that might not be reliable include arterial blood gas values if the sample is not read immediately if the patient has leukocytosis. Serum chemistry values may also be inaccurate depending on the quality of the sample, any delay in analysis, or the precision of the analysis.

Establishing and verifying the data collection and monitoring systems are important first steps in critical care judgment. The next step is establishing regular monitoring routines. Most critical care units have unit-specific routines for data collection, and some establish routines for monitoring particular types of clinical problems. These routines are important because a patient's status may change frequently in critical care, and regular monitoring allows the nurse to detect changes early, when intervention can prevent clinical deterioration. The nurse should consider, however, that each decision about data collection also has its own cost. For example, frequent blood draws over time can result in noticeable blood loss, particularly in pediatric settings. Awakening a patient hourly for days and nights in a row can result in sleep deprivation, which prevents healing and can lead to delirium. Sending samples for lab analysis costs the patient and the entire system financially as well.

The timing of data collection is one of the judgments that nurses should make by considering the entire situation of the patient. Additionally, unit protocols for assessment should be periodically reviewed after considering published reports and patient data. At which phase of recovery from major surgery is the patient most likely to have specific complications? When would data collection be appropriately timed to detect a specific complication? At what time should a sample be collected so that results are available for team rounds? Unit-level practice committees can address questions such as these.

Too often, data collection becomes a mindless routine. The numbers are generated and the flowsheet is filled in (either written or electronically), but no one really considers what the data mean. This situation represents a failure of the nurse to exert clinical judgment. It results in wasted energy and resources, and it does not protect the patient. Several ways that the CCN can be thoughtful about the data that are routinely collected are discussed next.

Trending and Knowing the Patient

Electronic or paper flowsheets are developed for specific critical care units to help organize data for processing purposes. By seeing how individual data bits change over time, "trends" can be detected. These trends are more important in determining the status of the patient than any individual piece of data would be. Has the blood pressure been making a slow decline over the past 2 hours? Is this patient's heart rate generally slower than baseline? Identifying such patterns helps to determine the clinical significance of a change in any data readings. For a patient with a normally slow heart rate, a new rate of 80 might

be worrisome; for another patient, a rate of 80 would not be a reason for clinical concern. Flowsheets also allow the nurse to see how readings of one parameter change along with other parameters. Blood pressure readings that are gradually decreasing but remain in the acceptable range might not be of concern. However, if the urine output is dropping during the same period, a condition of low cardiac output must be considered as a possible hypothesis. Additional data about recent fluid loss, rates of fluid replacement, and an assessment for crackles in lungs would be needed. Critical care nurses spend much of their time collecting data. This is not the end of task, however, but just the beginning. Taking time to reflect on the "movement" or trend of the data is essential for critical care clinical judgment.

Even in critical care, contextual patient-related factors are important in coming to know the patient. The AACN Synergy Model for Patient Care points out patient characteristics that are part of each encounter. Central to critical care are consideration of patient stability and the predictability of the course of recovery. Other key characteristics include patient resiliency, vulnerability, complexity, and resource availability. The Synergy Model also incorporates a consideration of the patient's ability to participate in decision making and care (Reed et al., 2007). Clearly, coming to know the patient involves more than just gathering physiologic data.

Common Trajectories

Making sense of data requires knowing the individual patient, but it also requires knowing pathophysiology and understanding the workings of the body's compensatory mechanisms for a variety of critical care conditions. Nurses know, for their own particular specialty unit—be it cardiovascular surgical, trauma, coronary care, neurosurgical, medical, transplant, or some other unit—the particular problems typically faced by patients in that unit. Critical care judgments are formed through a blend of knowing individual patients and knowing the trajectories that patients are likely to experience in a particular setting. In individual orientation programs or staff meetings, the particularities of units can be discussed and a common understanding developed by nurses or, even more powerfully, in an interdisciplinary perspective.

A trajectory is a predictable path or sequence of events that is commonly seen in a particular setting. For example, following open heart surgery for coronary revascularization with cardiopulmonary bypass, patients commonly require vasopressor administration to maintain blood pressure to support patency of newly implanted vessels. In addition, patients may experience tachycardia that can decrease cardiac output. Patients may be mechanically ventilated and have multiple chest tubes and pacing wires implanted directly in the myocardium. They will have central vascular access to facilitate fluid and medication administration. A common trajectory includes improvement in hemodynamic stability so that weaning the patient from vasopressors can occur on the first night following surgery. A decrease in the effects of anesthesia can lead to weaning from mechanical ventilation by the morning after surgery (if not extubated before), and a gradual reduction in chest tube drainage can be noted as blood vessels heal. Deviation from this expected trajectory, such as decreased oxygenation when weaning from mechanical ventilation is attempted or continued blood loss from chest tubes, indicates that this particular patient will require an individualized approach to support. Experienced CCNs recognize patients' progress along specific trajectories. A sense of how the patient is progressing down the predictable path of recovery is one way that the CCN sees patterns and senses the wholeness of the situation.

Surveillance

In critical care areas, nurses use a type of thinking that assesses for problems that do not yet exist. This is a different style of thinking than problem identification. It is a continual scanning for signs that a problem is developing. This method of thinking requires several kinds of knowledge, data collection, and processing. Critical care nurses who wait until a problem becomes obvious before they intervene have missed a chance to prevent a cascade of events.

Knowledge that supports effective surveillance includes a deep understanding of the physiologic responses to the critical care setting and to the particular patient problems being addressed. Knowing that tracheal intubation exposes a patient to risk of ventilator-associated conditions, the CCN with a high level of clinical judgment monitors arterial blood gas results, breath sounds, airway pressures, and vital signs. Waiting until pneumonia is fully evident would result in risk of hemodynamic instability and sepsis, both of which can lead to longer intensive care unit (ICU) stays or death.

Regular data collection for evidence of stability or signs of problems is essential to the process of surveillance. Most important, though, is the nurse's ability to recognize patterns that indicate deviation from the normal trajectory.

Investigating Problems

Experienced CCNs read their "gut" reactions. When patient responses indicate that things are going as predicted, nurses can alter their vigilance. Conversely, if the patient is not following the predicted trajectory, then the nurse appropriately considers other data sources, and discusses possible meanings of this divergent pattern with the treatment team. The nurse does not "rest" until the picture becomes clearer. Even "hunches" about what is going on can be explored and discussed until the patient's picture becomes clearer and data indicate an appropriate direction for decision.

One practice that CCNs use is that of "running possibilities." This process is a form of hypothesis generation, referred to earlier in this chapter. What could be a possible explanation for this finding? Could this person have an unusual presentation of a treatable problem? What if we try a treatment option for a while and see how the patient responds? This sort of thinking frequently happens in conversation with other nurses or healthcare providers (Chase, 1995).

Communicating Findings

Nurses in critical care have more autonomy than nurses in many other practice settings regarding data collection and treatment decisions, such as weaning from various types of support. Critical care nurses do not work in isolation, however, and they contribute to excellence in patient care by working collaboratively with a team of other healthcare providers. One of the skills that CCNs develop is effective communication of their impressions of the status of the patient to other members of the team. Many nurses have had the frustrating experience of believing that the patient needs to be managed in a certain way, but other members of the team do not agree. When the direction of the care and support differs, nurses are obligated to clarify, verify, and question the appropriateness of the treatment plan if they believe that harm will come to the patient. Learning to communicate data and impressions in ways that allow others to understand the basis for the CCN's judgment can minimize this source of frustration.

Assembly of data into patterns that have meaning will assist CCNs in communicating their overall impressions. Calling a healthcare provider and offering random bits of data will often not result in a positive response. The nurse can better organize this process by

coming to know the types of data that individual clinicians value. For example, even if the findings are not abnormal, the amount of chest tube drainage will be important to a cardiac surgeon. When working with new interdisciplinary teams of providers, an anticipatory question can help to establish communication, such as, "Is there any particular parameter that you want us to pay special attention to this evening?" or "I've noticed a downward trend in blood pressure. Is there a level at which you want us to notify you?" Then, should a call be necessary, it has a context. This kind of communication requires "thinking forward."

One method that has been established in healthcare settings to assist with the assembly of data into meaningful patterns is the SBAR (Situation–Background–Assessment–Recommendation) technique. This framework facilitates communication among healthcare providers by providing a focused approach for communicating essential patient information in a usable context so that accurate care decisions can be made (Institute for Healthcare Improvement, 2008).

By understanding the competing hypotheses for the patient's condition, the CCN will be better able to present data in a way that assists the entire team in making good decisions. One kind of data that must be considered is "pertinent negative" data—that is, showing that certain data are normal to reduce the likelihood of one of the diagnostic options. For example, if the blood pressure is trending down, but breath sounds and arterial blood gas results are normal, that combination of findings would decrease the likelihood of left ventricular failure and increase the likelihood that the patient is volume depleted. The breath sounds and arterial blood gas results should be reported even though they are normal, because they assist the other clinicians to understand the whole picture; they are "pertinent" even though they are normal.

Mobilizing the Team

Sometimes a CCN may detect that the patient's condition is changing rapidly and must assemble the necessary team members to respond appropriately. To do so, the nurse may need to page respiratory therapy, anesthesia, or other airway management teams, as well as the primary provider. Making the decision to mobilize the team can be a daunting one for new CCNs. Experienced nurses and leaders can assist the new CCN in making this decision in a timely fashion. On the one hand, waiting until the situation becomes obvious would be dangerous for the patient. On the other hand, if the nurse calls the team in unnecessarily, that decision has costs, both financial and personal. It is possible that the CCN's clinical judgment was at a lower level in the AACN Synergy Model and that the call came prematurely or in error.

To deal with such issues, CCNs can discuss the process of mobilizing the team on individual units and reflect on how the process went: Did the nurse assemble sufficient data to generate the calls? Was the potential patient problem severe enough to warrant the call? Was the presentation of findings sufficiently clear? Did other members of the team respond appropriately? In hindsight, would any aspect of the patient's care be managed differently?

Team Decision Making

Ultimately, the critical care process is a team process. Data support the idea that good communication on a unit results in better patient outcomes (AACN, 2005; Arford, 2005; Estabrooks, Midodzi, Cummings, Ricker, & Giovannetti, 2005; Flicek, 2012; Schmalenberg & Kramer, 2009). Units vary widely in how effectively communication occurs. Several possible problems can occur that the CCN should be aware of and try to correct.

The first consideration is nurse-to-nurse communication. Are experienced nurses helpful to new orientees, or do they require the new nurses to "pay their dues"? This kind of bullying should be recognized as such and dealt with by other observing staff and unit leadership. Other nurse-to-nurse difficulties can come at change-of-shift report, where one shift does not help establish the new shift nurses' understanding of patient baselines due to emotionally charged communication.

Other issues that arise may relate to whether the patient unit is orderly, with supplies on hand and with essential data already assembled. Small things like this can lead to difficult communication and ultimately can result in poor nursing care.

Additional nurse-to-nurse difficulties can happen at the time of patient transfer. It is essential to the clinical judgment process that open and clear communication be established between patient care areas. By sharing with healthcare providers in the new unit what the patient's clinical course or trajectory has been, how this patient is unique, and which approaches have worked best, better clinical judgment is promoted on the new unit.

The healthcare team involves many disciplines and individual technicians. These teams can come to decisions for action using different processes and standards. It sometimes seems as if different disciplines use different languages to describe patient data and situations. Critical care nurses need to learn to be flexible in communication so that essential meaning of data can be communicated to support patient care (Chase, 1995).

Choosing Interventional Approaches

Much of our consideration thus far has focused on clinical judgment as it relates to the status of the patient, patient stability, patient movement along a recovery trajectory, or the identification of problems. Judgment is also required regarding how best to respond to the issues that are identified in the assessment process. All management choices should be goal oriented and contextually appropriate. The AACN Synergy Model provides for a way of matching the CCN's competencies to the patient's needs. "Synergy results when the needs and characteristics of a patient, clinical unit, or system are matched with a nurse's competencies" (Hardin & Kaplow, 2005, p. 4). Even given the same medical condition, the CCN's response to the patient should reflect numerous factors, including those described in the Synergy Model. For example, a patient who has high levels of resiliency, as evidenced by return to baseline data after treatments, can be expected to recover more quickly and need less aggressive support than a patient who, because of longstanding concurrent conditions, might not be capable of rallying. A patient with few external resources might require aggressive advocacy on the part of the CCN.

Goal-Oriented Decisions

In line with the concept of trajectory, CCNs should always have a goal in mind when planning specific nursing actions. If the goal is stability, then support of basic physiologic functioning will support that goal. If the goal is to increase participation in care so as to support the patient–family unit, then adjusting visiting times to allow for prolonged contact might be chosen, provided that patient stability is not compromised. The CCN can then reflect on the effectiveness of those interventions in accomplishing the goal.

Critical care nurses can actively support the unit in developing documentation systems that include goals and nursing actions. If a patient is anxious about how the family is responding to critical illness, for example, being able to see and be with a family member can reduce stress and the related

catecholamine release that can have negative effects on the cardiovascular system. Nursing actions can have real effects on overall patient status. Promoting comfort and dignity for patients is a requirement for humanistic care and healing.

Supporting the Dying

As discussed earlier, the experienced CCN develops a sense of the big picture of the patient's condition and the direction of the trajectory. Often, critically ill patients have life-threatening conditions that can result in death. Death sometimes happens during aggressive resuscitative efforts. Frequently, however, an impending death is recognized by at least one member of the team. The goals of care may then shift to allow for patient comfort and family communication. The transition to caring for the dying patient can be one that provides the ultimate meaningful contribution on the part of the staff. Too often, however, an impending death is a time of competing goals, shifting direction of care, and difficult communication among team members.The CCN can assist in the dying process by maintaining a consideration of "Where are we going?" Asking that question during team meetings can assist the entire team in addressing the futility of care. The patient's and family members' goals will also need to be determined as part of this process, and it is often the nurse who assists in clarifying these values (Hiltunen, Medich, Chase, Peterson, & Forrow, 1999).

A review (Kryworuchko, Hill, Murray, Stacey, & Fergusson, 2013) of studies using the shared decision-making (SDM) intervention (Makoul & Clayman, 2006) for end-of-life situations in critical care units showed that few studies included all elements of SDM, which include understanding the problem, hearing options, and considering values, among other elements. Two studies showed that ICU length of stay was reduced after offering SDM. The study points out that even when the healthcare team and the family understand the gravity of the situation, time may be required to clarify options and come to acceptance. More research needs to be done on how to support patients, families, and healthcare teams through this difficult process. Critical care nurses are key players in this conversation.

SUMMARY

A critical care nurse is not a technician. As a professional nurse, the CCN's focus of care is on the whole person and family at a vulnerable time. The focus of care on the physical problems patients face in critical care is obvious. More is known by clinicians about the functioning of the human body of patients in a critical care unit than by providers in almost any other environment of the healthcare system. Critical care nurses learn over time, however, that more is going on in a critical care unit than simply the care of physical bodies. Critically ill patients are whole human beings. Their fear or trust, their will to live, their ability to participate in care, and family support can make a real difference in patient outcomes. Ultimately, the clinical judgments made by CCNs are pivotal to providing care to acutely and critically ill patients. Nurses are essential to the process of providing care by virtue of their perspective on meeting the needs of the whole patient. These needs can be based on the eight patient characteristics outlined in the Synergy Model. Nurses' constant presence provides for a way of seeing and knowing the person who is experiencing critical illness. Growing in ability to form exquisitely appropriate clinical judgments is a lifetime challenge—but it is one that is rewarding to both patient and nurse.

REFERENCES

American Association of Critical-Care Nurses. (2002). *Competency level description for nurse characteristics*. Aliso Viejo, CA: AACN Certification Corporation.

American Association of Critical-Care Nurses. (2005). *AACN standards for establishing and sustaining healthy work environments: A journey to excellence*. Retrieved from http://www.aacn. org/wd/hwe/docs/hwestandards.pdf

Arford, P. H. (2005). Nurse–physician communication: An organizational accountability. *Nursing Economic$, 23*(2), 55, 72–77.

Chase, S. K. (1995). The social context of critical care clinical judgment. *Heart & Lung, 24*(2), 154–162.

Chase, S. K. (2004). *Clinical judgment and communication in nurse practitioner practice*. Philadelphia, PA: F. A. Davis.

Estabrooks, C. A., Midodzi, W. K., Cummings, G. G., Ricker, K. L., & Giovannetti, P. (2005). The impact of hospital nursing characteristics on 30-day mortality. *Nursing Research, 54*, 74–84.

Flicek, C. L. (2012). Communication: A dynamic between nurses and physicians. *MEDSURG Nursing, 21*(6), 385–387.

Hardin, S. R., & Kaplow, R. (Eds.). (2005). *Synergy for clinical excellence: The AACN Synergy Model for Patient Care*. Sudbury, MA: Jones and Bartlett.

Hiltunen, E., Medich, C., Chase, S., Peterson, L., & Forrow, L. (1999). Family decision making for end of life treatment: The SUPPORT nurse narratives. *Journal of Clinical Ethics, 10*(2), 126–134.

Institute for Healthcare Improvement. (2008). *SBAR techniques for communication: A situational briefing model*. Retrieved from http://www.ihi. org/IHI/Topics/PatientSafety/SafetyGeneral/ Tools/SBARTechniqueforCommunication-ASituationalBriefingModel.htm

Kryworuchko, J., Hill, E., Murray, M. A., Stacey, D., & Fergusson, D. A. (2013). Interventions for shared decision-making about life support in the intensive care unit: A systematic review. *Worldviews on Evidence-Based Nursing, 10*, 3–16.

Makoul, G., & Clayman, M. L. (2006). An integrative model of shared decision-making in medical encounters. *Patient Education &Counseling, 60*, 301–312.

Reed, K. D., Cline, M., & Kerfoot, K. M. (2007). Implementation of the Synergy Model in critical care. In R. Kaplow & S. R. Hardin (Eds.), *Critical care nursing: Synergy for optimal outcomes* (pp. 3–12). Sudbury, MA: Jones and Bartlett.

Schmalenberg, C., & Kramer, M. (2009). Nurse–physician relationships in hospitals: 20,000 nurses tell their story. *Critical Care Nurse, 29*(1), 74–83.

Thompson, C., & Dowding, D. (2002). *Clinical decision making and judgment in nursing*. Philadelphia, PA: Churchill Livingstone.

WEB RESOURCES

Synergy Concept Map: https://www.youtube.com/watch?v=Z-M3VsFnD64

Use the Synergy Model in Nursing Practice: https://www.youtube.com/watch?v=FH4oPWvf0jA

Chapter 2

Cardiovascular Anatomy and Physiology

Susan K. Chase

INTRODUCTION

The heart is a muscular organ located beneath the sternum, between and slightly anterior to the lungs, in a section of the thorax known as the mediastinum. The mediastinum also contains the great blood vessels—the vena cavae, the pulmonary artery, and the aorta—as well as the esophagus and (in children) the thymus gland. **Figure 2-1** illustrates the location of the heart.

The heart is surrounded by the pericardium, a dual-layer sac that is minimally elastic. This sac allows for smooth movement of

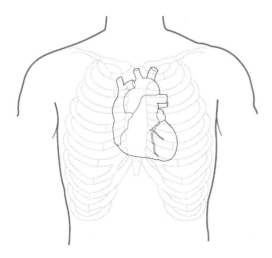

Figure 2-1 The heart and its location in the thoracic cavity.

Source: Illustrated by James R. Perron

the cardiac muscle within the pericardium. If fluid or blood fills the pericardium, it puts pressure on the heart from the outside and prevents normal filling of heart chambers. The main function of the heart is to pump blood throughout the body, thereby allowing for the delivery of oxygen and nutrients to the body cells and for the transport of waste products to processing or removal of organs. Other functions of the cardiovascular system flow from the blood itself. The blood consists of cells that support the body's ability to fight off infection as well as chemicals such as hormones that control processes of bodily systems. In addition, the heart releases hormones that assist in controlling blood flow and pressure.

CHAMBERS AND VALVES OF THE HEART

The structure of the heart supports its functions. The heart consists of four chambers, each with muscular walls (**Figure 2-2**). It also has four valves that control the direction of the blood flow through these chambers. The two upper chambers of the heart are the atria; the two lower chambers are the ventricles. Actually, the terminology of "upper" and "lower" refers to a conceptual picture of the heart, with the most anterior chambers of the heart being the right and left ventricles.

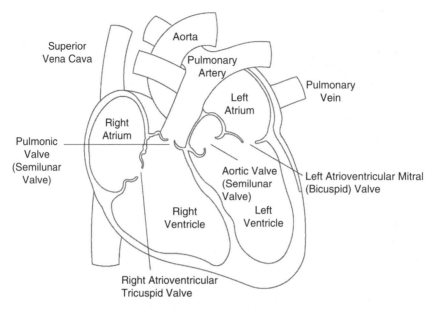

Figure 2-2   Chambers of the heart and valves.
Source: Illustrated by James R. Perron

The muscle walls of the four chambers vary widely in thickness. Because the left ventricle must pump blood into the systemic circulation, which has relatively higher pressure than the pulmonary system, the wall of the left ventricle is the thickest (13–15 mm). The right ventricle is only 3–5 mm thick. The atria have the thinnest walls (2–5 mm).

POINT OF MAXIMAL IMPULSE

The tip of the left ventricle is positioned anterior and to the left in the mediastinum. When the left ventricle contracts, its tip is forced even more anteriorly toward the chest wall. This movement can be palpated as the "point of maximal impulse" (PMI). The PMI is normally located in the midclavicular line at the fifth intercostal space, but can sometimes vary. Abnormalities in the shape and size of the heart, for example, can alter the position and location of the heart itself. A distended abdomen can flatten and elevate the level of the heart. Hyperextended lungs can depress the level of the heart. Enlargement of the heart can cause the PMI to shift to the left in the chest. Noting the position of the PMI can, therefore, give some indication of the size or position of the heart (Woods, Froelicher, Motzer, & Bridges, 2009).

Although most of the heart tissue is muscle, this organ also has a fibrous band that separates the atria from the ventricles and contains the four cardiac valves, which are themselves made up of connective tissue. The cardiac valves consist of fibrous rings to which valve leaflets are attached. The tricuspid valve contains three flat valve leaflets. The mitral valve has two flat leaflets that resemble the pointed shape of a bishop's miter. The pulmonic and aortic valves each have three leaflets that are termed "semilunar" because of their crescent-like shape. The tricuspid and mitral valves (collectively termed the *atrioventricular [AV] valves* because of their location) are attached to chordae tendineae, which are connected on their opposite ends to papillary muscles in the ventricles. The muscles prevent the valve leaflets from being pushed backward into the atria when pressure rises in the ventricular chambers during ventricular contraction. Proper functioning of the valves depends on all these features being intact. The valves themselves are covered with epithelial tissue.

The right and left sides of the heart are divided by the septa. The interatrial septum consists of the fossa ovalis (the sealed foramen ovale that normally closes in the postpartum period) and the muscular walls of the right and left atria. The interventricular septum is formed by the ventricular muscle in the lower portions and by the upper membranous section (Woods et al., 2009).

BLOOD FLOW THROUGH THE HEART AND MAJOR BLOOD VESSELS

Blood flow is determined by a pressure gradient. It flows from areas of higher pressure to those of relatively lower pressure. The valves support "one-way" flow of blood through the heart. The right atrium receives blood from the body through the superior and inferior vena cavae as well as from the coronary sinus, which returns the blood that has circulated through the heart muscle itself. Blood enters the right atrium during atrial relaxation (and ventricular systole). When the pressure in the right ventricle decreases during its resting phase (ventricular diastole), the tricuspid valve opens, allowing the blood flow from the right atrium to the right ventricle. Contraction of the right atrium at near the end of ventricular diastole forces additional blood into the right ventricle. After the right ventricle fills with blood, the muscle wall contracts, increasing the pressure in its chamber, which

in turn forces the tricuspid valve to close. As pressures continue to increase, blood is forced out of the right ventricle across the pulmonic valve and into the pulmonary artery. The pulmonary artery transports the still unoxygenated blood into the pulmonary vascular system. At the end of right ventricular systole, the pressures in the right ventricle decrease and the pulmonic valve closes, preventing blood in the pulmonary artery from returning to the right ventricle. Blood from the right atrium then refills the ventricle for the next systole.

In the pulmonary system, the blood circulates through a series of arteries, capillaries, and veins. In the thin-walled capillaries of the pulmonary circuit, red blood cells exchange carbon dioxide for oxygen. The oxygenated blood then returns to the left atrium, driven by the pressure differential: Pressures in the left ventricle are lower than in the pulmonary vascular system. Oxygenated blood returning from the pulmonary vein enters the resting left atrium. When the left atrium pressure rises higher than the pressure in the resting left ventricle, the mitral valve opens. Blood then passes to the left ventricle across the mitral valve. The contraction of the left atrium forces additional blood into the left ventricle. Finally, as the left ventricle contracts, the pressure there increases and forces the mitral valve closed and the aortic valve open. Blood passes from the left ventricle to the systemic circulation across the aortic valve. It flows to the cardiac muscle itself through the right and left coronary arteries, which arise from the lower aorta, just above the aortic valves. At the end of left ventricular systole, with decreased pressure in the left ventricle, the aortic valve closes.

Each of the cardiac chambers has its own range of normal fluid pressures, which depend on the force of contraction of the muscle walls and the position of the cardiac valves in that chamber. Each chamber has a phase when its walls are contracting (systole)

Box 2-1   Murmur Differentiation

Valve	Stenosis	Insufficiency
Tricuspid and Mitral	Diastolic	Systolic
Pulmonic and Aortic	Systolic	Diastolic

and a phase when the muscle is resting (diastole). Most of the time, the words "systole" and "diastole" are used to refer to the phases of the ventricles. Under normal circumstances, due to the electrical control system of the heart, the atria contract together and the ventricles contract together.

It is useful to be able to picture the heart during systole and diastole when interpreting heart sounds (see **Box 2-1**). During ventricular systole, the AV valves are closed and the semilunar valves are open; blood flows through the latter valves into the pulmonary and systemic circulation. During ventricular diastole, the semilunar valves close and the AV valves open, with blood flowing through the latter valves from the atria to the ventricles. Unexpected sounds heard during ventricular systole could result from tight or "stenotic" semilunar valves (aortic or pulmonic) or from incompetent or regurgitant AV valves (mitral or tricuspid). These sounds are best heard between heart sounds S_1 and S_2. Unexpected sounds heard during ventricular diastole are heard between S_2 and the following S_1 heart sound. These sounds can be related to mitral/tricuspid stenosis or aortic/pulmonic insufficiency (regurgitation). Obstruction to forward flow can be called "stenotic," and backward flow of blood is due to an incompetent valve and can be called "regurgitant." This also causes an unexpected sound. Heart sounds can further be differentiated by noting the area on the chest wall where they are heard most prominently. For example, a sound can be referred to as a "systolic aortic murmur" when it is heard between S_1 and S_2

in the upper right border of the sternum. Such a murmur is often caused by aortic stenosis.

Cardiac surgery often involves the replacement or repair of cardiac valves. The heart and lungs of patients with long-term valve disorders have often adapted to changes in pressure and blood flow and may result in dysfunction even after the valve has been repaired. Patients may need support until physiology returns to more normal responses.

Being able to think spatially will assist the nurse in making sense of cardiovascular assessment data. The diagram of the cardiac cycle in **Figure 2-3** shows the simultaneous events of cardiac function, including pressure changes in individual vessels and chambers and electrical activity.

CORONARY ARTERIES

Normally we think of tissue perfusion as occurring during systole, but because the pressure in the muscle tissue during ventricular systole is so high, the coronary arteries are perfused during ventricular diastole. The left main coronary artery divides fairly quickly into the left anterior descending (LAD) artery and the circumflex artery (CA) (**Figure 2-4**). The right coronary artery (RCA) supplies most of the right atrium and ventricle and the sinoatrial (SA) node (in 60% of people), the AV node (in 80–90% of people), and part of the bundle branches. The LAD artery supplies the left atrium and ventricle, including the ventricular septum. The circumflex artery supplies the posterior portion of the left ventricle and the left atrium. The blood supply to the SA node of 40% of the population is received through the left circumflex artery. The venous return of the heart leads to the great coronary vein, which parallels the circumflex artery and eventually returns to the right atrium.

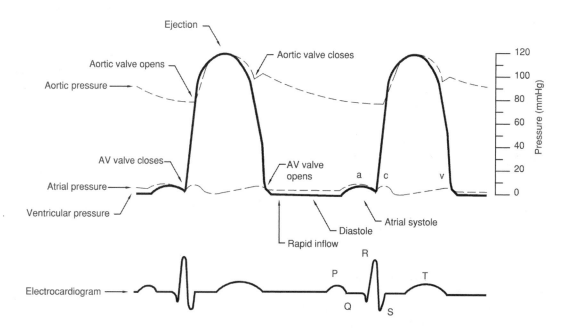

Figure 2-3   The cardiac cycle.

Source: Illustrated by James R. Perron

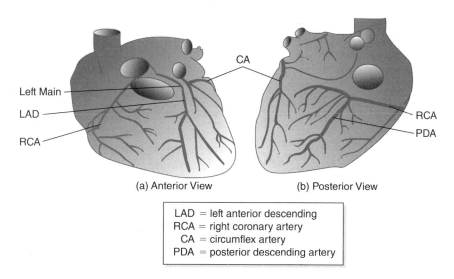

LAD = left anterior descending
RCA = right coronary artery
CA = circumflex artery
PDA = posterior descending artery

Figure 2-4   Diagram of coronary circulation.

People can vary somewhat in terms of the arrangement and area that the coronary arteries supply. Coronary angiography can reveal the individual's unique configuration. With age, vessels may become narrowed due to plaque and thickening of the arterial walls. Collateral circulation may then develop, as blood is drawn from nearby arterioles to supply areas that might otherwise not be perfused adequately because of blockages to primary blood sources. If collateral circulation is well developed, blockage of a major artery may not cause as much damage as it would for a person with no collateral circulation (Woods et al., 2009).

CARDIAC LYMPHATIC SYSTEM

The heart produces a certain amount of lymphatic drainage that flows through the pretracheal lymph node and eventually empties into the superior vena cava. Blockage of lymph flow can affect pressures in the heart itself related to venous congestion. The return of lymph to the systemic circulation is critical to prevent interstitial edema. Also of importance is that cardiac lymph fluid contains hormones (atrial natriuretic peptide) and adrenergic neurons (norepinephrine) that can be used as markers for myocardial edema, reperfusion injury, and myocardial damage (Konuralp, Idiz, & Unal, 2001).

People can vary somewhat in terms of the arrangement and area that the coronary arteries supply. Coronary angiography can reveal the individual's unique configuration.

PRESSURE OF BLOOD IN MAJOR BLOOD VESSELS

Major blood vessels experience variations in their pressures related to cardiac events. Pressure waves in the great veins and the right atrium are given codes (letters) to assist in the interpretation of waveforms (**Figure 2-5**). For example, the "A" wave represents increased

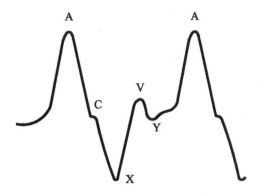

Figure 2-5   Pressure waveforms.
Source: Illustrated by James R. Perron

right atrial pressure caused by atrial contraction and follows the P wave on the ECG tracing. The "C" wave represents the slight increase in RA pressure coming from the ventricle that causes the tricuspid valve to close. The "C" wave immediately follows the R wave on the ECG tracing. The "X" descent follows the "C" wave and represents change in shape of the atrium as a result of ventricular systole and corresponding displacement of the tricuspid valve during ventricular systole. The "V" wave represents filling of the atrium from systemic veins and corresponds to the area immediately following the T wave on the ECG tracing. The "Y" descent represents opening of the tricuspid valve and follows the "V" wave.

Arterial pressure increases rapidly with ventricular systole and attains the pressure represented by the systolic blood pressure. The dicrotic notch of the arterial waveform represents the closure of the aortic valve. This closure maintains the pressure of the system circuit at the level represented by the diastolic blood pressure.

ELECTRICAL CONTROL OF CARDIAC MUSCLE

Cardiac muscle cells are unique in the body for a number of reasons. First, unlike skeletal muscle cells, they are capable of automaticity.

That is, cardiac muscle cells do not require stimulation from an outside force such as a nerve to initiate an action potential, which causes contraction. Second, cardiac muscle cells are interconnected in a web-like fashion with separation only by intercalated discs, which allows for impulses to pass through the entire section of the heart like a wave.

Action potentials occur when the polarity (i.e., electrical charges) across the cell membrane changes rapidly. In the resting state, there are more positive ions (sodium ions, which are present in the largest number, but also calcium and magnesium ions) outside the cell membrane as compared with the positive charges inside the cell. Potassium is the chief intracellular cation (positive ion), and there exist relatively more anions (negative ions) inside the cell from proteins and other sources.

The cell membrane is therefore "polar"—similar to the scheme used to power a flashlight battery, which has more positive ions on one side than on the other. An action potential spreads to neighboring cardiac cells like a wave.

The atria and ventricles are separated by thick fibrous tissue that supports the four heart valves. This fibrous tissue prevents action potentials from being transmitted between the atria and ventricles. The exception to this barrier occurs in the AV junction, or the AV node. Electrical impulses pass from atria to ventricles across this specialized set of tissues (**Figure 2-6**). To support simultaneous contraction of the thick ventricular muscle walls, specialized conduction tissue transmits electrical impulses through the bundle branches and the Purkinje fibers; the atria have similar transmission fibers. The

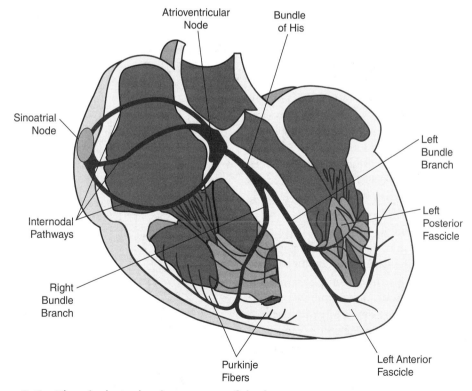

Figure 2-6   Electrical conduction system of the heart.

Box 2-2   Action Potential Phases

Phase 0: Depolarization. Sodium ions cross the cell membrane rapidly through sodium channels, causing the polarity of the cell membrane to change rapidly.

Phase 1: Rapid Repolarization. Potassium ions "leak" outside the cell.

Phase 2: Plateau. Opening of slower calcium channels allows cations to enter the cell, balancing the loss of potassium ions.

Phase 3: Rapid Repolarization. At the end of the action potential, the channels close and the cell returns to its resting state by pumping sodium ions out of the cell and bringing potassium ions back inside.

Phase 4: Resting State. This phase is diastole where cells remain resting until an electrical impulse occurs.

electrical impulse is slowed at the AV node, a delay that allows for the atria to contract and empty blood into the ventricles before the action potential moves through the ventricles.

Each cell of the heart is capable of initiating an action potential, but different areas of the heart have different basic rates of discharging. Under normal conditions, the SA node, which is located in the right atrium, has the fastest rate; depolarization occurs there approximately 60 to 100 times per minute. Cells of the AV node can depolarize 40 to 60 times per minute unless a more frequent impulse, such as from the SA node, is transmitted through them. Ventricular cells can initiate an action potential 20 to 40 times per minute. This activity is protective to the heart: If something happens to prevent normal action potentials from reaching the ventricle, the heart will still beat. Thus, the SA node is normally in control of the heart rate because it has the fastest intrinsic rate.

Box 2-2 provides a closer look at the various phases of action potentials to help explain these events and explain how certain medications can affect them. Action potentials for the SA and AV nodes are somewhat different from the pattern depicted in **Figure 2-7**, which allows the SA node to operate more independently. These impulses are more tightly controlled by the slow calcium channels than the sodium channels. Calcium channel blockers can slow heart rate by slowing the

transport of calcium across the cell membrane (McCance & Huether, 2006).

A refractory period occurs after the action potential before the resting concentrations have fully returned to normal. New impulses that reach the tissue during this period will not be transmitted, or potentially can establish abnormal rhythm patterns. Because reestablishing the normal concentration gradient of electrolytes requires working against the concentration gradient, it requires the expenditure of energy. As much as two-thirds of the cardiac cell's energy is spent in supporting the sodium–potassium pump. Any loss in energy

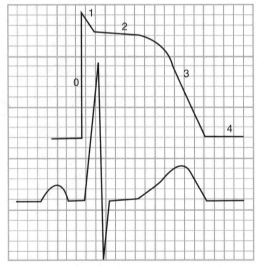

Figure 2-7   Action potential diagram.
Source: Illustrated by James R. Perron

for the cardiac cell results in interruption of this essential pump fairly quickly. Such a disruption affects the cell's ability to return to normal polarity. Without sodium–potassium pump activity, sodium ions build up in the cell. Water (a polar molecule) is attracted to the sodium ion. As a result, internal structures of the cardiac cell swell, resulting in the release of internal cell enzymes. Electrolyte abnormalities can make cardiac cells more prone to develop an action potential and more likely to initiate a transmittable impulse, which causes an abnormal cardiac rhythm.

Electrical events precede mechanical events. When a cardiac cell experiences an action potential, it contracts. As the wave of electrical activity passes through the cardiac muscle wall, the muscle contracts in a wavelike fashion. For this reason, cardiac function is often monitored by electrocardiography. The nurse must be aware that damaged cardiac muscle may not respond with full-force contraction even if the electrocardiogram tracings appear normal.

CARDIAC OUTPUT, PRELOAD, AND AFTERLOAD

As mentioned earlier, the heart functions to pump oxygenated blood to cells, organs, muscles, and tissues and deoxygenated blood back from the systemic circulation. Some concepts have been developed that assist clinicians in understanding overall cardiac function. Cardiac output (CO) is a measure of the amount of blood that is ejected by the heart each minute. Stroke volume (SV) represents the amount of blood that is ejected from the left ventricle with one contraction. Cardiac output, then, is the product of the stroke volume and the heart rate (HR):

$$CO = SV \times HR$$

Stroke volume is influenced by the amount of blood in the ventricle and by the force of contraction of the ventricle. It can also be affected if the aortic valve restricts flow out of the left ventricle. The ejection fraction (EF) is the percentage of the volume of the left ventricle that is ejected with each contraction. A normal ejection fraction is in the range of approximately 65% to 70%, where this value reflects the efficiency of the left ventricle in pumping blood forward into the systemic circulation.

Preload (sometimes referred to as left ventricular end-diastolic pressure) is the pressure found in the left ventricle at the end of diastole. The Frank-Starling law states that stretched muscle fibers produce a more powerful contraction; thus, when the left ventricle is fully filled, a more powerful contraction becomes possible. Conditions that prevent filling of the ventricle with blood—such as hypovolemia, dehydration, or external pressure on the heart from fluid in the pericardium—will reduce the volume of blood in the ventricle and its ability to pump blood forward. Nevertheless, the Frank-Starling law reaches its limit when cardiac chambers are overstretched: The resulting contraction is not as effective as it would have been with slightly less stretch. The overstretching can eventually result in a lower cardiac output. Preload can also be affected by blood that was not ejected during the previous systole. A low ejection fraction can increase preload and overstretch the ventricle.

Afterload is the resistance against which the left ventricle must pump to move blood forward. The pressure of the arterial systemic circulation produces afterload. Smooth muscle tone in arterioles can increase the resistance to blood flow and increase afterload. Medications can also alter the amount of resistance that arteriolar smooth muscle generates. For example, arterial vasodilators decrease afterload, whereas vasoconstrictor agents increase preload, afterload, or both. Chronic, uncontrolled hypertension can lead to left ventricular hypertrophy, a thickening of the ventricle wall due to increased workload (Huether & McCance, 2012).

EXTERNAL CONTROL OF THE HEART

Nervous system control of the heart comes through the autonomic nervous system and can cause rapid changes in heart activity. The autonomic nervous system consists of sympathetic and parasympathetic nerve fibers. The sympathetic nervous system controls the body's "fight or flight" mechanisms, quickly preparing the total organism to resist an attack.

The parasympathetic system governs the "rest and refresh" responses to stress and has nerves that function more individually. The vagus nerve has the chief parasympathetic influence on the heart by affecting primarily the SA and AV nodes, slowing the heart rate and increasing the conduction block at the AV node. Parasympathetic nerve fibers release acetylcholine, which slows the heart—a function sometimes termed "cholinergic."

Sympathetic stimulation increases heart rate and contractility, affecting all parts of the heart. Sympathetic nerve fibers release norepinephrine, which has a profound effect by increasing cardiac contractility and vascular resistance. Additionally, the medulla of the adrenal glands is part of the sympathetic nervous system and can stimulate the release of epinephrine into the systemic circulation—a function sometimes termed "adrenergic." Receptors for adrenergic neurotransmitters can be classified as either alpha (α) or beta (β) receptors. Receptors can be further subclassified as α_1 and α_2, or as β_1 and β_2. Dopamine is another neurotransmitter that affects the cardiovascular system. **Table 2-1** summarizes the locations and actions of the various receptors.

Table 2-1   Autonomic Receptors and Cardiovascular Function

Location	Adrenergic Receptor Type	Adrenergic Effect	Vagus Nerve Cholinergic Effect
Sinoatrial (SA) node	β_1	Increased rate	Decreased rate, arrest
Atrial tissue	β_1	Increased contractility and conduction velocity	Decreased contractility, shorter action potential
Atrioventricular (AV) node	β_1	Increased automaticity and conduction velocity	Decreased conduction velocity and automaticity
Purkinje fibers	β_1	Increased automaticity and conduction velocity	No receptors
Ventricles	β_1	Increased contractility	No receptors
Coronary	α_1, β_1	Constriction, dilation	Dilation
Skin	α_1, β_2	Constriction	Dilation
Skeletal muscle	α_1, β_2	Constriction, dilation	No receptors
Cerebral	α_1	Constriction (slight)	No receptors
Pulmonary	α_1, β_2	Constriction, dilation	
Renal	$\alpha_1, \beta_1, \beta_2$	Constriction, dilation	

The activity of the sympathetic neurotransmitters is determined by the location and type of receptors in various tissues. In this way, the same chemical can have different effects in different locations. The heart is rich in β receptors, so that effect is most prevalent for the heart. The systemic circulation has relatively more α receptors, so that effect is more predominant there. Epinephrine stimulates all types of adrenergic receptors, but norepinephrine has little effect on $β_2$ receptors. Dilation of $α_2$ coronary blood vessels is promoted by epinephrine, but not norepinephrine (McCance & Huether, 2006).

SYSTEMIC CIRCULATION

Blood is pumped from the left ventricle into the aorta, the largest artery in the body. The aorta rises from the aortic valve and heads superiorly and to the right, which explains why one listens for aortic valve heart sounds at the first intercostal space on the right sternal border. Arteries branch from the aorta beginning at the aortic arch and continue until the aorta itself branches into the two iliac arteries. Multiple systemic arteries branch off from the aorta as it passes through the body. Arteries then branch into a series of increasingly smaller units until they become the smallest of all blood vessels, the capillaries. The capillaries eventually collect into venules, which combine to form veins, which return blood to the heart through the inferior and superior vena cavae.

The entire circulatory system is lined with endothelial cells that are active in controlling local conditions through the release of chemicals. The types of blood vessels have unique characteristics that affect their function. Arteries have thicker walls containing three layers, including a smooth muscle layer. The constriction of the smooth muscle surrounding the arteries is controlled by the action of chemicals such as epinephrine or norepinephrine. The outer layer of the artery consists of connective tissue. Veins have narrower walls with a thinner muscle layer. Venous blood is squeezed up from the legs through skeletal muscle contraction; the large veins of the leg have internal valves that prevent blood from flowing down by gravity.

The endothelial layer of cells constitutes the capillary wall. Capillaries have incredibly thin walls; the varying spaces between the cells that line them allow for fluid and blood cells to pass through the capillary cell membranes or through the spaces between the cells. In the brain, however, the extremely tight junctions between the endothelial cells force all fluid to go through these cells. In contrast, capillaries found in other parts of the body have relatively more open spaces between endothelial cells that allow for easier exchange of fluid and dissolved chemicals; this kind of openness is found in the liver, for example. Certain conditions, such as inflammation or sepsis, can result in widened spaces, leading to a condition euphemistically called "leaky" capillaries. Precapillary sphincters—smooth muscle cells that control the smallest arterioles—control blood flow to capillary networks. Under normal circumstances, local acidosis causes opening of a precapillary sphincter to an area, thereby increasing its blood supply.

Pressures in the arterial system can be measured by use of a sphygmomanometer or by direct arterial cannulation. Pressures in the capillary network are lower than arteriolar pressures; venous pressures are even lower, supporting venous return. As with blood flow through the heart, blood flow in the periphery is determined by control of pressures and resistance to flow. Resistance to blood flow comes in the form of pressure in vessels, which is partly determined by smooth muscle tone and length of the blood vessels. In general, the key principle governing blood flow can be summarized as "the greater the resistance, the lower the flow." Resistance to flow can also be increased if the blood is more viscous, such as occurs with polycythemia.

Blood flow can also be affected by the shape and internal smoothness of the blood vessels.

Blockage of arteries can cause decreased blood flow to areas of the body normally supplied by these arteries. Blockage can be caused by gradual increase in formation of smooth muscles from hyperinsulinism or by the accumulation of plaque from hypercholesterolemia. When plaques rupture, they cause a break in the endothelial lining of the vessel and a blood clot forms, further blocking the artery. Cardiac surgery often involves revascularization of arteries that have been blocked over time.

SYSTEMIC CONTROL OF BLOOD PRESSURE

In addition to acting through the sympathetic nervous system, which can increase the blood pressure by increasing vascular resistance, the body can control blood pressure through other chemical pathways. The kidneys autoregulate their blood flow so that pressures at the glomerulus are sufficiently high to maintain filtration. If the kidneys detect decreased blood flow, they also release renin. Renin leads to production of angiotensin I, which is later converted to angiotensin II. Angiotensin II increases systemic vascular resistance by causing vasoconstriction. It also stimulates the release of aldosterone from the adrenal glands. Aldosterone, a mineralocorticoid, causes sodium—and therefore water—retention. If the cause of renal blood flow decrease is blood loss, these compensatory mechanisms are helpful. Conversely, if low cardiac output is caused by pump failure, then these mechanisms actually work against cardiac function by increasing afterload and water retention. Angiotensin-converting enzyme (ACE) inhibitors block this pathway, and guidelines now recommend their use both for heart failure and following myocardial infarction.

The body's water levels are regulated by antidiuretic hormone (ADH), a chemical released from the posterior pituitary gland. When diuresis slows, the amount of free body water increases. This effect then reduces the concentration (osmolality) of dissolved substances in the body. Baroreceptors in the left atrium, the aortic arch, and the carotid artery are sensitive to fluid volume and will send messages to increase ADH production when pressures are low.

Natriuretic peptides are released by parts of the body in response to plasma volume changes. Atrial natriuretic protein is released by atrial monocytes if they detect increased pressure in the right atrium. Atrial natriuretic protein inhibits ADH, thereby causing a loss of body water, and ultimately reducing the pressure in the right atrium. Brain natriuretic protein was first discovered in the brain but is also released from the heart cells; the level of this protein can reflect overall ventricular function (McCance & Huether, 2006).

DISORDERS OF MAJOR BLOOD VESSELS

Sometimes, as a result of longstanding pressure inside arteries or because of turbulent flow caused by irregularities in the internal shape of the artery, weaknesses may develop in the arterial wall. An aneurysm is a widening in an artery that can completely surround the artery or that can consist of an outpouching at one part of the circumference of the artery. When aneurysms rupture, they cause rapid blood loss from the artery into surrounding tissues and a reduction in blood flow to areas normally supplied by the artery.

The aorta is prone to aneurysm development because it sustains the highest pressures in the vascular system. When an aneurysm involves all three levels of the arterial wall, it is termed a "true aneurysm." This type of aneurysm typically involves the entire circumference of the vessel. Other aneurysms form between the layers of the artery, particularly following vascular surgery. In this case, blood leaks through the endothelial and tunica media layers and collects under the adventitia.

Aneurysms are usually undetectable until they threaten to rupture or actually do rupture. Symptoms depend on the location of the aneurysm. A widening aneurysm can result in decreased blood flow to small arteries in the area. A ruptured aneurysm causes pain, which can often be referred, meaning the pain is perceived in an area of the body different from where the actual injury is located. Thoracic aneurysms can cause dyspnea or dysphagia due to pressure on the esophagus and lung tissue. An abdominal aortic aneurysm can result in ischemia to tissues normally supplied by blood from the area below the aneurysm.

Diagnosis of aneurysms may be made through ultrasonography and by using imaging technologies such as computed tomography or magnetic resonance imaging. The goals of treatment are to reduce blood loss by reducing blood pressure until surgical repair can be accomplished. Asymptomatic aneurysms are sometimes detected on chest radiograph or by abdominal palpation of a pulsatile mass.

The decision to make a surgical repair depends on the relative risk of the repair itself compared with the risk of the aneurysm's rupture. If, for example, the renal arteries are compromised by the location of the aneurysm, then the intravascular repair may not be possible. The age of the patient and the size of the aneurysm are factored into this decision. Intravascular approaches to supporting the integrity of the artery have been developed that allow for much quicker recovery by patients. The location of the aneurysm is key to understanding the symptoms produced by the arterial defect.

SUMMARY

By understanding the anatomy and physiology of the cardiovascular system, the nurse is able to make reasoned responses to patient problems. Concepts such as CO and electrophysiology will be daily concerns of the critical care nurse. Accurate assessment of cardiovascular function and early detection of problems are essential to providing high-quality care. Cardiovascular conditions remain the leading cause of death in the United States. Nurses caring for acutely and critically ill patients who are expert in the care of patients with these conditions will be needed.

SELF-ASSESSMENT QUESTIONS

1. Which of the following effects do hyperinflated lungs have on the heart?
   a. Elevated level of the heart
   b. Shift of the PMI to the left
   c. Depressed level of the heart
   d. Shift of the PMI to the right

2. Blood enters the right atrium during which of the following phases?
   a. Atrial diastole
   b. Atrial systole
   c. Ventricular diastole
   d. Ventricular systole

3. Which of the following is associated with a diastolic murmur?
   a. Tricuspid insufficiency
   b. Aortic stenosis
   c. Mitral insufficiency
   d. Mitral stenosis

4. Which of the following is associated with a systolic murmur?
   a. Pulmonary insufficiency
   b. Tricuspid stenosis
   c. Aortic insufficiency
   d. Mitral stenosis

5. Which area of the heart does the circumflex coronary artery supply?
   a. Bundle branches
   b. Purkinje fibers
   c. Posterior portion of the left atrium
   d. Atrioventricular node

6. The LAD artery supplies blood to which area of the heart?
   a. Ventricular septum
   b. SA node
   c. AV node
   d. Bundle branches

7. The wave of a right atrial pressure waveform represents which of the following?
   a. Ventricular emptying
   b. Atrial contraction
   c. Filling of the atrium from systemic circulation
   d. Tricuspid valve opening

8. How often do AV node cells typically initiate an action potential?
   a. 20–40 times/minute
   b. 60–100 times/minute
   c. 40–60 times/minute
   d. 100–150 times/minute

9. What occurs during Phase 4 of an action potential?
   a. Sodium ions are pumped out of the cells and potassium ions are pumped back in
   b. Potassium ions leak out of cells
   c. Diastole cells rest until electrical impulse occurs
   d. Opening of slower calcium channels

10. Preload is defined as:
    a. the amount of work the heart must do to eject blood.
    b. force of contractions of heart muscle.
    c. pressure in the ventricle at the end of filling.
    d. amount of blood ejected by the heart each minute.

Answers to Self-Assessment Questions

1. c	6. a
2. d	7. c
3. d	8. c
4. c	9. c
5. c	10. c

REFERENCES

Huether, S. E., & McCance, K. L. (2012). *Understanding pathophysiology* (5th ed.). St. Louis, MO: Elsevier Mosby.

Konuralp, C., Idiz, M., & Unal, M. (2001). Importance of the cardiac lymphatic system in open heart surgery. *European Journal of Cardio-Thoracic Surgery, 19*(3), 372–373.

McCance, K. L., & Huether, S. E. (2006). *Pathophysiology: The biologic basis for disease in adults and children* (5th ed.). St. Louis, MO: Elsevier Mosby.

Woods, S. L., Froelicher, E. S., Motzer, S. A., & Bridges, E. (Eds.). (2009). *Cardiac nursing* (6th ed.). Philadelphia, PA: Lippincott Williams & Wilkins.

WEB RESOURCES

St. Jude Medical presents an informational video about the anatomy of the human heart and how it pumps blood throughout the body: http://health.sjm.com/heart-valve-answers/videos-and-animations

"Heart Anatomy: Interior View" is an interactive photograph that allows the learner to point to any structure for highlighted identification on the picture (provided by GateWay Community College, Phoenix, AZ): http://www.gwc.maricopa.edu/class/bio202/cyberheart/hartint0.htm

"Heart Anatomy: Posterior View" is an interactive photograph that allows the learner to point to any structure for highlighted identification on the picture (provided by GateWay Community College, Phoenix, AZ): http://www.gwc.maricopa.edu/class/bio202/cyberheart/hartbak.htm

The Auscultation Assistant provides heart sounds, heart murmurs, and breath sounds to help medical students and others improve their physical diagnosis skills: http://www.med.ucla.edu/wilkes/inex.htm

The University of Washington Department of Medicine provides "Demonstrations: Heart Sounds and Murmurs" at: http://depts.washington.edu/physdx/heart/demo.html

Basic cardiac assessment: http://www.youtube.com/watch?v=dp5m2tXHDmA

Second Life: Heart Murmur Sim: http://www.youtube.com/watch?v=xJY2Iwbzop4

Chapter 3

Indications for Cardiac Surgery

Kristine J. Peterson

INTRODUCTION

The heart has fascinated human beings for centuries as the seat of life and emotions. Although the idea of operating on the heart is not new, it was only in the mid-20th century that such surgery became practical. With the development of cardiopulmonary bypass came the ability to create a bloodless surgical field and a motionless target for surgical therapies. Since that time, multiple advances in surgical techniques, patient management, technology, and pharmacotherapy have resulted in the emergence of cardiac surgery as a dynamic and very successful medical and nursing specialty.

The ability to operate on the heart saves thousands of lives each year. These surgeries present exciting and varied challenges for the critical care nurse and interdisciplinary team. The purpose of this chapter is to review the types of cardiac surgery and their indications.

SURGERY FOR ISCHEMIC HEART DISEASE

An estimated 83.6 million adult Americans have one or more types of cardiovascular disease, with approximately 15.4 million having coronary heart disease (CHD) (Go et al., 2014). Once significant coronary artery stenosis is established, the three major treatment strategies used to prevent further ischemic damage are medical therapy, percutaneous revascularization, and surgical revascularization. Revascularization is the process of restoring blood flow and oxygen delivery to the myocardium. Its dual purposes are to alleviate angina symptoms and prolong life. Percutaneous transluminal coronary angioplasty (PTCA) uses an arterial catheter and various mechanical means to increase the diameter of diseased coronary arteries, thereby improving blood flow. Surgical revascularization, also known as coronary artery bypass grafting (CABG), uses arterial or venous vessels to create a new pathway for blood to reach the coronary arteries, thus "bypassing" the stenosis. In 2004, 427,000 coronary artery bypass graft procedures were performed on 249,000 patients in the United States (American Heart Association [AHA], 2007). It is estimated that inpatient bypass procedures in the United States in 2010 declined to 397,000 (Go et al., 2014). With advances in percutaneous strategies such as drug-eluting stents (DESs), the number of percutaneous revascularizations has increased while the number of surgical revascularizations has declined (Go et al., 2014). Decisions regarding whether coronary revascularization is indicated for an individual patient now include which type of revascularization is indicated.

Medical Therapy Versus Surgical Revascularization

Coronary artery bypass grafting is an extensively studied procedure. Early trials consistently indicated the greatest benefits of CABG over medical therapy in those patients at highest risk (Brown, Sundt, & Gersh, 2008; Hueb et al., 1995; Yusuf et al., 1994). High-risk patients were defined based on the severity of their angina or ischemia, the number of diseased vessels, and the presence of left ventricular (LV) dysfunction. Yusuf and colleagues (1994), in a meta-analysis, demonstrated significantly higher survival at 5, 7, and 10 years after CABG for patients at high and moderate risk, but not for low-risk patients. However, CABG has not been shown to be of more benefit than medical therapy for patients with single-vessel disease (Brown et al., 2008). The 2011 American College of Cardiology Foundation (ACCF)/AHA guideline for CABG recommends against CABG in patients with single-vessel disease without proximal left anterior descending (LAD) involvement (Hillis et al., 2011).

Percutaneous Versus Surgical Revascularization

A large number of clinical trials have compared short- and long-term outcomes from percutaneous coronary intervention (PCI) and surgical revascularization (Goy et al., 1999; Goy et al., 2000; Hannan et al., 2005; Hoffman et al., 2003; Hueb et al., 1995; Serruys et al., 2001). In the Arterial Revascularization Therapy Study (ARTS—the largest of these trials), 1- and 5-year follow-up data indicated no differences in major adverse cardiac and cerebrovascular events (MACCE) between CABG and stent placement (Serruys et al., 2001). A CABG resulted in fewer revascularizations, but PCI provided substantial cost savings (Gruberg, 2005). Other data suggest that CABG resulted in reduced 5-year mortality,

less angina, and fewer revascularization procedures than PCI (Hoffman et al., 2003). Adding stents to PCI reduced revascularizations, but the need for such follow-up procedures remained significantly lower in CABG patients (Hannon et al., 2005; Hoffman et al., 2003). Mercado and colleagues (2005) demonstrated that PCI and CABG resulted in no differences in 1-year death, myocardial infarction (MI), and stroke rates, but higher revascularization rates than found with PCI. It should be noted that these studies were all conducted prior to 2003, when DESs were first introduced.

The ARTS II registry compared outcomes with a sirolimus-eluting stent and PCI to those in the PCI and CABG arms of the ARTS I study (Gruberg, 2005). ARTS II registry patients had a higher incidence of diabetes, hypertension, and hypercholesterolemia than did members of the ARTS I group, but included fewer smokers than in the original study. Rates of stable versus unstable angina were similar in the two groups, although the patients enrolled in ARTS II had more complex lesions than those in the first registry. The MACCE-free survival at 1 year was not significantly different between the two groups, probably due to the higher revascularization rate in ARTS II patients.

In a meta-analysis comparing DESs with bare metal stents, Babapulle, Joseph, Belisle, Brophy, and Eisenberg (2004) found no differences in survival or MI. Placement of a DES resulted in fewer restenoses and major cardiac events. Since that time, PCI and CABG techniques have significantly advanced; PCI is increasingly being used for more complex lesions.

The SYNTAX Score (SS) is an anatomically based tool that uses angiographic findings to define the complexity of coronary artery disease. Developed over several years from other tools to define the severity of coronary disease, the SS was evaluated in the landmark SYNTAX trial (Farooq, Brugaletta, & Serruys, 2011). The score has since established itself as an independent predictor of MACCE following PCI (Farooq et al., 2011; Valgimigli et al., 2007).

In a meta-analysis of 11,148 patients, Alam and colleagues (2012) concluded that when using DESs, PCI for unprotected left main coronary disease (ULMD) has comparable mortality and MI, lower stroke rates, and higher revascularization to CABG. The SYNTAX trial (Serruys et al., 2009) compared CABG with PCI for patients with left main coronary disease or 3-vessel disease. In this multi-center trial, the local cardiac surgeon and interventional cardiologist jointly determined the optimal treatment strategy. They randomized 1,800 patients for PCI or CABG. Those patients suitable for only one treatment were entered into a nested PCI or CABG registry. The investigators concluded that CABG remains the standard of care for these patients, with significantly less MACCE at 12 months in the CABG patients. This was due in large part to significantly higher revascularization rates in the PCI group (p = 0.002). Stroke was higher in CABG patients.

Morice and colleagues (2010) analyzed the results of a pre-specified subgroup of 705 randomized patients with left main disease. This analysis indicated that, for patients with left main disease, the safety and efficacy outcomes at 1 year were comparable for both treatment strategies. Kappetein and colleagues (2011), in a 3-year follow up of the SYNTAX trial, and Mohr and colleagues (2013), in a 5-year follow up of the same trial, corroborated that CABG should be the standard of care for patients with complex lesions (per SS score), but either treatment is acceptable for those with less complex or left main disease. In another SYNTAX follow up, Farooq and colleagues (2013) analyzed stent thrombosis and graft occlusion at 5 years. They found the incidence of stent occlusion and graft thrombosis to be similar at 5 years, but stent thrombosis had a greater clinical implication with increased short-term and long-term mortality.

Deb and colleagues (2013) conducted a systematic review of 13 randomized controlled trials and 5 meta-analyses and concluded that PCI and CABG are both reasonable in patients with extensive coronary disease. They recommended CABG for patients with complex disease and ULMD, multi-vessel disease, or LV dysfunction. A PCI should be considered for less complex disease or for those who have surgical risk. A CABG is also recommended for patients with diabetes and multi-vessel disease. The same researchers validated earlier conclusions that revascularization is higher after PCI, while incidence of stroke is higher after CABG.

The 2013 ACCF/AHA ST-segment elevation myocardial infarction (STEMI) guidelines recommend a limited role for CABG in the acute phase of STEMI (O'Gara et al., 2013). They recommend CABG for failed PCI and for anatomy not amenable to PCI in the setting of STEMI with high risk factors such as ongoing or recurrent ischemia, severe heart failure, or cardiogenic shock. The guidelines also recommend CABG for STEMI at the time of surgical repair of mechanical defects (e.g., a ventricular septal defect or mitral valve repair [MVR]). The same guidelines also recommend considering emergency CABG for STEMI in patients who are not in cardiogenic shock and who are also not candidates for PCI or fibrinolytic therapy (O'Gara et al., 2013).

INDICATIONS FOR CORONARY ARTERY BYPASS GRAFTING

The ACCF/AHA Task Force on Practice Guidelines has established recommendations for CABG surgery with the goals to improve survival and to relieve symptoms. Hillis and colleagues (2011) have published recommendations for CABG surgery for each patient population, including recommendation levels.

The recommendations are categorized into three classes: I, II, and III. Class I indicates that evidence or general agreement exists that the intervention is effective, or both. Class II indicates that conflicting evidence or a divergence of opinion exists about the efficacy of the intervention, or both. Class II is further divided into Class IIa and Class IIb: Class IIa indicates that evidence/opinion is in favor of the intervention's efficacy, whereas Class IIb interventions have less efficacy as established by evidence/opinion. For Class III interventions, evidence, general opinion, or both suggest that the intervention is not effective or is harmful.

The strength of the level of evidence for specific interventions is also identified according to the type or presence of research. For example, Level of Evidence A indicates that findings from multiple randomized clinical trials or meta-analyses supported use of an intervention. Level of Evidence B indicates that a single randomized trial or a series of nonrandomized trials supported an intervention. Level of Evidence C is assigned to those interventions supported by consensus opinion of experts, case studies, or standard of care (Hillis et al., 2011).

CABG in Diabetics

The connection between diabetes mellitus and CHD is well established. Diabetes produces prothrombotic, inflammatory, and proliferative states in the vascular endothelium and carries a higher risk for restenosis. Individuals with diabetes tend to have more diffuse coronary disease—a state that favors use of a procedure that can produce complete revascularization. Regardless of the revascularization procedure used, diabetics have a higher risk of adverse outcomes (BARI Investigators, 2000). For persons with diabetes, there is a trend toward lower mortality and fewer revascularizations with CABG than with PCI. As yet, no studies have compared the outcomes from PCI with DES with the outcomes from CABG in patients with diabetes.

The 2011 ACCF/AHA guideline for CABG surgery recommends CABG over PCI for diabetics with multi-vessel disease (Hillis et al., 2011).

CABG in Patients with Concomitant Carotid Disease

Perioperative stroke rate is reported to be twice as high for patients with bilateral versus unilateral carotid atherosclerotic disease (Mohler & Fairman, 2014). In a review of 350 patients, Shishehbor and colleagues (2013) compared three treatment strategies: staged carotid endarterectomy (CEA)-open heart surgery (OHS), combined CEA and OHS, and staged carotid artery stenting (CAS)-OHS. They concluded that short-term mortality, stroke, and MI were similar for staged CAS-OHS and combined CEA-OHS, and both were better than staged CEA-OHS. However, at 12 months, the same outcomes favored staged CAS-OHS. Aydin, Ozen, Sarikaya, and Yukseltan (2014) reported a case series of 110 patients who underwent simultaneous CEA and CABG. They concluded that this strategy can be used with low morbidity and mortality. Authors of another cohort study reported a small risk of ipsilateral stroke in isolated CABG patients with both carotid and coronary disease (Kassaian et al., 2013). They concluded that staged CAS-CABG may be the preferred option for bilateral carotid disease in symptomatic patients, but this would require experienced operators. Controversy remains for this subset of patients.

Minimally Invasive Myocardial Revascularization

Approaches to CABG other than the traditional median sternotomy with CPB include the minimally invasive direct coronary artery bypass (MIDCAB), which uses an entry other than a median sternotomy; the off-pump (or beating heart surgery) approach; and newer hybrid approaches to CABG.

Early data on off-pump coronary artery bypass (OPCAB) indicated patency rates and survival rates equivalent to those seen with traditional CABG (Puskas et al., 2003; Sharony et al., 2004), although many studies were very small. The U.S. Department of Veterans Affairs randomized on/off bypass study randomized 2,203 patients to on- or off-pump CABG; endpoints were composite death or complications at 30 days and 1 year following surgery (Shroyer et al., 2009). No difference was reported in the composite endpoints at 30 days; however, at 1 year off-pump patients had poorer outcomes and lower graft patency than did the on-pump patients. Møller and colleagues (2010) reported a 3-year follow up of a randomized trial of off-pump versus on-pump CABG for 341 patients. They found no differences in MACCE and coronary re-intervention at 3 years. Nardi and colleagues (2014) retrospectively analyzed data at 4-year follow up for 166 OPCAB patients and 203 on-pump CABG patients. They concluded that MACCE and repeat revascularization were similar in both groups but freedom from cardiac death is better after on-pump CABG. Brewer and colleagues (2014) reached the same conclusion. The 2011 ACCF/AHA guideline for CABG (Hillis et al., 2011) concludes that either approach is reasonable. The use of OPCAB has steadily declined over the last several years—from 23% in 2002 to fewer than one in five CABG procedures in 2012 (Bakaeen et al., 2014). OPCAB is discussed in more detail in Chapter 6.

The MIDCAB approaches appear to offer no advantage over the traditional sternotomy approach and may result in less complete revascularization. Also, MIDCAB is currently recommended for those with cosmetic reasons to prefer a MIDCAB or those who require a reoperation and for whom a repeat sternotomy carries a high risk (Stulak, 2014).

Hybrid approaches include a MIDCAB using the left internal thoracic artery to the LAD coronary artery combined with PCI for other vessels with or without valvular or other procedures. There is little evidence to guide the use of these approaches (Stulak, 2014).

TRANSMYOCARDIAL LASER REVASCULARIZATION

A substantial number of patients with diffuse CHD have refractory angina despite maximal medical and interventional therapy (Horvath & Zhou, 2008). Severe, diffuse CHD is often not amenable to complete revascularization, leaving the myocardium at risk even after such a procedure is attempted. Incomplete revascularization is a predictor of adverse events (Horvath & Zhou, 2008).

Options to treat refractory CHD include angiogenesis, genetic therapies, and transmyocardial revascularization. These strategies involve various means of creating new pathways for blood to reach the myocardium. Transmyocardial laser revascularization (TMR) is a procedure whereby transmyocardial channels are created from the epicardium into the ventricle via a laser. The new channels then allow blood from the ventricle to reach the myocardium directly. Results of trials have failed to show sustained symptom relief with TMR; therefore, it is not recommended (Laham & Simons, 2014; Schofield & McNab, 2010).

SURGERY FOR VALVE DISEASE

Valve disease can occur due to congenital or acquired factors. Decisions regarding medical or surgical management (repair or replacement) are made by weighing the risks and benefits of each treatment modality. Valve surgery is discussed in detail in Chapter 5.

SURGICAL MANAGEMENT OF ARRHYTHMIAS

Durrer, Schoo, Schuilenburg, and Wellens (1967) first reported the successful initiation and termination of a tachycardia in 1967, when they induced and successfully terminated atrioventricular reentrant tachycardia (AVRT). Advancements in understanding of arrhythmia initiation and propagation as well as surgical techniques created a role for surgical ablation for tachyarrhythmias (Eckart & Epstein, 2008). The need for open heart surgery limited this role and spurred the development of catheter ablation techniques. Many arrhythmias—including atrioventricular nodal reentrant tachycardia (AVNRT), AVRT, atrial tachycardia, atrial flutter, atrial fibrillation (AF), and ventricular tachycardia (VT)—have been mapped and ablated using catheter techniques with varying degrees of success (Eckart & Epstein, 2008). For persistent or recurring dysrhythmias, surgical management remains an option.

Atrial Fibrillation

Atrial fibrillation is increasing in prevalence, with more than 6 million Americans having this dysrhythmia. It increases in frequency with age, and it is estimated that more than 12 million people in the United States will have AF by 2050 (Oral & Latchamsetty, 2014). There are four classifications of atrial fibrillation, based on duration: paroxysmal, persistent, long-standing persistent, and permanent. Treatment approaches differ with classification. The most important goals of therapy for AF are symptom alleviation and reducing the risk of stroke and tachycardia-related cardiomyopathy (Padanilam & Prystowsky, 2009).

First-line therapy is usually antiarrhythmic therapy. However, pharmacologic therapy is limited by its inconsistent efficacy and side effects. For this reason, strong interest remains in nonpharmacologic approaches to AF. Treatment of AF is discussed in detail in Chapter 15.

Atrial fibrillation is a complex, multifactorial arrhythmia, involving both arrhythmogenic triggers and altered atrial substrate that maintains the arrhythmia. In addition, AF leads to remodeling in the atria, which will perpetuate AF (Oral & Latchamsetty, 2014). The pulmonary veins are frequent triggers for AF, which has led to the development of catheter-based and surgical techniques to isolate them.

Thromboembolic risk in AF is multifactorial as well. It involves left atrial mechanical dysfunction, blood stasis in the left atrial appendage, a hypercoagulable state, and elevated C-reactive protein levels (Oral & Latchamsetty, 2014). Surgery for AF is indicated when maximal medical therapy does not relieve symptoms that interfere with lifestyle or ability to work. It can also be performed in conjunction with mitral valve surgery with documented evidence of AF (Kouchoukos, Blackstone, Hanley, & Kirklin, 2013). The original surgical technique for AF, the Maze procedure, was introduced by James Cox in 1987 (Zembala & Suwalski, 2013). The Maze procedure interrupts the reentrant pathways required for AF using surgical incisions. This procedure, and subsequent evolutions, involved a median sternotomy and CPB. Modifications to the original cut-and-sew procedure have evolved to include radiofrequency ablation (RFA) rather than cut-and-sew lesions, pulmonary vein isolation, left atrial appendage exclusion, modified lesion patterns, autonomic ganglia ablation, endoscopic surgical approaches, and combinations of catheter-based and surgical interventions. The Cox Maze IV procedure uses radiofrequency, cryoablation to create the Maze III lines of ablation, or both, and can be done with a thoracoscopic approach. Procedures that involve both atria have been most effective in controlling AF (Kouchoukos et al., 2013). The purposes of the surgical approach are to isolate the pulmonary veins, modify the left atrial substrate, and decide the fate of the left atrial appendage (Zembala & Suwalski, 2013).

The FAST trial was the first randomized trial comparing catheter ablation and minimally invasive surgical ablation of AF (Boersma et al., 2012). The investigators randomized 124 patients to catheter ablation or surgical ablation. Surgical ablation included RFA of pulmonary veins, ablation of the ganglionic plexi (GP), and left atrial appendage exclusion. Freedom from atrial arrhythmias without pharmacotherapy at 12 months was significantly better with surgical ablation than catheter ablation, although procedural adverse events were higher with surgical ablation. Krul and colleagues (2011) reported on a series of 31 patients who underwent a total thoracoscopic procedure consisting of bilateral mapping and ablation of GP, pulmonary venous isolation, left atrial appendage exclusion, creation of ablation lines via bipolar radiofrequency ablation, and confirmation of the ablation lines via GP electrophysiology. They found that 86% of the patients were free of AF at 1 year. In a systematic review of surgical ablation versus catheter ablation, Kearney and colleagues (2014) reviewed seven studies and found significantly higher rates of freedom from AF after surgical ablation, with comparable rates of complications and higher rates for pacemaker implantation. Their systematic review examined randomized trials of surgical ablation at the time of mitral valve surgery. They found that adding surgical ablation significantly increases freedom from AF in mitral valve surgery patients with no difference in MACCE from mitral surgery patients without surgical ablation.

Ad, Suri, and Gammie (2012) analyzed data on surgical AF ablations using the Society of Thoracic Surgeons Adult Cardiac Surgery Database. There were 91,801 surgical ablations documented over the 5 years reviewed, and 4,893 (5.3%) were stand-alone procedures. Operative mortality and stroke rates were the same in both the on- and off-pump bypass groups. The off-pump bypass group had significantly less bleeding reoperations, shorter ventilation, and shorter hospital stays. There was a significant increase in stand-alone surgical ablations for AF over the 5 years reviewed. Ad and colleagues concluded that both on- and off-pump bypass approaches

were safe, and surgical ablation should be considered as a viable alternative to catheter-based ablation.

The 2014 American Heart Association/ American College of Cardiology/Heart Rhythm Society (AHA/ACC/HRS) Guideline for the Management of Patients with Atrial Fibrillation (January et al., 2014) recommends surgical ablation as reasonable for patients undergoing cardiac surgery for other reasons and stand-alone surgical ablation in patients who are not well managed by other treatments.

Surgical Management of Ventricular Tachycardia

Ventricular arrhythmias—particularly sustained VT—are not uncommon in patients who survive an acute myocardial infarction (AMI); the incidence in this patient population is approximately 3.5% (Podrid & Ganz, 2014). Surgery to eradicate ventricular tachyarrhythmias began in the 1970s with a technique called endocardial resection (Pagé, 2004) and evolved to include intraoperative mapping and ablation. Over time, the initial enthusiasm for the development of surgical therapies for VT waned as medical therapies such as mapping, catheter ablation, and implantable devices advanced.

Indications for surgery for VT are ill-defined and largely dependent on the surgeon's judgment. Consensus does exist that VT caused by ischemic heart disease is most amenable to surgical therapy. To date, surgical interventions for VT have failed to demonstrate a positive effect on long-term mortality (Kouchoukos et al., 2013). Hillis and colleagues (2011), in the ACCF/AHA Guideline for Coronary Artery Bypass Graft Surgery, list CABG as a class IIIC (harm) recommendation for patients with VT, scar, and no evidence of ischemia. Coronary artery bypass grafting is a class IB recommendation for patients with resuscitated cardiac arrest that is thought to be due to significant or multi-vessel coronary artery disease (CAD) and ischemia.

SURGICAL THERAPIES FOR HEART FAILURE

Following an MI, both the infarcted and non-infarcted areas undergo pathological changes such as thinning and fibrous replacement, which alter the size and shape of the ventricle and ultimately lead to heart failure. Medical therapy can improve symptoms and increase life span, but it cannot cure the condition. Mechanical support, such as a ventricular assist device, has been used as a bridge to transplant and occasionally as a bridge to recovery, but is not generally regarded as a feasible long-term therapy for heart failure. The treatment of choice for end-stage heart failure is cardiac transplantation, although the shortage of donor hearts renders this option available to only a few patients. Accordingly, other surgical options have been developed. Cardiac transplantation is discussed in detail in Chapter 19.

Coronary Revascularization as Treatment for Heart Failure

Coronary revascularization via CABG or PCI is known to improve ejection fraction (EF) when viable myocardium exists. Revascularization can be used even for patients with an EF as low as 10%. Coronary artery bypass grafting for ischemic cardiomyopathy results in improved quality of life and fewer hospitalizations compared with medical therapy alone, and in survival rates superior to transplant for the first 2 years. Revascularization for heart failure is indicated for those patients with documented viable myocardium and no evidence of right ventricular (RV) dysfunction. Revascularization is not a good option for heart failure patients with RV dysfunction,

signs of right-sided heart failure, or pulmonary hypertension (Spoor & Bolling, 2008).

MITRAL VALVE REPAIR IN DILATED CARDIOMYOPATHY

Ventricular failure and dilatation will eventually result in functional mitral regurgitation (MR). This increases LV work, and it increases hypertrophy and dilation, which in turn increase MR. Mitral regurgitation is often a pre-terminal event and is associated with a survival time of 6–24 months (Spoor & Bolling, 2008). To date, there is no demonstrated long-term survival benefit from mitral valve repair for functional MR in heart failure (Gaasch, 2014). Mitral valve repair is discussed in more detail in Chapter 5.

VENTRICULAR RECONSTRUCTION TECHNIQUES

Ventricular reconstruction techniques are based on the principle that the ventricular wall tension is proportional to the LV radius and pressure and inversely proportional to the wall thickness (Law of Laplace) (Spoor & Bolling, 2008). By changing the size and shape of the ventricle, these techniques seek to reduce wall tension and improve LV function. Specifically, surgical reconstruction techniques attempt to remove or isolate dysfunctional myocardium, reduce the diameter of the ventricle, and restore a more elliptical ventricular shape (Fang, 2014).

Partial Left Ventriculectomy

Batista and colleagues (1996) described a procedure to restore the proper mass-to-diameter ratio for the left ventricle. To do so, a section of the LV wall from the apex to the mitral annulus was removed, and the edges were reapproximated. The mitral valve was repaired or replaced as necessary. Early results were promising, indicating improved LV function, decreased heart size, and improved functional status in one-third of patients. Mortality did not improve, and this procedure is not currently used (Fang, 2014).

Geometric Ventricular Reconstruction

The Dor procedure, also known as endoventricular circular patch plasty repair, is a procedure whereby the left ventricle is reconstructed using a purse-string suture to isolate nonfunctional segments of myocardium (rather than excising them) and a circular patch to control the shape of the ventricle. The Dor procedure is usually performed concomitantly with a CABG (Di Donato et al., 2001). The first case series report demonstrated a significant improvement in left ventricular ejection fraction (LVEF), which was maintained at 1-year follow up. In addition, in those patients for whom data were available, 92% had improved New York Heart Association (NYHA) functional class, and 91% of patients with VT were free of VT at 1-year follow up (Dor, Saab, Coste, Sabatier, & Montiglio, 1998). Mickleborough, Merchant, Ivanov, Rao, and Carson (2004) reported that a similar LV reconstruction procedure improved patients' LVEF and NYHA functional class and had low perioperative mortality.

Another modification of the original Dor concept—the surgical anterior ventricular endocardial restoration (SAVER) procedure—has produced similar results. Studies have shown that SAVER leads to a significant reduction of LV volume and a significant increase in EF as well as significant reductions in hospitalizations for heart failure. Survival at 18 months was 89%. A majority of patients had concomitant CABG, and 23% had mitral valve replacement at the time of the procedure (Athanasuleas et al., 2004; Hernandez et al., 2006). Studies reported consistently favorable results with ventricular reconstruction (Athanasuleas et al., 2004; Mickleborough et al., 2004). In the STICH trial, 1,000 patients

with LVEF of 35% or lower and anterior LV dysfunction were randomly assigned to CABG alone or CABG plus reconstruction using the SAVER technique (Jones et al., 2009). Although there was a decrease in end-diastolic volume with CABG plus ventricular reconstruction, there was no impact on symptoms, exercise tolerance, death, or cardiac hospitalization. At this time, ventricular reconstruction is not recommended (Fang, 2014).

Dynamic Cardiomyoplasty

Dynamic cardiomyoplasty is an innovative technique whereby the latissimus dorsi muscle is wrapped around the heart. An implanted stimulator is then used to stimulate the muscle to contract in synchrony with ventricular contraction. Another technique is the ACORN Cardiac Support Device (Acorn Medical, Minneapolis, MN)—a polyester mesh fabric that is wrapped snugly around the ventricles. This device provides passive support to the ventricles, which should reduce wall stress and prevent further remodeling. Both of these procedures have been abandoned. There does not appear to be a role for ventricular reconstruction in the treatment of heart failure (Fang, 2014).

CARDIAC TRANSPLANTATION

Transplantation is considered the definitive therapy for end-stage heart failure, with a 5-year posttransplant survival of 71.7% (Yancy et al., 2013). The principal limitation to heart transplantation is the growing gap between the number of potential recipients and the number of available donor organs. Given this mismatch in supply and demand, selection of recipients becomes an ethical dilemma as well as a clinical issue.

To date, the best outcomes are seen in patients with reversible pulmonary hypertension and hypertrophic, peripartum, and restrictive cardiomyopathies (Yancy et al.,

2013). The 2013 ACCF/AHA guideline for the management of heart failure lists a IC indication for transplantation in patients who remain in Stage D despite optimal medical, device, and surgical therapies (Yancy et al., 2013). For more detail on cardiac transplantation, see Chapter 19.

Heart–Lung Transplantation

Introduced in 1982, heart–lung transplantation was used for patients with end-stage cardiopulmonary and septic lung disease (Sheikh, Pelletier, & Robbins, 2008). The procedure reached its peak in the 1990s. Since then, however, due to improvements in single- and double-lung transplant techniques as well as donor allocation to critically ill heart recipients, the number of procedures has declined substantially. The International Heart and Lung Transplantation Registry noted a 40% decrease in the number of centers performing such transplants since 1994 (Yusen et al., 2013). The three most common indications for heart–lung transplantation are currently congenital heart disease with Eisenmenger syndrome, idiopathic pulmonary arterial hypertension, and cystic fibrosis (Nador & Lien, 2014).

SURGERY FOR ADULT CONGENITAL HEART DISEASE

In 2000, it was estimated that about 800,000 Americans have congenital heart disease (Kouchoukos et al., 2013). There are two categories of adult congenital heart disease. The first is secondary congenital heart disease, which is disease that has previously been treated; it is more common than primary congenital heart disease. Primary congenital heart disease in the adult consists either of previously unknown and untreated disease or newly diagnosed anomalies. The most common of these are atrial septal defect (ASD) and bicuspid aortic valve congenital heart

disease (Kouchoukos et al., 2013). For the purposes of this chapter, this section focuses on management of ASDs.

Most ASDs of less than 8 mm close spontaneously in childhood. For those patients whose defects do not close, the primary cause of symptoms is left-to-right shunting. An ASD is most often asymptomatic until the individual reaches adulthood. By age 30 to 40 years, however, AF and reduced exercise tolerance as a result of the defect are usually evident. Chronic left-to-right shunting may cause RV failure, tricuspid regurgitation, atrial arrhythmias, paradoxical embolization, and cerebral abscesses. Ultimately, irreversible pulmonary hypertension and right-to-left shunting and hypoxia will develop (Laks, Marelli, Plunkett, & Myers, 2008; Wiegers & St. John Sutton, 2007). Atrial septal defects can also be the source of paradoxical emboli where a venous clot (usually lower extremity clot) passes through the ASD to the arterial system.

Atrial septal defects with a diameter of 5 mm or less usually do not require closure but should be followed closely due to the risk of paradoxical embolism. Surgical closure has been considered for patients with an ASD when the ratio of pulmonary flow to systemic flow is greater than 1.5:1 and pulmonary vascular resistance is less than 6–8 U/m^2 (Laks et al., 2008). However, there are no data to indicate a standard pulmonary/systemic flow ratio for closure (Connolly, 2014). The indications for closure of an ASD include paradoxical embolism or atrial arrhythmias, regardless of the size of the ASD, and RV enlargement (Kouchoukos et al., 2013). Atrial septal defects may be closed by patch under CPB or via percutaneous closure using a closure device.

Outcomes from surgical closure are good. Mortality appears to be associated with the degree of pulmonary artery hypertension (Humenberger et al., 2011; Kouchoukos et al., 2013). In a review of 236 consecutive patients having transcatheter closure of their ASD, Humenberger and colleagues

(2011) found that survival was better the less functional impairment was present and the lower the pulmonary artery pressure (PAP). They also found that closure at any age is followed by significant symptom decrease, decrease in RV size, and decrease in PAP. Given that PAP increases with age, an ASD should be closed when the diagnosis is made (Humenberger et al., 2011; Kouchoukos et al., 2013).

HYPERTROPHIC CARDIOMYOPATHY

Hypertrophic cardiomyopathy (HCM) is a common genetic cardiovascular disease characterized by abnormal myocytes leading to hypertrophy without dilatation and preserved systolic function (Padera & Schoen, 2008). Hypertrophy is most severe in the ventricular septum. This asymmetrical growth usually arises at the level of the LV outflow tract, leading to subaortic stenosis or asymmetrical HCM. In addition, abnormal systolic anterior motion of the mitral valve contributes to the outflow obstruction (Padera & Schoen, 2008; van der Lee et al., 2005).

Hypertrophic cardiomyopathy has a variable course, although two presentations commonly lead to treatment. Impaired diastolic filling due to massive hypertrophy is usually responsible for signs and symptoms of heart failure, although obstruction of the LV outflow tract also contributes (Maron, 2005; Padera & Schoen, 2008). In addition, HCM is the most common cause of sudden cardiac death in young adults (Padera & Schoen, 2008). Four approaches are employed for treatment of HCM: pharmacologic therapy, dual-chamber pacing, surgery, and chemical ablation (Maron, 2013). Pharmacologic therapy is usually the first approach to signs and symptoms of heart failure; indeed, it is often the only treatment needed in patients without outflow obstruction. Beta blockade is the standard first-line therapy, with verapamil (Calan®) and

disopyramide (Norpace®) often being added to the treatment regimen to take advantage of their negative inotropic properties (Gersh et al., 2011). A second treatment approach, dual-chamber pacing, was introduced in the 1990s. Pacing was thought to change the geometry of ventricular contraction and lead to reduced LV outflow tract obstruction and symptomatic improvement. Data failed to show significant reductions in the outflow tract obstruction or exercise tolerance. The 2011 ACCF/AHA Task Force on Practice Guideline for the Diagnosis and Treatment of Hypertrophic Cardiomyopathy lists IIbB recommendation for pacing in patients who are symptomatic despite medical therapy and who are not considered candidates for septal reduction surgery (Gersh et al., 2011). The guideline also states that if a patient has a dual-chamber pacemaker for non-HCM reasons, it is reasonable to use that device to reduce symptoms of outflow tract obstruction (IIaB). Permanent pacemakers are not indicated for patients who are asymptomatic or who respond to medical therapy (IIIC) and are not indicated as first-line therapy for patients who are candidates for septal reduction.

The mainstay of treatment for patients with HCM who develop significant drug-refractory LV outflow tract obstruction has been surgical LV myectomy, mitral valve replacement, or both (Gersh et al., 2011; Kouchoukos et al., 2013; Maron, 2005, 2013; Maron et al., 2004; McKenna, 2007; van der Lee et al., 2005; Woo et al., 2005). The myectomy procedure involves excision of a section of subaortic septal muscle with or without mitral valve replacement. The procedure is performed in conjunction with perioperative transesophageal echocardiography to precisely determine the amount of tissue to be removed. This procedure has a long history and experience and is well documented to be safe, provide excellent hemodynamic results, and improve quality of life (Gersh et al., 2011; Kouchoukos et al., 2013; Maron, 2013).

Systolic anterior motion (SAM) of the mitral valve has been shown to be a major determinant of the amount of outflow obstruction. Mitral valve replacement (MVR) is often added to the myectomy procedure, depending on the degree of SAM and obstruction. The 2011 guideline lists a IC recommendation for septal reduction in patients whose symptoms are refractory to pharmacologic therapy and who have demonstrated outflow tract obstruction (Gersh et al., 2011). The guideline further recommends that this procedure be done only by experienced surgeons in the context of a comprehensive HCM program. The guideline lists class IIIC (harm) recommendations against septal reduction surgery for patients who are asymptomatic and have normal exercise tolerance or in those who are controlled with medical therapy. Solo mitral valve replacement for relief of outflow tract obstruction has a class IIIC recommendation in patients who are candidates for septal reduction (Gersh et al., 2011).

Finally, a percutaneous alternative for relieving outflow obstruction is available. Ethanol septal ablation is accomplished by infusing ethanol into the first septal branch of the left anterior descending coronary artery via an angioplasty catheter (Maron, 2013). Studies of this approach indicate that ethanol ablation creates a myocardial scar and reduces outflow tract obstruction, increases exercise capacity, and improves symptoms (Maron, 2013). In an observational series of 177 patients who had ethanol septal ablation, long-term survival was no different from surgical septal myectomy (Sorajja et al., 2012). The 2011 HCM guideline lists a IIaB indication for ethanol septal ablation for NYHA Class III or IV patients who are high-risk surgical candidates (Gersh et al., 2011). It carries a IIbB (uncertain) indication as an alternative to myectomy in selected situations where there is a patient preference for ethanol ablation and when the septum is

greater than 30 mm. Ethanol ablation carries a Class IIIC (harm) indication for asymptomatic or medically controlled patients if the patient needs cardiac surgery for other reasons, if the patient is less than 21 years of age, and if it is not part of a comprehensive HCM program. It carries a IIIC indication for adults under 40 if myectomy is a viable option.

OTHER CARDIAC SURGERIES: PERICARDIAL SURGERY

Bleeding and cardiac tamponade are known complications after cardiac surgery. Typically, the surgeon leaves the pericardium open and places mediastinal chest tubes to manage any postoperative bleeding. Despite these precautions, it is still possible for blood and clots to accumulate in the mediastinal space and impair ventricular filling (cardiac tamponade).

Reexploration of the mediastinum is indicated for signs of tamponade, including a sudden decrease or cessation of chest tube output, tachycardia, narrowing pulse pressure, and decreased cardiac index. Partial resection of the pericardium is known as a pericardial window. In such a procedure, a portion of the pericardium is excised to allow fluid to drain into the pleural or peritoneal space and prevent reaccumulation of pericardial fluid.

CARDIAC TUMORS

Atrial myxoma is a benign tumor and is the most common primary cardiac tumor. About 80% of myxomas originate in the left atrium. These tumors cause obstruction of blood flow, which in turn leads to the clinical presentation of heart failure, signs of central nervous system embolization, and constitutional symptoms such as fever, weight loss, fatigue, weakness, arthralgia, and myalgia. Resection of the myxoma is the only effective therapy and should be performed as an elective procedure when the diagnosis is made. Mortality and complications from surgery are low. Recurrence can be serious but occurs in only about 1% to 3% of patients. Familial myxomas recur more frequently (Kouchoukos et al., 2013).

SUMMARY

This chapter described the various cardiac surgical procedures and their associated indications based on the most recent evidence.

CASE STUDY

C. P. is a 57-year-old male with a 4-year history of coronary artery disease. He underwent angioplasty and stenting to the left posterior descending artery and an obtuse marginal 2 years ago. He reports increased symptoms over the past 2 weeks, including more frequent episodes of chest pain on exertion that is relieved with rest. He underwent coronary angiography, which revealed proximal left anterior descending artery and right coronary artery occlusion of 95%. He also had diffuse atherosclerosis. Transesophageal echocardiogram revealed an ejection fraction of 40% with septal dyskinesis and LV hypokinesis. He has normal RV systolic function.

C. P.'s medical history is significant for end-stage renal disease secondary to polycystic kidney disease; he undergoes hemodialysis three times weekly. His medical history is also significant for hypertension and hypercholesterolemia. C. P.'s medications include daily aspirin, an angiotensin-converting enzyme inhibitor, and a statin.

C. P. underwent a CABG procedure with a left internal thoracic artery graft to the left anterior descending artery and a radial artery graft to the right coronary artery. The operation was uneventful, and the patient was transferred to the intensive care unit in stable condition. He had a smooth recovery. His only postoperative complication was self-limiting hyperglycemia. He was extubated within 4 hours and transferred to the progressive care unit the next morning. C. P. was discharged to home on postoperative day 6. His discharge instructions included consumption of a low-fat, low-cholesterol diet and outpatient cardiac rehabilitation. He was given an appointment for the hospital's "Living with Heart Disease" class and was discharged on his pre-admission medications. He was to follow up with his surgeon in 2 weeks and his primary care provider in 4 weeks.

Critical Thinking Questions

1. Why did the healthcare provider recommend CABG procedure instead of stenting?
2. What were the indications for CABG on this patient?
3. What was the likely etiology of self-limiting hyperglycemia?

Answers to Critical Thinking Questions

1. C. P. had contraindications for PTCA. Specifically, he had multi-vessel disease with diffuse atherosclerosis and impaired LV function.
2. Two-vessel disease with proximal left anterior descending artery disease.
3. The hyperglycemia was likely related to increased catecholamines.

SELF-ASSESSMENT QUESTIONS

1. For which of the following rhythms is the use of catheter ablation techniques indicated?
   a. Accelerated junctional rhythm
   b. Atrial tachycardia
   c. Second-degree AV Block Type II
   d. Ventricular fibrillation

2. For which of the following is transmyocardial laser revascularization indicated as a sole therapy?
   a. Ejection fraction 40% refractory to medical therapy or surgical revascularization
   b. Stage IV angina responsive to medical therapy
   c. Irreversible ischemia of the LV free wall
   d. Transmyocardial laser revascularization is no longer indicated

3. For which of the following patients with atrial fibrillation is a surgical intervention indicated? A patient who:
   a. doesn't want the risk of life-threatening side effects of pharmacotherapy
   b. has cardiomyopathy secondary to tachyarrhythmias
   c. has supraventricular tachycardia unresponsive to medical therapy
   d. is not compliant with pharmacotherapy

4. Which of the following patients is most likely to be successfully treated with surgical therapy for ventricular tachycardia? A patient with:
   a. diffuse myocardial damage
   b. cardiomyopathy
   c. irreversibly damaged myocardium
   d. frequent episodes of hyperkalemia

5. For which of the following patients with heart failure is revascularization indicated? A patient with:
   a. pulmonary hypertension
   b. RV dysfunction
   c. right-sided heart failure
   d. an ejection fraction 10%

6. For which of the following patients is percutaneous coronary intervention recommended? A patient with:
   a. diabetes and multi-vessel disease
   b. unprotected left main disease
   c. LV dysfunction
   d. surgical risk

7. Which of the following patients has an indication for cardiac transplantation? A patient with:
   a. pulmonary vascular resistance > 5 U/m^2
   b. diabetic neuropathy
   c. active sarcoidosis
   d. ischemic heart disease with intractable angina

8. For which of the following patients is a heart–lung transplant indicated? A patient with:
   a. bilirubin 2.6 mg/dL with glomerular filtration rate 40 mL/min
   b. cystic fibrosis
   c. body mass index 42 kg/m^2
   d. COPD with heart failure

9. Which of the following is a sequela of chronic right-to-left shunting?
   a. Mitral regurgitation
   b. LV failure
   c. Ventricular dysrhythmias
   d. Pulmonary hypertension

10. The nurse should anticipate that the initial treatment for hypertrophic cardiomyopathy with sinus node dysfunction is:
    a. beta blocker
    b. dual-chamber pacing
    c. calcium channel blocker
    d. mitral valve replacement

Answers to Self-Assessment Questions

1. d	6. d
2. d	7. d
3. b	8. b
4. c	9. d
5. d	10. a

Clinical Inquiry Box

Question: What is the effect of diabetes on graft patency 1 year following CABG?

Reference: Singh, S. K., Desai, N. D., Petroff, S. D., Deb, S., Cohen, E. A., Radhakrishnan, S., . . . Fremes, S. E. (2008). The impact of diabetic status on coronary artery bypass graft patency: Insights from the Radial Artery Patency Study. *Circulation, 118,* 5222–5225.

Objective: To determine the impact of diabetes on graft patency 1 year following CABG

Method: Multicenter randomized trial. Follow up with angiography was made 1 year following CABG.

Results: A total of 561 patients were enrolled. A comparison of the saphenous vein and radial artery was made. Thirty-three of 230 (14.4%) of the grafts were occluded in patients with diabetes. This compared to 63 of 650 (9.7%) of patients who did not have diabetes. Saphenous vein grafts were statistically more often occluded in patients with diabetes (19% versus 12%). Fewer radial artery grafts were occluded in patients with diabetes.

Conclusions: Occlusion occurred more often in patients with diabetes as compared to those without diabetes. This was attributed to more frequent saphenous vein graft failures in patients with diabetes.

REFERENCES

Ad, N., Suri, R. M., & Gammie, J. S. (2012). Surgical ablation of atrial fibrillation trends and outcomes in North America. *Journal of Thoracic and Cardiovascular Surgery, 144,* 1051–1060.

Alam, M., Huang, H. D., Shahzad, S. A., Kar, B., Virani, S. S., Rogers, P. A., . . . Jneid, H. (2012). Percutaneous coronary intervention vs. coronary artery bypass graft surgery for unprotected left main coronary artery disease in the drug-eluting stents era. *Circulation, 77,* 372–382.

American Heart Association (AHA). (2007). Heart disease and stroke statistics—2007 update. Retrieved from http://circ.ahajournals.org/content/115/5/e69.full

Athanasuleas, C. L., Buckberg, G. D., Stanley, A. W., Siler, W., Dor, V., Di Donato, M., . . . Accola, K. A. (2004). Surgical ventricular restoration in the treatment of congestive heart failure due to post-infarction ventricular dilation. *Journal of the American College of Cardiology, 44*(7), 1439–1445.

Aydin, E., Ozen, Y., Sarikaya, S., & Yukseltan, I. (2014). Simultaneous coronary artery bypass grafting and carotid endarterectomy can be performed with low mortality rates. *Cardiovascular Journal of Africa, 25,* 130–133.

Babapulle, M. N., Joseph, L., Belisle, P., Brophy, J. M., & Eisenberg, M. J. (2004). A hierarchical Bayesian meta-analysis of randomized clinical trials of drug-eluting stents. *Lancet, 364*(9434), 583–591.

Bakaeen, F. G., Shroyer, A. L., Gammie, J. S., Sabik, J. F., Cornwell, L. D., Coselli, J. S., . . . Puskas, J. D. (2014). Trends in use of off-pump coronary artery bypass grafting: Results from the Society of Thoracic Surgeons Adult Cardiac Surgery Database. *Journal of Thoracic and Cardiovascular Surgery, 148*(3), 856–864.

BARI Investigators. (2000). Seven-year outcome in the Bypass Angioplasty Revascularization Investigation (BARI) by treatment and diabetic status. *Journal of the American College of Cardiology, 35*(5), 1122–1129.

Batista, R. J., Santos, J. L., Takeshita, N., Bocchino, L., Lima, P. N., & Cunha, M. A. (1996). Partial left ventriculectomy to improve left ventricular function in end-stage heart disease. *Journal of Cardiac Surgery, 11*(2), 96–97.

Boersma, L. V., Castella, M., van Boven, W., Berruezo, A., Yilmaz, A., Nadal, M., . . . Mont, L. (2012). Atrial fibrillation catheter ablation versus surgical ablation treatment (FAST): A 2-center randomized clinical trial. *Circulation, 125*(1), 25–30.

Brewer, R., Theurer, P. F., Cogan, C. M., Bell, G. F., Prager, R. L., & Paone, G.; Membership of the Michigan Society of Thoracic and Cardiovascular Surgeons. (2014). Morbidity but not mortality is decreased after off-pump coronary artery bypass surgery. *Annals of Thoracic Surgery, 97,* 831–836.

Brown, M. L., Sundt, T. M., & Gersh, B. J. (2008). Indications for revascularization. In L. H. Cohn (Ed.), *Cardiac surgery in the adult* (3rd ed., pp. 551–572). New York, NY: McGraw-Hill Medical.

Connolly, H. W. (2014). Management of atrial septal defects in adults. Retrieved from http://www.uptodate.com/contents/management-of-atrial-septal-defects-in-adults

Deb, S., Wijeysundera, H. C., Ko, D. T., Tsubota, H., Hill, S., & Fremes, S. E. (2013). Coronary artery bypass graft surgery vs percutaneous interventions in coronary revascularization. A systematic review. *Journal of the American Medical Association, 310*(19), 2086–2095.

Di Donato, M., Sabatier, M., Dor, V., Gensini, G. F., Toso, A., Maioli, M., . . . Buckberg, G. (2001). Effects of the Dor procedure on left ventricular dimension and shape and geometric correlates of mitral regurgitation one year after surgery. *Journal of Thoracic and Cardiovascular Surgery, 121*(1), 91–96.

Dor, V., Saab, M., Coste, P., Sabatier, M., & Montiglio, F. (1998). Endoventricular patch plasties with septal exclusion for repair of ischemic left ventricle: Technique, results and indications from a series of 781 cases. *Japanese Journal of Thoracic and Cardiovascular Surgery, 46*(5), 389–398.

Durrer, D., Schoo, L., Schuilenburg, R. M., & Wellens, H. J. (1967). The role of premature beats in the initiation of and the termination of supraventricular tachycardia in the Wolff-Parkinson-White syndrome. *Circulation, 36*, 644–662.

Eckart, R. E., & Epstein, L. (2008). Interventional therapy for atrial and ventricular arrhythmias. In L. H. Cohn (Ed.), *Cardiac surgery in the adult* (3rd ed., pp. 1357–1374). New York, NY: McGraw-Hill Medical.

Fang, J. C. (2014). Surgical management of heart failure. Retrieved from http://www.uptodate.com/contents/surgical-management-of-heart-failure

Farooq, V., Brugaletta, S., & Serruys, P. (2011). The SYNTAX score and SYNTAX-based clinical risk scores. *Seminars in Thoracic and Cardiovascular Surgery, 23*(2), 99–105.

Farooq, V., Serruys, P. W., Zhang, Y., Mack, M., Ståhle, M., Holmes, D. R., . . . Mohr, F. W. (2013). Short-term and long-term clinical impact of stent thrombosis and graft occlusion in the SYNTAX trial at 5 years. *Journal of the American College of Cardiology, 62*, 2360–2369.

Gaasch, W. H. (2014). Functional mitral regurgitation. Retrieved from http://www.uptodate.com/contents/functional-mitral-regurgitation

Gersh, B. J., Maron, B. J., Bonow, R. O., Dearani, J. A., Fifer, M. A., Link, M. S., . . . Yancy, C. W. (2011). 2011 ACCF/AHA guideline for the diagnosis and treatment of hypertrophic cardiomyopathy: A report of the American College of Cardiology Foundation/American Heart Association Task Force on Practice Guidelines. *Circulation, 124*(24), e783–e831.

Go, A. S., Mozaffarian, D., Roger, V. L., Benjamin, E. J., Berry, J. D., Blaha, M. J., . . . Turner, M. B. (2014). Heart disease and stroke statistics—2014 update. A report from the American Heart Association. *Circulation, 129*(3), e28–e292.

Goy, J. J., Eeckhout, E., Moret, C., Burnand, B., Vogt, P., Stauffer, J. C., . . . Kappenberger, L. (1999). Five-year outcome in patients with isolated proximal left anterior descending coronary artery stenosis treated by angioplasty or left internal mammary artery grafting: A prospective trial. *Circulation, 99*(25), 3255–3259.

Goy, J. J., Kaufmann, U., Goy-Eggenberger, D., Garachemani, A., Hurni, M., Carrel, T., . . . Eeckhout, E. (2000). A prospective randomized trial comparing stenting to internal mammary artery grafting for proximal, isolated de novo left anterior coronary artery stenosis: The SIMA trial: Stenting vs. internal mammary artery. *Mayo Clinic Proceedings, 75*(11), 1116–1123.

Gruberg, L. (2005). *ARTS II: Arterial Revascularization Therapies Study Part II: The role of sirolimus-eluting stents in patients with unstable angina.* Retrieved from http://www.medscape.org/viewarticle/501424

Hannan, E. L., Racz, M. J., Walford, G., Jones, R. H., Ryan, T. J., Bennett, E., . . . Rose, E. A. (2005). Long-term outcomes of coronary artery bypass grafting versus stent implantation. *New England Journal of Medicine, 352*(21), 2174–2183.

Hernandez, A. F., Velazquez, E. J., Dullum, M. K., O'Brien, S. M., Ferguson, T. B., & Peterson, E. D. (2006). Contemporary performance of surgical ventricular restoration procedures: Data from the Society of Thoracic Surgeons' National Cardiac Database. *American Heart Journal, 152*(3), 494–499.

Hillis, L. D., Smith, P. K., Anderson, J. L., Bittl, J. A., Bridges, C. R., Byrne, J. G., . . . Winneford, M. D. (2011). 2011 ACCF/AHA guideline for coronary artery bypass graft surgery. *Journal of the American College of Cardiology, 58*(24), e123–e210.

Hoffman, S. N., TenBrook, J. A., Wolf, M. P., Pauker, S. G., Salem, D. N., & Wong, J. B. (2003). A meta-analysis of randomized controlled trials comparing coronary artery bypass graft with percutaneous transluminal coronary angioplasty: One- to eight-year outcomes. *Journal of the American College of Cardiology, 41*(8), 1293–1304.

Horvath, K. A., & Zhou, Y. (2008). Transmyocardial laser revascularization and extravascular angiogenetic techniques to increase myocardial blood flow. In L. H. Cohn (Ed.), *Cardiac surgery in the adult* (3rd ed., pp. 733–751). New York, NY: McGraw-Hill Medical.

Hueb, W. A., Bellotti, G., de Oliveira, S. A., Ariê, S., de Albuquerque, C. P., Jatene, A. D., . . . Pileggi, F. (1995). The Medicine, Angioplasty or Surgery Study (MASS): A prospective, randomized trial of medical therapy, balloon angioplasty or bypass surgery for single proximal left anterior descending artery stenoses. *Journal of the American College of Cardiology, 26*(7), 1600–1605.

Humenberger, M., Rosenhek, R., Gabriel, H., Rader, F., Heger, M., Klaar, U., . . . Baumgartner, H. (2011). Benefit of atrial septal defect closure in adults: Impact of age. *European Heart Journal, 32*(5), 553–560.

January, C. T., Wann, L. S., Alpert, J. S., Calkins, H., Cleveland, J. C. Jr, Cigarroa, J. E., . . . Yancy, C. W. (2014). 2014 AHA/ACC/HRS Guideline for the management of patients with atrial fibrillation: A report of the American College of Cardiology/American Heart Association task force on practice guidelines and the Heart Rhythm Society. *Circulation, 130*(23), e199–e267.

Jones, R. H., Velazquez, E. J., Michler, R. E., Sopko, G., Oh, J. K., O'Connor, C. M., . . . Lee, K. L. (2009). Coronary bypass surgery with or without surgical ventricular reconstruction. *New England Journal of Medicine, 360*(17), 1705–1717.

Kappetein, A. P., Mohr, F. W., Feldman, T. E., Morice, M. C., Holmes, D. R., Ståhle, E., . . . Colombo, A. (2011). Comparison of coronary bypass surgery with drug-eluting stenting for the treatment of left main and/or three-vessel disease: 3-year follow-up of the SYNTAX trial. *European Heart Journal, 17*, 2125–2134.

Kassaian, S. E., Abbasi, K., Hakki Kazazi, E., Soltanzadeh, A., Alidoosti, M., Karimi, A., . . . Razmjoo, K. (2013). Staged carotid artery stenting and coronary artery bypass surgery versus isolated coronary artery bypass surgery in concomitant coronary and carotid disease. *Journal of Invasive Cardiology, 25*(1), 8–12.

Kearney, K., Stephenson, R., Phan, K., Chan, W. Y., Huang, M. Y., & Yan, T. D. (2014). A systematic review of surgical ablation versus catheter ablation for atrial fibrillation. *Annals of Cardiothoracic Surgery, 3*(1), 15–29.

Kouchoukos, N. T., Blackstone, E. H., Hanley, F. L., & Kirklin, J. K. (2013). *Kirklin/Barratt-Boyes cardiac surgery* (4th ed.). Philadelphia, PA: Elsevier.

Krul, S. P., Driessen, A. H., van Boven, W. J., Linnenbank, A. C., Geuzebroek, G. S., Jackman, W. M., . . . de Groot, J. R. (2011). Thoracoscopic video-assisted pulmonary vein antrum isolation, ganglionated plexus ablation, and periprocedural confirmation of ablation lesions: First results of a hybrid surgical-electrophysiological approach for atrial fibrillation. *Circulation: Arrhythmia and Electrophysiology, 4*(3), 262–270.

Laham, R. J., & Simons, M. (2014). Transmyocardial laser revascularization for management of refractory angina. Retrieved from http://www.uptodate.com/contents/transmyocardial-laser-revascularization-for-management-of-refractory-angina

Laks, H., Marelli, D., Plunkett, M., & Myers, J. (2008). Adult congenital heart disease. In L. H. Cohn (Ed.), *Cardiac surgery in the adult* (3rd ed., pp. 1431–1463). New York, NY: McGraw-Hill Medical.

Maron, B. J. (2005). Surgery for hypertrophic obstructive cardiomyopathy: Alive and quite well. *Circulation, 111*(16), 2016–2018.

Maron, B. J., Dearani, J. A., Ommen, S. R., Maron, M. S., Schaff, H. V., Gersh, B. J., & Nishimura, R. A. (2004). The case for surgery in obstructive hypertrophic cardiomyopathy. *Journal of the American College of Cardiology, 44*(10), 2044–2053.

Maron, M. S. (2013). Nonpharmacologic treatment of outflow obstruction in hypertrophic cardiomyopathy. Retrieved from http://www.uptodate.com/contents/nonpharmacologic-treatment-of-outflow-obstruction-in-hypertrophic-cardiomyopathy

McKenna, W. J. (2007). Nonpharmacologic treatment of outflow obstruction in hypertrophic cardiomyopathy. Retrieved from www.uptodate.com

Mercado, N., Wijns, W., Serruys, P. W., Sigwart, U., Flather, M. D., Stables, R. H., . . . Boersma, E. (2005). One-year outcomes of coronary artery bypass graft surgery versus percutaneous coronary intervention with multiple stenting for multisystem disease: A meta-analysis of individual patient data from randomized clinical trials. *Journal of Thoracic and Cardiovascular Surgery, 130*(2), 512–519.

Mickleborough, L. L., Merchant, N., Ivanov, J., Rao, V., & Carson, S. (2004). Left ventricular reconstruction: Early and late results. *Journal of Thoracic and Cardiovascular Surgery, 128*(1), 27–35.

Mohler, E. R., & Fairman, R. M. (2014). Carotid endarterectomy. Retrieved from http://www.uptodate.com/contents/carotid-endarterectomy

Mohr, F. W., Marice, M. C., Kappetein, A. P., Feldman, T. E., Ståhle, E., Colombo, A., . . . Serruys, P. W. (2013). Coronary artery bypass graft surgery versus percutaneous coronary interventions in patients with three-vessel disease and left main coronary disease: 5-year follow up of the randomised clinical SYNTAX trial. *Lancet, 381*, 629–638.

Møller, C. H., Perko, M. J., Lund, J. T., Andersen, L. W., Kelbæk, H., Madsen, J. K., . . . Steinbrüchel, D. A. (2010). No major differences in 30-day outcomes in high-risk patients randomized to off-pump versus on-pump coronary bypass surgery: The best bypass surgery trial. *Circulation, 121*, 498–504.

Morice, M. C., Serruys, P. W., Kappetein, P., Feldman, T., Ståhle, E., Colombo, A., . . . Mohr, F. (2010). Outcomes in patients with de novo left main disease treated with either percutaneous coronary intervention using Paclitaxel-eluting stents or coronary artery bypass graft treatment in the Synergy Between Percutaneous Coronary Intervention With TAXUS and Cardiac Surgery (SYNTAX) Trial. *Circulation, 121*, 2645–2653.

Nador, R. G., & Lien, D. (2014). Heart-lung transplantation. Retrieved from http://www.uptodate.com/contents/heart-lung-transplantation

Nardi, P., Pellegrino, A., Bassano, C., Mani, R., Chiariello, G. A., Zeitani, J., . . . Chiariello, L. (2014). The fate at mid-term follow-up of the on-pump vs. off-pump coronary artery bypass grafting surgery. *Journal of Cardiovascular Medicine, 16*(2), 125–133.

O'Gara, P. T., Kushner, F. G., Ascheim, D. D., Casey, D. E., Jr., Chung, M. K., de Lemos, J. A., . . . Yancy, C. W. (2013). 2013 ACCF/AHA guideline for the management of ST-elevation myocardial infarction: A report of the American College of Cardiology Foundation/American Heart Association Task Force on Practice Guidelines. *Journal of the American College of Cardiology, 61*(4), e78–e140.

Oral, H., & Latchamsetty, R. (2014). Atrial fibrillation: Paroxysmal, persistent, and permanent. In D. P. Zipes & J. Jalife (Eds.), *Cardiac electrophysiology: From cell to bedside* (6th ed., pp. 739–754). Philadelphia, PA: Elsevier.

Padanilam, B. J., & Prystowsky, E. N. (2009). Atrial fibrillation: Goals of therapy and management strategies to achieve the goals. *Cardiology Clinics, 27*(1), 189–200.

Padera, R. F., & Schoen, F. J. (2008). Pathology of cardiac surgery. In L. H. Cohn (Ed.), *Cardiac surgery in the adult* (3rd ed., pp. 112–178). New York, NY: McGraw-Hill Medical.

Pagé, P. L. (2004). Surgery for cardiac arrhythmias. In D. P. Zipes & J. Jalife (Eds.), *Cardiac electrophysiology: From cell to bedside* (4th ed., pp. 1104–1115). Philadelphia, PA: Saunders.

Podrid, P. J., & Ganz, L. I. (2014). Pathogenesis of ventricular tachycardia and ventricular fibrillation during acute myocardial infarction. Retrieved from http://www.uptodate.com/contents/pathogenesis-of-ventricular-tachycardia-and-ventricular-fibrillation-during-acute-myocardial-infarction

Puskas, J. D., Williams, W. H., Duke, P. G., Staples, J. R., Glas, K. E., Marshall, J. J., . . . Guyton, R. A. (2003). Off-pump coronary artery bypass grafting provides complete revascularization with reduced myocardial injury, transfusion requirements and length of stay: A prospective, randomized comparison: SMART study. *Journal of Thoracic and Cardiovascular Surgery, 125*(4), 797–808.

Schofield, P. M., & McNab, D. (2010). National Institute for Health and Clinical. NICE evaluation of transmyocardial laser revascularisation and percutaneous laser revascularisation for refractory angina. *Heart, 96*, 312–313.

Serruys, P. W., Morice, M. C., Kappetein, A. P., Colombo, A., Holmes, D. R., Mack, M. J., . . . Mohr FW; SYNTAX Investigators. (2009). Percutaneous coronary intervention versus coronary-artery bypass grafting for severe coronary artery disease. *New England Journal of Medicine, 360*(10), 961–972.

Serruys, P. W., Unger, F., Sousa, J. E., Jatene, A., Bonnier, H. J., Schonberger, J. P., . . . van Hout, B. A. (2001). Comparison of coronary-artery bypass surgery and stenting for the treatment of multivessel disease. *New England Journal of Medicine, 344*(15), 1117–1124.

Sharony, R., Grossi, E. A., Saunders, P. C., Galloway, A. C., Applebaum, R., & Ribakove, G. H. (2004). Propensity case-matched analysis of off-pump coronary artery bypass grafting in patients with atheromatous aortic disease. *Journal of Thoracic and Cardiovascular Surgery, 127*(2), 406–413.

Sheikh, A. Y., Pelletier, M. P., & Robbins, R. C. (2008). Heart–lung and lung transplantation. In L. H. Cohn (Ed.), *Cardiac surgery in the adult* (3rd ed., pp. 1579–1608). New York, NY: McGraw-Hill Medical.

Shishehbor, M. H., Venkatachalam, S., Sun, Z., Rajeswaran, J., Kapadia, S. R., Bajzer, C., . . . Blackstone, E. H. (2013). A direct comparison of early and late outcomes with three approaches to carotid revascularization and open heart surgery. *Journal of the American College of Cardiology, 62*, 1948–1956.

Shroyer, A. L., Grover, F. L., Hattler, B., Collins, J. F., McDonald, G. O., Kozora, E., . . . Novitzky, D.; The ROOBY study group. (2009). On-pump versus off-pump coronary-artery bypass surgery. *New England Journal of Medicine, 361*, 1827–1837.

Sorajja, P., Ommen, S. R., Holmes, D. R., Jr., Dearani, J. A., Rihal, C. S., Gersh, B. J., . . . Nishimura, R. A. (2012). Survival after alcohol septal ablation for obstructive hypertrophic cardiomyopathy. *Circulation, 126*(20), 2374–2380.

Spoor, M. T., & Bolling, S. F. (2008). Nontransplant surgical options for heart failure. In L. H. Cohn (Ed.), *Cardiac surgery in the adult* (3rd ed., pp. 1639–1655). New York, NY: McGraw-Hill Medical.

Stulak, J. M. (2014). Off-pump and minimally invasive direct coronary bypass graft surgery: Outcomes. Retrieved from http://www.uptodate.com/contents/off-pump-and-minimally-invasive-direct-coronary-artery-bypass-graft-surgery-outcomes

Valgimigli, M., Serruys, P. W., Tsuchida, K., Vaina, S., Morel, M. A., van den Brand, M. J., . . . Parrinello, G. (2007). Cyphering the complexity of coronary artery disease using the Syntax score to predict clinical outcome in patients with three-vessel lumen obstruction undergoing percutaneous coronary intervention. *American Journal of Cardiology, 99*, 1072–1081.

van der Lee, C., ten Cate, F. J., Geleijnse, M. L., Kofflard, M. J., Pedone, C., van Herwerden, L. A., . . . Serruys, P. W. (2005). Percutaneous versus surgical treatment for patients with hypertrophic obstructive cardiomyopathy and enlarged anterior mitral leaflets. *Circulation, 112*(4), 482–488.

Wiegers, S. E., & St. John Sutton, M. (2007). Management of atrial septal defects in adults. Retrieved from www.uptodate.com

Woo, A., Williams, W. G., Choi, R., Wigle, D., Rozenblyum, E., Fedwick K., . . . Rakowski, H. (2005). Clinical and echocardiographic determinants of long-term survival after surgical myectomy in obstructive hypertrophic cardiomyopathy. *Circulation, 111*(16), 2033–2041.

Yancy, C. W., Jessup, M., Bozkurt, B., Butler, J., Casey, D. E., Jr., Drazner, M. H., . . . Wilkoff, B. L. (2013). 2013 ACCF/AHA Guideline for the management of heart failure: A report of the American College of Cardiology Foundation/American Heart Association Task Force on Practice Guidelines. *Journal of the American College of Cardiology, 62*(16), e147–e239.

Yusen, R. D., Christie, J. D., Edwards, L. B., Kucheryavaya, A. Y., Benden, C., Dipchand, A. I., . . . Stehlik, J. (2013). The Registry of the International Society for Heart and Lung Transplantation: Thirtieth adult lung and heart-lung transplant report—2013; focus theme: age. *Journal of Heart and Lung Transplantation, 32*(10), 965–978.

Yusuf, S., Zucker, D., Passamani, E., Peduzzi, P., Takaro, T., Fisher, L. D., . . . Chalmers, T. C. (1994). Effect of coronary artery bypass graft surgery on survival: Overview of 10-year results from randomized trials by the Coronary Artery Bypass Graft Surgery Trialists Collaboration. *Lancet, 344*(8922), 563–570.

Zembala, M. O., & Suwalski, P. (2013). Minimally invasive surgery for atrial fibrillation. *Journal of Thoracic Disease, 5*, S704–S712.

WEB RESOURCE

2011 ACCF/AHA Guideline for Coronary Artery Bypass Graft Surgery: http://content.online-jacc.org/article.aspx?articleid=1147818

Chapter 4

Preoperative Cardiac Surgery Nursing Evaluation

Roberta Kaplow and Sonya R. Hardin

INTRODUCTION

Preoperative evaluation and preparation of the patient for cardiac surgery affects postoperative outcomes and progress. The primary goal of a presurgical assessment is evaluation of perioperative risk. An in-depth assessment assists in minimizing surgical risk and potential morbidity and mortality. The literature supports the preoperative optimization of a patient's cardiovascular status as part of the effort to improve patient outcomes (Zambouri, 2007). An evaluative screening identifies special needs that may require modification of the patient's course of treatment before, during, and after surgery.

RISK FACTORS OF MORBIDITY AND MORTALITY FOLLOWING CARDIAC SURGERY

The major risk factors for adverse outcomes of cardiac surgery include factors in all three phases of hospitalization (pre-, intra-, and postoperative). A number of risk assessment tools (Parsonnet, Dean, & Bernstein, 1989; Tu, Jaglal, & Naylor, 1995; Tuman, McCarthy, March, Najafi, & Ivankovich, 1992) score risk factors for morbidity and mortality, such as advanced age, emergency surgery, previous cardiac surgery, dialysis dependency, creatinine level of 2 mg/dL or higher, and preoperative renal insufficiency (Bhukal et al., 2012). EuroSCORE factors include age, gender, chronic obstructive pulmonary disease (COPD), extracardiac arteriopathy, neurologic dysfunction, previous cardiac surgery, serum creatinine, active endocarditis, preoperative state, cardiac factors (i.e., unstable angina, left ventricular [LV] dysfunction, recent myocardial infarction [MI], and pulmonary hypertension), and procedure-related factors (i.e., emergency, other than isolated coronary artery bypass grafting [CABG], thoracic aorta, and postinfarct septal rupture) (EuroSCORE.org, n.d.; Kobayashi et al., 2009).

Numerous risk assessment tools have been developed to predict mortality in patients undergoing heart surgery. Some of these scoring tools include the Parsonnet, Cleveland Clinic, French, Euro, Pons, and Ontario Province Risk scores (Geissler et al., 2000). The Parsonnet score has been found to be predictive in the oldest of old individuals who require cardiac surgery (Chaturvedi, deVarennes, & Lachapelle, 2007). Prolonged hospital stays and increased mortality are associated with higher scores. Scoring is located in the Web Resource at the end of the chapter.

Research has demonstrated a decreased incidence of physical and psychological problems that adversely affect recovery when preoperative education of patients is completed. Evidence further indicates that preoperative patient education results in increased patient compliance, resulting in decreased length of hospital stay (Kaur, Verma, & Singh, 2007; Kramer et al., 2012; Marley, Calabrese, & Thompson, 2014).

NURSING ASSESSMENT

Nursing assessment prior to cardiac surgery typically begins during an outpatient visit, but may occur during an acute inpatient admission. The latter situation may occur in patients with conditions that increase their operative risk. The preoperative nursing assessment provides baseline information for the postoperative period, along with an opportunity to develop a relationship with the patient. Components of the preoperative assessment include information from the patient, family, and medical records, and the physical exam.

Preoperative Patient Interview

The purpose of a patient interview is to review past medical and surgical histories and to conduct a systems evaluation to identify processes that may affect the outcome of a patient's cardiac surgery. The interview helps the nurse evaluate patient and family knowledge as well as determine educational needs related to the planned procedure. Understanding of the underlying illness, planned surgical course, and willingness and ability to adhere to the surgical regimen are also evaluated. Put simply, the nurse is responsible for the overall assessment of the patient's physical and psychological readiness for surgery. Data suggest that cardiac surgery patients who receive preoperative education with or without coping strategies as opposed to routine preoperative preparation experience less emotional distress, have better physical and psychological recovery, and experience fewer hypertensive episodes postoperatively (Kramer et al., 2012).

Baseline information is obtained about the patient's clinical history, including the type of heart disease, associated symptoms, resource availability, stability, and ability to participate in care and decision making. The level of resilience is determined when the nurse ascertains the degree of compensation the patient has developed.

During the patient interview, the nurse should seek to discover any information that can affect perioperative risk and postoperative management. Several risk factors have been identified in the literature as influencing the mortality of cardiac surgery patients. **Table 4-1** lists many of these comorbid conditions.

The nurse should also inquire if the patient has any history of gastrointestinal bleeding, peptic ulcer disease, or bleeding diathesis. Any of these conditions may affect the antiplatelet regimen following revascularization or the choice of a valvular prosthesis. Likewise, the nursing evaluation should gather information on the presence of cardiac risk factors as well as presence of associated medical diseases, such as COPD, cerebrovascular or other peripheral arterial occlusive disease, and hypertension.

The patient's baseline sleep patterns should be determined. Patients who undergo CABG procedures are at risk of developing sleep disturbances postoperatively. The presence of anxiety and depression should be assessed as well, because these psychosocial conditions may develop in the postoperative cardiac surgery patient (Sveinsdóttir & Ingadóttir, 2012).

Obstructive Sleep Apnea

Presence of obstructive sleep apnea (OSA) is typically assessed for by surgery and anesthesia providers prior to surgery. The diagnosis of OSA can impact postoperative outcomes after cardiac surgery. In some instances providers may decide to offer elective surgery to treat OSA with continuous positive airway pressure (CPAP) several weeks prior to surgery. The literature supports OSA patients sleeping in the lateral, prone, or sitting

Table 4-1 Factors That May Affect Cardiac Surgery Patient Mortality	
Alcohol use	Tobacco use
Diabetes	Elevated serum creatinine (2 mg/dL or higher)
Chronic airway disease	Prior cardiac surgery
Recent MI	Low left ventricular ejection fraction
Chronic heart failure	Pulmonary hypertension
Unstable angina	Depression
Obesity	Hypoalbuminemia
Active endocarditis	Procedure urgency
Ventricular septal rupture	Critical preoperative condition
Dialysis	Advanced age
Preoperative GFR	African American race
Preoperative functional status	Left heart function
Aortic regurgitation	Atrial fibrillation
Coronary artery disease	Ascending aortic aneurysm
Aortic valve endocarditis	

GFR, glomerular filtration rate; MI, myocardial infarction

Sources: Data from Kouchoukos, N. T., Blackstone, E. H., Hanley, F. L., & Kirklin, J. K. (2013a). Aortic valve disease. In N. T. Kouchoukos, E. H. Blackstone, F. L. Hanley, & J. K. Kirklin (eds.) Kirklin/Barratt-Boyes cardiac surgery (4th ed., pp 541–643). Philadelphia, PA: Elsevier Saunders; Thakar, C. V., Arrigain, S., Worley, S., Yared, J. P., & Paganini, E. P. (2005). A clinical score to predict acute renal failure after cardiac surgery. Journal of the American Society of Nephrology, 16(1), 162–168.

position to improve apnea–hypopnea index scores. Nurses should be aware that concurrent administration of sedative agents increases the risk of respiratory depression and airway obstruction. Supplemental oxygen should be used postoperatively until peripheral capillary oxygen saturation (SpO_2) monitoring shows that individuals can maintain an airway with their CPAP as was used in the home environment (American Society of Anesthesiologists, 2014).

Nutrition Evaluation

The preoperative evaluation should also look for indicators of nutritional deficiency. In particular, malnutrition is a risk factor associated with significant morbidity and mortality in surgical patients. During the nursing evaluation, it is essential that all cardiac surgery patients undergo nutritional screening to identify malnourished or at-risk patients to ensure that an adequate nutritional plan is included as part of the patient's care.

The Malnutrition Universal Screening Tool (MUST) has been found to predict postoperative complications in cardiac surgery patients (Lomivorotov et al., 2013). The MUST tool includes the variables of body mass index (BMI), weight loss in last 3–6 months, and the effect of lack of nutritional intake for greater than 5 days due to acute disease process. A score of 3 or greater indicates malnutrition. Malnutrition is observed in 10% to 25% of patients having cardiac surgery (van Venrooij, van Leeuwen, de Vos, Borgmeijer-Hoelen, & de Mol, 2009).

In addition to the nutritional assessment screens available, unintentional weight loss, protein-calorie malnutrition, laboratory findings (e.g., anemia, hypoalbuminemia, prealbumin, vitamin B_{12} deficiency, other vitamin and mineral deficiency), and low BMI are among the variables suggesting nutritional deficiency (Centers for Disease Control and Prevention, 2012; Hengstermann, Nieczaj, Steinhagen-Thiessen, & Schulz, 2008). Patients with hypoalbuminemia (< 2.5 g/dL) should have their nutritional status optimized 1 to 4 weeks prior to cardiac surgery, because they are at greater risk for sepsis and respiratory failure. Enhanced nutrition is also essential to promote wound healing and meet postoperative metabolic demands (Daley, 2014). This can be accomplished with dietary enhancement or enteral feeding if no contraindications are present. Patients who are undergoing cardiac surgery and who have a low BMI (< 20 kg/m^2) and hypoalbuminemia (< 2.5 g/dL) are at increased risk of postoperative morbidity and mortality (Meneghini, 2009; Montazerghaem, Safaie, & Samiei, 2014). Further, patients with hypoalbuminemia are at increased risk for developing sternal wound infections, postoperative anemia, infection from the saphenous vein graft harvest site, renal failure, increased risk of postoperative atrial fibrillation (AF), increased hospital length of stay, and prolonged ventilatory support (Meneghini, 2009). Conversely, patients with a high percentage of body fat have a greater risk for sternal wound infections (Bojar, 2011; Ji et al., 2012).

Discharge Planning

To begin proactive discharge planning, the patient's living arrangements are assessed. Many patients need assistance at discharge owing to limited social and financial resources. Early discharge planning alleviates stressors and anxiety for both the patient and family (Carroll & Dowling, 2007). Discharge to rehabilitative units either in long-term care or subacute care units can be easily predicted. Strong predictors include use of an intra-aortic balloon pump (IABP), emergency surgery, older age, long postoperative stays, poor nutritional state, comorbidities, and descending thoracic aorta procedures (Pattakos, Johnston, Houghtaling, Nowicki, & Blackstone, 2012).

Physical Assessment

Cardiac Assessment

For patients undergoing cardiac surgery, the assessment of the cardiovascular system will likely be more extensive than the assessment of the other body systems. Blood pressure, temperature, assessment of peripheral pulses, and weight are recorded. Blood pressure

readings should be obtained from both arms. Blood pressure difference between arms is associated with increased morbidity and mortality (Clark et al., 2014) and subclavian artery stenosis (Ochoa & Yeghiazarians, 2010). This condition may eliminate the possibility of using the internal thoracic (formerly mammary) artery for grafting (Ochoa & Yeghiazarians, 2010). It has been suggested that stenting the subclavian artery will make the vessel suitable for CABG (George, O'Murchu, & Bashir, 2011).

Auscultation of the heart and carotid arteries will provide essential baseline information. Heart sounds should be evaluated in terms of their rate, rhythm, and presence of extra sounds, murmurs, gallops, or rubs. Identification of aortic regurgitation (AR) is a significant finding, because this condition may be exacerbated during cardiopulmonary bypass (CPB) and lead to acute LV distention (Hessel II, 2008). Aortic regurgitation is identified with the presence of an early diastolic murmur that can be heard at the second and third intercostal spaces (ICSs) at the right sternal border and at the second and fourth ICSs at the left sternal border. The murmur of AR usually decreases in intensity (decrescendo) and disappears before the S_1 heart sound (Jung & Lilly, 2011).

A carotid bruit is a sound associated with turbulent flow and may indicate arterial stenosis. Auscultation of the carotid arteries is performed from the base of the neck to the angle of the jaw while breath holding. A bruit is usually most audible in the upper third of the carotid near the bifurcation (Fitzgerald, 2014).

As noted in Chapter 3, perioperative stroke rate is reported to be twice as high for patients with bilateral versus unilateral carotid atherosclerotic disease (Mohler & Fairman, 2014). Accordingly, carotid endarterectomy is recommended before CABG in patients with high-grade carotid stenosis and for whom coronary revascularization is not urgent or concurrently with CABG in patients who have an urgent need for revascularization (i.e., those with severe left main coronary heart disease, diffuse coronary heart disease without satisfactory collateral circulation, or unstable angina) (Lazar, Wilson, & Messé, 2014).

Peripheral vascular assessment is performed to help determine the extent of peripheral perfusion. Components of this evaluation include determining the presence and strength of pulses in all extremities, capillary refill time, extremity and nail bed color, and temperature. Calculating the ankle-brachial index helps evaluate the arterial blood flow to the lower extremities; steps to determine this index appear in Chapter 10. The results of this calculation are then used to rate degree of peripheral artery disease and will help determine if the saphenous vein is suitable for use during cardiac surgery (Slovut & Lipsitz, 2012).

A cardiac assessment further entails determining presence of varicose veins. Presence of significant numbers of lower-extremity varicosities may indicate the need to use upper-extremity vessels (e.g., radial artery) as conduits during CABG.

Pulmonary Assessment

Postoperative pulmonary complications contribute significantly to morbidity and mortality. A thorough pulmonary assessment, including identification of associated risk factors, is pivotal so that implementation of strategies to mitigate complications can begin in a timely fashion or risk of complications can be anticipated (Adabag et al., 2010).

Lung auscultation provides information about respiratory rate and breath sounds, and the presence of crackles or wheezing. Presence of crackles indicates fluid in the alveoli, which may require diuresis prior to surgery. Presence of decreased breath sounds or adventitious sounds may be related to an undiagnosed condition that may increase the risk of postoperative pulmonary complications or to underlying

heart or lung disease. In either case, optimizing the patient's clinical condition preoperatively is indicated (Khan & Hussain, 2005).

A patient's smoking history should be determined. Some data suggest that patients who smoke are more likely to experience pulmonary adverse events following cardiac surgery (Jones, Nyawo, Jamieson, & Clark, 2011). Long-term effects of smoking following cardiac surgery are also emphasized in the literature. Patients should be counselled on smoking cessation 4 to 8 weeks prior to cardiac surgery to avoid these long-term effects. Quitting smoking a few days prior to cardiac surgery likely has no benefit and may result in increased secretions (Bojar, 2011). Preoperative cardiac surgery patients should be assessed for preexisting pulmonary disease to help anticipate potential postoperative conditions. Specifically, a history of pulmonary hypertension and COPD are two predictors of pulmonary complications following cardiac surgery (Bojar, 2011). Patients with COPD, bronchitis, poor control of asthma symptoms, productive cough, or lower respiratory tract colonization are also more likely to develop postoperative complications (Bojar, 2011). It is recommended that patients with COPD who are undergoing cardiac surgery have preoperative pulmonary function testing (Adabag et al., 2010).

Abdominal Assessment

A preoperative abdominal assessment is important to determine the presence of an abdominal aortic aneurysm (AAA), which is a potential contraindication of the use of an intra-aortic balloon pump (IABP—discussed in detail in Chapter 10) (Haddad & Robertson, 2013).

Ultrasound is the preferred method to screen for presence of an AAA. It has high sensitivity and specificity levels. Abdominal palpation is not recommended for determining presence of an AAA as it is not an accurate assessment (Agency for Healthcare Research and Quality, 2009)

Neurologic Assessment

A patient who is undergoing cardiac surgery may develop neurologic impairment during the intraoperative or postoperative period. A baseline assessment will help facilitate identification of changes in neurologic status. Baseline data can help prevent unnecessary testing that might otherwise be performed to evaluate postoperative neurologic symptoms, which, in fact, might have been present preoperatively. The risk for postoperative delirium has been reported to be 11.5% in cardiac surgery patients. Risk factors include longer cross-clamping time, diabetes, gastritis or ulcer problems, volume received in the operating room, amount of time on mechanical ventilation in the intensive care unit (ICU), highest postoperative temperature in the ICU, amount of sodium received in the ICU, AF, and advanced age (Andrejaitiene & Sirvinskas, 2012; Smulter, Lingehall, Gustafson, Olofsson, & Engström, 2013).

PREOPERATIVE ASSESSMENT OF HEART DISEASE

Typically, patients undergoing cardiac surgery have coronary artery disease (CAD). In fact, increasing numbers of patients who are undergoing cardiac surgery have several comorbid conditions and have a higher operative risk. Resource utilization after cardiac surgery is higher in patients with risk, especially in the elderly. In one study, elderly patients used more medications (e.g., inotropic agents, antimicrobials, anti-arrhythmic therapy), blood products, interventions (e.g., renal replacement therapies, re-sternotomy, or sternal rewiring), and implantation of devices (e.g., IABP, pulmonary artery catheter, permanent pacemaker, or ventricular assist device), and their ICU and hospital lengths of stay were also higher (Ngaage, Britchford, & Cale, 2011).

A baseline assessment of underlying heart function is essential to help identify those patients who are at risk during the intraoperative period. Data specific to heart function as well as the presence and extent of comorbidities such as diabetes and hypertension should be collected. The patient history should include determination of when cardiac comorbidities (e.g., MI) occurred and whether associated complications are present (e.g., heart failure, ischemia, dysrhythmias) (Moonesinghe & Kelleher, 2006).

The relationship between CAD and valvular disease is discussed in Chapter 5. Patients with valvular heart disease are vulnerable to additional intraoperative and postoperative risk. A preoperative cardiac assessment for these patients should evaluate the impact of valvular disease on ventricular function.

Cardiac History

Nursing evaluation includes assessment of the current level of symptoms. During the patient interview, any increase in intensity or frequency of symptoms should be relatively easy to uncover. The interview is used to identify the degree of the patient's associated functional impairment and to observe for indications that heart function is inadequate during exertion. Several classification systems can be used to assess the functional status of patients with heart disease; these systems evaluate angina, heart failure, and other aspects of heart disease. For example, the Canadian Cardiovascular Society's functional classification system is used for the evaluation of angina; the New York Heart Association's classification is used to evaluate heart failure (Heart Failure Society of America, 2011; Kaul et al., 2009).

Preoperative evaluation of a patient's current medical status should include a cardiac history. Specifically, the presence and severity of symptoms of CAD should be determined.

In addition to assessing presence of risk factors for CAD (e.g., tobacco, hypertension, diabetes, hyperlipidemia), obtaining a list of the patient's current medications and patient adherence will provide essential information. Severity of pain should be rated on a 0 to 10 scale. Characteristics of angina patterns should be described in terms of onset; location; duration; character; precipitating, aggravating, and alleviating factors; and frequency. From this information, healthcare providers can decide whether the patient has stable or unstable angina. Existence of a previous or recent MI and presence of dysrhythmias or palpitations are also essential pieces of information. Signs of pulmonary edema or pulmonary hypertension or other associated cardiovascular, peripheral vascular, or valvular heart disease should be identified as well. The surgeon should be notified of significant findings and if possible preoperative hospital admission is anticipated.

Dyspnea is another symptom of heart disease to be evaluated in the preoperative cardiac surgery patient; it usually results from inadequate tissue oxygen delivery. Patients may report difficult, labored, or uncomfortable breathing. Some of the more common causes of dyspnea include heart failure, cardiac ischemia, asthma, COPD, and pneumonia. If dyspnea is noted, determination of whether it has a cardiac or pulmonary etiology is vital. Indices of a cardiac etiology include a history of dyspnea on exertion, paroxysmal nocturnal dyspnea, orthopnea, and chest pain. Physical findings may include jugular venous distention, S_3 gallop, ascites, and peripheral edema. Radiologic studies may reveal cardiomegaly (McStay, 2007). Dyspnea is commonly observed in patients with valvular disease; it may also be experienced by patients with ventricular dysfunction.

Orthopnea is the sensation of breathlessness when the patient is lying in a position of rest. It is relieved by sitting or standing. With worsening cardiac disease, orthopnea often develops such that the patient needs to elevate the head of the bed with more than one pillow to breathe comfortably while recumbent.

Serological Testing

In addition to patient history, preoperative testing with serological and other diagnostic methods should be performed. Data from these tests will help determine surgical and postoperative risk and define the presence or extent of any new or known comorbid conditions.

Laboratory data that may be collected preoperatively include complete blood count; coagulation profile; liver, renal, and thyroid function; electrolytes; and albumin level. Identifying the presence of anemia or infection is an important consideration when evaluating cardiac patients, because there are always risks of intraoperative bleeding and dilutional effects with bypass procedures. Attaining and maintaining a hematocrit greater than 35% is recommended. In addition, CBC data will help suggest presence of an infection from an elevated white blood cell count. Preoperative treatment of infection should be implemented. It is recommended that surgery not be delayed because of the infection unless implantation of prosthetic material is planned (Johnson, 2009). Preoperative anemia is associated with increased risk of noncardiac complications and increased morbidity and mortality during cardiac surgery (Meneghini, 2009). If CBC results reveal thrombocytopenia, a decision as to whether the patient should receive heparin should be made, because thrombocytopenia may be an indication of heparin-induced thrombocytopenia (HIT). Further testing must be done to confirm HIT. If a patient tests positive for HIT, an alternative anticoagulation method should be considered for CPB. For example, bivalirudin (Angiomax®), a direct thrombin inhibitor, has been used in cardiac surgery patients requiring bypass (Coutre, 2014).

Patients will be heparinized during bypass procedures. Any coagulopathies should be corrected (e.g., with fresh frozen plasma or platelet transfusion, administration of vitamin K) prior to surgery to minimize risk of postoperative bleeding (O'Glasser, 2013).

Assessment of liver function should be conducted to help predict how medications, including anesthetic agents, will be metabolized. The value in optimizing a patient's nutritional status preoperatively was discussed earlier; albumin level is one component of that assessment.

Renal dysfunction is common in patients awaiting cardiac surgery and is a predictor of postoperative morbidity and mortality. Perioperative management includes minimizing use of nephrotoxic agents and maintaining perfusion to the kidneys (Meneghini, 2009). Sometimes a patient develops acute kidney injury (AKI) following cardiac surgery. The 30-day mortality rate increases dramatically with this complication. Risk factors for the development of AKI following cardiac surgery have been identified. These include female gender, COPD, diabetes, peripheral vascular disease, renal insufficiency, heart failure, left ventricular ejection fraction (LVEF) less than 35%, need for emergent surgery, presence of cardiogenic shock that requires use of an IABP, left main CAD, and total circulatory arrest (Gude & Jha, 2012). These data speak to the essential nature of a comprehensive patient assessment prior to cardiac surgery.

The overall mortality rate from AKI following cardiac surgery is reported to be as high as 80%, depending on development of multiple organ dysfunction, increase in serum creatinine, and need for renal replacement therapies. The high mortality rate is attributed primarily to infection; other factors such as immune dysregulation, platelet dysfunction, and issues related to being on hemodialysis (e.g., hemodynamic instability, infections of the vascular access devices, and ventricular

ectopy) have been implicated as well (Gude & Jha, 2012).

Although thyroid function tests are not part of the usual preoperative assessment, data suggest that hypothyroidism is overlooked in cardiac surgery patients. Postoperative cardiac surgery patients with hypothyroidism are reported to have a longer length of stay in the ICU and hospital, higher incidence of postoperative AF, and higher long-term mortality rates (Jyrala, Weiss, Jeffries, & Kay, 2012). These data provide justification for preoperative thyroid function testing.

Maintaining serum glucose levels within a normal range decreases the rate of cardiac surgery complications. Effective treatment and monitoring of these data for the cardiac surgery patient should begin in the preoperative setting. Data suggest that presence of hyperglycemia in cardiac surgery patients increases mortality, postoperative AF, length of stay, and infection rates (Haga et al., 2011; Lazar, 2012).

Diagnostic Studies

In addition to laboratory tests, a number of diagnostic procedures may potentially be performed for the preoperative cardiac surgery patient. Results of these tests will provide information about cardiac anatomical and physiologic issues and pulmonary status, help identify those patients who may be at higher risk (and the degree of risk) with surgery, alert the surgeon that preoperative "fine-tuning" may be necessary, or suggest that modifications of fluids or medications, or both, intraoperatively may be anticipated. Some of the diagnostic procedures that may be performed for these purposes include echocardiography, computed tomography (CT), magnetic resonance imaging (MRI), radionuclide scanning, cardiopulmonary exercise testing (CPET), cardiac catheterization, and pulmonary function tests (PFTs) (Moonesinghe & Kelleher, 2006).

Echocardiography may be performed to discover any cardiac anatomical irregularities that might affect surgery. Results of an echocardiogram may reveal conditions such as decreased ejection fraction (EF) or right ventricular (RV) function, presence of aortic stenosis (AS) or insufficiency, or mitral insufficiency. These data may be used to reevaluate the surgical plan, identify intraoperative risk, or devise a plan to optimize the patient's clinical status as much as possible prior to surgery. Data from echocardiography are important, because decreased EF is associated with poor survival following revascularization (Hamad et al., 2010).

Computed tomography may be performed to identify any cardiac anatomical irregularities that might affect the surgery outcome. A literature review suggested that use of preoperative CT has resulted in surgery being cancelled up to 13% of the time and use of preventive intraoperative strategies (e.g., not using a midline approach, initiating bypass procedures before re-sternotomy, and peripheral vascular exposure). A lower incidence of intraoperative injury is also reported with preoperative CT scanning (Khan & Yonan, 2009). As part of the preoperative evaluation, MRI may be performed to identify any cardiac anatomical irregularities, assess cardiac function and perfusion, and evaluate valves and blood vessels. Cardiac MRI creates cardiac images while the heart is beating, thereby providing both still and moving images of the heart and major blood vessels. Heart structure and function can be evaluated. Chamber size and damage from MI may be determined through use of this technology as well (National Heart, Lung, and Blood Institute, 2012a).

Cardiopulmonary exercise testing may be performed to determine a patient's fitness for surgery. It assesses the heart's functional reserve—that is, the amount of work the heart is able to do in extraordinary conditions (Bhagwat & Paramesh, 2010). During this noninvasive evaluation, concomitant cardiac and ventilatory effects of exercise are assessed. Gas exchange, heart rate, and blood pressure measurements, along with electrocardiogram evaluation, provide information on actual energy expenditure and stroke volume during exercise. The oxygen extraction from each beat is also measured at varying work intensities (Agnew, 2010; Bhagwat & Paramesh, 2010). Cardiopulmonary exercise testing is increasing in acceptance in Europe because of its precise evaluation of postoperative morbidity (Bhagwat & Paramesh, 2010).

Cardiac catheterization is considered the gold standard for the diagnosis of CAD. In the case of the cardiac surgery patient, it is performed to evaluate coronary anatomy and efficacy of cardiac contractility (National Heart, Lung, and Blood Institute, 2012b). Data such as baseline right atrial, pulmonary artery systolic, diastolic, and occlusive pressures, as well as pulmonary vascular resistance (PVR), EF, and cardiac output, will help determine LV and RV function, augment valve function data, and assist with intraoperative and postoperative hemodynamic management. Administration of fluids and vasoactive agents and the choice of the operative procedure itself are guided by these data. A cardiac catheterization may sometimes reveal the presence of an LV mural thrombus, which places the patient at risk for a stroke in the intraoperative or postoperative period. In patients with valvular heart disease, cardiac catheterization may be used to estimate the degree of regurgitation. Unlike echocardiography, which provides an indirect measurement of the pressure gradient, cardiac catheterization provides for a direct measurement of this parameter (Moonesinghe & Kelleher, 2006).

Pulmonary function tests may be performed on patients who have preexisting lung disease (e.g., COPD). As noted earlier in this chapter, patients with a history of

COPD are at greater risk for developing postoperative complications and requiring prolonged intubation. Data from a preoperative arterial blood gas sample can help guide postoperative weaning (Roekaerts & Heijmans, 2012).

Even patients with healthy lungs may have pulmonary complications after cardiac surgery. Issues include decreased functional residual capacity following general anesthesia and neuromuscular blocking agent administration; decreased vital capacity from sternotomy and intrathoracic manipulation, atelectasis, intravascular lung water, and increased capillary permeability leading to leakage; and increased extravascular lung water secondary to the inflammatory response associated with CPB. Lung function may also be compromised due to fluid overload from blood and fluid administration (Roekaerts & Heijmans, 2012).

Pulmonary function tests have been helpful to reclassify COPD before cardiac surgery. In one study, data provided from PFTs were used to determine prognosis after cardiac surgery (Adabag et al., 2010).

Given that carotid artery stenosis is a risk factor for stroke following CABG, a preoperative carotid ultrasound should be considered. Patients with a carotid bruit or a history of cerebrovascular accident are at greater risk for developing this complication. Assessment of the carotid arteries preoperatively may decrease the postoperative risk of stroke (Cornily et al., 2011).

Patients who are undergoing cardiac surgery should receive a preoperative dental examination. This is especially true of patients who will be receiving a prosthetic heart valve. These patients are at increased risk for infective endocarditis or prosthetic valvular endocarditis (Schmelzeisen & Varbroudi, 2008).

Other recent data suggest that delaying cardiac surgery to have dental work may be associated with adverse events or death. The authors of one study noted that patients who required dental work tended to be sicker (Smith et al., 2014). In that study, six patients (2.9%) died between dental surgery and the planned cardiac procedure; 10 (4.8%) had major adverse outcomes before cardiac surgery including acute coronary syndrome or stroke. Postoperatively, there was an increased time on mechanical ventilation and renal failure.

Medications

A comprehensive review of the patient's current medication profile and concomitant medical and surgical histories is essential to assist with preoperative planning and prevent intraoperative and postoperative complications. Although some medications may be withheld before cardiac surgery, many others are continued or adjusted during the preoperative period, particularly those used to manage hypertension or heart disease (Moonesinghe & Kelleher, 2006).

Nitrates

Nitrates should be continued up to the time of surgery to avoid an ischemic event (Saber, 2006). Further, preoperative administration of a nitrate or other vasodilator (e.g., prostacyclin, nitric oxide) may be indicated to decrease PVR (Sparacino-Watkins, Lai, & Gladwin, 2012).

Inotropes

If patients have a history of PVR that results in RV dysfunction, preoperative administration of an inotropic agent may be indicated. Agents such as dobutamine (Dobutrex®) or milrinone (Primacor®) may be used. Patients who are awaiting heart transplant may have low cardiac output (CO) preoperatively as well. Patients with low CO before transplant have higher mortality rates as compared to patients with acceptable hemodynamics. Preoperative administration of an inotrope improves hemodynamics before heart transplantation, bringing mortality statistics equal to other transplant recipients (Kouchoukos, Blackstone, Hanley, & Kirklin, 2013b).

Beta Blockers

Discontinuing beta-adrenergic-blocking agents can result in a hypersympathetic state that could precipitate myocardial ischemia, infarction, rebound hypertension, tachycardia, or dysrhythmias. As such, they should be continued in patients who are already taking these agents (Fleisher et al., 2009; Poldermans et al., 2009; Saber, 2006; Wiesbauer et al., 2007). As noted in Chapter 15, the incidence of AF following cardiac surgery varies with the procedure performed. In one study, of the patients who underwent aortic valve replacement, CABG, or off-pump coronary artery bypass (OPCAB), 74%, 44%, and 35%, respectively, developed postoperative AF (Helgadottir, Sigurdsson, Ingvarsdottir, Arnar, & Gudbjartsson, 2012). The patients who developed AF in this study were older, more often female, had a lower EF, and were less likely to be smokers. Other identified risk factors include greater age, history of hypertension or AF, and heart failure. Preoperative prophylactic administration of beta blockers has reportedly decreased the incidence of AF by 70% to 80% in patients who undergo CABG. Some researchers suggest that sympathetic tone, which is augmented during cardiac surgery, is diminished when beta blockers are taken.

It is further suggested that beta blockers not be initiated before surgery in patients who are not currently taking them as this practice has been found to be harmful. Worse cardiac outcomes occurred when beta blocker–naïve patients were started on therapy preoperatively (Ellenberger, Tait, & Beattie, 2011). If a beta blocker must be started, it is recommended that it be started several weeks before surgery to allow time for dose adjustments and to check for adverse events (Devereaux

et al., 2008; Fleisher et al., 2009; Poldermans et al., 2009). It has been further suggested that beta blockers be tapered or changed to short-acting agents to help patients avoid potential intraoperative myocardial depression (Wiesbauer et al., 2007).

Angiotensin-Converting Enzyme (ACE) Inhibitors and Angiotensin Receptor Blockers (ARBs)

While most cardiac medications are not held in the preoperative cardiac surgery patient, ACE inhibitors are typically held on the morning of surgery (Saber, 2006). Continuation of ACE inhibitors may result in intraoperative hypotension by augmenting the effects of anesthesia (Whinney, 2009). Data from one study suggest that ACE inhibitors be discontinued before CABG surgery. In this study, patients who continued on ACE inhibitor therapy experienced more hypotension upon anesthesia induction and the period immediately following bypass (Hasija et al., 2010). In a meta-analysis conducted by Rosenman and colleagues (2008), the increased risk of intraoperative hypotension was corroborated. Despite these data, some believe it may be wise to continue ACE inhibitor therapy unless the patient's indication is hypertension and the blood pressure is well controlled (Whinney, 2009). The key risks associated with ACE inhibitor discontinuation are arterial graft spasm and increased requirements for vasodilator therapy (Moonesinghe & Kelleher, 2006). It is further recommended that ARBs be held for 24 hours prior to surgery because of their long half-life (Whinney, 2009).

Calcium Channel Blockers (CCBs)

Patients should continue to take their CCB up to and including the day of surgery. One exception may be in cases of poor hemodynamics (i.e., hypotension, arrhythmias). A short-acting CCB may be substituted (e.g., diltiazem [Cardizem®]) (Saber, 2006; Smith & Jackson, 2010).

Anticoagulants

Medications affecting hemostasis or bleeding are discontinued in preparation for cardiac surgery. Specifically, warfarin (Coumadin®) is held 5 days prior to surgery so that the international normalized ratio (INR) reaches a level less than 2.0 (Meneghini, 2009). Patients who are at risk for developing thrombosis should receive intravenous heparin when the INR reaches subtherapeutic levels (Dunning et al., 2008).

Clopidogrel (Plavix®) is held 5–10 days before surgery to decrease the risk of excessive intraoperative bleeding, transfusion requirements, and reoperations (Dempsey, Limin, & Stacey, 2007; Meneghini, 2009; Moonesinghe & Kelleher, 2006; Saber, 2006). Clopidogrel is also associated with a two- to five-fold increase in risk for surgical reexploration and a 30% to 100% increase in blood loss from the chest tube (Dunning et al., 2008). Patients can be transfused with platelets if bleeding is a postoperative issue (Dempsey et al., 2007).

Aspirin irreversibly inhibits platelet function. Recent data suggest, however, that there is no difference in 30-day and 1-year mortality, or MI or stroke at 30 days in patients who continued aspirin therapy before CPB surgery (Guay & Ochroch, 2014). In another study, up to a 20% increase in bleeding was reported. There was no difference in severity of bleeding or mortality between patients taking aspirin and those who were not (Burger, Chemnitius, Kneissl, & Rücker, 2005; Ellenberger et al., 2011). It is recommended that low-dose aspirin be continued unless the risk of bleeding outweighs the benefit (Biondi-Zoccai et al., 2006; Burger et al., 2005; Fleisher et al., 2009; Holt, 2012; Poldermans et al., 2009).

Glycoprotein IIb/IIIa inhibitors (e.g., eptifibatide [Integrilin®], tirofiban [Aggrastat®]) are anti-platelet drugs. They should be discontinued 4–6 hours before surgery (Meneghini, 2009).

The use of heparin before CPB surgery has two rationales. First, heparin provides prophylaxis against development of a venous thrombotic event. Second, heparin can serve as a substitute for aspirin. Low-molecular-weight heparin (LMWH) may serve as a substitute for unfractionated heparin and as a bridging therapy to CPB surgery if aspirin is discontinued while the patient is nil per os (NPO—not allowed oral intake) (Renda et al., 2007). Some data suggest that LMWH does not increase postoperative blood loss when it is withheld shortly before cardiac surgery (Meneghini, 2009).

Bivalirudin, a short-acting direct thrombin inhibitor (DTI), should be discontinued 3 hours before cardiac surgery. Long-acting DTIs (e.g., hirudin [Refludan®, Revasc®] and argatroban [Acova®]), should be discontinued earlier and unfractionated heparin given in its place (Meneghini, 2009).

The American College of Chest Physicians (ACCP) has proposed guidelines for noncardiac surgical patients who are at risk for a venous thromboembolism. If patients are at low risk, warfarin should be held 4–5 days prior to surgery; no bridge with heparin is recommended for these patients. There is no consensus regarding optimal perioperative management for patients on long-term warfarin therapy. There are some suggestions for minor procedures only (Daley, 2012). The ACCP recommends heparin prophylaxis for high-risk groups. Other data suggest use of LMWH as a bridge for patients receiving chronic anticoagulation who are undergoing cardiac surgery (Dunning et al., 2008).

Hypoglycemics

Patients with diabetes are at increased risk of complications following surgery. This is due to hormonal and inflammatory stressors that can occur with surgery and anesthesia (Meneghini, 2009). Preoperatively, the patient's blood sugar should be made as stable as possible. This is typically accomplished with subcutaneous insulin. Patients who have not taken insulin in the past should be placed on a sliding scale to correct the blood sugar. Low-dose basal insulin may be added to patients with hyperglycemia. Basal insulin analogs are preferred because of their consistent action and decreased risk of hypoglycemia. For patients already receiving insulin, it is recommended that the basal insulin be continued with a possible decrease of 25% of the dose and sliding-scale insulin, as needed. Patients who take combination insulin or premixed insulin types should receive an estimate of the basal dose. Delivery of 40% to 50% of that dose can be administered as basal insulin. Sliding-scale insulin may be added as needed (Meneghini, 2009).

Patients who are taking oral hypoglycemic agents for type 2 diabetes should have these agents withheld preoperatively for several days because of the risks associated with them. This is especially true of metformin (Glucophage®), which is known to contribute to the development of postoperative lactic acidosis if there is a decrease in renal function (Evans, Ogston, Emslie-Smith, & Morris, 2006; Meneghini, 2009). Further, the combination of metformin and sulfonylureas is known to contribute significantly to postoperative morbidity and mortality (Evans et al., 2006; O'Riordan, 2013). Metformin should be held 1–2 days before surgery if administration of intravenous contrast is anticipated or if hemodynamic instability is anticipated (as this latter condition leads to decreased renal perfusion).

Thiazolidinediones (e.g., pioglitazone [Actos®], rosiglitazone [Avandia®]) induce fluid retention and should be discontinued a few days before surgery. Glucagon-like peptide 1 (GLP-1) agonists (e.g., exenatide [Byetta®]) have the potential to decrease gastric motility and delay gastrointestinal recovery following surgery. As such, it is recommended that GLP-1 agonists be held on the day of surgery. Gliptins or dipeptidyl peptidase 4 (DPP-4) inhibitors (e.g., alogliptin [NESINA®], linagliptin [Tradjenta®], saxagliptin [Onglyza®], sitagliptin [Januvia®]) may be continued as long as there are no associated significant side effects. However, because of their mechanism of action, these agents should not be needed if the patient is NPO (Meneghini, 2009).

Patients with type 1 diabetes must continue to receive their basal insulin replacement in the preoperative period. Sliding-scale insulin may be used to correct elevated blood sugar levels (Meneghini, 2009).

Long-acting insulin is usually discontinued preoperatively as well. In contrast, insulin glargine (Lantus®), a long-acting basal insulin, may be continued during the surgical period (Marks, 2003). Other patients who receive insulin therapy may have their dose withheld on the day of surgery, with medication levels being regulated based on blood glucose monitoring.

Statins

In addition to lowering lipids, statins decrease vascular inflammation, augment endothelial function, and stabilize atherosclerotic plaque (Meneghini, 2009). Data suggest that continuing statin therapy in patients undergoing cardiac or vascular surgery decreases cardiac risk (Meneghini, 2009; Winchester, Wen, Xie, & Bavry, 2010). Stopping statins abruptly results in a rebound effect. During this time, there is an increased cardiac risk (Holt, 2012; Whinney, 2009). Statins should be initiated several weeks before surgery to maximize their benefits (Holt, 2012). Data suggest that statin therapy should be continued through the day of surgery (Saber, 2006). Administration of a statin prior to cardiac surgery is associated with a 38% decrease in mortality, and decreased incidence of AF and stroke (Meneghini, 2009).

Herbal Remedies

Use of herbal remedies can cause increased risk of bleeding and drug interactions. While the medication profile obtained during the preoperative evaluation should include information about the use of herbal remedies, more is being learned about potential interactions between these supplements and other medications every day. As this growing knowledgebase has significant clinical implications for the cardiac surgery patient, no herbal remedies should be taken for at least 2 weeks prior to surgery. Garlic, ginseng, echinacea, ginkgo biloba, St. John's wort, valerian, kava, flavonoids, and grapefruit juice are all known to decrease platelet activity (Hodges & Kam, 2002). Ginseng may also cause hypoglycemia. Kava and valerian may cause an enhanced sedative effect of anesthetic agents. St. John's wort may cause increased metabolism of many of the drugs used in the perioperative period (Ang-Lee, Moss, & Yuan, 2001). Herbal remedies should be stopped at least 1 week before surgery (Whinney, 2009).

MANAGEMENT OF HIGH-RISK PATIENTS

Ventricular Dysfunction

Preoperative cardiac surgery patients with heart failure and a history of hypertension, ischemia, hypertrophic cardiomyopathy, or acute valvular dysfunction are at risk for, and should be assessed for, ventricular dysfunction. High morbidity and mortality rates are associated with cardiac surgery in patients who have severe LV dysfunction and clinically significant heart failure secondary to ischemic or valvular heart disease (Weisberg, Weisberg, Wilson, & Collard, 2009). Patients with LV dysfunction and valvular disease (e.g., mitral regurgitation, AS) require preoperative management of their hemodynamic status.

The presence of heart failure may cause surgery to be delayed while healthcare providers attempt to improve the patient's cardiac function and decrease surgical risk. Data suggest that patients who are undergoing a CABG procedure who had an LVEF less than 20% have almost four times the in-hospital mortality rates, were less likely to be discharged home, and had a higher incidence of postoperative respiratory failure, AKI, and sepsis than patients with an LVEF greater than 40%. A preoperative cardiac evaluation of these patients may include positive emission tomography, dobutamine echocardiogram, dobutamine MRI, or delayed enhancement MRI (Meneghini, 2009). Therapy focuses on maintaining adequate preload and afterload. Medication or the IABP may be used to augment afterload reduction. In such a case, the nursing evaluation focuses on identifying and optimizing the patient's unstable hemodynamic status.

CABG-associated mortality is higher in patients who had a recent (within the past 3 to 7 days) MI. It is recommended that surgery be delayed for at least that amount of time. Patients who sustained an anterior wall MI should be evaluated for presence of an LV thrombus with transesophageal echocardiogram. An inferior wall MI decreases RV function. These patients undergoing CPB may develop hemodynamic consequences exacerbated during CPB procedures. A recovery of 4 weeks is recommended (Meneghini, 2009).

Patients with peripheral vascular disease or a carotid bruit should be further evaluated with carotid Doppler to determine if and when carotid revascularization should be performed (Meneghini, 2009).

SUMMARY

Patients who present for cardiac surgery have higher levels of complexity than in the past. Often, because of comorbid or concomitant conditions, surgical procedures are combined, creating potentially higher levels of vulnerability and instability. An in-depth preoperative evaluation of the patient's history and cardiac status, along with collection of laboratory data and possibly invasive and noninvasive procedures, is critical to prevent poor outcomes postoperatively. Early detection of potential complications can improve outcomes and help ensure a successful recovery. Critical care nurses are in a unique position to utilize clinical inquiry techniques and critical thinking skills to uncover those risk factors and data that can redirect interventions to become more individual specific.

CASE STUDY

K. P. is a 72-year-old frail female with a history of hypertension, heart failure (with an LVEF of 20%), and 3-vessel disease. She is scheduled for CABG. She is admitted preoperatively for evaluation and to control her blood pressure. Her medication profile includes losartan 50 mg daily, enalapril 2.5 mg twice daily, and furosemide 40 mg daily. She reports that she also takes St. John's wort for depression and ginkgo biloba to help prevent memory loss. Both of these supplements were encouraged by her daughter. Her preoperative albumin level is 2.2 g/dL.

Critical Thinking Questions

1. Given the history of this patient, which potential postoperative problem might the nurse expect?
2. What medications should the nurse anticipate being administered and held in preparation for this patient's surgery?
3. What should the patient be told about taking herbal supplements?

Answers to Critical Thinking Questions

1. Given that K. P. is frail and her albumin level is low, she is showing indications of nutritional deficiencies that could affect her recovery.
2. K. P.'s ACE inhibitor will be held on the morning of surgery as its continuation may result in intraoperative hypotension by augmenting the effects of anesthesia. The ARB that K. P. is receiving will likely be discontinued 24 hours before surgery as these agents have a longer half-life. The furosemide will likely be held the day of surgery in order to prevent electrolyte depletion during and after surgery.
3. The St. John's wort and gingko biloba will need to be stopped immediately. Ideally, a week should pass prior to surgery. St. John's wort is of concern because of the numerous drug–drug interactions associated with this supplement; it is a known CYP3A4 inducer. As such, it will decrease levels of other drugs that are metabolized by this enzyme system. Gingko biloba is of concern because it inhibits platelet-activating factor; this puts K. P. at increased risk for bleeding.

SELF-ASSESSMENT QUESTIONS

1. Which of the following is the primary goal of an assessment before cardiac surgery?
   a. Select the best anesthetic agent
   b. Predict postoperative complications
   c. Determine perioperative risk
   d. Improve patient outcomes

2. Which of the following patients is at greatest risk for adverse outcomes of cardiac surgery? A:
   a. 55-year-old male with elevated low-density lipoproteins
   b. 48-year-old male with HbA1c 5.5%
   c. 70-year-old female with creatinine 2.1 mg/dL
   d. 61-year-old female with LVEF 45%

3. An 80-year-old patient is being evaluated for cardiac surgery. Presence of which of the following puts the patient at greatest mortality risk?
   a. Cardiogenic shock
   b. Acute kidney injury
   c. LV aneurysm
   d. Second reoperation required

4. Which of the following is evaluated during a nursing interview before cardiac surgery?
   a. Understanding of education materials provided
   b. Willingness to adhere to the surgical regimen
   c. Ability to pay the hospital bill after discharge
   d. Preference for type of procedure to be performed

5. A patient is to undergo emergent cardiac surgery. Preoperative evaluation revealed an albumin level of 2.1 g/dL and body mass index of 19 kg/m². For which of the following should the nurse anticipate having to monitor postoperatively?
   a. Excessive clotting
   b. Respiratory failure

   c. Ventricular dysrhythmias
   d. Sternal wound infection

6. Upon preoperative assessment for cardiac surgery, the nurse notes presence of an early diastolic murmur at the second and third intercostal spaces at the right sternal border. Which of the following should be anticipated in the postoperative period following cardiopulmonary bypass?
   a. Papillary muscle rupture
   b. LV distention
   c. Cardiogenic shock
   d. Right bundle branch block

7. Which of the following conditions puts the patient at greatest risk for cognitive impairment following cardiac surgery?
   a. Anxiety disorder
   b. COPD
   c. Abdominal aortic aneurysm
   d. Atrial fibrillation

8. Dyspnea is noted on cardiac assessment. Which of the following is most likely present?
   a. Valvular disease
   b. Pericardial effusion
   c. 2-vessel occlusion of 80%
   d. Aortic aneurysm

9. Which of the following sets of electrolytes places the patient at greatest risk for development of dysrhythmias following cardiac surgery?

Potassium (mEq/L)	Magnesium (mg/dL)
a. 5.2	1.6
b. 3.1	4.0
c. 3.2	1.5
d. 5.1	4.1

10. Which of the following medications should the nurse anticipate being discontinued at least a day before cardiac surgery?
    a. Nitroglycerin (Tridil®)
    b. Metoprolol (Lopressor®)
    c. Enalapril (Vasotec®)
    d. Milrinone (Primacor®)

Answers to Self-Assessment Questions

1. c   3. a
2. c   4. b

5. b   9. c
6. b   10. c
7. d
8. a

Clinical Inquiry Box

Question: How can undernutrition prior to cardiac surgery be assessed more accurately?

Reference: van Venrooij, L. M. W., Visser, M., de Vos, R., van Leeuwen, P. A. M., Peters, R. J. G., & de Mol, B. A. J. M. (2013). Cardiac surgery–specific screening tool identifies preoperative undernutrition in cardiac surgery. *Annals of Thoracic Surgery, 95,* 642–647.

Objective: To determine whether a revision in the nutritional screen of cardiac patients improves diagnostic accuracy

Methods: A prospective observational study was performed with 325 patients. Examination of the correlation of undernutrition as measured by bioelectrical impedance spectroscopy and/or unintended weight loss (UWL), decreased appetite, and low physical activity were data utilized to develop a new tool for screening for malnutrition in the cardiac surgery population.

Results: Reduced food intake and inactivity were associated with undernutrition. Reduced food intake and inactivity were integrated with BMI and UWL into a new scoring system: the Cardiac Surgery–Specific Undernutrition Screening Tool (CSSUST). Sensitivity in identification of undernourished patients was considerably higher with the CSSUST at 90%.

Conclusions: Results suggest that reduced food intake and inactivity partly explain undernutrition before cardiac operations. The new tool, CSSUST, is superior to existing tools in identifying undernutrition in cardiac surgery patients. This tool measures four factors: BMI, recent weight loss, decreased appetite, and admission preoperatively. A score greater than 2 equates with high risk for undernutrition.

REFERENCES

Adabag, A. S., Wassif, H. S., Rice, K., Mithani, S., Johnson, D., Bonawitz-Conlin, J., . . . Kelly, R. F. (2010). Preoperative pulmonary function and mortality after cardiac surgery. *American Heart Journal, 159*(4), 691–697.

Agency for Healthcare Research and Quality. (2009). *Screening for abdominal aortic aneurysm—aaa.* Retrieved from http://www.ahrq.gov/professionals/clinicians-providers/resources/aaaprovider.html

Agnew, N. (2010). Preoperative cardiopulmonary exercise testing. *Continuing Education in Anaesthesia, Critical Care & Pain, 10*(2), 33–37.

American Society of Anesthesiologists Committee on Standards and Practice Parameters and the Task Force on Perioperative Management of Obstructive Sleep Apnea. (2014). Practice guidelines for the perioperative management of patients with obstructive sleep apnea. *Anesthesiology, 120*(2), 1–19.

Andrejaitiene, J., & Sirvinskas, E. (2012). Early post-cardiac surgery delirium risk factors. *Perfusion, 27*(12), 105–112.

Ang-Lee, M. K., Moss, J., & Yuan, C.-S. (2001). Herbal medicines and perioperative care. *Journal of the American Medical Association, 286*(2), 208–216.

Bhagwat, M., & Paramesh, C. (2010). Cardiopulmonary exercise testing: An objective approach to pre-operative assessment to define level of perioperative care. *Indian Journal of Anaesthesia, 54*(4), 286–291.

Bhukal, I., Solanki, S. L., Ramaswamy, S., Yaddanapudi, L. N., Jain, A., & Kumar, P. (2012). Perioperative predictors of morbidity and mortality following cardiac surgery under cardiopulmonary bypass. *Saudi Journal of Anaesthesia, 6,* 242–247.

Biondi-Zoccai, G., Lotrionte, M., Agostoni, P., Abbate, A., Fusaro, M., Burzotta, F., . . . Sangiorgi, G. (2006). A systematic review and meta-analysis on the hazards of discontinuing or not adhering to aspirin among 50279 patients at risk for coronary artery disease. *European Heart Journal, 27*(22), 2667–2674.

Bojar, R. M. (2011). Post-ICU care and other complications. In R. M. Bojar (Ed.), *Manual of perioperative care in adult cardiac surgery* (pp. 641–726). Hoboken, NJ: Blackwell.

Burger, W., Chemnitius, J. M., Kneissl, G. D., & Rücker, G. (2005). Low-dose aspirin for secondary cardiovascular prevention—cardiovascular risks after its perioperative withdrawal versus bleeding risks with its continuation—review and meta-analysis. *Journal of Internal Medicine, 257*(5), 399–414.

Carroll, A., & Dowling, M. (2007). Discharge planning: Communication, education, and patient participation. *British Nursing Journal, 16*(14), 882–886.

Centers for Disease Control and Prevention. (2012). *Second national report on biochemical indicators of diet and nutrition in the U.S. population. Executive summary.* Retrieved from http://www.cdc.gov/nutritionreport/pdf/exesummary_web_032612.pdf

Chaturvedi, R. K., deVarennes, B., & Lachapelle, K. (2007). Preoperative cardiac surgery risk assessment by Parsonnet score in octogenarians: Correlation with survival and lifestyle study. *Chest, 132*(4), 440a.

Clark, C. E., Steele, A. M., Taylor, R. S., Shore, A. C., Ukoumunne, O. C., & Campbell, J. L. (2014). Interarm blood pressure difference in people with diabetes: Measurement and vascular mortality implications. *Diabetes Care, 10.* Retrieved from http://care.diabetesjournals.org/content/early/2014/03/13/dc13-1576

Cornily, J.-C., LeSaux, D., Vinsonneau, U., Bezon, E., Le Ven, F., Le Gal, G., . . . Blanc, J. J. (2011). Assessment of carotid stenosis before coronary artery bypass surgery: Is it always necessary? *Archives of Cardiovascular Diseases, 104*(2), 77–83.

Coutre, S. (2014). *Management of heparin-induced thrombocytopenia.* Retrieved from http://www.uptodate.com/contents/management-of-heparin-induced-thrombocytopenia

Daley, B. J. (2012). *Perioperative anticoagulation management.* Retrieved from http://emedicine.medscape.com/article/285265-overview

Daley, B. J. (2014). *Wound care treatment and management.* Retrieved from http://emedicine.medscape.com/article/194018-treatment

Dempsey, C. M., Limin, S., & Stacey, S. G. (2007). A prospective audit of blood loss and blood transfusion in patients undergoing coronary artery bypass grafting after clopidogrel and aspirin therapy. *Critical Care and Resuscitation, 6,* 248–282.

Devereaux, P. J., Yang, H., Yusuf, S., Guyatt, G., Leslie, K., Villar, J. C., . . . Choi, P. (2008). Effects of extended-release metoprolol succinate in patients undergoing non-cardiac surgery (POISE trial): A randomized controlled trial. *Lancet, 371*(9627), 1839–1847.

Dunning, J., Versteegh, M., Fabbri, A., Pavie, A., Kolh, P., Lockowandt, U., . . . Nashef, S. A. (2008). Guideline on antiplatelet and anticoagulation management in cardiac surgery. *European Journal of Cardio-Thoracic Surgery, 34*(1), 73–92.

Ellenberger, C., Tait, G., & Beattie, W. S. (2011). Chronic β blockade is associated with a better outcome after elective noncardiac surgery than acute β blockade: A single-center propensity-matched cohort study. *Anesthesiology, 114*(4), 817–823.

EuroSCORE.org. (n.d.). *EuroSCORE scoring system.* Retrieved from http://www.euroscore.org/euroscore_scoring.htm

Evans, J. M., Ogston, S. A., Emslie-Smith, A., & Morris, A. D. (2006). Risk of mortality and adverse cardiovascular outcomes in type 2 diabetes: A comparison of patients treated with sulfonylureas and metformin. *Diabetologia, 49*(5), 930–936.

Fitzgerald, K. (2014). Cerebrovascular disease. In C. R. Christensen & P. A. Lewis (Eds.), *Core curriculum for vascular nursing* (pp. 201–214). Philadelphia, PA: Lippincott Williams & Wilkins.

Fleisher, L., Beckman, J. A., Brown, K. A., Calkins, H., Chaikof, E. L., Fleischmann, K. E., . . . Robb, J. F. (2009). 2009 ACCF/AHA focused update on perioperative beta blockade incorporated into the ACC/AHA 2007 guidelines on perioperative cardiovascular evaluation and care for non-cardiac surgery: A report of the American College of Cardiology Foundation/American

Heart Association task force on practice guidelines. *Circulation, 120*(21), e169–e276.

Geissler, H. J., Hölzl, P., Marohl, S., Kuhn-Régnier, F., Mehlhorn, U., Südkamp, M., . . . de Vivie, E. R. (2000). Risk stratification in heart surgery: Comparison of six score systems. *European Journal of Cardio-Thoracic Surgery, 17*(4), 400–406.

George, J. C., O'Murchu, B., & Bashir, R. (2011). Endovascular management of subclavian artery stenosis using balloon expandable covered stents. *Journal of Cardiology Cases, 3*(3), e159–e162.

Guay, J., & Andrew, O. E. (2014). Continuing antiplatelet therapy before cardiac surgery with cardiopulmonary bypass: A meta-analysis on the need for reexploration and major outcomes. *Journal of Cardiothoracic and Vascular Anesthesia, 28*, 1, 90–97.

Gude, D., & Jha, R. (2012). Acute kidney injury following cardiac surgery. *Annals of Cardiac Anaesthesia, 15*, 279–286.

Haddad, E. V., & Robertson, C. H. (2013). *Intra-aortic balloon counterpulsation*. Retrieved from http://emedicine.medscape.com/article/1847715-overview

Haga, K. K., McClymont, K. L., Clarke, S., Grounds, R. S., Ng, K. Y. B., Glyde, D. W., . . . Alston, R. P. (2011). The effect of tight glycaemic control, during and after cardiac surgery, on patient mortality and morbidity: A systematic review and meta-analysis. *Journal of Cardiothoracic Surgery, 6*. Retrieved from http://www.cardiothoracicsurgery.org/content/6/1/3

Hamad, M. A. S., van Straten, A. H. M., Schönberger, J. P. A. M., ter Woorst, J. F., de Wolf, A. M., Martens, E. J., . . . van Zundert, A. A. J. (2010). Preoperative ejection fraction as a predictor of survival after coronary artery bypass grafting: Comparison with a matched general population. *Journal of Cardiothoracic Surgery, 5*. Retrieved from http://www.cardiothoracicsurgery.org/content/5/1/29

Hasija, S., Makhija, N., Choudhury, M., Hote, M., Chauhan, S., & Kiran, U. (2010). Prophylactic vasopressin in patients receiving the angiotensin-converting enzyme inhibitor ramipril undergoing coronary artery bypass graft surgery. *Journal of Cardiothoracic and Vascular Anesthesia, 24*(2), 230–238.

Heart Failure Society of America. (2011). *NYHA classification—The stages of heart failure*. Retrieved from http://www.hfsa.org/hfsa-wp/wp/stages-of-heart-failure/

Helgadottir, S., Sigurdsson, M. I., Ingvarsdottir, I. L., Arnar, D. O., & Gudbjartsson, T. (2012). Atrial fibrillation following cardiac surgery: Risk analysis and long-term survival. *Journal of Cardiovascular Surgery, 7*(87), 1749–1753.

Hengstermann, S., Nieczaj, R., Steinhagen-Thiessen, E., & Schulz, R. J. (2008). Which are the most efficient items of mini nutritional assessment in multimorbid patients? *Journal of Nutrition, Health & Aging, 12*(2), 117–122.

Hessel II, E. A. (2008). Circuitry and cannulation techniques. In G. P. Gravlee, R. F. Davis, A. H. Stammers, & R. M. Ungerleider (Eds.), *Cardiopulmonary bypass: Principles and practice* (3rd ed., pp. 63–113). Philadelphia, PA: Lippincott Williams & Wilkins.

Hodges, P. J., & Kam, P. C. (2002). The perioperative implications of herbal medicines. *Anaesthesia, 57*(9), 889–899.

Holt, N. F. (2012). Perioperative cardiac risk reduction. *American Family Physician, 85*(3), 239–246.

Ji, Q., Duan, Q., Wang, X., Cai, J., Zhou, Y., Feng, J., . . . Mei, Y. (2012). Risk factors for ventilatory dependency following coronary artery bypass grafting. *International Journal of Medical Sciences, 9*(4), 306–310.

Johnson, R. G. (2009). *Preoperative evaluation*. Retrieved from http://www.merckmanuals.com/professional/special_subjects/care_of_the_surgical_patient/preoperative_evaluation.html

Jones, R., Nyawo, B., Jamieson, S., & Clark, S. (2011). Current smoking predicts increased operative mortality and morbidity after cardiac surgery in the elderly. *Interactive Cardiovascular and Thoracic Surgery, 12*(3), 449–453.

Jung, H., & Lilly, L. S. (2011). The cardiac cycle: Mechanisms of heart sounds and murmurs. In L. S. Lilly (Ed.), *Pathophysiology of heart disease* (5th ed., pp. 28–43). Philadelphia, PA: Lippincott Williams & Wilkins.

Jyrala, A., Weiss, R. E., Jeffries, R. A., & Kay, G. L. (2012). Is hypothyroidism overlooked in cardiac surgery patients? *Open Journal of Thoracic Surgery, 2*, 29–35.

Kaul, P., Naylor, C. D., Armstrong, P. W., Mark, D. B., Theroux, P., & Dagenais, G. R. (2009). Assessment of activity status and survival according to the Canadian Cardiovascular

Society angina classification. *Canadian Journal of Cardiology, 25*(7), e225–e231.

Kaur, N., Verma, P., & Singh, S. (2007). Effectiveness of planned preoperative teaching on self-care activities for patients undergoing cardiac surgery. *Nursing and Midwifery Research Journal, 3*(1), 36–42.

Khan, M. A., & Hussain, S. F. (2005). Pre-operative pulmonary evaluation. *Journal of Ayub Medical College: Abbottabad, 17*(4), 82–86.

Khan, N. U., & Yonan, N. (2009). Does preoperative computed tomography reduce the risks associated with re-do cardiac surgery? *Interactive Cardiovascular and Thoracic Surgery, 9*, 119–123.

Kobayashi, K. J., Williams, J. A., Nwakanma, L. U., Weiss, E. S., Gott, V. L., Baumgartner, W. A., . . . Conte, J. V. (2009). EuroSCORE predicts short- and mid-term mortality in combined aortic valve replacement and coronary artery bypass patients. *Journal of Cardiac Surgery, 24*, 637–643.

Kouchoukos, N. T., Blackstone, E. H., Hanley, F. L., & Kirklin, J. K. (2013a). Aortic valve disease. In N. T. Kouchoukos, E. H. Blackstone, F. L. Hanley, & J. K. Kirklin (Eds.), *Kirklin/Barratt-Boyes cardiac surgery* (4th ed., pp. 541–643). Philadelphia, PA: Elsevier Saunders.

Kouchoukos, N. T., Blackstone, E. H., Hanley, F. L., & Kirklin, J. K. (2013b). Cardiac transplantation. In N. T. Kouchoukos, E. H. Blackstone, F. L. Hanley, & J. K. Kirklin (Eds.), *Kirklin/Barratt-Boyes cardiac surgery* (4th ed., pp. 809–872). Philadelphia, PA: Elsevier Saunders.

Kramer, J. B., Howard, P. A., Barnes, B. J., Bashar, A., Mukhopadhyay, P., Biria, M., . . . Vacek, J. L. (2012). Secondary prevention following coronary artery bypass surgery: A pilot study for improved patient education. *International Journal of Clinical Medicine, 3*, 286–294.

Lazar, H. L. (2012). Glycemic control during coronary artery bypass graft surgery. *International Scholarly Research Notices, 2012*, Article ID 292490. Retrieved from http://www.hindawi.com/journals/isrn/2012/292490/

Lazar, H. L., Wilson, C. A., & Messé, S. R. (2014). *Coronary artery bypass grafting in patients with cerebrovascular disease*. Retrieved from http://www.uptodate.com/contents/coronary-artery-bypass-grafting-in-patients-with-cerebrovascular-disease

Lomivorotov, V. V., Efremov, S. M., Boboshko, V. A., Nikolaev, D. A., Vedernikov, P. E., Lomivorotov, V. N., & Karaskov, A. M. (2013). Evaluation of nutritional screening tools for patients scheduled for cardiac surgery. *Nutrition, 29*, 436–442.

Marks, J. B. (2003). Perioperative management of diabetes. *American Family Physician, 67*(1), 93–100.

Marley, R. A., Calabrese, T., & Thompson, K. J. (2014). Preoperative evaluation and preparation of the patient. In J. J. Nagelhout & K. L. Plaus (Eds.), *Nurse anesthesia* (4th ed., pp. 335–381). Philadelphia, PA: Elsevier Saunders.

McStay, L. H. (2007). Cardiomegaly. In P. M. Paulman, A. A. Paulman, & J. D. Harrison (Eds.), *Taylor's 10-minute diagnosis manual* (2nd ed., pp. 125–128). Philadelphia, PA: Lippincott Williams & Wilkins.

Meneghini, L. F. (2009). Perioperative management of diabetes: Translating evidence into practice. *Cleveland Clinic Journal of Medicine, 76*(Suppl. 4), S53–S59.

Mohler III, E. R., & Fairman, R. M. (2014). Carotid endarterectomy. Retrieved from http://www.uptodate.com/contents/carotid-endarterectomy

Montazerghaem, H., Safaie, N., & Samiei, N. V. (2014). Body mass index or serum albumin levels: Which is further prognostic following cardiac surgery? *Journal of Cardiovascular and Thoracic Research, 6*(2), 123–126.

Moonesinghe, S. R., & Kelleher, A. A. (2006). Preoperative assessment for cardiac surgery. *Anaesthesia & Intensive Care Medicine, 7*(8), 267–270.

National Heart, Lung, and Blood Institute. (2012a). *What is cardiac MRI?* Retrieved from http://www.nhlbi.nih.gov/health/health-topics/topics/mri/

National Heart, Lung, and Blood Institute. (2012b). *What is cardiac catheterization?* Retrieved from http://www.nhlbi.nih.gov/health/health-topics/topics/cath/

Ngaage, D. L., Britchford, G., & Cale, A. R. J. (2011). The influence of an ageing population on care and clinical resource utilisation in cardiac surgery. *British Journal of Cardiology, 17*(6), 28–32.

Ochoa, V. M., & Yeghiazarians, Y. (2010). Subclavian artery stenosis: A review for the vascular medicine practitioner. *Vascular Medicine, 16*(1), 29–34.

O'Glasser, A. Y. (2013). *Perioperative management of the patient with liver disease.* Retrieved from http://emedicine.medscape.com/article/284667-overview#aw2aab6b4

O'Riordan, M. (2013). *Sulfonylurea use increases all-cause mortality risk.* Retrieved from http://www.medscape.com/viewarticle/811641

Parsonnet, V., Dean, D., & Bernstein, A. D. (1989). A method of uniform stratification of risk for evaluating the results of surgery in acquired adult heart disease. *Circulation, 79*(Suppl. I), I3–I12.

Pattakos, G., Johnston, D. R., Houghtaling, P. L., Nowicki, E. R., & Blackstone, E. H. (2012). Preoperative prediction of non-home discharge: A strategy to reduce resource use after cardiac surgery. *Journal of the American College of Surgeons, 214*(2), 140–147.

Poldermans, D., Bax, J. J., Boersma, E., De Hert, S., Eeckhout, E., Fowkes, G., . . . Vermassen, F. (2009). Guidelines for pre-operative cardiac risk assessment and perioperative cardiac management in non-cardiac surgery. *European Heart Journal, 30*(22), 2769–2812.

Renda, G., Di Pillo, R., D'Alleva, A., Sciartilli, A., Zimarino, M., De Candia, E., . . . De Caterina, R. (2007). Surgical bleeding after pre-operative unfractionated heparin and low molecular weight heparin for coronary bypass surgery. *Haematologica, 92,* 366–373.

Roekaerts, M. M. H. J., & Heijmans, J. H. (2012). Early postoperative care after cardiac surgery, perioperative considerations in cardiac surgery. Retrieved from http://www.intechopen.com/books/howtoreference/perioperative-considerations-in-cardiac-surgery/-early-postoperative-care-after-cardiac-surgery-

Rosenman, D. J., McDonald, F. S., Ebbert, J. O., Erwin, P. J., LaBella, M., & Montori, V. M. (2008). Clinical consequences of withholding versus administering renin-angiotensin-aldosterone system antagonists in the preoperative period. *Journal of Hospital Medicine, 3*(4), 319–325.

Saber, W. (2006). Perioperative medication management: A case-based review of general principles. *Cleveland Clinic Journal of Medicine, 73*(1), S82–S87.

Schmelzeisen, R., & Varbroudi, F. (2008). Pre- and post-operative dental focus of patients with prosthetic heart valves. *Internet Journal of Cardiovascular Research, 6*(1). Retrieved from http://ispub.com/IJCVR/6/1/11186

Slovut, D. P., & Lipsitz, E. C. (2012). Peripheral artery disease. *Circulation, 126,* 1127–1138.

Smith, I., & Jackson, I. (2010). Beta-blockers, calcium channel blockers, angiotensin converting enzyme inhibitors, and angiotensin receptor blockers: Should they be stopped or not before ambulatory anaesthesia? *Current Opinion in Anaesthesiology, 23*(6), 687–690.

Smith, M. M., Barbara, D. W., Mauermann, W. J., Viazz, C. F., Dearani, J. A., & Grim, K. J. (2014). Morbidity and mortality with dental extractions before cardiac operation. *Annals of Thoracic Surgery, 97*(3), 838–844.

Smulter, N., Lingehall, H. C., Gustafson, Y., Olofsson, B., & Engström, K. G. (2013). Delirium after cardiac surgery: Incidence and risk factors. *Interactive Cardiovascular and Thoracic Surgery, 17*(5), 790–796.

Sparacino-Watkins, C. E., Lai, Y.-C., & Gladwin, M. T. (2012). Nitrate-nitrite-nitric oxide pathway in pulmonary arterial hypertension therapeutics. *Circulation, 125,* 2824–2826.

Sveinsdóttir, H., & Ingadóttir, B. (2012). Predictors of psychological distress in patients at home following cardiac surgery: An explorative panel study. *European Journal of Cardiovascular Nursing, 11*(3), 339–348.

Tu, J. V., Jaglal, S. B., & Naylor, C. D. (1995). Multicenter validation of a risk index for mortality, intensive care unit stay, and overall hospital length of stay after cardiac surgery. Steering committee of the Provincial Adult Care Network of Ontario. *Circulation, 91,* 677–684.

Tuman, K. J., McCarthy, R. J., March, R. J., Najafi, H., & Ivankovich, A. D. (1992). Morbidity and duration of ICU stay after cardiac surgery. A model for preoperative risk assessment. *Chest, 102,* 36–44.

van Venrooij, L. M., van Leeuwen, P. A., de Vos, R., Borgmeijer-Hoelen, M. M., & de Mol, B. A. (2009). Preoperative protein and energy intake and postoperative complications in well-nourished, non-hospitalized elderly cardiac surgery patients. *Clinical Nutrition, 28,* 117–121.

Weisberg, A. D., Weisberg, E. L., Wilson, J. M., & Collard, C. D. (2009). Preoperative evaluation and preparation of the patient for cardiac surgery. *Anesthesiology Clinics, 27,* 633–648.

Whinney, C. (2009). Perioperative medication management: General principles and practical applications. *Cleveland Clinic Journal of Medicine, 76*(4), S126–S132.

Wiesbauer, F., Schlager, O., Domanovits, H., Wildner, B., Maurer, G., Muellner, M., . . . Schillinger, M. (2007). Perioperative beta-blockers for preventing surgery-related mortality and morbidity: A systematic review and meta-analysis. *Anesthesia & Analgesia, 104,* 27–41.

Winchester, D. E., Wen, X., Xie, L., & Bavry, A. A. (2010). Evidence of pre-procedural statin therapy a meta-analysis of randomized trials. *Journal of the American College of Cardiology, 56*(14), 1099–1109.

Zambouri, A. (2007). Preoperative evaluation and preparation for anesthesia and surgery. *Hippokratia, 11*(1), 13–21.

WEB RESOURCE

General Practice Notebook (delineates risk factors based on the Parsonnet risk score): http://www.gpnotebook.co.uk/simplepage.cfm?ID=-1811546076

Chapter 5

Heart Valve Surgery

Kristine J. Peterson

INTRODUCTION

Heart valve surgery is performed to either repair or replace a failing valve. Cardiac valves allow for one-way, low-resistance blood flow. The opening and closing of a valve occur according to pressure gradients between each side of the valve. The valves must open widely to allow for rapid blood movement and minimal cardiac work; conversely, they must remain tightly closed to prevent backward flow of blood. Proper functioning of cardiac valves depends on normal fibroelastic tissue of the valve leaflets, proper number of cusps of the valve, ability to open and close rapidly, normal-sized ring or annulus, and proper function of chordae tendineae and papillary muscles (mitral and tricuspid) (Fann, Ingels, & Miller, 2008; Mihaljevic, Sayeed, Stamou, & Paul, 2008). This chapter describes the various valve surgery procedures and their associated care implications.

VALVULAR HEART DISEASE

Valvular heart disease (VHD) is defined according to the valve or valves affected and the type of functional alteration. Abnormality of the valve is identified as either stenosis (narrowing or constriction that creates a pressure gradient) or regurgitation (incomplete closure of the valve leaflets resulting in a backflow of blood).

Valvular heart disease may be caused by either congenital or acquired factors. Congenital factors include a bicuspid rather than tricuspid valve, and other congenital malformations, such as Marfan syndrome (discussed further in Chapter 21). Acquired causes of valve disease include ischemic coronary artery disease (CAD), degenerative changes associated with aging, heart failure (HF), rheumatic changes, infective endocarditis (IE) from a bacterial infection, neoplasm, and thrombus (Fann et al., 2008; Mihaljevic et al., 2008).

The relationship between ischemic CAD and VHD is bidirectional. Myocardial infarction (MI) due to CAD can result in ventricular remodeling (a pathological change in the shape and size of the ventricle). Chordae tendineae, papillary muscle, and the valve annulus may be affected, leading to impaired valve function. A malfunctioning valve will cause an increase in myocardial workload and can eventually lead to ischemia as a symptom of valve disease.

Decisions about whether to pursue medical or surgical management and which type of surgical management to use, if necessary, are based on the goals of maximizing the life of the valve and minimizing complications of treatment (Shemin, 2008). Often the decision to repair or replace a valve is made once the surgeon has an opportunity to visualize the valve. Nevertheless, patients are educated on both repair and replacement procedures. Pros and cons exist for both mechanical and biological valves. Mechanical valves are believed to be more durable than bioprosthetic valves, but require that patients receive life-long anticoagulation therapy. In recent years, use of bioprosthetic valves has increased significantly, while use of mechanical valves has decreased. The percentage of aortic replacement devices changed from 57% mechanical in 1995 to 84% bioprosthetic in 2010 (Kouchoukos, Blackstone, Hanley, & Kirklin, 2013). The surgeon and the patient together decide which type of valve will be used for replacement. All patients, regardless of valve prosthesis used, will require anticoagulation for some period following surgery. The American College of Cardiology (ACC)/American Heart Association (AHA) provide guidelines for anticoagulation following valve intervention.

AORTIC STENOSIS

Aortic stenosis (AS) due to age-related calcific disease (formerly known as degenerative or senile AS) is the most common adult valve lesion in the United States (Otto & Bonow, 2012). Bicuspid aortic valve disease is another cause of aortic stenosis and is believed to be present in about 1% to 2% of the population (Otto & Bonow, 2012). Given that the U.S. population is aging, the incidence of AS is increasing. Long thought to be a disease of stress and degenerative changes, the calcification of aortic stenosis is now regarded as an active proliferative and inflammatory process, similar to atherosclerosis (Mihaljevic et al., 2008; Otto & Bonow, 2012).

Aortic stenosis, in which the aortic valve does not open completely, creates a left ventricular outflow tract obstruction and increases workload and afterload of the left ventricle (LV). The increase in afterload is the etiology of the signs and symptoms associated with AS (Otto & Bonow, 2012).

Factors involved in grading the severity of AS include the mean systolic gradient across the valve, blood velocity, valve area, left ventricular function, and severity of symptoms (Otto & Bonow, 2012). Normally, the pressures in the LV and the aorta are virtually equal during systole, meaning there is no aortic systolic gradient. As the valve opening narrows, however, the pressure required to eject blood—and therefore the pressure in the LV—increases, creating a gradient. The normal aortic valve area is 2.6–3.5 cm^2 (Mihaljevic et al., 2008). As the valve area narrows and the gradient increases, blood velocity increases. Mild AS is associated with a mean gradient of less than 25 mmHg, valve area of less than 1.5 cm^2, and jet velocity of less than 3 m/sec. Severe aortic stenosis is associated with jet velocity of more than 4 m/sec, mean systolic gradient greater than 40 mmHg, and a valve area of less than 1.0 cm^2 (Kouchoukos et al., 2013).

Classic signs and symptoms of AS include angina, syncope, exertional dyspnea, sudden cardiac death, and heart failure. Typically, these conditions appear only after a prolonged latent period when the disease is already severe, usually evident by age 50–70 for a bicuspid valve and after age 70 with age-related calcific stenosis. Heart failure symptoms are thought to be due to diastolic failure (Otto & Bonow, 2012).

Once patients become symptomatic, the outcome is poor if obstruction is not relieved (Nishimura et al., 2014; Otto & Bonow, 2012). In patients with HF, time from onset of symptoms to death is 2 years; in those with angina, time from onset of symptoms to death is 5 years (Otto & Bonow, 2012). Medical therapy may improve symptoms of heart failure but is not effective long-term therapy for AS (Nishimura et al., 2014). With the addition of transcatheter aortic valve replacement (TAVR), surgeons can choose replacement via median sternotomy, minimally invasive aortic valve replacement, or TAVR. The choice is based on patient factors, surgical risk, and surgeon/patient preference. Transcatheter aortic valve replacement is discussed in more detail in Chapter 7. **Table 5-1** outlines the

Table 5-1   Indications for Aortic Valve Replacement in Aortic Stenosis

Class IA

1. Patients who meet an indication for AVR with low or intermediate surgical risk. Indications for AVR include decreased systolic opening of aortic valve, aortic velocity of 4.0 m/sec or greater, mean pressure gradient 40 mmHg or higher, or symptoms.

Class IB

1. Symptomatic patients with severe AS with:
   a. Decreased systolic opening of a calcified or congenitally stenotic aortic valve; and
   b. An aortic velocity 4.0 m/sec or greater or mean pressure gradient 40 mmHg or higher; and
   c. Symptoms of heart failure, syncope, exertional dyspnea, angina, or pre-syncope by history or on exercise testing.
2. Asymptomatic patients with severe AS and LVEF less than 50% with a decreased systolic opening, aortic velocity of 4 m/sec or greater, and mean pressure gradient of 40 mmHg or higher.
3. Severe AS when undergoing cardiac surgery for other indications when there is decreased systolic opening, aortic velocity of 4 m/sec or greater, and mean pressure gradient of 40 mmHg or higher.
4. TAVR is recommended for patients who meet an indication for AVR, have a prohibitive surgical risk, and have a predicted post-TAVR survival of more than 12 months.

Class IIaB

1. Asymptomatic patients with severe AS with:
   a. Decreased systolic opening of a calcified valve;
   b. An aortic velocity 5.0 m/sec or greater or mean pressure gradient 60 mmHg or higher; and
   c. A low surgical risk.
2. Apparently asymptomatic patients with severe AS and:
   a. A calcified aortic valve;
   b. An aortic velocity of 4.0 m/sec to 4.9 m/sec or mean pressure gradient of 40 mmHg to 59 mmHg; and
   c. An exercise test demonstrating decreased exercise tolerance or a fall in systolic BP.
3. Symptomatic patients with low-flow/low-gradient severe AS with reduced LVEF with:
   a. Calcified aortic valve with reduced systolic opening;
   b. Resting valve area 1.0 cm^2 or less;
   c. Aortic velocity less than 4 m/sec ec or mean pressure gradient less than 40 mmHg;
   d. LVEF less than 50%; and
   e. A low-dose dobutamine stress study that shows an aortic velocity 4 m/sec or greater or mean pressure gradient 40 mmHg or higher with a valve area 1.0 cm^2 or less at any dobutamine dose.
4. TAVR is reasonable for patients who meet an indication for AVR and have a high surgical risk.

Class IIaC

1. Symptomatic patients with low-flow/low-gradient severe AS with an LVEF 50% or greater, a calcified aortic valve with significantly reduced leaflet motion, and a valve area 1.0 cm^2 or less only if clinical, hemodynamic, and anatomic data support valve obstruction as the most likely cause of symptoms and data recorded when the patient is normotensive (systolic BP less than 140 mmHg) indicate:
   a. An aortic velocity less than 4 m/sec or mean pressure gradient less than 40 mmHg; and
   b. A stroke volume index less than 35 mL/m^2; and
   c. An indexed valve area 0.6 cm^2/m^2 or less.
2. Patients with moderate AS (stage B) with an aortic velocity between 3.0 m/sec and 3.9 m/sec or mean pressure gradient between 20 mmHg and 39 mmHg who are undergoing cardiac surgery for other indications.

Continued

Table 5-1   Indications for Aortic Valve Replacement in Aortic Stenosis *(Continued)*

Class IIbC

   1. Asymptomatic patients with severe AS and rapid disease progression and low surgical risk

Class IIIB

   1. TAVR not recommended for patients with comorbidities so severe they would not be expected to benefit from AVR.

AS, aortic stenosis; AVR, aortic valve replacement; BP, blood pressure; LVEF, left ventricular ejection fraction; TAVR, transcatheter aortic valve replacement
Source: Data from Nishimura, R. A., Otto, C. M., Bonow, R. O., Carabello, B. A., Erwin, J. P. 3rd, Guyton, R. A., . . . Yancy, C. W. (2014). 2014 AHA/ACC guideline for the management of patients with valvular heart disease: A report of the American College of Cardiology/American Heart Association Task Force on Practice Guidelines. *The Journal of Thoracic and Cardiovascular Surgery, 148*(1), e1–e132.

2014 ACC/AHA recommendations for aortic valve replacement (AVR) in the presence of aortic stenosis. These guidelines apply to all of the replacement modalities.

As discussed in Chapter 3, the AHA classifies recommendations based on the degree of agreement and type and/or amount of available evidence. The level of recommendation is classified as Class I, II, or III. Class I indicates that evidence and/or general agreement exists that the intervention is effective. Class II refers to conflicting evidence and/or a divergence of opinion about the efficacy. Class II is further subdivided into Class IIa and Class IIb: Class IIa indicates that evidence/opinion is in favor of efficacy, whereas Class IIb recommendations have less efficacy as established by evidence/opinion. Class III refers to evidence and/or general opinion that an intervention is not effective or is harmful.

The strength of the level of evidence is also identified according to the type and/or presence of research. For example, Level of Evidence A indicates that findings from multiple randomized clinical trials or meta-analyses support the use of an intervention. Level of Evidence B indicates that a single randomized trial or nonrandomized trials support an intervention. Level of Evidence C refers to consensus opinion of experts, case studies, or standard of care (Nishimura et al., 2014).

Aortic stenosis results in development of a hypertrophied and noncompliant LV. Postoperatively, while symptoms improve rapidly, the hypertrophy and stiffness remain. Such a ventricle is dependent on adequate filling volumes. The nurse must monitor filling volumes and blood pressure closely, control heart rate, and maintain sinus rhythm. Patients may require atrioventricular (AV) pacing at rates of 90–100 per minute and cardioversion of atrial fibrillation (AF) to maintain adequate cardiac output (CO). In addition, the aortic valve is located very near to the AV node so some degree of AV block may occur due to edema, inflammation, hemorrhage, or suturing near the node. Epicardial pacing and/or implantation of a permanent pacemaker may be necessary if the block fails to resolve within a few days (Bojar, 2011; Jacobson, Marzlin, & Webner, 2014). More detailed discussion of postoperative nursing management for all valve surgeries is provided in later chapters.

AORTIC REGURGITATION

When aortic regurgitation (AR) is present, there is a reflux of blood from the aorta into the LV during diastole, because the valve leaflets fail to close completely and to remain tightly closed during diastole. Symptoms of

AR depend on the acuity of onset, severity of regurgitation, and left ventricular function. Acute AR imposes a large-volume load that a normal LV cannot accommodate. The sudden increase in end-diastolic volume (preload) will result in increased left ventricular end-diastolic pressure (LVEDP) and decreased CO. Patients with acute aortic regurgitation will rapidly develop hemodynamic instability and LV failure. Early diagnosis and intervention are critical. Patients with concomitant CAD may develop left ventricular dilation and cardiac failure. Such patients often present with HF.

Like chronic AS, chronic AR has a slow, insidious onset and progression. Aortic regurgitation may be well tolerated for years. Because it develops slowly, the LV compensates with hypertrophy and an increase in sympathetic tone to keep the LVEDP relatively low and maintain CO. This change results in a characteristic sign of aortic regurgitation, a widened pulse pressure (Mihaljevic et al., 2008). If left untreated, this process will lead eventually to myofibril slippage, ventricular remodeling, and irreversible changes in LV function. In chronic AR, left ventricular dilation develops over time and patients may be asymptomatic for long periods. Dyspnea on exertion, orthopnea, and paroxysmal nocturnal dyspnea will develop gradually, along with feelings of heart pounding and awareness of every heartbeat. Later in its course, angina and palpitations will develop (Otto & Bonow, 2012).

The most common causes of AR in developed countries are bicuspid valve, age-related calcific aortic valve disease, traumatic tears of the aorta, and aortic root disease (Otto & Bonow, 2012; Nishimura et al., 2014). Other causes of AR include chronic systemic hypertension, aortitis of various etiologies, and connective tissue disease such as Marfan syndrome, Reiter disease, Ehlers-Danlos syndrome, and rheumatoid arthritis (Otto & Bonow, 2012). Most commonly, AR is seen concomitantly with AS (e.g., aortic disease, rheumatoid disease, or degenerative disease (Mihaljevic et al., 2008).

Indications for Aortic Valve Replacement in Aortic Regurgitation

Surgical intervention for AR consists largely of valve replacement. Some specialized centers perform aortic valve repair; however, there are insufficient data on repair to gauge the durability of repair compared with replacement (Nishimura et al., 2014). For the purposes of this chapter, surgical intervention will consist of valve replacement. While acute AR should be treated with early valve replacement, valve replacement is not recommended for asymptomatic patients with chronic aortic regurgitation and good left ventricular function (Nishimura et al., 2014). Left ventricular size, as measured by left ventricular end-systolic diameter (LVESD) of greater than 50 mm, or indexed LVESD of greater than $25mm/m^2$, is a measure of the degree of LV volume overload and remodeling. It is an independent predictor of outcome (Otto & Bonow, 2012; Nishimura et al., 2014). Deteriorating left ventricular function, as indicated by an ejection fraction (EF) less than 50% to 55% and an end-diastolic dimension greater than 70 mm or an end-systolic dimension greater than 50 mm, would indicate need for surgery (Mihaljevic et al., 2008). **Table 5-2** lists the indications for surgery for aortic regurgitation.

Aortic regurgitation results in both volume and pressure overload for the LV. The result is a dilated LV with some degree of hypertrophy. Postoperative considerations will be similar following AVR to those for AS including consideration of filling volumes, heart rate, AV blocks, and maintaining sinus rhythm. Most patients will be vasodilated in the immediate postoperative period and may require a vasopressor such as norepinephrine or phenylephrine (Bojar, 2011).

Table 5-2   Indications for Aortic Valve Replacement in Aortic Regurgitation

Class IB
1. Symptomatic patients with severe AR irrespective of left ventricular function
2. Asymptomatic patients with chronic, severe AR and left ventricular systolic dysfunction (EF < 50%) at rest if no other cause for systolic dysfunction is identified

Class IC
1. Chronic pure, severe AR while undergoing cardiac surgery for other reasons

Class IIaB
1. Asymptomatic patients with pure, severe AR and normal LV systolic function (LVEF > 50% but with severe left ventricular dilatation (LVESD > 50 mm or indexed LVESD > 25 mm/m^2)

Class IIaC
1. Patients with moderate AR while undergoing surgery on the ascending aorta
2. Patients with moderate AR while undergoing other cardiac surgery

Class IIbC
1. Asymptomatic patients with severe AR and normal left ventricular function at rest (EF ≥ 50%) when evidence of progressive LV dilatation (end-diastolic dimension > 65 mm, decreasing exercise tolerance, or abnormal hemodynamic response to exercise if surgical risk is low)

AR, aortic regurgitation; CABG, coronary artery bypass grafting; EF, ejection fraction; LV, left ventricle; LVESD, left ventricular end-systolic diameter.

Source: Data from Nishimura, R. A., Otto, C. M., Bonow, R. O., Carabello, B. A., Erwin, J. P. 3rd, Guyton, R. A., . . . Yancy, C. W. (2014). 2014 AHA/ACC guideline for the management of patients with valvular heart disease: A report of the American College of Cardiology/American Heart Association Task Force on Practice Guidelines. *The Journal of Thoracic and Cardiovascular Surgery*, *148*(1), e1–e132.

MITRAL STENOSIS

Mitral stenosis (MS), like aortic stenosis, is a condition where the valve leaflets do not open completely, creating resistance to the forward flow of blood into the LV during diastole. Mitral stenosis is predominantly caused by rheumatic heart disease. Other causes, which are less common, include left atrial myxoma, thrombus, annular calcification, endocarditic vegetation, malignant carcinoid syndrome, and metabolic disorders (Otto & Bonow, 2012).

Most commonly, rheumatic disease is acquired in childhood; however, MS does not usually become symptomatic until decades later. Time from initial episode of rheumatic fever to appearance of symptoms varies from a few years to more than 20 years. The valve leaflets gradually become thickened and calcified. Often, the chordae and commissures fuse (Fann et al., 2008). Left atrial pressure rises as the disease worsens, and a progressively higher gradient develops across the mitral valve. Pulmonary artery systolic pressure increases as the valve area narrows. Defining characteristics of severe MS include a gradient of greater than 10 mmHg, leukocyte alkaline phosphatase (LAP) greater than 15 mmHg, valve area less than 1.5 cm^2, and pulmonary artery systolic pressure greater than 50 mmHg (Otto & Bonow, 2012; Nishimura et al., 2014).

Because of the resistance to the forward flow of blood, patients with MS will not develop volume overload in the LV and will likely have satisfactory left ventricular function. These individuals, however, have pulmonary hypertension, right ventricular failure, and tricuspid insufficiency. Symptoms of low CO and pulmonary venous congestion develop as left atrial and pulmonary pressures rise. At first, symptoms may occur only on exertion. As the valve area narrows, symptoms occur with less exertion, emotional stress, or AF. Dyspnea on exertion, fatigue, and decreased exercise tolerance are the first symptoms to occur, followed by orthopnea and episodes of pulmonary edema—especially with any increases in heart rate. Once pulmonary hypertension develops, right-sided heart failure with edema, hepatomegaly, ascites, and tricuspid regurgitation (TR) are seen. Atrial fibrillation is common (Otto & Bonow, 2012).

Intervention depends on the stage of the disease, as defined by valve characteristics, hemodynamic effects, and symptoms (Nishimura et al., 2014). Close follow up is necessary for asymptomatic patients. Anticoagulation is a class IB recommendation for patients with MS and AF, prior embolic event, or left atrial thrombus (Nishimura et al., 2014). Heart rate control, if necessary, is a class IIaB recommendation for patients in AF and a class IIbB recommendation for patients in normal sinus rhythm with exertional symptoms. Once symptoms develop, outcome is poor without intervention. First-line intervention is the percutaneous balloon mitral valvotomy (PBMV). It is indicated for symptomatic patients with moderate or severe MS. This is defined as a mitral valve area less than 1 cm^2/m^2 body surface area of less than 1.5 m^2 for a normal-sized adult (Otto & Bonow, 2012). Closed mitral commissurotomy had limited effectiveness and has been replaced by PBMV. Open commissurotomy has good results and low mortality; however, it has mostly been replaced by the percutaneous balloon valvotomy procedure. Open commissurotomy is not recommended for patients with a left atrial clot or concomitant mitral regurgitation (MR) (Bojar, 2011). Mortality and complications from PBMV are very low with acceptable improvement in hemodynamics (Kouchoukos et al., 2013). Percutaneous balloon mitral valvotomy and commissurotomy are not curative. Late

mortality is usually due to thromboembolism or from complications of surgery. In general, mitral valve repair is better suited to treating MR than as a therapy for MS (Gudbjartsson, Absi, & Aranki, 2008). The Web Resources section at the end of this chapter provides the 2014 ACC/AHA guideline recommendations for MS.

Patients with MS will have pulmonary hypertension, small LV cavity, and normal left ventricular function. Pulmonary hypertension decreases markedly in the immediate postoperative period and may continue to do so for some time. Even so, the degree of pulmonary hypertension present preoperatively will have a great effect on postoperative status. Because of pulmonary hypertension, patients will require careful monitoring of fluids, hydration status, and filling volumes to maintain CO. Ventilator times may be longer. In addition, hemodynamic support for the right ventricle (RV) is often necessary. A transesophageal echocardiogram is often used postoperatively to assist in assessing right and left ventricular function. Administration of dobutamine or milrinone in combination with norepinephrine (Levophed®) may be indicated to enhance contractility of the RV and decrease pulmonary vascular resistance (right-sided afterload). Mitral stenosis patients are frequently diuretic-dependent and will require diuretics to return to their preoperative weight—another reason to carefully monitor for adequate filling volumes. Use of a right ventricular assist device may be indicated in the immediate postoperative period (Khalpey, Ganim, & Rawn, 2008).

MITRAL REGURGITATION

In MR, the valve leaflets do not close tightly, resulting in a backward jet of blood into the left atrium during ventricular systole. Proper function of the mitral valve depends on a complicated interaction between the mitral leaflets, annulus, chordae tendineae, papillary muscles, and the left atrium and ventricle (Fann et al., 2008).

The most common causes of MR include ischemic CAD, mitral valve prolapse syndrome, IE, rheumatic heart disease, mitral annular calcification, and dilated cardiomyopathy (Otto & Bonow, 2012).

A sudden cause—such as ruptured papillary muscle or chordae tendineae—will result in acute and severe MR, and surgical repair is usually indicated (Nishimura et al., 2014). Alternatively, chronic MR may progress slowly over time, with symptoms appearing only when the disease is very advanced.

Mitral regurgitation causes an increase in LVEDP because forward CO is decreased and the regurgitant flow is added to LVEDP. An enlarged left atrium is likely as well. If MR develops suddenly, CO will decrease. Patients may present with signs of severe HF, and the electrocardiogram may reveal findings consistent with ischemia. Patients may also have AF and associated decrease in CO related to the enlarged left atrium. The CO achieved during exercise is the most important determinant of patient functional capacity (Otto & Bonow, 2012). The left atrium may be normal sized with decreased compliance and high atrial pressure. In long-standing MR, however, the atrium is usually significantly enlarged with only slightly elevated pressures.

The decision to perform corrective surgery is based on a number of factors. These include degree of mitral regurgitation, severity of symptoms, left ventricular function, feasibility of valve repair, presence of AF, presence and degree of pulmonary hypertension, and patient expectations (Kouchoukos et al., 2013. Severe MR is characterized by the following findings (Nishimura et al., 2014):

- Central jet MR greater than 40% left atrium or holosystolic eccentric jet
- Regurgitant volume 60 mL or greater
- Regurgitant fraction 50% or greater

- Effective regurgitant orifice 0.40 cm² or greater
- Angiographic grade 3−4+ regurgitation

Asymptomatic patients with severe MR can be safely followed for some time (Otto & Bonow, 2012).

Mitral valve repair, rather than replacement, is the preferred approach to MR because it provides better outcomes for most patients and avoids potential complications of anticoagulation and valve prostheses (Kouchoukos et al., 2013). In addition, mitral valve repair or replacement can be accomplished via minimally invasive approaches. The Web Resources section provides information on the 2014 ACC/AHA guideline for surgical management of mitral regurgitation.

A number of devices and techniques are in use or in clinical trials for percutaneous mitral valve repair. Among these are the MitraClip (Abbott Vascular, Santa Clara, CA). This device was approved by the U.S. Food and Drug Administration in 2013 and is used in patients with very high surgical risk. The largest database to date for this registry is the ACCESS-EU study registry, which confirms that the device is safe, has a high implant success rate, low rates of mortality and adverse events, and provides clinically meaningful functional improvement (Maisano et al., 2013).

Care in the immediate postoperative period may be challenging. Mitral regurgitation can mask LV dysfunction because of "unloading" through the regurgitant valve. Upon repair of the mitral valve for mitral regurgitation, the left atrium will no longer be receiving regurgitant blood from the LV and the patient will experience an immediate increase in afterload (systemic vascular resistance). Left ventricular dysfunction that was masked by the regurgitant valve may become apparent, requiring inotropic support or vasodilators. Further compounding the potential for cardiac dysfunction postoperatively are pulmonary hypertension and effects of myocardial hibernation (discussed in Chapter 13) that take time to be reversed. Patients, therefore, are at risk for the development of right ventricular failure. Patients should be monitored for right ventricular failure. If they develop decreased blood pressure, decreased CO, elevated central venous pressure, decreased cardiac volumes, and variable pulmonary artery pressures, suspect right ventricular failure (Bojar, 2011).

The efficacy of medical therapy for asymptomatic MR is the topic of ongoing debate; however, diuretics, digoxin, and arterial vasodilators may be used to decrease ventricular size, regurgitant orifice size, and regurgitant volumes. To date, there is a lack of data that medical therapy will improve outcomes, and it is not recommended for chronic primary MR unless the patient carries a high surgical risk. Patients with AF should be anticoagulated. For MR secondary to other causes, such as LV dilatation, treatment of the underlying cause is sometimes effective in reducing MR. For patients with indications, biventricular pacing may improve MR as well (Otto & Bonow, 2012).

Increased mortality after mitral valve surgery has been found among perimenopausal women. The higher mortality rate is thought to be associated with a state of estrogen withdrawal that may trigger inflammatory responses (Novella, Heras, Hermenegildo, & Dantas, 2012); these responses may in turn potentiate ischemia-reperfusion injury (Song et al., 2008).

Choice of Valve Prosthesis

Prosthetic valves are categorized as mechanical or biologic (tissue) valves. Mechanical valves are manufactured from manmade materials such as metal alloys, pyrolite carbon, and polyethylene terephthalate (Dacron). Biologic valves are constructed from bovine, porcine, or human cardiac tissue, although they may contain some manmade materials.

Mechanical prosthetic valves are more durable and last longer than biologic valves, but they carry an increased risk of venous thrombotic events, necessitating long-term anticoagulation therapy. Biologic valves do not require life-long anticoagulation therapy, but they are less durable due to their tendency toward early calcification, tissue degeneration, and stiffening of the leaflets.

Advantages and disadvantages of valve replacement with either a prosthetic or mechanical valve must be carefully weighed by the patient. Indications for either type of valve vary by patient characteristics and surgeon preference (Kouchoukos et al., 2013).

TRICUSPID VALVE DISEASE

The tricuspid valve has an annular ring and three leaflets connected via chordae tendineae to papillary muscles that are integrated with the RV. It is located between the right atrium and ventricle, near the AV node, right coronary artery, and coronary sinus. Its function is to maintain forward flow of blood between the right atrium and the RV.

Tricuspid Regurgitation

The functional defects that are seen in tricuspid disease are classified as either primary or secondary. Primary valve disease is caused by conditions that affect valve anatomy—for example, congenital abnormalities, rheumatic disease, infective endocarditis, toxicities, tumor, and blunt trauma. Secondary tricuspid disease can result from right ventricular pathology, pulmonary hypertension, increased right ventricular systolic pressure (especially if greater than 55 mmHg), mitral or aortic valve disease (that results in elevated LAP and LVEDP), left-sided HF, dilated cardiomyopathy, tricuspid annular dilatation, or pulmonary embolism (Kouchoukos et al., 2013; Otto & Bonow 2012). Occasionally, wires inserted through the valve such as an automatic implantable cardioverter defibrillator or pacemaker may cause TR (Shemin, 2008). The most common cause of TR is right ventricular dilatation, causing secondary, or functional, TR. Other causes of TR are rheumatic disease and MR (Kouchoukos et al., 2013; Nishimura et al., 2014; Otto & Bonow, 2012).

If the patient does not have pulmonary hypertension, TR is generally well tolerated. Patients with pulmonary hypertension will have signs and symptoms of right ventricular failure such as reduced CO, fatigue, ascites, painful congested hepatomegaly, abnormal venous pulsations, and significant peripheral edema. Weight loss, cachexia, cyanosis, and jaundice may be present, and AF is common (Nishimura et al., 2014; Otto & Bonow, 2012).

Primary TR is generally a progressive disease, as is other valve disease. Secondary TR is often present with mitral disease. Diuretics and therapies to reduce pulmonary vascular resistance may be used for severe TR (Nishimura et al., 2014). Because the most common cause of TR is mitral valve disease, decisions about tricuspid repair or replacement will be influenced by the degree of mitral disease. Data now indicate that TR in the presence of mitral repair or replacement should be repaired as well due to the risk of needing reoperation to repair progressive TR (Kouchoukos et al., 2013; Nishimura et al., 2014). Various repair techniques and tricuspid valve replacement are available. The Web Resources section has a link that discusses the indications for surgery for patients with TR.

Tricuspid Stenosis

Patients with tricuspid stenosis have an obstruction to blood flow from the right atrium to the RV. The most common etiology for tricuspid stenosis is rheumatic heart disease, and it almost always occurs in conjunction with mitral valve disease (Otto & Bonow, 2012). Other conditions associated with tricuspid stenosis include carcinoid syndrome, endocarditis, and intracardiac tumors. The clinical presentation of tricuspid stenosis is logically consistent with right-sided HF, decreased CO, fatigue, anasarca, hepatomegaly, and ascites out of proportion to the degree of dyspnea (Otto & Bonow, 2012).

Surgery for Tricuspid Stenosis

Surgical options for tricuspid stenosis (TS) include annuloplasty, bicuspidization, other repair techniques, percutaneous balloon tricuspid commissurotomy, and valve replacement. The Web Resource section has a link for the indications for surgery for TS.

INFECTIVE VALVE ENDOCARDITIS

Infective valve endocarditis is a complex and serious disease with a high mortality rate even with appropriate antimicrobial therapy. In-hospital mortality is 15% to 20% and 1-year mortality is as high as 40% (Nishimura et al., 2014). The characteristic sign of IE is a vegetation. This is an amorphous mass of fibrin, platelets, microorganisms, and inflammatory cells. *Staphylococcus aureus*, streptococci, and enterococci are the causative agents in most cases (Karchmer, 2012). Causes of IE include hemodynamically significant mitral valve prolapse, congenital heart disease, human immunodeficiency virus, and intravenous drug abuse. Prosthetic valve endocarditis alone accounts for as high as 30% of cases (Karchmer, 2012). Diagnosis is made by using the Duke criteria and transesophageal echocardiogram (Nishimura et al., 2014).

Signs and symptoms are often nonspecific and may come from a complication rather than IE itself. Maintaining a high degree of suspicion is important, especially in a patient who presents with fever, a predisposing cardiac lesion, bacteremia, embolic events, new prosthetic valve dysfunction, or evidence of an active endocardial process (Karchmer, 2012).

Treatment has two arms. First, eradication of the infective organism is paramount to prevent recurrence. Second, invasive complications must be resolved. Antimicrobial therapy specific to the causative agent is critical. Complications may require surgical intervention (Karchmer, 2012).

Indications for surgery differ (see **Table 5-3**). Mortality has been reduced since antimicrobial therapy has been supplemented with earlier surgical intervention (Gaasch, 2014). Early surgery is more likely to result in a successful repair and reduces the risk of infection of the prosthesis (Karchmer, 2012).

Table 5-3   Indications for Surgical Intervention for Infective Endocarditis

Class	Recommendation	Level of Evidence
I	Early surgery (during initial hospitalization before completion of a full course of antibiotics) for patients with IE who present with valve dysfunction resulting in symptoms of HF	B
I	Early surgery for patients with left-sided IE caused by *S. aureus*, fungal, or other highly resistant organisms	B
I	Early surgery for patients with IE complicated by heart block, annular or aortic abscess, or destructive penetrating lesions	B
I	Early surgery for patients with evidence of persistent infection as manifested by persistent bacteremia or fevers lasting longer than 5 to 7 days after onset of appropriate antimicrobial therapy	B
I	Surgery is recommended for patients with prosthetic valve endocarditis and relapsing infection (defined as recurrence of bacteremia after a complete course of appropriate antibiotics and subsequently negative blood cultures) without other identifiable source for portal of infection	C
I	Complete removal of pacemaker or defibrillator systems, including all leads and the generator, is indicated as part of the early management plan in patients with IE with documented infection of the device or leads	B
I	Complete removal of pacemaker or defibrillator systems, including all leads and the generator, is reasonable in patients with valvular IE caused by *S. aureus* or fungi, even without evidence of device or lead infection	B
IIa	Complete removal of pacemaker or defibrillator systems, including all leads and the generator, is reasonable in patients undergoing valve surgery for valvular IE	C
IIa	Early surgery for patients with IE who present with recurrent emboli and persistent vegetations despite appropriate antibiotic therapy	B
IIb	Early surgery for patients with NVE who exhibit mobile vegetations greater than 10 mm in length (with or without clinical evidence of embolic phenomenon)	B

HF, heart failure; IE, infective endocarditis; NVE, native-valve infective endocarditis
Sources: Data from Gaasch, W. H. (2014). *Complications of prosthetic heart valves.* Retrieved from http://www.uptodate.com/contents/complications-of-prosthetic-heart-valves; Prendergast, B. D. & Tornos, P. (2010). Surgery for infective endocarditis: Who and when? *Circulation, 121,* 1141–1152; and O'Gara, P. T. (2007). Infective endocarditis 2006: Indications for surgery. *Transactions of the American Clinical and Climatological Association, 118,* 187–198.

COMPLICATIONS OF HEART VALVE SURGERY

While complications of heart valve surgery are rare, the intensive care unit nurse should be aware of the possibility of their development and implement measures to try to prevent their development. Complications of heart valve surgery reported in the literature include the following conditions:

- Venous thrombotic events (Gaasch, 2014)

- Atrial dysrhythmias (Gaasch, 2014; Ngaage, Cowen, Griffin, Guvendik, & Cale, 2008)

- Renal insufficiency (Gaasch, 2014; Ngaage et al., 2008)

- Heart failure (Gaasch, 2014)

- Neurological complications, stroke, or transient ischemic attack (Filsoufi, Rahmanian, Castillo, Bronster, & Adams, 2008; Gaasch, 2014; Ngaage et al., 2008)

- Respiratory insufficiency (Gaasch, 2014; Ngaage et al., 2008; Tabata et al., 2008)

- AV block (Gaasch, 2014)

- Myocardial infarction (Gaasch, 2014; Ngaage et al., 2008)

- Sternal wound infection (Rahmanian et al., 2007; Tabata et al., 2008)

- Bleeding—requiring reexploration in most cases (David, Armstrong, Maganti, & Ihlberg, 2008; Gaasch, 2014; Ngaage et al., 2008; Tabata et al., 2008)

- Circulatory failure (Haddad et al., 2007)

- Low cardiac output state (Ngaage et al., 2008)

- Gastrointestinal complications (Ngaage et al., 2008)

Two case reports of uncommon complications—left ventricular–right atrial communication (Frigg, Cassina, Siclari, & Mauri, 2008) and an immobilized prosthetic mitral valve (Murugesan, Banakal, & Muralidhar, 2008)—following valve surgery have also been described.

SUMMARY

Selection of a mechanical or biologic prosthetic valve has lifelong implications. These patients may require lifestyle modification and medication therapy for the rest of their lives. Advances in technology in the area of heart valve surgery offer more options, facilitate less invasive techniques, and potentially may improve outcomes. Vigilant postoperative nursing care is critical to help ensure a good outcome for the patient who undergoes valve surgery.

CASE STUDY

A 73-year-old male patient with a history of hypertension is admitted. He leads an active life. His hobbies include line dancing. Three weeks ago, he developed shortness of breath that has been gradually increasing with severity. He sought care from his cardiologist and was diagnosed with aortic stenosis. He was admitted to the hospital for an aortic valve replacement. He underwent on-pump surgery and received a porcine valve; he was admitted to the cardiovascular intensive care unit postoperatively. His postoperative infusions included norepinephrine (Levophed®), insulin, and dexmedetomidine (Precedex®). His initial blood glucose level was 186 mg/dL. Admitting vital signs were as follows: temperature 35.6°C; B/P 100/70, heart rate 92; central venous pressure 5; pulmonary artery pressure 21/8, cardiac index 2.1 L/min/m². He was given a 500 mL bolus of normal saline and placed on a warming blanket. His norepinephrine infusion was titrated up for a systemic vascular resistance of 770 dynes/sec/cm^{-5}. Two hours later, he was awake and responsive on dexmedetomidine, his temperature was 36.4°C, and CI was 2.5 L/min/m^2. A spontaneous breathing trial was conducted; the patient was weaned and extubated.

Critical Thinking Questions

1. Does this patient need to receive anticoagulation as part of his postoperative management?
2. Why was this patient hypothermic postoperatively?
3. Why was norepinephrine required in the immediate postoperative period?

Answers to Critical Thinking Questions

1. Anticoagulation is not required with porcine valves.
2. The patient was cooled in the operating room to decrease myocardial oxygen demand.
3. Norepinephrine was required because the patient was vasodilated from anesthesia and as he began to warm.

SELF-ASSESSMENT QUESTIONS

1. Which of the following is true regarding artificial valves?
   a. Bioprosthetic valves require the patient to remain on anticoagulant therapy throughout their lifetime.
   b. Mechanical valves are less durable.
   c. Mechanical valves are associated with an increased risk of venous thromboembolic events.
   d. Bioprosthetic valves are associated with an increase in thromboembolic complications.

2. Which of the following is a possible sequela of aortic stenosis?
   a. Increased systemic vascular resistance
   b. Increased oxygen delivery
   c. Decreased pulmonary vascular resistance
   d. Decreased myocardial oxygen consumption

3. Which of the following types of murmurs is associated with aortic stenosis?
   a. Continuous murmur
   b. Diastolic murmur
   c. Mid/late diastolic murmur
   d. Systolic murmur

4. Your patient underwent surgery for aortic stenosis. For which of the following should the nurse assess in the immediate postoperative period?
   a. Increased afterload
   b. Left ventricular hypertrophy
   c. Hypertension
   d. Noncompliant LV

5. For which of the following should the nurse observe when caring for a patient with left ventricular hypertrophy from aortic stenosis?
   a.

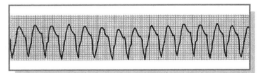

b.

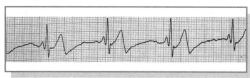

c.

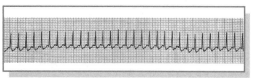

d.

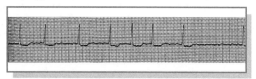

6. Which of the following sets of hemodynamic parameters is consistent with a patient with acute aortic regurgitation?

	PAOP*	CO	HR
a.	6	3.0	120
b.	16	8.2	62
c.	5	9.7	55
d.	20	3.5	116

*pulmonary artery occlusion pressure

7. Following surgery to repair aortic regurgitation, the nurse should anticipate administration of which of the following in the immediate postoperative period?
   a. Norepinephrine (Levophed®)
   b. Milrinone (Primacor®)
   c. Vasopressin (Pitressin®)
   d. Losartan (Cozaar®)

8. Which of the following sets of hemodynamic parameters is consistent with severe mitral stenosis?

	Left atrial pressure	Pulmonary artery systolic pressure
a.	15	40
b.	16	55
c.	12	35
d.	18	45

9. Your patient has mitral stenosis. Which of the following should the nurse anticipate being present?
   a. LV overload
   b. RV failure
   c. Aortic insufficiency
   d. Normal pulmonary artery pressure

10. A patient is admitted immediately following mitral valve repair. Which of the following sets of hemodynamic parameters should the nurse anticipate?

	SVR	PAP
a.	1600	33/21
b.	750	24/10
c.	1750	24/11
d.	700	40/25

Answers to Self-Assessment Questions

1. c	6. d
2. a	7. a
3. d	8. b
4. c	9. b
5. b	10. a

Clinical Inquiry Box

Question: Is minimally invasive mitral valve surgery safe and effective?

Reference: Perier, P., Hohenberger, W., Lakew, F., Batz, G., & Diegeler, A. (2013). Rate of repair in minimally invasive mitral valve surgery. *Annals of Cardiothoracic Surgery, 2*(6), 751–757.

Objective: To determine if minimally invasive surgery for valve repair is safe and effective

Method: Retrospective review

Clinical Inquiry Box (*Continued*)

Results: Over 6 years, 842 patients with degenerative mitral valve regurgitation and anterior, posterior, and bileaflet prolapses had minimally invasive surgery. 99.3% had concomitant ring annuloplasty; 0.7% had valve replacement. Two patients had re-repair secondary to mitral regurgitation progression of infective endocarditis. The 30-day mortality was 0.2% (2 patients); 7.1% (60 patients) had major adverse events.

Conclusion: Minimally invasive procedures can be used for essentially all degenerative valves with good short-term outcomes.

REFERENCES

Bojar, R. M. (2011). *Manual of perioperative care in adult cardiac surgery* (5th ed.). Hoboken, NJ: Wiley-Blackwell.

David, T. E., Armstrong, S., Maganti, M., & Ihlberg, L. (2008). Clinical outcomes of combined aortic root replacement with mitral valve surgery. *Journal of Thoracic and Cardiovascular Surgery,* 136(1), 82–87.

Fann, J. I., Ingels, N. B., & Miller, D. C. (2008). Pathophysiology of mitral valve disease. In L. H. Cohn (Ed.), *Cardiac surgery in the adult* (3rd ed., pp. 973–1012). New York, NY: McGraw-Hill Medical.

Filsoufi, F., Rahmanian, P. B., Castillo, J. G., Bronster, D., & Adams, D. H. (2008). Incidence, imaging analysis, and early and late outcomes of stroke after cardiac valve operation. *American Journal of Cardiology,* 101(10), 1472–1478.

Frigg, C., Cassina, T., Siclari, F., & Mauri, R. (2008). Unusual complication after aortic valve replacement. *Interactive Cardiovascular and Thoracic Surgery,* 7(1), 149–150.

Gaasch, W. H. (2014). *Complications of prosthetic heart valves.* Retrieved from http://www.uptodate.com/contents/complications-of-prosthetic-heart-valves?source=search_result&search=Complications+of+prosthetic+heart+valves.&selectedTitle=1%7E150

Gaasch, W. H., & Sexton, D. J. (2014). *Surgery for native valve endocarditis.* Retrieved from http://www.uptodate.com/contents/surgery-for-native-valve-endocarditis

Gudbjartsson, T., Absi, T., & Aranki, S. (2008). Mitral valve replacement. In L. H. Cohn (Ed.), *Cardiac surgery in the adult* (3rd ed., pp. 1032–1068). New York, NY: McGraw-Hill Medical.

Haddad, F., Denault, A. Y., Couture, P., Cartier, R., Pellerin, M., Levesque, S., . . . Tardif, J. C. (2007). Right ventricular myocardial performance index predicts perioperative mortality or circulatory failure in high-risk valvular surgery. *Journal of the American Society of Echocardiography,* 20(9), 1065–1072.

Jacobson, C., Marzlin, K., & Webner, C. (2014). *Cardiovascular nursing practice* (2nd ed.). Burien, WA: Cardiovascular Nursing Associates.

Karchmer, A. W. (2012). Infective endocarditis. In R. O. Bonow, D. L. Mann, D. P. Zipes, & P. Libby (Eds.), *Braunwald's heart disease: A textbook of cardiovascular medicine* (9th ed., pp. 1540–1560). Philadelphia, PA: Elsevier.

Khalpey, Z. I., Ganim, R. B., & Rawn, J. D. (2008). Postoperative care of cardiac surgery patients. In L. H. Cohn (Ed.), *Cardiac surgery in the adult* (3rd ed., pp. 465–486). New York, NY: McGraw-Hill Medical.

Kouchoukos, N. T., Blackstone, E. H., Hanley, F. L., & Kirklin, J. K. (2013). *Kirklin/Barratt-Boyes cardiac surgery* (4th ed.). Philadelphia, PA: Elsevier.

Maisano, F., Franzen, O., Baldus, S., Schäfer, U., Hausleiter, J., Butter, C., . . . Schillinger, W. (2013). Percutaneous mitral valve interventions in the real world: Early and 1-year results from the ACCESS-EU, a prospective, multicenter, nonrandomized post-approval study of the MitraClip therapy in Europe. *Journal of the American College of Cardiology,* 62(12), 1052–1061.

Mihaljevic, T., Sayeed, M. R., Stamou, S. C., & Paul, C. (2008). Pathophysiology of aortic valve disease. In L. H. Cohn (Ed.), *Cardiac surgery in the adult* (3rd ed., pp. 826–840). New York, NY: McGraw-Hill Medical.

Murugesan, C., Banakal, S., & Muralidhar, K. (2008). An unusual complication following mitral valve surgery and use of intra-operative transoesophageal echocardiography. *Annals of Cardiac Anaesthesia, 11*(2), 127–128.

Ngaage, D. L., Cowen, M. E., Griffin, S., Guvendik, L., & Cale, A. R. (2008). Early neurological complications after coronary artery bypass grafting and valve surgery in octogenarians. *European Journal of Cardio-Thoracic Surgery, 33*(4), 653–659.

Nishimura, R. A., Otto, C. M., Bonow, R. O., Carabello, B. A., Erwin, J. P. 3rd, Guyton, R. A., . . . Yancy, C. W. (2014). 2014 AHA/ACC guideline for the management of patients with valvular heart disease: A report of the American College of Cardiology/American Heart Association Task Force on Practice Guidelines. *The Journal of Thoracic and Cardiovascular Surgery, 148*(1), e1–e132.

Novella, S., Heras, M., Hermenegildo, C., & Dantas, A. P. (2012). Effects of estrogen on vascular inflammation. A matter of timing. *Arteriosclerosis, Thrombosis and Vascular Biology, 32*, 2035–2042.

O'Gara, P. T. (2007). Infective endocarditis 2006: Indications for surgery. *Transactions of the American Clinical and Climatological Association, 118*, 187–198.

Otto, C. M., & Bonow, R. O. (2012). Valvular heart disease. In R. O. Bonow, D. L. Mann, D. P. Zipes, & P. Libby (Eds.), *Braunwald's heart disease: A textbook of cardiovascular medicine* (9th ed., pp. 1469–1539). Philadelphia, PA: Elsevier.

Prendergast, B. D., & Tornos, P. (2010). Surgery for infective endocarditis: Who and when? *Circulation, 121*, 1141–1152.

Rahmanian, P. B., Adams, D. H., Castillo, J. G., Chikwe, J., Bodian, C. A., & Filsoufi, F. (2007). Impact of body mass index on early outcome and late survival in patients undergoing coronary artery bypass grafting or valve surgery or both. *American Journal of Cardiology, 100*(11), 1702–1708.

Shemin, R. J. (2008). Tricuspid valve disease. In L. H. Cohn (Ed.), *Cardiac surgery in the adult* (3rd ed., pp. 1111–1127). New York, NY: McGraw-Hill Medical.

Song, H. K., Grab, J. D., O'Brien, S. M., Welke, K. F., Edwards, F., & Ungerleider, R. M. (2008). Gender differences in mortality after mitral valve operation: Evidence for higher mortality in perimenopausal women. *Annals of Thoracic Surgery, 85*(6), 2040–2045.

Tabata, M., Umakanthan, R., Cohn, L. H., Bolman, R. M., Shekar, P. S., Chen, F. Y., . . . Aranki, S. F. (2008). Early and late outcomes of 1000 minimally invasive aortic valve operations. *European Journal of Cardio-Thoracic Surgery, 33*(4), 537–541.

WEB RESOURCES

American Association of Cardiovascular and Pulmonary Rehabilitation: http://www.aacvpr.org

American College of Cardiology: http://www.acc.org

American Heart Association: http://www.americanheart.org

Mended Hearts: http://www.mendedhearts.org

National Heart, Lung, and Blood Institute: http://www.nhlbi.nih.gov

The Society of Thoracic Surgeons: http://www.sts.org

Aortic Valve Stenosis: Minimally Invasive Valve Replacement Video: http://www.youtube.com/watch?v=-miuqi1iyrw

Mitral Valve Repair: http://www.youtube.com/watch?v=zTHPLWBNjCU

Life after heart valve replacement surgery: http://www.youtube.com/watch?v=_hUG8Np9yk8

Understanding Heart Valve Replacement Choices: What you Need to Know: http://www.youtube.com/watch?v=4xN-c8k7IPs

2014 ACC/AHA Guideline recommendations for MS: http://cardioaragon.com/web/pdf/GUIDELINESValvularHeartDisease.AHA.ACC2014.pdf

2014 ACC/AHA guideline for surgical management of mitral regurgitation: http://cardioaragon.com/web/pdf/GUIDELINESValvularHeartDisease.AHA.ACC2014.pdf

Indications for surgery for patients with TR: http://cardioaragon.com/web/pdf/GUIDELINESValvularHeartDisease.AHA.ACC2014.pdf

Indications for surgery for TS: http://cardioaragon.com/web/pdf/GUIDELINESValvularHeartDisease.AHA.ACC2014.pdf

Chapter 6

Cardiopulmonary Bypass and Off-Pump Coronary Artery Bypass

Julie Miller and Shelley K. Welch

INTRODUCTION

For years, nurses have cared for patients who have undergone traditional coronary artery bypass grafting (CABG) surgery, in which the patient is placed on a cardiopulmonary bypass (CPB) circuit. Since 1990, however, nurses have seen an increase in the number of patients undergoing off-pump coronary artery bypass (OPCAB) surgery, in which the surgeon sews the grafts onto the beating heart. Nursing care of patients who have received the CABG and OPCAB procedures has a number of similarities and differences.

Care of the coronary bypass surgery patient has evolved over the years. Previously, patients spent 2 to 3 days on a ventilator, sedated, with a pulmonary artery catheter (PAC) in place and multiple vasoactive drips infusing to maintain optimal hemodynamic status. Today, a patient undergoing CABG or OPCAB may be discharged from the operating room without a PAC, extubated, and transferred from the intensive care unit (ICU) to a progressive care unit within 12 hours of surgery. Regardless of the short stay, patients remain critically ill when transferred from the ICU. Nurses are often faced with the challenge of patients and families who are anxious over the potential for death throughout the course of hospitalization.

Anxiety during the preoperative and postoperative periods has been correlated with poor outcomes such as increased pain levels (Navarro-Garcia et al., 2011; Viars, 2009) and more readmissions (Tully, Baker, Turnbull, & Winefield, 2008). Factors predictive of increased anxiety include being female, having to wait for surgery, pain prior to surgery, concerns over returning to work, prior anxiolytic or antidepressant use, and difficulty sleeping (Chocron et al., 2013). Nurses must assess patients' anxiety levels throughout the hospitalization and seek to understand the best patient-specific approach in countering their stress. The provision of realistic information about what to expect through every step of the care delivered and effective pain management are crucial in decreasing anxiety levels. Additionally, recent research suggests that patients with preoperative depression may benefit from administration of antidepressant therapy (Chocron et al., 2013).

Despite the need to address anxiety levels, the hemodynamic challenges, constant observation for potential complications, and need for the astute critical care nurse remain the same. This chapter explores the similarities and differences in the care of the traditional on-pump coronary artery bypass (ONCAB, or CABG) patient compared to the patient who undergoes OPCAB.

POTENTIAL COMPLICATIONS OF BYPASS SURGERY

Stroke, infection, bleeding, dysrhythmias, myocardial infarction (MI), gastrointestinal dysfunction, renal failure, and death are all potential complications for the bypass surgery patient, whether the procedure is performed with the on- or off-pump technique. The risk for atrioventricular heart block is present in both types of bypass procedures, and both types of patients should have epicardial pacing wires placed. Nursing challenges for bypass surgery patients include ensuring hemodynamic stability, monitoring for and treating cardiac dysrhythmias, balancing the need to adequately medicate for pain while guarding against oversedation and respiratory complications, and monitoring for and intervening to prevent the myriad of potential postoperative complications.

On-pump coronary artery bypass patients undergo surgery while their heart is not beating. In this procedure, through a median sternotomy incision, the heart is stopped using cardioplegia solution. Oxygen needs are met by cannulating the aorta and placing the patient on the CPB circuit. On-pump coronary artery bypass carries a higher risk of aortic dissection and embolization because of the cannulation and cross-clamping of the aorta for bypass procedures (Puskas et al., 2011).

Heparin is utilized to maintain patency of the CPB circuit and to reduce the risk of microemboli formation. Heparin-induced thrombocytopenia (HIT) and bleeding are potential complications for all patients receiving heparin. In addition, the CPB circuit can contribute to the development of systemic inflammatory response syndrome (SIRS) and microemboli (Hattler et al., 2012). Moderate hypothermia is utilized during the ONCAB procedure to decrease myocardial oxygen demand. The postoperative rewarming process contributes to vasodilation and can worsen the effects of SIRS.

As part of the ONCAB procedure, the bypass grafts are sewn onto the heart and aorta while the heart is not beating. When the surgery is completed, the heart is restarted and the CPB circuit withdrawn. There is a risk that the patient will not be able to be weaned from CPB and may require an intra-aortic balloon pump (IABP) or pacemaker postoperatively. Intra-aortic balloon pump therapy is discussed in detail in Chapter 10. On rare occasions, a patient's heart does not restart following CPB.

OFF-PUMP CORONARY ARTERY BYPASS

Off-pump coronary artery bypass is performed either through a median sternotomy incision or via a thoracotomy incision, also known as minimally invasive direct coronary artery bypass (MIDCAB). Robotic-assisted coronary artery bypass (ROBOCAB) surgery is another type of off-pump procedure that is done through a minimally invasive approach. Minimally invasive surgery is discussed in detail in Chapter 7.

In OPCAB, the surgeon sews the grafts onto the beating heart using specialized instruments to stabilize the myocardial tissue where the surgeon is sewing the graft (St. Andre & DelRossi, 2005). These instruments, known as stabilizers, are similar in shape to the sewing foot for a sewing machine (see **Figure 6-1**).

Off-pump coronary artery bypass techniques gained popularity in the 1990s in efforts to

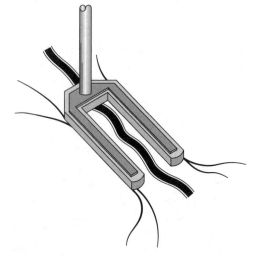

Figure 6-1 Stabilizer used in OPCAB.
Source: Illustrated by James R. Perron

reduce the complications associated with the CPB circuit. Recent studies have noted that OPCAB procedures have higher reocclusion rates than ONCAB, and outcomes at 1 year are worse for the OPCAB than the ONCAB patient (Hattler et al., 2012). However, a study conducted in 2009 notes that patients who have Society of Thoracic Surgeon (STS) preoperative predicted risk of mortality (PROM) scores greater than 2.5% to 3% have better operative mortality rates with OPCAB than ONCAB (Puskas et al., 2009). Studies have noted that patients undergoing OPCAB receive fewer grafts than those undergoing ONCAB. This pattern may lead to a higher reintervention rate for OPCAB patients (Hattler et al., 2012; Sedrakyan, Wu, Parashar, Bass, & Treasure, 2006). The risk for aortic dissection with OPCAB is less than traditional CABG, however (Shekar, 2006). Approximately 50 of 1,000 (5%) patients undergoing off-pump bypass procedures may need to be converted to on-pump procedures (Sedrakyan et al., 2006). This possibility should be discussed with the patient and family during preoperative teaching.

Off-pump coronary artery bypass is performed on a patient with either mild hypothermia or normothermia. Hypothermia contributes to postoperative bleeding by causing impairment in the clotting cascade. It is theorized that less bleeding occurs with mild hypothermia as compared to the moderate hypothermia (30–34°C) utilized in the ONCAB procedure. Mild hypothermia does help reduce myocardial oxygen demand and may be beneficial to both ONCAB and OPCAB patients. Data suggest that moderate hypothermia protects against intraoperative mortality for on-pump patients (Greason, Kim, Suri, Wallace, & Englum, 2014). Other data from a systematic review suggest no difference in safety between normothermia and hypothermia in cardiopulmonary bypass grafting. One difference reported was the increasing need for blood transfusions in patients with mild hypothermia (Ho & Tan, 2011).

COMPLICATIONS OF ON-PUMP SURGERY VERSUS OFF-PUMP SURGERY

Off-pump coronary artery bypass grafting, also known as a beating heart procedure, was developed partly to offset the risk of postoperative alterations associated with on-pump procedures. Specifically, patients who undergo OPCAB are felt to be less likely to develop cerebral hypoperfusion, embolization, and inflammatory response associated with on-pump procedures (Hattler et al., 2012). Recent work has found that the cytokine and chemokine production is similar in ONCAB and OPCAB, but biomarkers such as eotaxin, macrophage inflammatory protein-1 beta (MIP-1β), and interleukin-12 (IL-12) were found to be more prevalent in the setting of ONCAB. Although more research needs to be conducted on the inflammatory response most often seen in ONCAB, OPCAB does appear to produce less of an inflammatory response, which may improve cardiopulmonary outcomes (Castellheim et al., 2008).

Assessment for postoperative bleeding is essential, especially given that mediastinal reexploration rates for bypass surgery patients are as high as 5% (Yetkin, Yürekil, & Gürbüz, 2008). Bleeding in these patients can be attributed to CPB, hypothermia, fibrinolytic agents administered during the procedure, heparin reversal, and loose anastomoses. As OPCAB was developed, concern was voiced that these patients would have more bleeding due to the risk of sewing onto the beating heart. In fact, data from randomized controlled trials suggest that OPCAB patients experience less bleeding postoperatively than ONCAB patients (Hattler et al., 2012).

In all post-bypass patients, assessment for bleeding is necessary. The mediastinal and pleural tubes must be monitored hourly for amount and quality of drainage, including assessment for clots. Monitoring for narrowing of pulse pressure is performed, as this finding could indicate cardiac tamponade in the post-bypass patient.

Heparin is utilized to maintain vessel patency and prevent thrombus formation during OPCAB, but the amount is about one-third to one-half the dose used in traditional CABG. Because heparin is utilized in both on- and off-pump procedures, it is imperative that the nurse assess all post-bypass patients for bleeding, check lab data for presence of a coagulopathy, and assess for HIT.

Protamine is a protein that occurs in salmon sperm (DailyMed.gov, 2014). It is utilized in both on- and off-pump procedures to bind heparin and reverse its anticoagulant effect (Bollinger et al., 2010). In one study, researchers estimated that protamine caused adverse events in approximately 2.6% of cardiac surgery patients (Lee, Cheng, & Ko, 2013). Risk factors for protamine reactions include being a diabetic patient who uses protamine-containing insulin (most commonly NPH) (Nybo & Madsen, 2008), previous drug reaction, and allergy to protamine or fish. An estimated 39% of bypass surgery patients have these risk factors (Levy & Adkinson, 2008).

A minor protamine reaction may result in hypotension and an increase in pulmonary artery pressure (PAP) (Lee et al., 2013). This effect is more common in patients who have diabetes, perhaps related to their use of protamine-containing insulin. Anaphylaxis has been associated with administration of protamine, and the affected patient may suffer cardiac arrest. Any adverse reaction to protamine increases the risk of mortality for both ONCAB and OPCAB patients (Welsby et al., 2005).

The critical care nurse must be vigilant in monitoring for protamine reactions, including assessing the patient for different presentations of these reactions. Massive systemic vasodilation is manifested by hypotension, decreased systemic vascular resistance (the amount of work the heart must do to eject blood), and increased cardiac output (CO) (the amount of blood ejected by the heart every minute). This syndrome, referred to as vasoplegia, if not responding to administration of fluid and vasopressors, may respond to an intravenous infusion of methylene blue (Lutjen & Arndt, 2012). Acute pulmonary vasoconstriction will lead to an increase in PAP with subsequent right ventricular failure. The hemodynamic profile in this type of reaction will reveal bradycardia, decreased CO, elevated PAP, systemic vascular resistance (SVR), and pulmonary vascular resistance.

In recent years, studies have tested new drugs suggested as candidates to replace protamine for reversing heparin and improve the safety of the bypass procedure for all CABG patients. Unfortunately, none of these drugs has demonstrated a superior safety profile as compared to protamine during clinical trials (Stafford-Smith et al., 2005). As a consequence, heparin–protamine remains the only drug combination approved for use in the CPB circuit.

Recent studies have evaluated a direct thrombin inhibitor, bivalirudin (Angiomax®), as a replacement for heparin anticoagulation for CPB and OPCAB. These studies indicate that bivalirudin can be used safely in patients with heparin allergy or increased risk for HIT (Kashyap et al., 2010). Nursing care for a patient receiving bivalirudin includes astute monitoring of lab data and for bleeding. Specific tests that may be used to evaluate the efficacy of bivalirudin include activated clotting time, activated partial thromboplastin time (aPTT), international normalized ratio, and thromboelastogram (Nikolaidis, Velissaris, & Ohr, 2007).

Patients who undergo bypass procedures may develop postoperative temporary metabolic, hemodynamic, and neurohormonal changes (Puskas et al., 2011). For example, in one study, on- and off-pump cardiac surgery patients were evaluated at 24-hour intervals. Both groups of patients had elevated cardiac markers and white blood cell, neutrophil, and monocyte counts postoperatively; the levels were consistently and significantly higher in the on-pump group. In addition, the hematologic abnormalities persisted longer in the on-pump group. Patients who underwent OPCAB had less of a rise in serum lactate levels. Those whose peak lactate level was greater than 4.0 mmol/L were more likely to develop postoperative morbidities, including those hemodynamic, pulmonary, and renal in nature as well as MI. The same group of patients had a greater tendency for hypoxic episodes, were intubated longer, had a higher length of stay, and consumed more hospital resources. Three patients in the on-pump group required postoperative use of the IABP (Warang et al., 2007).

Hemodynamic alterations may occur after cardiac surgery. These alterations may include a decrease in CO/cardiac index from intraoperative myocardial ischemia, tachycardia, bradycardia, increased SVR, or decreased myocardial contractility; hypotension due to decreased preload, contractility, or SVR; hypertension from a disrupted surgical anastomosis; and myocardial depression, vasoconstriction, or ventricular dysrhythmias from hypothermia (Martin & Turkelson, 2006).

HEMODYNAMIC MONITORING

In the initial postoperative period for both ONCAB and OPCAB patients, the primary focus is hemodynamic stability. The first 6 hours postoperatively tend to be when the patient is the most vulnerable and unstable.

Cardiac dysfunction tends to manifest as decreased compliance and contractility from the pressure-overloaded myocardial tissue. A pressure-overloaded ventricle will have reduced compliance and be stiff, which will result in a decreased ejection fraction, CO, and contractility.

Preoperative ischemia and duration of the operative procedure contribute to instability in patients who undergo either on- or off-pump procedures. In the ONCAB patient, hemodynamic instability is related to effects from the CPB circuit and the cold potassium cardioplegia used to reduce myocardial oxygen demand. In contrast, manipulation of the beating heart for OPCAB leads to decreased compliance and contractility (Puskas et al., 2011).

A patient who has had valve replacement is typically volume overloaded (Gaasch & Meyer, 2008). In both ONCAB and OPCAB surgeries, fluid needs may be higher than expected; thus, the critical care nurse will need to assess all interventions for their effect on hemodynamics to ensure adequate preload. Hemodynamic profiles of cardiac surgery patients are discussed in detail in Chapter 9.

RISKS OF ON-PUMP SURGERY VERSUS OFF-PUMP SURGERY

A number of risks are associated with coronary artery bypass surgery, whether it is performed on an on- or off-pump basis. Specifically, stroke, atrial fibrillation (AF), acute renal failure, acute liver failure, bleeding, infection, and death have all been associated with on- and off-pump surgery.

The ONCAB procedure and the CPB circuit have been shown to increase the risk for development of acute renal failure, stroke, liver failure, AF, and bleeding (Puskas et al., 2011). Use of the CPB circuit has also been associated with the development of microemboli and SIRS, which occurs in OPCAB patients, albeit to a lesser degree than in ONCAB patients (Bilgin & van de Watering, 2013). The risk of death for both OPCAB and ONCAB is variable by gender and procedure. In one study, 30-day mortality with ONCAB was 5.2% in women and 2.5% in men. At 1 year, mortality rates were 8.7% for women and 4.8% for men. Conversely, OPCAB 30-day and 1-year mortality was 1.7% for women. For men who received an OPCAB procedure, the 30-day mortality was 2.1%; at 1 year, mortality rate was 3.7% (Eifert et al., 2010). However, patients who have PROM scores greater than 2.5% to 3% may have lower operative mortality with OPCAB (Puskas et al., 2009). Nursing interventions for both OPCAB and ONCAB patients include assessment for and prevention of these adverse events and preoperative teaching that includes a discussion of these potential risks.

Off-pump coronary artery bypass was developed to try to minimize the risks of the CPB circuit (Verma et al., 2004). A meta-analysis revealed a reduced incidence of stroke, AF, and infections with OPCAB as compared to ONCAB (Sedrakyan et al., 2006). These data are not consistent. Women undergoing bypass surgery are at a higher risk for complications. Data also suggest that OPCAB benefits women by reducing their intraoperative and postoperative morbidity and mortality rates (Puskas et al., 2007). The off-pump bypass is technically more challenging than ONCAB. Critics cite this difference as a factor that complicates the process of setting up randomized controlled studies and comparing outcomes for on- and off-pump procedures. The ROOBY trial conducted from February 2002 to May 2008 by the U.S. Department of Veterans Affairs randomized 2,203 patients to either OPCAB or ONCAB using a standard median sternotomy approach. This trial, the largest to date, showed patients in the low to moderate risk category who underwent OPCAB had higher 1-year mortality and higher arterial and saphenous vein reocclusion rates (Shroyer et al., 2009). Also, long-term survival has been shown to be better in elective CABG surgery patients undergoing ONCAB (Kim et al., 2014).

Cognitive Decline

Cognitive decline has been noted in patients who have undergone coronary artery bypass. It had been theorized that this decline in function was related to the CPB circuit. In recent studies comparing ONCAB, OPCAB, and healthy patients, however, researchers determined that the rate of cognitive decline in both types of surgery was the same. Off-pump coronary artery bypass proponents had theorized there would be less cognitive decline without CPB. Demographic data revealed that cognitive decline was present prior to surgery in both the ONCAB and OPCAB groups at a higher level than in the healthy patients (Farhoudi et al., 2010; Kozova et al., 2010). At this time, the decline in cognitive function does not appear to be related to CPB. The ROOBY trial noted similar neuropsychological outcomes in both OPCAB and ONCAB (Shroyer et al., 2009). Cognitive decline in patients undergoing coronary artery bypass surgery will require more study to determine the contributing factors.

Graft Occlusion

Both on- and off-pump procedures utilize the saphenous vein and arterial conduits for grafts. Saphenous vein harvesting is accomplished endoscopically, which reduces the pain and scarring associated with the historical harvest approach of an inner thigh to ankle incision (Kurfirst, Candayoua, & Mokracek, 2012). Vein grafts are implanted in a reverse direction relative to their valves and have a higher occlusion rate when compared to the left internal thoracic artery grafts (Hu & Zhao, 2011).

Arterial grafts include the left internal thoracic artery, radial artery, and, less commonly, the right internal thoracic artery. The intrathoracic arteries, formerly known as mammary arteries, are used to bypass the anterior coronary circulation and require only one anastomosis. The elimination of anastomosis to the ascending aorta may reduce emboli, which might otherwise cause stroke (Vallely, Edelman, & Wilson, 2013). Arterial grafts have been shown to decrease the need for revascularization and reduce short- and long-term mortality; approximately 80% of these grafts are still patent 8 years after implantation (Taboulis, 2013).

The radial artery, which was first utilized as a graft in the 1970s, has regained popularity as a graft in recent years due to its long patency duration (Barner et al., 2012). Improved harvest techniques for radial artery grafts and the use of calcium channel blockers intraoperatively and postoperatively (e.g., diltiazem [Cardizem®]) for 6 months have produced patency rates similar to those for other arterial grafts at 5 years (Hayward, Hare, Gordon, Matalanis, & Buxton 2007; Voucharas, Bisbos, Moustakidis, & Tsilimingas, 2010).

Patient Assessment

Ongoing preoperative and postoperative assessments are crucial for patients undergoing radial artery harvest. In the preoperative phase, the nurse performs a detailed assessment of the patient's history, activity level, and collateral ulnar blood flow to the affected hand(s). Collateral blood flow to the hand is most commonly assessed by using the Allen test. Specifically, the Allen test is used to assess the adequacy of blood supply to the hand through the ulnar artery. **Table 6-1** outlines the performance and evaluation criteria included on the Allen test. The literature varies in interpretation of an Allen test, with 5 to 9 seconds being considered a positive result (Hayward et al., 2007; Voucharas et al., 2010). The recommended contraindication for radial graft harvest is a positive Allen test (the red color of the palm returns) in greater than 6 seconds (Asif & Sarkar, 2007). A positive Allen test has been reported to have a predictive value of 53%, which means there is a need to investigate collateral flow further.

Techniques to more closely examine collateral flow include the use of Doppler flow measurements, thumb systolic pressure, finger-pulse plethysmography, and pulse oximetry (Asif & Sarkar, 2007). Some sources suggest that the Allen test could give a

Table 6-1　Steps for Performing the Allen Test
Step 1: Simultaneously locate the radial and ulnar artery; palpate and compress them with three digits. Step 2: Maintaining compression on the radial and ulnar arteries, ask the patient to clench and unclench the hand 10 times. Step 3: Release pressure from the ulnar artery and monitor the time it takes for flushing to return to the palm, thumb, and nail beds. Step 4: If the amount of time it takes for flushing to return is greater than 6 seconds, this means that collateral flow is impaired. The radial artery should not be used as a graft.
Source: Data from Asif, M., & Sarkar, P. K. (2007). Three digit Allen test. *Annals of Thoracic Surgery, 84,* 686–687.

false-negative result. Regardless of the result, it is always mandatory to have a preoperative ultrasound study if radial artery harvesting is being considered (Sajja, 2008).

Patients who perform manual labor, are physically active with their hands, have suffered a stroke with upper limb involvement, have peripheral vascular disease or Raynaud's disease, or have experienced a traumatic injury to the affected side should not be considered candidates for radial artery harvest (Hayward et al., 2007; Shah et al., 2007). Additionally, smoking, diabetes, hypertension, and hyperlipidemia have been associated with diminished radial artery graft patency rates. Data suggest that patients with peripheral vascular disease are more likely to have early occlusion of a radial artery graft (Cheng & Slaughter, 2013).

Data suggest that radial artery graft patency rates are decreased in the OPCAB population (Shroyer et al., 2009). Desai and colleagues (2007) report that women are more likely to have longer graft patency with radial artery grafts when compared to saphenous vein grafts for non-left anterior descending bypasses. Puskas and colleagues (2007) report women have better outcomes when using OPCAB. Although more studies on this topic are necessary, the current evidence points to women benefiting from complete arterial revascularization instead of vein grafting and to patients with peripheral vascular disease benefiting from vein grafts.

Radial Artery Harvesting

In the early development of radial artery harvesting, it was recommended that the non-dominant hand be the site of harvest owing to fear of hand ischemia. Shah and colleagues (2007) suggest that harvesting of radial arteries from the dominant hand can be accomplished safely with minimal adverse effects for the patient, as hand ischemia is actually a rare occurrence. Depending on surgeon preference, the radial artery donor site may or may not have a drain placed. If a drain is placed, it is usually removed when drainage is less than 20 mL for 8 hours. The incision will be covered loosely with a sterile gauze dressing and wrapped with a compressive wrap for 24 hours (Blitz, Osterday, & Brodman, 2013).

Postoperative assessment of the affected extremity includes the amount and quality of drainage, signs and symptoms of infection, and the "six Ps" for diminished arterial blood flow (i.e., pain, pulselessness, pallor, paresthesia, paralysis, and polar [cold]). Patients should be made aware that they may experience loss of motor strength and numbness on the affected extremity. These symptoms usually resolve in most patients 6 months postoperatively. Patients who smoke report higher levels of sensory loss but no difference in motor function compared to nonsmokers (Shah et al., 2007).

Compartment Syndrome

The literature reports a rare occurrence of compartment syndrome in the vein donor limbs for coronary artery bypass (Kolli, Au, Lee, Klinoff, & Ko, 2010). Nursing assessment of the donor limb should include assessment for diminished blood flow. Like their counterparts undergoing radial artery harvesting, vein graft donors should have the six Ps assessed. Early symptoms of compartment syndrome include severe pain and tenderness on passive stretch. This assessment may be masked by the use of sedation and narcotic analgesia in the early postoperative period.

Off-pump coronary artery bypass was developed to reduce the complications associated with the ONCAB procedure. Recent evidence suggests that OPCAB has higher 1-year mortality rates, lower 1-year arterial and saphenous vein patency rates (Hattler et al., 2012), and shorter long-term survival (Kim et al., 2014). However, other studies suggest that patients who have higher operative mortality risk benefit from the OPCAB procedure (Puskas et al., 2009). Off-pump coronary artery bypass has been associated with a reduction in cost. Factors contributing to the reduction in cost for OPCAB are shorter lengths of stay in the ICU, shorter intubation times, decreased risk of stroke, reoperations for bleeding, and use of blood products due to diminished blood loss (Brewer et al., 2014). The majority of bypass surgeries performed in the United States remain on-pump procedures.

SUMMARY

Nursing care of both on- and off-pump coronary artery bypass patients continues to advance as evidence mounts regarding the risks and advantages of each procedure. On- and off-pump patients remain at risk for myriad complications. Patients who undergo off-pump procedures tend to experience a lower incidence of stroke, infection, and atrial fibrillation; a notable cost savings with the use of off-pump procedures has also been documented. As the techniques and utilization of off-pump surgery continue to evolve, so will the skill and practice of the expert cardiac surgery nurse. Care of these patients will continue to be highly challenging and rewarding.

CASE STUDY

A 68-year-old patient with a history of hypertension, diabetes mellitus, and hyperlipidemia underwent an on-pump 3-vessel bypass procedure for the left anterior descending and right proximal coronary arteries. Postoperatively, he was transferred to the cardiovascular ICU on epinephrine, insulin, milrinone, and propofol infusions. His blood sugars increased over the first 6 hours; the epinephrine infusion was changed to dobutamine. As the patient was warmed from 35.6°C to 37.5°C, his SVR changed from 1,400 to 874 dynes/sec/cm^{-5}. His filling pressures decreased, for which he received volume resuscitation and, ultimately, an infusion of norepinephrine. His chest tube draining was 300 mL the first hour and 310 mL the second hour. Protamine sulfate and blood and blood products were administered. The chest tube volume decreased.

Critical Thinking Questions

1. Why was epinephrine changed to a dobutamine infusion?
2. Why was the patient hypothermic upon admission to the cardiovascular ICU?
3. Why was protamine sulfate administered for the chest tube drainage?

Answers to Critical Thinking Questions

1. The epinephrine was changed to dobutamine because of the difficulty controlling the patient's blood glucose from the epinephrine and his history of diabetes mellitus.
2. The patient was hypothermic postoperatively from the cardioplegia and from being kept cool in the operating room to decrease myocardial oxygen demand.
3. Protamine was administered to ensure complete reversal of heparin administered when on the bypass circuit.

SELF-ASSESSMENT QUESTIONS

1. For which of the following complications is a patient more at risk when having cardiac surgery on cardiopulmonary bypass as compared to a patient having the procedure off-pump?
   a. Renal failure   c. Infection
   b. Embolization   d. Myocardial infarction

2. Your on-pump cardiac surgery patient has the following labs:

	On admission	Postoperative Day 1
Hgb	9.8 g/dL	9.5 g/dL
Hct	28.6%	27.5%
Platelets	140,000	70,000
PT	12.5 sec	12.8 sec
aPTT	36.5 sec	36.8 sec

Which of the following should the nurse suspect?
   a. Postoperative bleeding
   b. Red blood cell hemolysis
   c. Disseminated intravascular coagulation
   d. Heparin-induced thrombocytopenia

3. Your patient has undergone on-pump coronary artery bypass grafting. For which of the following sets of data is the patient at risk for complications?

	HR	Temp	RR	WBC
a.	114	37.8°C (100°F)	16	10,000
b.	73	36.1°C (97°F)	14	2,000
c.	98	35.8°C (96.4°F)	22	3,000
d.	84	37.6°C (99.7°F)	18	14,000

4. Which of the following statements by a nurse new to the cardiac surgery unit

indicates that additional education is required?

a. Patients who have off-pump procedures are more likely to need future interventions.

b. With both on- and off-pump bypass, the heart is not beating for part of the procedure.

c. There is less risk of aortic dissection with off-pump procedures.

d. There is greater risk of bleeding with on-pump procedures.

5. Which of the following patients is at greatest risk for a protamine reaction? A patient with a history of:
   a. Heparin-induced thrombocytopenia
   b. Diabetes
   c. Other drug allergies
   d. Asthma

6. Which of the following sets of hemodynamic parameters is consistent with a patient experiencing a protamine reaction?

	B/P	HR	CO	PAP
a.	146/94	55	10	14/8
b.	70/52	108	3	40/28
c.	150/90	116	3.5	16/6
d.	88/50	50	9	38/25

7. Which of the following patients is most likely to be at risk for postoperative on-pump complications? A patient with:
   a. WBC $12.1/mm^3$
   b. Elevated cardiac markers
   c. Elevated monocyte count
   d. Lactate 4.2 mmol/L

8. Your patient underwent off-pump coronary artery bypass surgery. For which of the following is the patient at greatest risk?
   a.

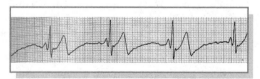

b.

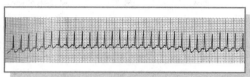

c.

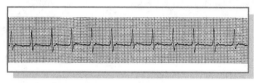

d.

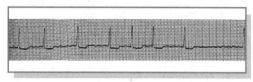

9. Which of the following statements about an Allen Test is true?
   a. Prior to compressing the arteries, the patient should clench and unclench the hand 10 times.
   b. If color is not restored after 3 seconds, a radial artery graft should not be done.
   c. The radial and ulnar arteries are compressed in sequence and compared for time to color restoration.
   d. Each artery should be kept compressed for 30 seconds and then released.

10. Which of the following is an early sign of compartment syndrome?
    a. Severe pain
    b. Polar (cold)
    c. Pallor
    d. Paresthesia

Answers to Self-Assessment Questions

1. b	6. d
2. d	7. d
3. c	8. d
4. b	9. b
5. b	10. a

Clinical Inquiry Box

Question: Are there differences in the incidence of adverse events in patients undergoing on-pump versus off-pump coronary artery bypass grafting?

Reference: Polomsky, M., He, X., O'Brien, S. M., & Puskas, J. D. (2013). Outcomes of off-pump versus on-pump coronary artery bypass grafting: Impact of preoperative risk. *Journal of Thoracic and Cardiovascular Surgery, 145*(5), 1193–1198.

Objective: To determine if there are differences in the incidence of adverse events in patients undergoing on-pump versus off-pump coronary artery bypass grafting

Methods: Multi-center evaluation. Patients who had a Predicted Risk of Mortality Score who underwent nonemergent isolated coronary artery bypass procedures between January 2005 and December 2010 were queried. A total of 210,469 patients underwent surgery at one of the participating sites. Data were analyzed using logistic models.

Results: Over the 6 years, there was a significant decrease in risk of death, stroke, acute renal failure, morbidity, mortality, and length of stay in patients who underwent off-pump coronary artery bypass grafting after adjustment for 30 patient risk factors ($p < .05$).

Conclusion: Off-pump procedures were associated with fewer adverse events when compared to patients undergoing on-pump procedures after adjustment for 30 patient risk factors.

REFERENCES

Asif, M., & Sarkar, P. K. (2007). Three digit Allen test. *Annals of Thoracic Surgery, 84,* 686–687.

Barner, H. B., Bailey, M., Guthrie, T. J ., Pasque, M. K., Moon, M. R., Damiano Jr., R., . . . Lawton, J. S. (2012). Surgery for coronary artery disease. *Circulation, 126,* 5140–5144.

Bilgin, Y. M., & van de Watering, L. M. G. (2013). Complications after cardiac surgery due to allogeneic blood transfusions. *Journal of Clinical & Experimental Cardiology, S7.* doi: 10.4172/2155-9880.S7-005. Retrieved from http://omicsonline.org/complications-after-cardiac-surgery-due-to-allogeneic-blood-transfusions-2155-9880-S7-005.php?aid=17752

Blitz, A., Osterday, R. M., & Brodman, R. F. (2013). Harvesting the radial artery. *Annals of Cardiothoracic Surgery, 2*(4). Retrieved from http://www.annalscts.com/article/view/2418/3284

Bollinger, D., Szlam, F., Azran, M., Koyama, K., Levy, J. H., Molinaro, R., . . . Tanaka, K. A. (2010). The anticoagulant effect of protamine sulfate is attenuated in the presence of platelets or elevated factor VIII concentrations. *Anesthesia & Analgesia, 11*(3), 601–608.

Brewer, R., Theurer, P. F., Cogan, C. M., Bell, G. F., Prager, R. L., & Paone, G. (2014). Morbidity but not mortality is decreased after off-pump coronary artery bypass surgery. *Annals of Thoracic Surgery, 97*(3), 831–836.

Castellheim, A., Hoel, T. N., Videm, V., Fosse, E., Pharo, A., Svennevig, J. L., . . . Mollnes, T. E. (2008). Biomarker profile in off-pump and on-pump coronary artery bypass grafting surgery in low-risk patients. *Annals of Thoracic Surgery, 85*(6), 1994–2002.

Cheng, A., & Slaughter, M. S. (2013). How I choose conduits and configure grafts for my patients—rationales and practices. *Annals of Cardiothoracic Surgery, 2*(4). Retrieved from http://www.annalscts.com/article/view/2417/3283

Chocron, S., Vandel, P., Durst, C., Laluc, F., Kaili, D., Chocron, M., . . . Etievent, J. P. (2013). Antidepressant therapy in patients undergoing coronary artery bypass grafting: The MOTIV-CABG trial. *Annals of Thoracic Surgery, 95,* 1609–1618.

DailyMed.gov. (2014). *Protamine sulfate.* Retrieved from http://dailymed.nlm.nih.gov/dailymed/drugInfo.cfm?setid=7a31fc4c-579f-45cc-9559-39cfad9a57b3

Desai, N. D., Naylor, C. D., Kiss, A., Cohen, E. A., Feder-Elituv, R., Miwa, S., . . . Fremes, S. E. (2007). Impact of patient and target-vessel characteristics on arterial and venous bypass graft patency: Insight from a randomized trial. *Circulation, 115*(6), 684–691.

Eifert, S., Killian, E., Beiras-Fernandez, A., Juchem, G., Reichart, B., & Lamm, P. (2010). Early and mid term mortality after coronary artery bypass grafting in women depends on the surgical protocol: Retrospective analysis of 3441 on- and off-pump coronary artery bypass grafting procedures. *Journal of Cardiothoracic Surgery, 5*, 90. doi: 10.1186/1749-8090-5-90

Farhoudi, M., Mehrvar, K., Afrasiabi, A., Parvizi, R., Khalili, A. A., Nasiri, B., . . . Ghabili, K. (2010). Neurocognitive impairment after off-pump and on-pump coronary artery bypass graft surgery—an Iranian experience. *Neuropsychiatric Disease Treatment, 6*, 775–778.

Gaasch, W. H., & Meyer, T. E. (2008). Valvular heart disease: Changing concepts in disease management. *Circulation, 118*, 2298–2303.

Greason, K. L., Kim, S., Suri, R. M., Wallace, A. S., & Englum, B. R. (2014). Hypothermia and operative mortality during on-pump coronary artery bypass grafting. *Journal of Thoracic and Cardiovascular Surgery, 148*(6), 2712–2718.

Hattler, B., Messenger, J. C., Shroyer, A. L., Collins, J. F., Haugen, S. J., Garcia, J. A., . . . Grover, F. L. (2012). Off-pump coronary artery bypass surgery is associated with worse arterial and saphenous vein graft patency and less effective revascularization: Results from the Veterans Affairs Randomized On/Off Bypass (ROOBY) trial. *Circulation, 125*(23), 2827–2835.

Hayward, P. A., Hare, D. L., Gordon, I., Matalanis, G., & Buxton, B. F. (2007). Which arterial conduit? Radial artery versus free right internal thoracic artery: Six year clinical results of a randomized controlled trial. *Annals of Thoracic Surgery, 84*(2), 493–497.

Ho, K. M., & Tan, J. A. (2011). Benefits and risks of maintaining normothermia during cardiopulmonary bypass in adult cardiac surgery: A systematic review. *Cardiovascular Therapeutics, 29*(4), 260–279.

Hu, X., & Zhao, Q. (2011). Systematic comparison of the effectiveness of radial artery and saphenous vein or right internal thoracic artery coronary bypass grafts in non-left anterior descending coronary arteries. *Journal of Zhejiang University SCIENCE, 12*(4), 273–279.

Kashyap, V. S., Bishop, P. D., Bena, J. F., Rosa, K., Sarac, T. P., & Ouriel, K. (2010). A pilot, prospective evaluation of a direct thrombin inhibitor, bivalirudin (Angiomax), in patients undergoing lower extremity bypass. *Journal of Vascular Surgery, 52*(2), 369–374.

Kim, J. B., Yun, S. C., Lim, J. W., Hwang, S. K., Jung, S. H., Song, H., . . . Choo, S. J. (2014). Long-term survival following coronary artery bypass grafting off-pump versus on-pump strategies. *Journal of the American College of Cardiology, 63*(21), 2280–2288.

Kolli, A., Au, J. T., Lee, D. C., Klinoff, N., & Ko, W. (2010). Compartment syndrome after endoscopic harvest of the great saphenous vein during coronary artery bypass grafting. *Annals of Thoracic Surgery, 89*(1), 271–273.

Kurfirst, V., Candayoua, J., & Mokracek, A. (2012). Endoscopic versus bridging technique of saphenous vein graft harvesting-one year results. *Cor et Vasa, 54*, e93–e96.

Lee, C.-H., Cheng, H.-C., & Ko, L. W. (2013). Successful treatment of anaphylactic shock after protamine administration. Report of a case. *Emergency Medicine, 3*. doi:10.4172/2165- 7548.1000157

Levy, J. H., & Adkinson, N. F. (2008). Anaphylaxis during cardiac surgery: Implications for clinicians. *Anesthesia & Analgesia, 106*, 392–403.

Lutjen, D. L., & Arndt, K. L. (2012). Methylene blue to treat vasoplegia due to a severe protamine reaction: A case report. *AANA Journal, 80*(3), 170–173.

Martin, C. G., & Turkelson, S. L. (2006). Nursing care of the patient undergoing coronary artery bypass grafting. *Journal of Cardiovascular Nursing, 21*(2), 109–117.

Navarro-Garcia, M. A., Marin-Fernandez, B., de Carlos-Alegre, V., Martinez-Oroz, A., Martorell-Gurucham, A., & Ordoñez-Ortigosa, E. (2011). Preoperative mood disorders in patients undergoing cardiac surgery: Risk factors and postoperative morbidity in the intensive care unit. *Revista Española de Cardiologia, 64*, 1005–1010.

Nikolaidis, N., Velissaris, T., & Ohr, S. K. (2007). Bivalirudin anticoagulation for cardiopulmonary bypass: An unusual case. *Texas Heart Institute Journal, 34*(1), 115–118.

Nybo, M., & Madsen, J. S. (2008). Serious anaphylactic reactions due to protamine sulfate: A systematic literature review. *Basic & Clinical Pharmacology & Toxicology, 103*(2), 192–196.

Puskas, J. D., Kilgo, D. D., Kutner, M., Pusca, S. V., Lattouf, O., & Guyton, R. (2007). Off-pump techniques disproportionately benefit women and narrow the gender disparity in outcomes after coronary artery bypass surgery. *Circulation, 116*(Suppl. I), I192–I199.

Puskas, J. D., Thourani, V. H., Kilgo, P., Cooper, W., Vassiliades, T., Vega, J. D., . . . Lattouf, O. M. (2009). Off-pump coronary artery bypass disproportionately benefits high-risk patients. *Annals of Thoracic Surgery, 88,* 1142–1147.

Puskas, J. D., Williams, W. H., O'Donnell, R., Patterson, R. E., Sigman, S. R., Smith, A. S., . . . Guyton, R. A. (2011). Off-pump and on-pump coronary artery bypass grafting are associated with similar graft patency, myocardial ischemia, and freedom from reintervention: Long-term follow-up of a randomized trial. *Annals of Thoracic Surgery, 91,* 1836–1843.

Sajja, L. R. (2008). Assessment of ulnar collateral circulation by the Allen test in patients undergoing radial artery harvest. *European Journal of Cardio-Thoracic Surgery, 33*(4), 755–756.

Sedrakyan, A., Wu, A. W., Parashar, A., Bass, E. B., & Treasure, T. (2006). Off-pump surgery is associated with reduced occurrence of stroke and other morbidity as compared with traditional coronary artery bypass grafting: A meta-analysis for systematically reviewed trials. *Stroke, 37*(11), 2759–2769.

Shah, S. A., Chark, D., Williams, J., Hessheimer, A., Huh, J., Wu, Y., . . . Drinkwater, D. C. (2007). Retrospective analysis of local sensorimotor deficits after radial artery harvesting for coronary artery bypass grafting. *Journal of Surgical Research, 139*(2), 203–208.

Shekar, P. S. (2006). Cardiology patient page: On-pump and off-pump coronary artery bypass grafting. *Circulation, 113*(4), e51–e52.

Shroyer, A. L., Grover, F. L., Hattler, B., Collins, J. F., McDonald, G. O., Kozora, E., . . . Novitzky, D. (2009). On-pump versus off-pump coronary-artery bypass surgery. *New England Journal of Medicine, 361,* 1827–1837.

Stafford-Smith, M., Lefrak, E. A., Qazi, A. G., Welsby, I. J., Barber, L., Hoeft, A., . . . Newman, M. F. (2005). Efficacy and safety of heparinase I versus protamine in patients undergoing coronary artery bypass grafting with and without cardiopulmonary bypass. *Anesthesiology, 103*(2), 229–240.

St. Andre, A. C., & DelRossi, A. (2005). Hemodynamic management of patients in the first 24 hours after cardiac surgery. *Critical Care Medicine, 33*(9), 2082–2093.

Taboulis, N. (2013). Total arterial coronary revascularization—patient selection, stenosis, conduits, targets. *Annals of Cardiothoracic Surgery, 2*(4). Retrieved from http://www.annalscts.com/article/view/2414/3280

Tully, P. J., Baker, R. A., Turnbull, D., & Winefield, H. (2008). The role of depression and anxiety in hospital readmissions after cardiac surgery. *Journal of Behavioral Medicine, 31*(4), 281–290.

Vallely, M. P., Edelman, J. B., & Wilson, M. K. (2013). Bilateral internal mammary arteries: Evidence and technical considerations. *Annals of Cardiothoracic Surgery, 2*(4). Retrieved from http://www.annalscts.com/article/view/2423/3289

Verma, S., Fedak, P. W., Weisel, R. D., Szmitko, P. E., Badiwala, M. V., & Bonneau, D. (2004). Off-pump coronary artery bypass surgery: Fundamentals for the clinical cardiologist. *Circulation, 109*(10), 1206–1211.

Viars, J. (2009). Anxiety and open heart surgery. *MEDSURG Nursing, 18*(5), 283.

Voucharas, C., Bisbos, A., Moustakidis, P., & Tsilimingas N. (2010). Open versus tunneling radial artery harvest for coronary artery grafting. *Journal of Cardiac Surgery, 25,* 504–507.

Warang, M., Waradkar, A., Patwardhan, A., Agrawal, N., Kane, D., Parulkar, G., & Kandeparkar, J. (2007). Metabolic changes and clinical outcomes in patients undergoing on and off pump coronary artery bypass surgery. *Indian Journal of Thoracic and Cardiovascular Surgery, 23*(1), 9–15.

Welsby, U., Newman, M. F., Phillips-Bute, B., Messier, R. H., Kakkis, E. M., & Stafford-Smith, M. (2005). Hemodynamic changes after protamine administration: Association with mortality after coronary artery bypass surgery. *Anesthesiology, 102*(2), 308–314.

Yetkin, U., Yürekli, I., & Gürbüz, A. (2009). Revision for postoperative bleeding: Timing and decision making. *Internet Journal of Thoracic and Cardiovascular Surgery*, *13*(1). Retrieved from http://ispub.com/IJTCVS/13/1/8856

WEB RESOURCES

Off-Pump Videos: http://www.cts.usc.edu/videos-mpeg-offpumpcoronaryarterybypassgrafting.html

Heart Online: Off-pump coronary artery bypass (OPCAB) Animation Video: http://www.yourpracticeonline.com.au/opcab-surgery-3dvideo.html

CABG 3D video: http://www.yourpracticeonline.com.au/cabg-surgery-3dvideo.html

Chapter 7

Minimally Invasive Cardiac Surgery

Tamara S. Goda, Brianna Gee, and Becky Dean

INTRODUCTION

After almost a decade of laparoscopic procedures being performed, cardiac surgeons began to accept the concept of minimally invasive cardiac surgery (MICS) in the mid-1990s (Mack, 2006). While no official definition of MICS has been established, it is often defined as cardiac surgery without the use of cardiopulmonary bypass (CPB), without a median sternotomy, or both. Since the late 1990s, MICS has become much more popular. Like other surgical specialties, advances in minimally invasive procedures have been largely driven by the desire to reduce pain and surgical healing time. However, in cardiac surgical operations, the desire to minimize or avoid the use of CPB and all of the potential complications associated with it has been a primary endpoint. In addition, reducing the potential for both respiratory dysfunction and the morbidity associated with deep sternal wound infection (SWI) prompted the use of alternative surgical incisions in order to avoid the use of a median sternotomy (Iribarne et al., 2011). Improvements in MICS have progressed to such a degree that it has become common to perform coronary artery bypass grafting (CABG) without the use of CPB. However, since the early 2000s, perhaps the greatest advances in MICS have been appreciated in the area of valve repair/replacement surgery. This chapter describes a variety of MICS procedures for coronary revascularization, valve repair/replacement, and atrial fibrillation (AF) surgery. In addition, the relatively new procedure for percutaneous valve repair/replacement is discussed.

MINIMALLY INVASIVE CORONARY REVASCULARIZATION

Since 1967, traditional CABG surgery has entailed creating a median sternotomy incision, creating cardiac standstill with a cardioplegia solution, and being connected to a bypass machine to maintain oxygenation and perfusion during cardiac standstill (Ley, 2006). Cardiopulmonary bypass refers to the temporary rerouting of blood from the right atrium to the aorta via an oxygenator (bypass machine), such that blood flow is circumvented around the heart and lungs during the surgical procedure. During a CABG, a bypass conduit is harvested, and new avenues for oxygenated blood are created from the aorta to the targeted blood vessel, "bypassing" the diseased segment of coronary artery.

Traditional CABG surgery is associated with a prolonged ventilation time (initially days; now 8–12 hours), prolonged intensive care unit (ICU) stay (initially 1 week; now 24 hours if the case is uncomplicated), prolonged hospitalization (initially several weeks; now 1 week), a prolonged rehabilitation phase (now 8–12 weeks), and potential SWI. Other complications associated with traditional CABG and their associated etiologies are listed in **Table 7-1**. These and other complications associated with CABG provided the impetus to develop procedures to perform CABG in a less invasive way.

Several different MICS procedures for coronary revascularization have been developed, each of which has its own patient selection criteria. Two approaches that can be used for these procedures are: (1) anterior mini-thoracotomy incisions or (2) an endoscopic approach. The major types of

Table 7-1 Pathophysiologic Changes Associated with a Traditional CABG Procedure and CPB	
Pathophysiologic Change	**Etiology**
Bleeding and thrombotic complications: disseminated intravascular coagulation, heparin-induced thrombocytopenia, and thrombosis	• Activation of platelets and plasma proteins • Patients are heparinized and given supplementary doses during bypass, titrated against clotting studies • Bleeding times after full reversal of heparin do not become normalized for as long as 12 hours after bypass
Considerable interstitial fluid shifts	• Increased systemic venous pressure • Volume loading • Decreased plasma protein concentration (secondary to dilution and absorption onto the bypass circuit, and the inflammatory response increasing capillary permeability)
Increased levels of cortisol, epinephrine, and norepinephrine (remain elevated for at least 24 hours)	• Stress of surgery • Hypothermia • Cardiopulmonary bypass • Nonpulsatile flow
Hyperglycemia	• Stress of surgery • Hypothermia • Cardiopulmonary bypass • Nonpulsatile flow
Decreased circulating triiodothyronine (T3)	• Stress of surgery • Hypothermia • Cardiopulmonary bypass • Nonpulsatile flow
Decreased myocardial compliance and contractility	• Myocardial stunning • Ischemia • Edema
Decreased myocardial function related to cardioplegia and surgical arrest (for 6 to 8 hours postoperatively)	• Ischemia-reperfusion injury
Progressive need for volume resuscitation	• Vasodilation • Capillary leak

Table 7-1 Pathophysiologic Changes Associated with a Traditional CABG Procedure and CPB (*Continued*)	
Pulmonary edema	• Activation of complement system • Sequestration of neutrophils in pulmonary vasculature (can mediate increase in capillary permeability, which is compounded by fluid shifts)
Pulmonary dysfunction	• Cardiopulmonary bypass decreases the effect of surfactant • General anesthesia • Median sternotomy • Cardiopulmonary bypass increases shunts, decreases compliance and functional residual volume, and can cause acute lung injury
Ischemic stroke	• Emboli released during the cannulation and clamping of the aorta
Hemorrhagic stroke	• Anticoagulation necessary for bypass
Impaired renal function	• Hemodilution • Microemboli • Catecholamines • Low perfusion pressure • Diuretics • Hypothermia • Hemolysis
Peptic ulceration	• Stress response
Endotoxin translocation, adding to the inflammatory response	• Greater permeability of gut mucosa

Sources: Data from Chikwe, J., Donaldson, J., & Wood, A. J. (2006). Minimally invasive cardiac surgery. *British Journal of Cardiology, 13*(2), 123–128; and Ley, S. J. (2006). Postoperative management of the cardiac surgery patient. In H. M. Schell & K. A. Puntillo (Eds.), *Critical care nursing secrets* (2nd ed., pp. 113–121). St. Louis, MO: Mosby.

MICS procedures that are currently performed include off-pump coronary artery bypass (OPCAB), minimally invasive direct coronary artery bypass (MIDCAB), or totally endoscopic or robot-assisted coronary artery bypass (TECAB). Both MIDCAB and TECAB can be performed with or without the use of CPB support. A number of alternative names for these various MICS procedures appear in the literature.

Off-Pump Coronary Artery Bypass (OPCAB)

Coronary artery bypass grafting done without the use of CPB—"off pump"—is also referred to as beating heart surgery and is commonly and routinely utilized for full coronary revascularization. Either internal thoracic artery (ITA) or both, the saphenous vein, and radial arteries, harvested in typical fashion, can be utilized for this procedure. It is typically performed using the median sternotomy incision to gain full access for all vessels, including those on the back of the heart, for revascularization. Special equipment has been developed that allows the surgeon to position the heart to isolate the diseased vessel and stabilize the localized region of epicardium for anastomosis without cardioplegic arrest—while the heart is beating. The stabilizer (see Chapter 6) provides a direct view, dampens the movement of the epicardium, and permits a nontraumatic grip on the beating heart (Edgar, Ebersole, & Mayfield, 1999). In addition to specific surgeon skill, OPCAB surgery requires meticulous attention by cardiac anesthesia as heart rate and blood pressure are extremely labile with manipulation of the beating heart.

The International Society of Minimally Invasive Cardiac Surgery recently developed several recommendations regarding the use of OPCAB, noting OPCAB should be utilized as a means to reduce perioperative mortality, neurocognitive dysfunction, and hospital length of stay (LOS) (Iribarne et al., 2011). Additionally, patients particularly at high risk because of renal disease, cirrhosis of the liver, and calcific disease of the ascending aorta may benefit from avoidance of aortic cross-clamping and exposure to CPB (Iribarne et al., 2011). Additional information regarding OPCAB is covered in detail in Chapter 6.

Minimally Invasive Direct Coronary Artery Bypass (MIDCAB)

Minimally invasive direct coronary artery bypass, which is an alternative approach to traditional CABG, has been performed since 1996 (Chen-Scarabelli, 2002). In lieu of a median sternotomy, a left lateral thoracotomy incision is made; there are a variety of incision sizes and variations, but most typically a 5–6 cm incision is created along the fourth intercostal space. Rib spreaders are used to spread and elevate the rib cage to provide ample space to dissect the ITA. The left mini-thoracotomy approach provides direct visualization of the left anterior descending (LAD) artery and the anastomotic site when a left internal thoracic artery (LITA) to the LAD is being performed. Off-pump coronary artery bypass can be applied to a MIDCAB approach (Iribarne et al., 2011).

Minimally invasive direct coronary artery bypass surgery is now utilized for full multivessel revascularization; however, patient

selection criteria—body habitus, presence of comorbidities, location and size of the diseased vessels—and surgeon expertise play into the equation when MIDCAB is being considered as a surgical option. Differences between MIDCAB and traditional CABG are primarily related to the incision size and associated surgical trauma. During this procedure, the patient is intubated with a double-lumen endotracheal tube, thereby allowing for ventilation of the right lung and deflation of the left lung, providing more room to manipulate the heart. In addition to the incision size being much smaller, a left lateral incision 4 to 6 inches in length is made between the ribs, thereby avoiding a full sternotomy. Importantly, because MIDCAB is typically a beating heart procedure, no cardioplegia or CPB are utilized, thereby avoiding the issues related to the pump and myocardial arrest. Documented advantages of MIDCAB include decreased pain secondary to a less invasive surgical approach, earlier mobilization secondary to decreased pain, shorter ICU and hospital LOS, decreased infection rates, especially with SWIs, earlier return to baseline physical activities, and reduced transfusion requirements (Iribarne et al., 2011). In addition and most importantly, preliminary data on the long-term patency of MIDCAB grafts show that it appears to be comparable to traditional CABG (Iribarne et al., 2011).

Table 7-2 lists additional advantages and disadvantages of the MIDCAB approach.

Robotic-Assisted or Totally Endoscopic Coronary Artery Bypass Grafting (TECAB)

There has been a growing body of research around the use of robotics in coronary artery revascularization surgery since the introduction of surgical robotics in the 1990s (Iribarne et al., 2011). Minimally invasive equipment had reached its limits; laparoscopic instruments were rigid and were only able to move

Table 7-2 Advantages and Disadvantages of the MIDCAB Approach	
Advantages	**Disadvantages**
Faster recovery/return to routine ADLs	Limited access and exposure to the operative area
Long-term graft patency appears to be similar to that of traditional CABG	Technical difficulty with beating heart
No risk of SWI	Steep learning curve; need experienced surgeon to perform
LITA/RITA more resistant to atherosclerosis/ increased longevity of patency	Increased risk of incomplete revascularization
No adverse effects related to CPB	Unable to access/visualize posterior heart for revascularization
Cosmetic results; no sternotomy	MIDCAB limits target vessels
Shorter hospital stay	Acute graft occlusion and incomplete revascularization risk increased
Decreased blood loss and transfusion requirements	Thoracotomy incision can be painful
No aortic manipulation	Decreased exposure to coronary vasculature
Capable of revascularization of multiple-vessel lesions	Less choice of vessels that can be grafted (usually only the internal thoracic artery to the LAD)
Decreased risk of musculoskeletal injury	More trauma to costal cartilage
Can be used for primary or redo procedures	
No risk of SIRS, coagulopathies, thromboembolic events, endothelial dysfunction, dysrhythmias, or MODS associated with CPB	
No risk of aortic dissection or neurologic consequences associated with aortic cross-clamping	
Decreased risk of stroke	
Decreased OR time	
Decreased incidence of AF	
Decreased need for transfusions	

ADLs, activities of daily living; AF, atrial fibrillation; CABG, coronary artery bypass grafting; CPB, cardiopulmonary bypass; LAD, left anterior descending; LITA, left internal thoracic artery; MIDCAB, minimally invasive direct coronary artery bypass; MODS, multiple organ dysfunction syndrome; OR, operating room; RITA, right internal thoracic artery; SIRS, systemic inflammatory response syndrome; SWI, sternal wound infection.

Sources: Data from Bojar, R. (2011). *Manual of perioperative care in adult cardiac surgery* (5th ed.). Hoboken, NJ: Wiley-Blackwell; Bojar, R. M., & Warner, K. G. (1999). Cardiovascular management. In R. M. Bojar & K. G. Warner. *Manual of perioperative care in cardiac surgery* (3rd ed., pp. 213–334). Malden, MA: Blackwell; Borger, M. A., & Rao, V. (2002). Temperature management during cardiopulmonary bypass: Effect of rewarming rate on cognitive dysfunction. *Seminars in Cardiothoracic and Vascular Anesthesia*, 6(1), 17–20; Caimmi, P., Fossaceca, R., Lanfranchi, M., Kapetanakis, E. I., Verde, A., Panella, A., . . . Micalizzi, (2004). Cardiac angio-CT scan for planning MIDCAB. *Heart Surgery Forum*, 7(2), E113–E116; Calafiore, A., Teodori, G., Di Giammarco, G., Vittola, G., Iaco, A., Iovino, T., . . . Gallina, S. (1997). Minimally invasive coronary bypass grafting on a beating heart. *Annals of Thoracic Surgery*, 63(Suppl 6), 572–575; Chen-Scarabelli, C. (2002). Beating-heart coronary artery bypass graft surgery: Indication, advantages, and limitation. *Critical Care Nurse*, 22(5), 44–58; Iribarne, A., Easterwood, R., Chan, E., Yang, J., Soni, L., Russo, M., . . . Argenziano, M. (2011). The golden age of minimally invasive cardiothoracic surgery: Current and future perspectives. *Future Cardiology*, 7(3), 333–346; and Pike, R. D. B. (2015). Off pump coronary artery bypass and minimally invasive direct coronary artery bypass. In M. J. Murray, R. A. Harrison, J. T. Mueller, S. H. Rose, C. T. Wass, & D. J. Wedel (Eds.), *Faust's anesthesiology review* (4th ed., pp. 341–342). Philadelphia, PA: Elsevier Saunders.

along two axes—up and down, clockwise and counterclockwise. The need for a more manipulative surgical intervention was realized with the introduction of the ROBODOC® (Integrated Surgical Systems) and the more developed da Vinci® Surgical System (see **Figure 7-1**) and Computer Motion AESOP and ZEUS systems (Intuitive Surgical).

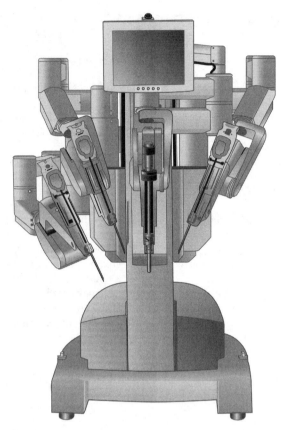

Figure 7-1 da Vinci® Surgical System.
Source: Courtesy of Intuitive Surgical Inc.

The first robotic-assisted CABG was performed in 1998 using the da Vinci surgical robot. The da Vinci surgical system allows the surgeon to access the heart through four half-inch incisions made in the intercostal spaces; these incisions are used to introduce instruments and a videoscope. The surgical robot consists of a collection of wristed tools called manipulators. The manipulators receive digital instructions from an interfaced computer. The (real-life) surgeon stays seated at a computer console with a three-dimensional display and acts as the "driver" of the computer. The surgeon initiates the digital instructions by controlling the hand grips. By using the hand grips, the surgeon's hand movements at the console are then duplicated by the robot,

with software filtering out physiologic hand tremors.

Currently, the term TECAB is primarily used when the LITA is harvested and used to graft a diseased LAD graft. Through a series of instrument exchanges, the LITA can be harvested, the pericardium opened, the LAD identified and stabilized, and the LITA to LAD anastomosis performed (Iribarne et al., 2011). There are, however, reports describing multi-vessel revascularizations where the surgeon performs a robotic-assisted takedown of the LITA followed by a MIDCAB—done either off pump or through cannulation of the femoral artery and vein for institution of CPB (Iribarne et al., 2011). Despite successful reports of TECAB, this operation has not become widely accepted mainly because of the increased time and personnel requirements of the surgical robot and a traditional approach is easier when multiple grafts are needed.

HYBRID CORONARY REVASCULARIZATION

Hybrid coronary revascularization is a new approach to treating multi-vessel coronary artery disease (CAD). It utilizes a minimally invasive LITA to LAD bypass graft. The other diseased vessels are then treated with percutaneous coronary intervention (PCI). This provides patients with the survival benefits of the LITA graft, which has a proven patency rate of 10-15 years or more (Iribarne et al., 2011). Currently, hybrid revascularization has been reserved for those patients that are too high risk for more traditional procedures because of the high rate of re-intervention that is required following PCI. However, as drug-eluting stent technology evolves and the need for re-intervention becomes less, hybrid revascularization may quickly become a viable option for many patients with multi-vessel CAD who desire a less invasive procedure (Iribarne et al., 2011).

Endoscopic technology has also been applied to the procedure used to harvest the greater saphenous vein. Instead of a long incision spanning the thigh to the lower leg, the vein can be dissected out using the endoscope and various instruments that may also cut or burn branches of the vein while it is still in the leg. This technology has also been adopted and applied to assist with removal of the radial artery from the forearm (Navia et al., 2013). Utilization of additional arterial conduits—bilateral ITAs and the radial arteries—has been recommended to improve long-term graft patency and outcomes (Bojar, 2011). An Allen test must be performed prior to radial artery removal to guarantee adequate collateral circulation in the extremity. (The Allen test is described in Chapter 6.)

Endoscopic procedures for both saphenous vein and radial artery harvest are performed through much smaller incisions, thereby reducing surgical trauma, pain, and recovery time. However, endoscopic conduit harvest, as with any minimally invasive procedure, carries with it a steep learning curve. Highly skilled operators and a standardized harvesting technique are necessary to maintain quality of the conduit and to avoid neurologic or infectious complications (Navia et al., 2013).

MINIMALLY INVASIVE VALVE SURGERY

Perhaps the greatest advances in MICS have been realized in the area of valve repair and replacement procedures. With the advent of new surgical instrumentation, including robotics, MICS has become widely accepted for certain surgical conditions, specifically valve repair/replacement (mitral, aortic, or tricuspid), pulmonary vein isolation and the Maze procedure to treat AF, congenital cardiac defects (e.g., atrial septal defects), and descending thoracic aortic aneurysm disease treatment (Mack, 2006). Unlike coronary revascularization, aortic and mitral valve surgeries always require CPB and cardioplegia; however, various alternate approaches have allowed for these procedures to be performed minimally invasively.

Minimally Invasive Mitral Valve Surgery (MIMVS)

The first MIMVS was performed in the mid 1990s through a parasternal incision. Since then, various pioneers—including Drs. Cosgrove, Carpentier, and Chitwood—developed and refined procedures that allowed for port access, video assistance and direction, transthoracic aortic cross-clamping, and retrograde cardioplegia. In 1998, the first minimally invasive mitral valve repair was performed using the da Vinci surgical system

(Iribarne et al., 2011). Currently, many institutions are performing MIMVS. Although robotic-assisted mitral valve surgery is being performed at various centers of excellence throughout the country, it has been limited by the rigorous training of the surgeon and the financial backing of the institution in terms of the cost of a dedicated robotic surgical system.

Various incisions can be utilized for MIMVS, but the most common approach is a right anterior mini-thoracotomy incision. This approach allows the surgeon to gain access to the mitral valve through the left atrium. The valve can either be repaired or replaced. During a repair, the valve leaflets are brought back together and the annulus reinforced with a ring to prevent further dilatation. During a replacement, the native valve is removed and fully replaced with either a bioprosthetic or mechanical implant.

The second most common approach is the robotic-assisted MIMVS. A small right anterolateral incision combined with two or three 1.5–2-cm robotic access port incisions make for "improved surgical cosmesis and patient satisfaction" (Mandal, Alwair, Nifong, & Chitwood, 2013). During robotic-assisted procedures, the surgeon sits at the control and looks through two lenses (like a microscope) that display the image from the camera. The computer generates a three-dimensional image of the surgical site. As the surgeon moves, the robotic arms mimic his multidirectional movements that may be even more precise than the surgeon's natural hand movement (Chitwood, 2011). Various instruments are utilized and exchanged through the access ports to allow the surgeon to repair or replace the valve. Additionally, specially designed titanium clips (The Cor-Knot™) are used to secure the valve sutures rather than tying knots (Mandal et al., 2013).

Various access techniques have been developed for cannulation and the institution of CPB to assist with MIMVS.

Typical cannulation for MIMVS involves cannulation of the femoral vasculature. However, central cannulation using the superior/inferior vena cava and the aorta can also be utilized in MIMVS to avoid the potential complications associated with lower extremity cannulation (Iribarne, 2011). Improvements in both CPB equipment and technique now allow for percutaneous cannulation of the lower extremities, making femoral cannulation less risky.

Regardless of the approach, the primary benefit of MIMVS is the avoidance of a median sternotomy. Decreased hospital LOS and reduced pain and potential for complications, combined with increased patient satisfaction and earlier return to full activity, have propelled MIMVS to popularity. Recent data suggest that robotic-assisted MIMVS is quickly becoming the "gold standard" with outcomes, morbidity, and mortality that appear to be equivalent to traditional valve surgery (Mandal et al., 2013). The various incisions utilized for mitral valve surgery are shown in **Figure 7-2**.

Endoscopic procedures have another benefit: They assist in making reentry into the sternum safer. Using this approach, the surgeon can readily visualize structures behind the sternum. Adhesions can form between the heart and the sternum, which can cause damage to the heart if reentry is required. Now the adhesions can be cut with the assistance of the scope prior to a second sternotomy, thereby reducing the risk of damaging the heart.

Table 7-3 outlines procedures that can be performed with robotic assistance.

Minimally Invasive Aortic Valve Replacement

The first minimally invasive aortic valve replacement (MIAVR) was described in 1996. Since that time, there has been significant evolution and acceptance of this procedure (Iribarne et al., 2011). The most commonly

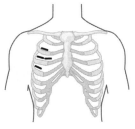
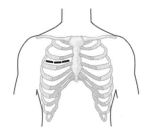
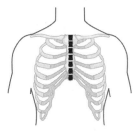

Robotic-Assisted
Heart Surgery
(Closed Surgery)

Less than 2 inch incision and
four (4) robotic ports

Right Thoracotomy

3–4 inch incision on side of chest

Median Sternotomy
(Open Surgery)

6–8 inch incision in
middle of chest

Figure 7-2   Mitral valve repair surgical comparison.

seen incision for MIAVR is a mini- or hemi-sternotomy; a right anterior thoracotomy can also be utilized. Both of these approaches allow the surgeon to gain access while maintaining the stability of the ribcage. In addition to the smaller incision, several cannulation methods for institution of CPB have also been described for MIAVR; femoral cannulation or a combination of femoral/atrial or atrial/axillary is commonly used (Iribarne et al., 2011). Morbidity and mortality outcomes of MIAVR and traditional AVR have been compared and have been found to be comparable; this includes transfusion rates and hospital LOS; however, post-discharge pain medication use has been lower for MIAVR (Iribarne et al., 2011).

Table 7-3   Robotic Surgery Procedures
• Single- and multiple-vessel CABG • Mitral valve repair and replacement • Aortic valve repair and replacement • ASD repair • VSD repair • Removal of cardiac tumors • Ablation for treatment of atrial fibrillation (Maze procedure)
ASD, atrial septal defect; CABG, coronary artery bypass grafting; VSD, ventricular septal defect.

Transcatheter Aortic Valve Replacement (TAVR)

One of the most recent breakthroughs in MICS is that of transcatheter aortic valve replacement (TAVR). The first TAVR performed on an adult occurred in Europe in early 2002 by the French interventional cardiologist, Alain G. Cribier (Hu, 2012). The driving force behind this innovation was the need to provide a suitable and effective alternative to surgical aortic valve replacement (SAVR) in select patients with severe aortic stenosis for whom a surgical intervention was deemed to be too high risk. Since then, minimally invasive valve replacement methods have rapidly evolved. Transcatheter aortic valve replacements have been performed in the United States since 2007 as part of clinical trials, most notably the PARTNER (Placement of AoRTic TraNscathetER) trial utilizing the Edwards Lifesciences SAPIEN bioprosthetic stent heart valve (see **Figure 7-3**) that received U.S. Food and Drug Administration approval for commercial use in nonsurgical candidates in 2011, and later in 2012 for high-risk surgical candidates (Hu, 2012; Tang et al., 2013; Thourani et al., 2013). Today, new-generation transcatheter heart valves (THVs), such as the Edwards Lifesciences SAPIEN XT and Medtronic CoreValve, are available to both high-risk nonsurgical and

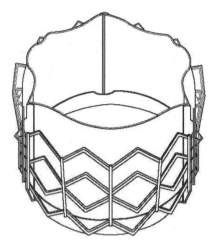

Figure 7-3   The SAPIEN transcatheter heart valve.

Source: Illustrated by James R. Perron.

surgical candidates alike. These minimalist procedures, especially transfemoral TAVRs, are quickly becoming the "standard of care" among the high-risk surgical population (Webb & Wood, 2012).

Access routes for TAVRs include transfemoral (TF), transapical (TA), transaortic, transaxillary or trans-subclavian, and transcarotid (Tang et al., 2013; Thourani et al., 2013). Determination of the best access route is made based on a multitude of factors including vessel size and integrity, previous sternotomies, comorbid conditions, and ejection fraction (Feldman, Sanborn, & O'Neill, 2005; Thourani et al., 2013). The TF route has become the most common and preferred access site for TAVR. Transfemoral TAVR is contraindicated in patients who have small vessel diameter and highly calcified or tortuous vessels (Masson et al., 2009; Thourani et al., 2013). In these cases, alternative entry sites are chosen.

Transcatheter aortic valve replacements can be performed either totally percutaneously or via a small right anterior thoracotomy incision. In the TF approach, a delivery catheter is threaded up the femoral artery via an introducer sheath and reaches the aortic valve in a retrograde fashion by way of the descending and ascending aorta. Sheath sizes vary from 16- to 19-French delivery systems for newer generation THVs. The THV is guided into position under echocardiography and fluoroscopy, and, once in place, the new valve is deployed against the orifice of the native valve. A transvenous pacer lead wire is placed in the right ventricle via the right femoral vein (Cheung & Lichtenstein, 2012). A 6- or 7-French venous sheath is typically used for this purpose. Pacing may be required should conduction problems occur during the procedure. Also, depending on the type of valve being placed (SAPIEN versus CoreValve), deployment of the valve is done during rapid ventricular pacing. Rapid ventricular pacing reduces forward blood flow and pulse pressure, and provides for optimal stability of the valve during expansion and deployment (Thourani et al., 2013).

The transapical approach requires a mini-thoracotomy. The aortic valve is accessed through the apex of the left ventricle (Thourani et al., 2013; Webb & Wood, 2012). The transaortic access is achieved with either a mini-sternotomy or mini-thoracotomy (Tang et al., 2013; Webb & Wood, 2012), and the aortic valve is reached through the ascending aorta (Thourani et al., 2013; Webb & Wood, 2012). Axillary or subclavian TAVRs also provide for a shorter and more direct pathway to the aortic valve; however, a surgical cutdown may be required to access the vessel (Webb & Wood, 2012). Other access sites, such as with transcarotid, are being evaluated as possible options for select patients who are not candidates for any of the other TAVR methods (Guyton, Block, Thourani, Lerakis, & Babaliaros, 2013).

The traditional SAVR remains the standard of care for patients with severe aortic stenosis if they are good surgical candidates. However, because aortic stenosis is a disease that occurs more frequently in the aging population, a large number of these patients are inoperable due not only to advanced age but also frailty and other comorbid conditions. Patients with severe aortic stenosis are evaluated using specific criteria: an aortic valve area of less than 1.0 cm^2 and either a mean gradient greater than 40 mmHg or a jet velocity of greater than 4 meters/sec (Nishimura et al., 2014). All patients being evaluated for TAVR must be seen by two cardiac surgeons, both agreeing that TAVR is a better option than SAVR (Smith et al., 2011).

Transcatheter aortic valve replacement centers nationwide perform these procedures in a hybrid operating room (OR) or specially outfitted catheterization lab where CPB is readily available if and when it is needed (Guyton et al., 2013). However, a few TAVR centers in the United States are performing TF TAVRs in the catheterization lab using moderate sedation. In all procedural areas, TAVRs are performed in collaboration with a dedicated heart valve/structural heart team that includes, but is not limited to, cardiac surgeons, interventional cardiologists, heart valve coordinators, echocardiographers, and a multitude of other highly specialized staff members (Mack et al., 2013). These practitioners help with everything from the

initial evaluation to post-procedure care. Most TAVR centers also have a valve clinic dedicated to the evaluation and workup of these patients. Once a patient is determined to be a potential candidate for TAVR, multiple pre-op studies are obtained prior to the procedure in order to rule out contraindications to the procedure, accurately size the aortic annulus, and evaluate access vessels to determine the approach for the procedure (Mack et al., 2013). Frailty parameters are also obtained as is a 5-meter walk test and a quality of life questionnaire (most commonly used is the Kansas City Cardiomyopathy Questionnaire).

The TAVR procedure is done most commonly using either the TF or TA approach. It can also be deployed directly via the transaortic approach (see **Figure 7-4**). Traditionally the procedure is done under general anesthesia with CPB standby should the patient need that level of support during the procedure. Recent data reveal that clinical benefits of transcatheter replacement included significantly shorter stays in the ICU and hospital (Mack et al., 2013; Smith et al., 2011). Currently, transcatheter valves are approved only for use in the aortic position. In certain populations, these valves are being inserted

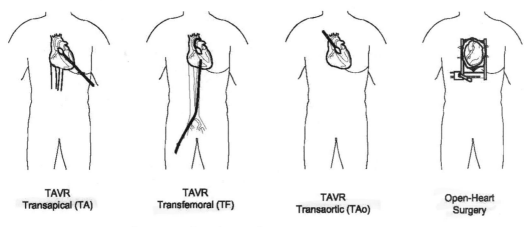

TAVR
Transapical (TA)   TAVR
Transfemoral (TF)   TAVR
Transaortic (TAo)   Open-Heart
Surgery

Figure 7-4   Transcatheter aortic valve replacement.

Source: Illustrated by James R. Perron.

under investigation in the mitral position. Long-term follow up on these valves and the efficacy of their use in the intermediate-risk population is ongoing (Mack et al., 2013).

Post-Procedure Nursing Care

Post-procedure nursing care varies depending on the access route of the intervention. Patients receiving general anesthesia, experiencing significant intraoperative complications, or both are recovered in the postanesthesia care unit and then transferred to a coronary care unit or ICU.

Barring any post-procedure complications, the patient is stepped down from the ICU on postoperative day (POD) 2 to an intermediate-care telemetry nursing floor before being discharged to home on POD 3. Length of stay varies among TAVR centers and ranges from 3 to 8 days.

Post-Procedure Complications

Transcatheter aortic valve replacement complications of particular concern to nursing staff during the post-procedure period are presented in the following subsection and include stroke, arrhythmias, and bleeding. Discussion of vascular complications is more extensively presented in the General Nursing Care section following this section.

STROKE

Stroke in post-TAVR patients is commonly related to athero, calcific, device or air emboli (Hu, 2012; Masson et al., 2009; Webb & Wood, 2012) and may be more common depending on the access method used. Thus, post-TAVR nursing care involves conducting frequent neurologic checks, recognizing signs and symptoms of stroke, and initiating and escalating treatment in the event of a stroke diagnosis.

ARRHYTHMIAS

New-onset AF and heart block are two of the most common arrhythmias seen in post-TAVR patients. Heart block can occur as a result of the atrioventricular conduction system and intermodal branches being inadvertently manipulated and compressed during balloon valvuloplasty and subsequent valve implantation (Masson et al., 2009; Webb & Wood, 2012). Valve type and shape, such as the CoreValve, also affect the development of heart block. Valves extending further into the ventricle (Masson et al., 2009; Tang et al., 2013; Webb & Wood, 2012) are associated with higher occurrence of heart block. Temporary or permanent pacemaker placement may be required in these patients.

New-onset AF is a common post-TAVR complication. This significantly increases the risk of cardioembolic stroke (Tang et al., 2013). In some cases, AF may spontaneously resolve. For persistent cases, treatment goals include rate and rhythm control with antiarrhythmic medication or synchronized cardioversion (Holmes et al., 2012).

Other arrhythmias that develop are bradycardia and junctional rhythms. Temporary pacing may be required to stabilize the patient. With persistent bradyarrhythmias, permanent pacemaker placement may be required.

BLEEDING

Bleeding is a complication of any surgical intervention. Transcatheter aortic valve replacement patients are at high risk for post-procedure bleeding mostly related to vascular access with large-diameter catheters. Arterial sheaths are generally 24-French, and even though the arterial incision is closed via a vascular closure device, once the sheath is removed, oozing or failure of the closure site is not uncommon (Tang et al., 2013). Frequent assessment of the incision site is necessary to monitor for oozing, bleeding, and hematoma formation.

Retroperitoneal hemorrhage is a life-threatening complication related to vascular injury during the procedure, but may not present until after the sheath has been removed and the patient has been transferred to the unit or floor. A sudden drop in blood pressure and intractable back or flank pain are telltale signs of a retroperitoneal bleed. Fluid resuscitation should be started immediately, emergent computed tomography scan should be performed to confirm the bleed, and the patient should be transferred back to the OR or catheterization lab for surgical or percutaneous repair.

General Nursing Care

Post-procedural care varies among TAVR centers. In all cases, TAVR patients are cared for in specially designated units where the nursing staff is well trained and highly skilled in providing care for this patient population.

Post-TAVR care includes the following:

1) Patients who have had general anesthesia should be extubated either immediately in the procedure area or within a few hours after arriving to the ICU (Holmes et al., 2012). Many of these patients have a history of chronic obstructive pulmonary disease (COPD). Combined with immobility and pain, they are at high risk for developing respiratory complications. This can be avoided with good pulmonary toileting, including the regular use of an incentive spirometer, coughing, deep breathing, and frequent turning.

2) Pain management is important for patient comfort and safety. For TF TAVRs, a low-dose oral narcotic analgesic may suffice to achieve good pain control. With any TAVR necessitating a mini-thoracotomy or vascular cutdown, more aggressive pain management regimens with higher potency narcotics that are given more frequently are required to manage the incisional pain and pain related to chest tube placement, drainage, and removal (Holmes et al., 2012). Chest tubes are removed when drainage output is less than 150 mL in a 24-hour period, there is no air leak, and the patient is ambulatory.

3) Vital signs are monitored every 30 minutes for the first 2 hours post-procedure and then either hourly in the ICU or every 4 hours thereafter on the intermediate-care telemetry floor. In addition, all TAVR patients require 24-hour telemonitoring as arrhythmias frequently develop 24–48 hours post-procedure. Early recognition and appropriate treatment of any arrhythmias are part of the standard post-TAVR nursing care.

4) Optimal blood pressure control should be maintained and hypertensive and hypotensive states must be avoided. Significantly elevated systolic blood pressure can stress the new valve and increase the risk of bleeding (Holmes et al., 2012). Hypertension can be controlled with oral or intravenous (IV) antihypertensive medications as needed (Gaasch, Brecker, & Aldea, 2014). Hypotension can be related to decreased volume status, and intraoperative and postoperative bleeding, or any combination of these. Patients who are volume depleted generally respond well to IV fluid administration. If hypotension is related to bleeding, the source must be investigated and quickly remedied. In severe cases, blood transfusions may be necessary to stabilize the patient.

5) Indwelling urinary catheters are removed POD 1. Urine output and daily serum creatinine levels should be closely monitored for indications of renal stress or injury.

6) Surgical sites must be assessed for appropriate healing and possible infection. Dressings stay in place through POD 2 unless saturated with blood or drainage, or are otherwise soiled or not intact. On assessment, surgical incisions should be well approximated and free of unusual swelling, erythema, and purulent and malodorous discharge.

7) Transfemoral TAVRs will have at least two groin punctures (one arterial and

one venous) and in some cases three (one arterial and two venous). The large sheaths are pulled in the procedure area, but patients may arrive to the unit with a smaller venous sheath still in place. This smaller sheath is pulled by the nurse according to specific coagulation parameters. Patients must lie supine with both legs kept straight until the sheath is removed and hemostasis is achieved. Afterward, the patient remains on bed rest in the same position for at least 4 hours. Should complications arise in the groin site after sheath removal, such as bleeding or hematoma formation, bed rest may be extended. Groin sites must be assessed for oozing, bleeding, hematoma, and new bruit. In addition, pedal and tibial pulses must be monitored and confirmed either by palpation or Doppler. Absent pulses indicate blood flow problems and must be reported to the provider immediately.

8) Preoperative medications should be resumed as soon as the patient is hemodynamically stable, alert and responsive, and able to tolerate oral intake. Mechanical venous thromboembolism prophylaxis should be initiated within the first 24 hours post-TAVR. Any subcutaneously administered low-molecular-weight heparin is avoided within the first 48 hours after the procedure. Typically, dual antiplatelet therapy is initiated with aspirin and clopidogrel (Plavix®) prior to discharge if the patient is not already on anticoagulation therapy (Holmes et al., 2012; Hu, 2012).

9) Antibiotic prophylaxis is started preoperatively and should be continued postoperatively as ordered. Avoiding infection is paramount. Diligent monitoring for changes in temperature, relevant labs such as white blood cell and platelet counts, and signs and symptoms of inflammation are required after TAVR.

Focusing care on early mobility, toileting, and nutrition (Harris, Dean, Babaliaros, & Keegan, 2014) plays an important part in boosting an already compromised immune system and averting secondary infections from other nonsurgical sources.

10) On POD 2, the patient is typically stable enough to transfer to a step-down telemetry floor if not already there. Prior to transfer out of the ICU, central lines are removed and a peripheral IV is placed. The patient may be transferred to the floor with the chest tube in place if criteria for removing it have not been met, but the patient is otherwise stable. Continuous cardiac monitoring will continue until discharge. Once on the floor, the emphasis is on ambulation, toileting, and nutrition (Harris et al., 2014). Although patients are transitioned to a solid-food diet once the sheath is removed on POD 1, eating may be hampered by bed rest and other factors while in the ICU. Early ambulation is prognostic for uncomplicated recovery so patients are ambulated once bed rest is complete at the earliest or by POD 2 the latest. Lack of movement and food as well as narcotic pain medication can result in constipation. Conversely, early ambulation and eating help support elimination. Stool softeners or laxatives may be indicated if normal bowel function is not restored by POD 2.

Discharge

Patients are instructed to follow up with their heart valve/structural heart team provider at 30 days, 6 months, and 1 year post-TAVR and annually thereafter (Holmes et al., 2012). Dual antiplatelet therapy is initiated in the hospital and continued for up to 6 months following the procedure with aspirin continuing for life (Gaasch et al., 2014; Holmes et al., 2012; Hu, 2012). Otherwise, discharge instructions and patient education are center specific. In general, all TAVR patients should be educated on what problems to report and what precautions to take should problems arise; how to care for wounds and incisions; activity and exercise limitations, if any; self-care requirements; and any equipment, supplies, or safety aids that might be needed for home recovery.

Innovation in Nursing Practice

As centers nationwide continue to hone their processes, patients are benefiting from both the technological advancements with TAVR and patient-care innovations being made at these facilities. One TAVR center has shown that patients undergoing TF TAVR can be successfully and safely managed on an intermediate-care cardiac floor post-procedure. This is possible due to 1) careful patient selection pre-procedure, 2) the experience level of the center and structural heart team, 3) the procedural technique used and the use of moderate sedation for select TF cases, 4) optimal staffing ratios of the floor, and 5) the skill level of the nursing staff with "sheath management and femoral access patients" (Harris et al., 2014). Avoiding the ICU when possible and nursing care that focuses on early ambulation, good nutrition, effective toileting and bowel management, and family involvement have provided the model upon which standards of nursing care for TF TAVRs have been developed at TAVR centers. As such, this innovation in nursing practice has emerged by putting into place new clinical guidelines for post-procedure care of TAVR patients. By following these guidelines, nursing staff have contributed significantly to positive patient outcomes that include shortened recovery times and LOS (Harris et al., 2014). Lastly, the financial impact of recovering TF TAVR patients on the cardiac inpatient floor rather than the ICU cannot be ignored, because a floor bed is less costly than that of an ICU bed.

Ongoing developments in TAVR will have implications for nurses caring for TAVR patients. New frontiers in valve replacement procedures are occurring at lightning speed. Transcatheter aortic valve replacements are still being perfected and new-generation THVs are enabling implants through smaller and smaller delivery systems. This has provided the groundwork for ongoing developments and research with valve replacement procedures and new-generation bioprosthetic heart valves. Nurses are ideally positioned to significantly impact the future of transcatheter valve replacement by standardizing patient care that is linked to evidence-based outcomes. This will pave the way for other centers seeking to take advantage of the benefits that highly skilled nurses can provide to these patients.

MitraClip®

Although there is not a percutaneous mitral valve available for use in the United States yet, there is a catheter-based therapy available for those patients who are ineligible for traditional mitral valve surgery. The MitraClip® (Abbott Vascular) was developed to treat patients with symptomatic degenerative mitral regurgitation (MR) ≥ 3+ who are too high risk for surgery. Approved for commercial use in the United States in October 2013, the MitraClip delivery system is introduced via the femoral vein. Once deployed, the MitraClip approximates the valve leaflet edges, mimicking a surgical mitral valve repair (Wan et al., 2013). Although these patients still have residual MR post-procedure, recent data reveal patients have symptomatic relief of symptoms, fewer hospitalizations, and improved quality of life (Wan et al., 2013). Similar to TAVR, a heart team approach is essential to the evaluation and management of these critically ill patients. These patients are most often in heart failure and have multiple comorbid conditions. The MitraClip will not be successful without aggressive heart failure medical management prior to and following the procedure. MitraClip patients also require close follow up in the valve clinic, with regularly scheduled post-procedure echocardiograms and outpatient visits.

MINIMALLY INVASIVE ATRIAL FIBRILLATION ABLATION

Atrial fibrillation is the most common arrhythmia reported, with an anticipated prevalence of 12.1 million in 2030 (from 5.2 million in 2010) (Colilla et al., 2013). Costs of treatment of AF were estimated at $26 billion per year (American Heart Association, 2011). In addition, the complications of AF—embolic stroke and anticoagulation-associated hemorrhage—make it a very morbid condition, particularly for the elderly who are often the affected. For these reasons, surgery for AF (covered in Chapter 3) has become increasingly popular. The original Cox-Maze III procedure, however, required full sternotomy and CPB. Minimally invasive approaches have been pursued. A majority of the time, the Maze procedure is being performed in conjunction with another cardiac procedure (e.g., mitral valve repair/replacement). As a standalone procedure, several methods have emerged to describe the minimally invasive approach: bilateral or single-sided thoracotomies, video-assisted thoracoscopic approach, and a robotic Maze procedure (Iribarne et al., 2011). The complete Maze operation involves isolation of both the left and right pulmonary veins. Because the left atrium is typically the focus of AF re-entry, a left-sided Maze is the most commonly performed procedure (Bojar, 2011). A variety of energy sources—radiofrequency, high-frequency ultrasound, or cryoablation—are used to create the lesions (i.e., myocardial scars), which block the micro re-entrant circuits causing AF (Bojar, 2011; Iribarne, 2011). In addition to ablation, the basic Maze procedure also involves ligation of the left atrial appendage to remove

the thromboembolic source in AF patients. Because the procedure is performed on a beating heart, atrial function can be monitored during treatment. Patients may convert to normal sinus rhythm during the procedure or it may take up to 12 weeks. The minimally invasive or robotic Maze procedure is associated with less postoperative pain due to smaller incisions and results in fewer complications because CPB is not required.

NURSING CARE AND SPECIAL CONSIDERATIONS FOR MICS

Preoperative teaching and education should be provided to all patients and families prior to cardiac surgery. However, any time a minimally invasive procedure is being planned, there may be unforeseen circumstances in which MICS may turn into a traditional CABG. Teaching should include the participation of not only the patient, but also any caregivers, because unforeseen activity restrictions may result from the need for a full sternotomy. Preoperative teaching for the intended procedure should also include a review of the potential complications associated with CPB and the standard of care employed by the facility.

Although emphasis should be placed on the decreased amount of postoperative pain experienced with MICS, patients should be encouraged to report pain levels honestly to help avoid complications and improve patient satisfaction. Specifically, patients should be encouraged to volunteer information regarding pain level and efficacy of treatment. Such is not always the case, however, and pain perception and subsequent management may be inadequate as a result (Watt-Watson, Stevens, Garfinkel, Streiner, & Gallop, 2004). The value of aggressive pulmonary toilet and early ambulation cannot be overemphasized despite a minimally invasive approach. Expectations for coughing and deep breathing as well as the use of incentive spirometry should be taught in the preoperative period similar to that of traditional cardiac procedures.

Immediate postoperative care of patients who have undergone MICS will, for the most part, follow the same path as care for those who required a sternotomy; however, there are a few specific issues that warrant discussion. Approximately 1 hour prior to the patient's arrival to the ICU, the OR nurse usually calls in a report to the admitting ICU nurse. After receiving the initial brief report, the patient's family should be updated. Early contact establishes a rapport with family and provides time to obtain information for the admission assessment and emergency contact names and numbers. The family should be notified where they will be contacted and the anticipated time until visitation after the patient arrives in the ICU. If the patient was not in the hospital prior to surgery and did not receive preoperative education, the family should be prepared for what to expect with the ICU environment and visitation guidelines to help reduce their stress level. Questions should be addressed, and any anticipated resources (e.g., pastoral care) may be provided at this time.

Admission to the ICU: The First 15 Minutes

Patients who are intubated will be sedated. The intraoperative paralytics are often reversed to assist with early extubation. Depending on the facility, the anesthesia provider will start a sedation infusion to promote comfort, decrease myocardial oxygen consumption, and enhance tolerance to the ventilator until weaning commences. The anesthesia provider will provide a more in-depth report including, but not limited to, the patient's past medical history, allergies, intraoperative course, last set of pertinent lab results, volume of crystalloids and colloids given, antibiotics administered and times, urinary output, and, if CPB was required, the

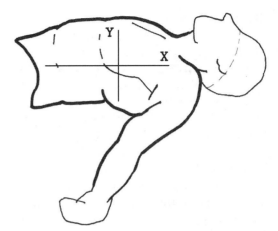

Figure 7-5 The phlebostatic axis (intersection of the X and Y reference lines).
Source: Illustrated by James R. Perron.

length of time on bypass and the length of time the aorta was cross-clamped.

While settling the patient after surgery, maintaining hemodynamic stability is essential. Baseline vital signs should be obtained and all pressure lines zeroed and leveled to the phlebostatic axis (see **Figure 7-5**). In addition to vital signs, an initial hemodynamic assessment should include a review of IV access, current medications, cardiac rhythm, and central venous pressure (CVP). If the patient has a pulmonary artery catheter in place, pulmonary artery pressure (PAP) and pulmonary artery occlusive pressure (PAOP) should be measured. Data should be obtained to allow for calculation of cardiac output (CO), SvO_2, and systemic vascular resistance (SVR) (Khalpey, Ganim, & Rawn, 2008). Pulmonary artery pressure readings and waveforms should be confirmed with the anesthesia provider to assess any changes and the pulmonary artery (PA) catheter location should be noted. Fluid and medication infusion rates should be titrated to maintain hemodynamic stability.

Among patients who did not have CPB, hypothermia is uncommon. A temperature less than 35° C (95° F) is considered hypothermic; in such a case, warming techniques should be implemented. Patients who have undergone MICS are routinely hypovolemic and have labile blood pressure, requiring volume repletion to achieve hemodynamic stability. The frequency with which vital signs and a hemodynamic profile are obtained depends on the facility guidelines and the patient's condition.

The patient's height and weight should be entered into the monitoring system database to ensure accurate calculations based on body surface area (e.g., cardiac index [CI]). If the patient is hypothermic, CI values will be skewed and reflect "cold numbers." A true hemodynamic picture will not be reflected until the patient is normothermic.

Lab specimens should be collected as prescribed by unit protocol or as indicated by the patient's clinical status. Baseline postoperative labs will likely include an arterial blood gas (ABG), ionized calcium, serum chemistries, coagulation profile, and a complete blood count (CBC). If the patient is bleeding, a fibrinogen level may be obtained as well. The patient should also have a portable chest radiograph and an electrocardiogram (ECG) performed.

An ECG after MICS is imperative because of the potential complications related to myocardial ischemia and graft patency. Early graft closure and arterial graft spasm may be manifested the same way that in traditional cardiac surgery, ST-segment elevation, T-wave inversion, and Q waves present in the leads, which is reflective of the revascularized myocardium (Edgar et al., 1999).

Placement of chest tubes may be less than ideal because of the limited exposure in MICS (Bojar, 2011). Chest tubes are typically left in place to drain the mediastinum and the pleural space similar to that in traditional cardiac surgery. It is common for Blake drains to be used in lieu of regular chest tubes, particularly in the pleural cavity,

because they are softer and presumably more pliable. All chest drains, regardless of type, should be connected to –20 cm suction and should be assessed regularly for amount and type of drainage, patency, and presence of clots. If a patient's blood pressure permits, the head of the bed should be elevated to facilitate chest tube drainage and to avoid accumulation in an undrained pleural space. Additionally, access to the right ventricle for the application of traditional epicardial pacing wires is often a challenge in MICS. The use of a PA catheter that contains a right ventricular pacing port is common. Additional options for pacing perioperatively would require placement of external pacing pads, which are often uncomfortable for patients (Bojar, 2011).

Secondary Assessment: The Next 15 Minutes

After initial stabilization of the MICS patient is achieved and a preliminary patient assessment for clinically significant issues (e.g., bleeding, hypotension, hypertension, agitation, dysrhythmias) is performed, a more focused head-to-toe assessment is completed. The neurologic assessment is ongoing and more complete as the patient emerges from anesthesia. Skin is assessed for temperature, color, and location of incisions (procedure-based).

Pain should be anticipated, and its level should be assessed with a scale appropriate for the cognitive status of the patient. Despite a minimally invasive incision being made, pain remains an expected finding; good pain control is essential to recovery. Measures to relieve the thoracotomy incision pain should be implemented immediately. Frequently, intercostal injections, epidural analgesia, or catheters left in the subcutaneous tissue and then tunneled out through the skin are used to achieve adequate pain control when rib-spreading procedures have been performed to optimize pulmonary function (Bojar, 2011;

Mandal et al., 2013). In the initial postoperative period, patients will primarily receive opioid analgesics. They should also be premedicated prior to potentially painful procedures (e.g., chest tube removal) (Puntillo & Ley, 2004). As discussed in Chapter 14, inadequate analgesia can result in tachycardia, increased peripheral vascular resistance, imbalance between oxygen supply and demand, hypoxemia, pneumonia, and atelectasis. Lower levels of pain are typically encountered with a minimally invasive procedure; chest tubes are frequently a source of pain regardless of the minimally invasive nature of the procedure.

Although many MICS procedures are done without the use of CPB, many procedures continue to require bypass; therefore, alternative cannulation sites are utilized. Minimally invasive mitral valve surgery done with or without robotic assistance frequently utilizes both femoral artery and vein. Because of the high incidence of concomitant aortoiliac and femoral disease, it is absolutely essential that distal perfusion of those extremities be assessed at the conclusion of the procedure and frequently in the ICU (Bojar, 2011). Axillary cannulation may also be utilized in certain situations when the femoral vessels have been determined inappropriate. Establishing a baseline for the presence of peripheral pulses is critical to recognition of the development of extremity vascular and motor function complications (Bojar, 2011).

Hemodynamic Monitoring

Successful hemodynamic monitoring begins with knowing the normal range for hemodynamic values. "Normal" in this case is a relative term, because normal values are based on healthy individuals with healthy hearts. The values most commonly monitored are identical to those utilized for traditional cardiac surgery patients; they are covered in more detail in Chapter 9.

Managing a patient's hemodynamic profile entails evaluating the patient's clinical condition and past medical and surgical histories so the correct decision is made about how to optimize preload, afterload, and contractility. Depending on comorbidities, hemodynamic values may be skewed. For example, a patient with pulmonary hypertension may have elevated pulmonary artery pressures and CVP secondary to lung disease. A valuable source for a patient's baseline hemodynamic values is the cardiac catheterization lab report. Trying to maintain a patient with underlying disease within the standard norms is unrealistic and can even be detrimental to the patient. For example, a patient with hypertension may not have adequate kidney perfusion with a mean arterial pressure (MAP) of 80 mmHg, but instead may need a slightly higher MAP of 90–95 mmHg to maintain end-organ perfusion.

The key to hemodynamic stability starts with maintaining and normalizing heart rate and stroke volume (SV). This goal may be accomplished through the administration and titration of fluids and medications. Stroke volume is affected by preload, afterload, and contractility (Zellinger, 2007); these variables are described further in Chapter 9.

Some of the more common etiologies of hemodynamic compromise are myocardial ischemia, hypothermia, and postoperative dysrhythmias (Khalpey et al., 2008). These are discussed in detail in Chapters 13 and 15. The goal of therapy is optimal end-organ perfusion with hemodynamic stability. Although hemodynamic parameter goals should be individualized, suggested minimum values for most patients will likely include an SvO_2 near 60%, a MAP greater than 65 mmHg, and CI greater than 2 L/min/m² (Khalpey et al., 2008).

Postoperative Complications

Postoperative complications of cardiac surgery in general are discussed in detail in Chapter 13. It is essential for the ICU nurse to monitor patients who have undergone MICS procedures for development of complications, intervene to prevent them from occurring, and promptly recognize and treat any complications that develop.

MICS-Specific Complications

Some of the complications related to MICS specifically are felt to be related to the more technically challenging nature of these procedures and to procedure-related stress on the heart. Because there is a learning curve associated with these operations, CPB time is often prolonged—more than 4 hours (Bojar, 2011). All of the complications discussed in Chapter 13 apply to MICS, with the primary offending factor being non-pulsatile blood flow for those procedures requiring CPB. Additionally, single-lung ventilation, which is often routinely required for these procedures, often results in atelectasis, lung parenchyma injury, pleural effusion, and hemothorax.

Dysrhythmias

Dysrhythmias are a common occurrence following cardiac surgery. Data have yet to show there to be a reduced rate of AF among MIC procedures (Iribarne et al., 2011). Atrial fibrillation can occur in patients with no prior history from electrolyte imbalances, volume overload, surgical manipulation, or acid–base imbalance. Patients undergoing minimally invasive Maze procedures may be loaded with IV amiodarone coming out of the OR to obtain or maintain normal sinus rhythm. Additionally, patients undergoing valve surgery or a Maze procedure may develop bradycardia or heart block as a result of intraoperative manipulation around the conduction system; this may require a period of temporary pacing postoperatively and eventual placement of a permanent pacemaker.

Lethal arrhythmias, such as ventricular tachycardia or ventricular fibrillation (VF), can also occur in the immediate postoperative period of MICS. Electrolyte imbalance, cardiac irritability from the surgery, and acidosis may be contributing factors to their development. Resuscitation of these dysrhythmias should follow the American Heart Association recommendations. Development of VF may require opening the patient's chest at the bedside. Postoperative dysrhythmias are discussed in more detail in Chapter 15.

Bleeding

Postoperative bleeding is a risk with any cardiac surgery, including MICS. The risk increases if the procedure is performed on CPB, as higher doses of heparin are administered. As with traditional cardiac surgery, hemodilution, fibrinolysis, and hypothermia are risk factors for postoperative bleeding. As previously stated, chest tube patency and evaluation of chest radiograph are very important, because chest tube placement and drainage of the pleural cavity can be challenging when working via limited incisions. Postoperative bleeding is discussed in more detail in Chapter 13.

Postoperative Ventilatory Support

Patients who undergo MICS may be extubated in the OR or very shortly after arrival to the ICU (within 2–3 hours). Patients may be weaned from mechanical ventilation when certain criteria, which may vary among facilities, are met. In general, these conditions may include the patient being awake and cooperative, dissipation of neuromuscular blocking agent effects (usually manifested with a sustained head lift), hemodynamic stability, absence of dysrhythmias, ABG values within physiologic range, normal chest radiograph findings, normothermia, chest tube drainage less than 100 mL/hr, and urine output more than 1 mL/kg/hr (Chikwe, Donaldson, & Wood, 2006; Kapoor et al., 2008). In addition, other factors should be considered while weaning the patient off ventilatory support, such as patient age, comorbidities, length of time in the OR, and intraoperative course. Weaning from mechanical ventilation following cardiac surgery is discussed in detail in Chapter 11.

Recovery from MICS

Patients who undergo MICS procedures traditionally have a quicker and less complicated recovery than patients who undergo conventional surgical procedures. Generally, patients are intensively monitored in the OR; for OPCAB, transesophageal echocardiogram and in-line mixed oxygen saturations are necessary to avoid decompensation during the procedure (Bojar, 2011). These patients typically return to the ICU hemodynamically stable, but often require inotrope or pressor support intraoperatively during the cardiac positioning necessary for OPCAB (Bojar, 2011).

Minimally invasive cardiac surgery patients, like all cardiac surgery patients, should have an ECG immediately upon return from the OR. Procedures performed through small incisions are often limited by full surgical exposure of the heart (Bojar, 2011). Because of this lack of direct visualization and the lack of full revascularization, graft patency and ischemia may be an issue postoperatively. The ICU nurse plays a key role in detection of ECG changes that may be an early sign of a problem with an anastomosis. There should be a low threshold for these patients to have additional testing—echocardiogram to assess for wall motion abnormalities and coronary angiography if postoperative ischemia is suspected (Bojar, 2011).

As previously stated, the lack of traditional epicardial pacing wires following MIDCAB and MIMVS may pose problems in the early postoperative period. Patients may return to the ICU with a right ventricular pacing lead as part of a special pulmonary artery catheter, which means catheter position may be a factor in pacing wire capture. Additionally, external pacing may be required, which is often less than optimal if the patient is awake.

Postoperative pain management is crucial for patients who have undergone rib-spreading procedures. In addition to epidural and intercostal analgesia, use of nonnarcotic medications can be helpful in preventing pulmonary complications following thoracotomy procedures. Ketorolac (Toradol®) and IV acetaminophen (Tylenol®) have both been used as adjunctive therapy to narcotics to accomplish early extubation.

Despite specific concerns related to the recovery of patients undergoing MICS, these patients often require less time in the ICU. Additionally, in a recent systematic review, eight out of 14 studies reported decreased hospital LOS for MIMVS, with one center reporting a 2-day LOS reduction when compared to traditional sternotomy patients (Iribarne et al., 2011).

SUMMARY

Minimally invasive cardiac surgery, with all of its benefits, provides a viable option for the patient who meets the criteria established for this type of procedure. The major benefits of MICS are the decreased level of pain and faster recovery. Additionally, decreased incidence of postoperative complications related to CPB and aortic cross-clamping, intraoperative anticoagulation, cardioplegia, and sternal wound infections have all been documented. Cardiac surgery centers of excellence with teams who have mastered the learning curve for MIMVS have achieved equivalent morbidity and mortality when compared to standard mitral valve surgery (Mandal et al., 2013). The cardiac surgery ICU nurse is a part of that important multidisciplinary team, taking on many roles when caring for this type of patient: educator, advocate for the patient and family, and collaborator with the multidisciplinary team. While MICS is not an innovative new treatment for cardiac disease, it is certainly an attractive approach to a traditional procedure.

CASE STUDY

A 73-year-old patient presented to the emergency department with reports of chest pain, shortness of breath, and nausea. He reported having multiple similar episodes over the last month, with the symptoms normally resolving with rest after 30 minutes. Today, the symptoms continued for more than 2 hours. He rated his pain as an 8 on a scale of 0 to 10. He also reported a history of COPD, a 50 pack-year smoking history, and diet-controlled diabetes.

Upon admission, the catheterization lab was notified. Prior to transfer, the patient received O_2 via nasal cannula at 2 L/min for an SpO_2 of 93% on room air. IV access was obtained and laboratory studies (CBC, chemistries, coagulation profile, and troponin) were drawn.

Sublingual nitroglycerin was administered 3 times with no relief of pain; 2 mg of IV morphine was given, which decreased the patient's pain from an 8 to a 6. A 12-lead ECG revealed ST-segment elevation in leads II, III, and aVF, indicating an inferior wall myocardial infarction.

The patient was taken to the catheterization lab. Cardiac catheterization revealed a 10% occlusion of the LAD and circumflex arteries. The right coronary had 90% occlusion, and the patient's ejection fraction was 40%. He was deemed not to be a candidate for angioplasty or stent placement because of a tortuous arterial anatomy.

A MIDCAB procedure was scheduled owing to the patient's comorbidities. Preoperative education was performed by the ICU nurse on the evening before surgery was scheduled.

Early the next morning, the patient underwent a MIDCAB procedure with a minithoracotomy approach under general anesthesia. The surgeon anastomosed the LITA to the LAD; no cardiopulmonary bypass was required.

The patient was transported to the ICU, attached to the cardiac monitor, and placed on a ventilator. He had an intra-arterial catheter, left pleural chest tube to a drainage-collection device at –20 cm suction, and urinary catheter. Initial labs were obtained and the assessment completed. Hemodynamic data were as follows: heart rate 90, sinus rhythm with no ectopy, BP 112/64 (80), PA 32/20 (24), CVP 13, CO 3.5, CI 1.9, SVR 1554, SvO_2 70%, SpO_2 100%, temperature 36.0 °C, urinary output 180 mL, and CT drainage 50 mL. A portable chest radiograph and ECG were obtained. The patient was extubated within 2 hours after his arrival to the ICU.

A postoperative angiography revealed a patent graft. The patient's postoperative course was uneventful, and he was discharged home on postoperative day 5.

Critical Thinking Questions

1. Which postoperative test will provide the necessary information about this patient's graft status, including the patency of the graft?
2. If graft occlusion has occurred, which ECG findings will be present in this case?
3. Why is diltiazem ordered postoperatively?

Answers to Critical Thinking Questions

1. 12-lead ECG
2. The patient will likely manifest ST-segment elevation, T-wave inversion, and the presence of Q waves in leads II, III, and aVF, indicating changes to the inferior wall—that is, the area of the heart that was revascularized.
3. One of the causes of graft closure is ITA graft vasospasm. Administration of a calcium channel blocker helps to prevent postoperative spasm of the graft vessel.

SELF-ASSESSMENT QUESTIONS

1. The family of a patient who just returned from the OR for a coronary artery bypass grafting procedure asked why the patient's heart is not functioning as well as it should be. The nurse's best response is:
   a. "It is related to the decrease in body temperature in the operating room."
   b. "Some of the body fluid is leaking from his vessels."
   c. "The patient received anticoagulants for the procedure."
   d. "Ischemia-reperfusion injury can occur."

2. Hemorrhagic stroke can occur after traditional coronary artery bypass grafting due to which of the following?
   a. Hypothermia
   b. Anticoagulants
   c. Red blood cell hemolysis
   d. Clamping of the aorta

3. The family of a patient who just returned from the OR for a coronary artery bypass grafting procedure asked why the patient's blood sugar is elevated. The nurse's best response is:
   a. "It could be related to the steroids given during surgery."
   b. "He might have had a fever in the operating room; I will check."
   c. "You can get higher blood sugars from being on bypass."
   d. "During surgery, there is activation of the complement system."

4. A patient is told that minimally invasive cardiac surgery was not feasible and that traditional cardiac surgery would be required. Which of the following conditions does this patient likely have?
   a. Atrial septal defect
   b. Multi-vessel coronary artery disease
   c. Aortic stenosis
   d. Atrial fibrillation

5. A nurse is asked to explain minimally invasive direct coronary artery bypass. Which of the following statements demonstrates an understanding of the procedure?
   a. "Cardioplegia is instilled for this procedure."
   b. "Patients with 3- or more vessel disease can be treated with this procedure."
   c. "There is minimal time spent on cardiopulmonary bypass."
   d. "There are smaller but more incisions than with traditional CABG."

6. Which of the following is true during minimally invasive direct coronary artery bypass?
   a. The heart's movement is limited throughout the procedure.
   b. It is commonly used in patients requiring single-vessel bypass.
   c. The left lung is deflated during the procedure.
   d. Because of the multiple lesions, early mobility is more challenging than with traditional bypass.

7. Which of the following is an advantage of minimally invasive direct coronary artery bypass?
   a. Limited circulatory support
   b. Minimal manipulation of the aorta
   c. Limited amount of cardioplegia instilled
   d. Decreased blood loss

8. Which of the following is a difference between minimally invasive direct coronary artery bypass and off-pump bypass?
   a. Number of vessels that can be repaired
   b. Amount of cardioplegia instilled
   c. Time the heart is not beating during the procedure
   d. Degree of postoperative inflammatory response

9. Which of the following is true regarding a minimally invasive direct view procedure?
   a. It entails use of robotics.
   b. It can be used for tricuspid valve replacement.
   c. It cannot be performed on a patient who has had a median sternotomy in the past.
   d. The patient will have an 8-cm incision.

10. Which of the following patients will likely be excluded from having a minimally invasive direct coronary artery bypass procedure? A patient with a:

   a. HbA1c 8%
   b. BMI 41 kg/m^2
   c. Troponin 0.4 ng/mL
   d. Serum creatinine 1.5 mg/dL

Answers to Self-Assessment Questions

1. d	6. c
2. b	7. d
3. c	8. a
4. a	9. d
5. d	10. b

Clinical Inquiry Box

Question: Can a patient's experience with heart valve replacement surgery be improved?

Reference: Jackson, K., Cook, L., Jackson, M., Simbodyal, R., Carver, K., Greig-Midlane, H., . . . Ponsonby, M. (2014). Evaluating patients' experiences of heart valve replacement surgery. *British Journal of Cardiac Nursing, 9*(5), 224–230.

Objective: The aims of this initiative were to critically assess current patient-reported experience measures (PREMs) frameworks to establish whether they are fit for purpose in today's healthcare environment and aligned to the NHS Constitution and the NICE Quality Standard for patient experience and to develop a PREMs questionnaire for adults undergoing heart valve replacement surgery.

Method: A seven-stage process was utilized with patients and patient organizations to develop items of importance for patient experience.

Results: A series of PREMs for heart valve replacement surgery were developed. An updated patient experience framework was also developed with two additional components (patient choice and financial burden) being added to the existing framework developed by the Picker Institute. Key components included respect for patient-centered values, coordination and integration of services, increased communication on clinical status, physical comfort during recovery, emotional support postoperatively, family involvement in care, and transition and continuity.

Conclusion: Patient-reported experience measures can have quantitative and qualitative methodologies to drive service improvement and can be used alongside patient-reported outcome measures to produce a rounded picture of patients' views on both the process and the outcome of care.

REFERENCES

American Heart Association. (2011). *Treating atrial fibrillation patients costs U.S. $26 billion annually.* Retrieved from http://newsroom.heart.org/news/1329

Bojar, R. (2011). *Manual of perioperative care in adult cardiac surgery* (5th ed.). Hoboken, NJ: Wiley-Blackwell.

Chen-Scarabelli, C. (2002). Beating-heart coronary artery bypass graft surgery: Indication, advantages, and limitation. *Critical Care Nurse, 22*(5), 44–58.

Cheung, A., & Lichtenstein, M. (2012). Illustrated techniques for transapical aortic valve implantation. *Annals of Cardiothoracic Surgery, 1*(2), 231–239. doi:10.3978/j.issn.2225-319X.2012.07.12

Chikwe, J., Donaldson, J., & Wood, A. J. (2006). Minimally invasive cardiac surgery. *British Journal of Cardiology, 13*(2), 123–128.

Chitwood, W. R. (2011). Robotic cardiac surgery by 2031. *Texas Heart Institute Journal, 38*(6), 691–693.

Colilla, A., Crow, A., Petkun, W., Singer, D. E., Simon, T., & Liu, X. (2013). Estimates of current and future incidence and prevalence of atrial fibrillation in the U.S. adult population. *American Journal of Cardiology, 112*(8), 1142–1147.

Edgar, W. F., Ebersole, N., & Mayfield, M. G. (1999). MIDCAB. *American Journal of Nursing, 99*(7), 40–46.

Feldman, T. E., Sanborn, T. A., & O'Neill, W. W. (2005). Balloon aortic and pulmonic valvuloplasty. In H. C. Hermann (Ed.), *Contemporary cardiology: Interventional cardiology: Percutaneous noncoronary intervention* (pp. 29–48). Totowa, NJ: Humana Press.

Gaasch, W. H., Brecker, S. J. D., & Aldea, G. S. (2014). Transcatheter aortic valve replacement. Retrieved from http://www.uptodate.com/contents/transcatheter-aortic-valve-replacement

Guyton, R. A., Block, P. C., Thourani, V., Lerakis, S., & Babaliaros, V. (2013). Carotid artery access for transcatheter aortic valve replacement [Electronic version]. *Catheterization and Cardiovascular Interventions, 82,* E583–E586. doi:10.1002/ccd.24596

Harris, A., Dean, A., Babaliaros, V., & Keegan, P. (2014). TAVR patients on an intermediate care unit: Direct from the cath lab to the floor. Poster session presented at the 10th annual conference of the American Association of Heart Failure Nurses, Los Angeles, CA.

Holmes, D. R., Mack, M. J., Kaul, S., Agnihotri, A., Alexander, K. P., Agnihortri, A., . . . Thomas, J. D. (2012). ACCF/AATS/SCAI/STS expert consensus document on transcatheter valve replacement [Electronic version]. *The Journal of Thoracic and Cardiovascular Surgery, 144*(3), e29–e84.

Hu, P. P. (2012). TAVR and SAVR: Current treatment of aortic stenosis. *Clinical Medicine Insights: Cardiology, 6,* 125–139. doi:10.4137/CMC.S7540

Iribarne, A., Easterwood, R., Chan, E., Yang, J., Soni, L., Russo, M., . . . Argenziano, M. (2011). The golden age of minimally invasive cardiothoracic surgery: Current and future perspectives. *Future Cardiology, 7*(3), 333–346.

Jackson, K., Cook, L., Jackson, M., Simbodyal, R., Carver, K., Greig-Midlane, H., . . . Ponsonby, M. (2014). Evaluating patient's experiences of heart valve replacement surgery. *British Journal of Cardiac Nursing, 9*(5), 224–230.

Kapoor, P. M., Kakani, M., Chowdhury, U., Choudhury, M., Lakshmy, R., & Kiran, U. (2008). Early goal-directed therapy in moderate to high-risk cardiac surgery patients. *Annals of Cardiac Anaesthesia, 11*(1), 27–34.

Khalpey, Z. I., Ganim, R. B., & Rawn, J. D. (2008). Postoperative care of cardiac surgery patients. In L. H. Cohn (Ed.), *Cardiac surgery in the adult* (pp. 465–486). New York, NY: McGraw-Hill.

Ley, S. J. (2006). Postoperative management of the cardiac surgery patient. In H. M. Schell & K. A. Puntillo (Eds.), *Critical care nursing secrets* (2nd ed., pp. 113–121). St. Louis, MO: Mosby.

Mack, M., Brennan, M., Brindis, R., Carroll, J., Edwards, F., Grover, F., . . . Holms, D. (2013). Outcomes following transcatheter aortic valve replacement in the United States. *Journal of the American Medical Association, 310*(19), 2069–2077.

Mack, M. J. (2006). Minimally invasive cardiac surgery. *Surgical Endoscopy, 20*(Suppl. 2), S488–S492.

Mandal, K., Alwair, H., Nifong, W. L., & Chitwood, W. R. Jr. (2013). Robotically assisted minimally invasive mitral valve surgery. *Journal of Thoracic Disease, 5*(6S), S694–S703.

Masson, J.-B., Kovac, J., Schuler, G., Ye, L., Cheung, A., Kapadia, S., . . . Webb, J. G. (2009). Transcatheter aortic valve implantation: Review of the nature, management, and avoidance of procedural complications. *Journal of the American College of Cardiology: Cardiovascular Interventions, 2*(9), 811–820.

Navia, J., Olivares, G., Ehasz, P., Gillinov, M., Svensson, L., Brozzi, N., & Lytle, B. (2013). Endoscopic radial artery harvesting procedure for coronary artery bypass grafting. *Annals of Cardiothoracic Surgery, 2*(4), 557–564.

Nishimura, R. A., Otto, C. M., Bonow, R. O., Carabello, B. A., Erwin, J. P., Guyton, R. A., . . . Thomas, J. D. (2014). Guidelines for the management of patients with valvular heart disease: A report of the American College of Cardiology/American Heart Association task force on practice guidelines. *Journal of the American College of Cardiology, 63*(22), e57–e185.

Pike, R. D. B. (2015). Off pump coronary artery bypass and minimally invasive direct coronary artery bypass. In M. J. Murray, R. A. Harrison, J. T. Mueller, S. H. Rose, C. T. Wass, & D. J. Wedel (Eds.), *Faust's anesthesiology review* (4th ed., pp. 341–342). Philadelphia, PA: Elsevier Saunders.

Puntillo, K., & Ley, S. J. (2004). Appropriately timed analgesics control pain during chest tube removal. *American Journal of Critical Care, 13*(4), 292–301.

Smith, C., Leon, M., Mack, M., Miller, C., Moses, J., Svensson, L., . . . Pocock, S. J. (2011). Transcatheter versus surgical aortic-valve replacement in high-risk patients. *New England Journal of Medicine, 364,* 2187–2198.

Tang, G. H. L., Lansman, S. L., Cohen, M., Spielvogel, D., Cuomo, L., Ahmad, H., . . . Dutta, T. (2013). Transcatheter aortic valve replacement: Current developments, ongoing issues, future outlook. *Cardiology in Review, 21*(2), 55–76.

Thourani, V. N., Gunter, R. L., Neravetla, S., Block, P., Guyton, R. A., Kilgo, P., . . . Babaliaros, V. (2013). Use of transaortic, transapical, and transcarotid transcatheter aortic valve replacement in inoperable patients. *Annals of Thoracic Surgery, 96,* 1349–1357.

Wan, B., Rahnavardi, M., Tian, D., Phan, K., Munkholm-Larsen, S., Bannon, P., & Yan, T. D. (2013). A meta-analysis of MitraClip system versus surgery for treatment of severe mitral regurgitation. *Annals of Cardiothoracic Surgery, 2*(6), 683–692.

Watt-Watson, J., Stevens, B., Garfinkel, P., Streiner, D., & Gallop, R. (2004). Relationship between nurses' knowledge and pain management outcomes for their postoperative cardiac patients. *Journal of Advanced Nursing, 36*(4), 535–545.

Webb, G. J., & Wood, D. A. (2012). Current status of transcatheter aortic valve replacement. *Journal of the American College of Cardiology, 60*(6), 483–492.

Zellinger, M. (2007). Cardiac surgery and heart transplant. In R. Kaplow & S. R. Hardin (Eds.), *Critical care nursing: Synergy for optimal outcomes* (pp. 229–242). Sudbury, MA: Jones and Bartlett.

WEB RESOURCES

Aortic Stenosis: Minimally Invasive: http://www.youtube.com/watch?v=-miuqi1iyrw

Robotic-Assisted Single-Vessel Coronary Artery Bypass Surgery: http://www.youtube.com/watch?v=YIRP3vS4zV0

Minimally Invasive Direct Coronary Artery Bypass (MIDCAB): http://www.youtube.com/watch?v=Iq4HXtDYxS8

Hybrid Maze procedure: http://www.youtube.com/watch?v=XRGLCmkSqso

Chapter 8

Recovery from Anesthesia

Toni Patrice Johnson

INTRODUCTION

Nearly 7.5 million cardiovascular operations and procedures were performed in the United States in 2010; of these, approximately 395,000 were coronary artery bypass grafting procedures (Go et al., 2014). Thousands of cardiac surgery patients have enjoyed speedy recovery times thanks to advances in surgical techniques, anesthetic agents, and postoperative medications. More importantly, improvements in anesthetic techniques have allowed patients to transition quickly from the intensive care unit (ICU) for the immediate postoperative period to a cardiac surgery unit and then home in increasingly shorter periods of time. Given these trends, ICU nurses must be assiduous in the care of these patients. This chapter focuses on care in the immediate postoperative period.

HAND-OFF COMMUNICATION

Postoperative care begins immediately after the patient is transferred from the operating room (OR). Following cardiac surgery, patients are typically transferred to the ICU for monitoring, hemodynamic stabilization, assessment for complications, and possibly extubation. Vital information is exchanged in the hand-off communication (also known as SBAR, or situation-background-assessment-recommendation) between the anesthesia provider and the ICU nurse. Data should include pertinent information regarding the surgical procedure, any intraoperative complications or events, hemodynamic and ventilatory status, cardiopulmonary bypass (CPB) time, recent laboratory data, type and amount of intravenous fluids and blood products administered, reversal of anticoagulants, pertinent medical and surgical history, preoperative status, location of intravenous lines and invasive catheters, vasopressor and inotropic agents used, and current infusion rates. Additional information includes use of mechanical cardiac assist devices, presence of pacing wires, length of surgery, estimated blood loss, intraoperative intake and output, patient position on the OR table, location of drains and dressings, and anesthetic and reversal agents administered. **Table 8-1** lists the more common anesthetic agents used.

In addition to the information provided by the anesthesia provider, an extensive preoperative evaluation is conducted prior to cardiac surgery. Details of this evaluation are described in Chapter 4. Information about existing comorbidities, cardiac disease, tobacco use, nutritional status, medication history, preoperative cardiac status, and any optimizing that might have taken place prior to surgery will help the ICU nurse anticipate the patient's immediate postoperative course and potentially required interventions. By way of illustration, as discussed in Chapter 5, the hemodynamic profile and resultant

Table 8-1   Anesthetic Agents/ Adjuncts Commonly Used in Cardiac Surgery

Intravenous Induction Agents

Propofol (Diprivan®)

Etomidate (Amidate®)

Thiopental sodium (Pentothal®)

Neuromuscular Blocking Agents

Rocuronium (Zemuron®)

Vecuronium (Norcuron®)

Succinylcholine (Anectine®)

Atracurium besylate (Tracrium®)

Mivacurium chloride (Mivacron®)

Cisatracurium (Nimbex®)

Rapacuronium (Raplon®)

Pancuronium (Pavulon®)

Tubocurarine

Metocurine

Analgesics/Sedatives

Fentanyl (Sublimaze®)

Sufentanil (Sufenta®)

Alfentanil (Alfenta®)

Remifentanil (Ultiva®)

Morphine sulfate

Midazolam (Versed®)

Lorazepam (Ativan®)

Dexmedetomidine (Precedex®)

Inhalation Agents

Isoflurane (Forane®)

Sevoflurane (Ultane®)

Enflurane (Ethrane®)

Halothane (Fluothane®)

Sources: Data from Bojar, R. (2011). Cardiovascular management. In R. Bojar (Ed.), *Manual of perioperative care in adult cardiac surgery* (5th ed). Hoboken, NJ: Blackwell; and Faulk, S. A., Fleisher, L. A., Jones, S. B., & Nussmeier, N. A. (2014). Overview of anesthesia and anesthetic choices. Retrieved from http://www.uptodate.com/contents/overview-of-anesthesia-and-anesthetic-choices?source=machineLearning&search=anesthetic+agents&selectedTitle=1%7E150&sectionRank=1&anchor=H6#H28

interventions indicated for patients who undergo cardiac surgery for valvular disease will vary with the pathophysiology of each of the respective disorders.

A patient's comorbidities may also help the ICU nurse anticipate problems in the immediate postoperative period. For example, patients with a history of conditions such as valvular disease, recent myocardial infarction (MI), arterial hypertension, diabetes, previous cardiac surgery, chronic peripheral vascular disease, involvement of three or more vessels, elevated serum creatinine, ejection fraction less than 40%, or chronic obstructive pulmonary disease (COPD) are more likely to require prolonged mechanical ventilation (Gutsche et al., 2014).

If the patient underwent CPB, the potential for a systemic inflammatory response with associated hemodynamic effects should be anticipated. As described in Chapter 13, the inflammatory response may be related to the surface of the CPB circuit being in contact with blood or reperfusion injury associated with aortic cross-clamping (Gil-Gomez et al., 2014; Landis et al., 2010).

IMMEDIATE POSTOPERATIVE CARE

The foremost objectives when caring for a cardiac surgery patient in the immediate postoperative period are maintenance of cardiac perfusion and maximization of tissue perfusion (Sanders et al., 2011). Goals of the first hour of care include stabilization of hemodynamic, oxygenation, and thermoregulatory status. Postoperative care requires assessment of physiologic parameters and hemodynamic monitoring, as well as assessment, prompt recognition, and treatment of potential complications that are related to either patient comorbidities, effects of anesthesia, or the surgical procedure itself.

Control of the cardiac surgery patient's blood pressure in the immediate postoperative period is important. In fact, variability in perioperative blood pressure is associated with an increase in 30-day mortality. The ICU nurse should monitor for hypertension to avoid associated complications such as bleeding, myocardial ischemia, dysrhythmias, stroke, or graft dehiscence. Initial management of hypertension may entail administration of opioids, sedatives, or both. However, infusion of a vasodilator may be required if initial therapies are not effective in controlling hypertension (Aronson et al., 2011).

ASSESSMENT

The nurse completes a detailed physical assessment. Electrocardiogram (ECG) monitoring of heart rate and rhythm is performed. The patient's hemodynamic profile (e.g., blood pressure, pulmonary artery pressures, pulmonary artery occlusive pressure [PAOP], central venous pressure [CVP], cardiac output [CO]/index, and systemic vascular resistance [SVR]), temperature, and pulse oximetry are evaluated. Additional invasive monitoring (e.g., mixed venous oxygen saturation) may be monitored as well. The ICU nurse can then correlate these findings with an assessment of peripheral perfusion. If temporary pacing wires are present, they should be checked to ensure proper function for emergent temporary pacing. A baseline postoperative ECG should be attained to determine presence of ischemia, infarction, conduction abnormalities, or graft spasm (Silvestry, 2014).

Assessment of neurologic status typically includes level of consciousness, degree of orientation, pupil size and reaction, and ability to move extremities. A more in-depth neurologic assessment may follow later in the postoperative period. Inherent in a neurologic assessment is an initial and ongoing assessment of pain. If the patient is able to self-report the level of pain, that is the most reliable indicator. The ICU nurse should differentiate incisional pain from anginal pain. If the patient is cognitively impaired and cannot self-report, use of a valid and reliable behavioral pain rating scale should be used. Management of pain in the postoperative cardiac surgery patient is discussed in detail in Chapter 14.

An initial respiratory assessment typically includes auscultation of breath sounds; oxygen delivery mode; presence of symmetrical chest expansion; and respiratory rate, depth, effort, and rhythm. If the patient remains on mechanical ventilation, assessment of tube placement by the markings on the endotracheal tube should be noted, and ventilator settings (e.g., mode, fractional inspired oxygen [FiO_2], rate, tidal volume, positive end-expiratory pressure [PEEP], pressure support, alarm settings) should be verified as applicable. Typical ventilator settings in the immediate postoperative period following cardiac surgery are discussed in Chapter 11. Once these data are obtained, the patient's respiratory status can be correlated with pulse oximetry and arterial blood gas (ABG) results. A baseline chest radiograph should be obtained to verify placement of the endotracheal tube (2 to 3 cm above the carina), catheters, wires, or any other devices that were inserted in the OR. The presence of any postoperative atelectasis, pneumothorax, or other common respiratory complication following cardiac surgery can also be determined (Silvestry, 2014).

Types and number of drainage catheters will vary based on the operative procedure and approach used. If a minimally invasive approach is used, a small-diameter catheter will be noted. If the patient had a sternotomy but the pleural space is not opened, the patient will have a mediastinal chest tube, or a chest tube in the mediastinal and pleural spaces will be present (Bojar, 2011).

Tubes are connected to -20 cm of wall suction. The ICU nurse should assess the amount, color, and viscosity of initial operative and subsequent drainage. Patency of the catheters must be maintained at all times. If the patient is experiencing bleeding, then volume repletion, treatment of the underlying cause (if possible), and monitoring of the patient's coagulation profile are indicated

(Bojar, 2011). Surgical reexploration may be indicated if blood loss exceeds 200 mL/hr for 4 hours, 300 mL/hr for 3 hours, 400 mL/hr for 2 hours, or 500 mL/hr for 1 hour (Bojar, 2011).

If a mediastinal chest tube becomes clotted, cardiac tamponade may ensue. Signs and symptoms may include sudden decrease or cessation of mediastinal bleeding, dyspnea, decreased CO and hypotension, tachycardia, low-voltage QRS on ECG, increased CVP, altered mental status, cyanosis or pallor, and anxiety (Reid et al., 2011). Other signs and symptoms are described in Chapter 13.

Preventive measures include positioning the patient on the side with the head of the bed elevated 30 degrees to facilitate drainage of the catheters. Until the condition is treated, the ICU nurse should administer volume to help counteract the decrease in preload from the associated decrease in diastolic filling pressures of the tamponade. Administration of afterload reducers (i.e., vasodilators) may help promote contractility (Silvestry, 2014). Cardiac tamponade management is discussed in detail in Chapter 13.

An initial assessment of the patient's fluid and electrolyte status should be performed upon admission to the ICU. In addition to the output from drains, a correlation between the patient's hemodynamic status and the intraoperative intake and output of fluids should be made. The ICU nurse should anticipate third spacing of fluid in the immediate postoperative period (Morin et al., 2011). Evaluation of serum electrolytes should be included in the initial assessment, as imbalances may be anticipated. Anticipated alterations and management of fluid and electrolytes in the postoperative cardiac surgery patient are discussed in detail in Chapter 17.

ANESTHETIC AGENTS

"Balanced" anesthesia or "fast-tracking" is generally employed to facilitate early extubation of the cardiac surgery patient while concomitantly decreasing anxiety, pain, length of ICU stay, and complications; minimizing mechanical ventilation time; and promoting a quicker, uneventful recovery from anesthesia. Typically, shorter acting agents—although more costly—result in earlier extubation and reduced postoperative stays (Salhiyyah et al., 2011). It is important for the ICU nurse to recognize signs and symptoms, multisystem effects, and postoperative nursing implications of commonly used anesthetic agents administered during surgery.

Induction Agents

Combinations of intravenous agents are administered to augment the effects of inhalation agents. Classifications of these agents include barbiturates (e.g., thiopental sodium, methohexital), nonbarbiturates (e.g., etomidate, propofol), and tranquilizers (e.g., midazolam, lorazepam) (Drain, 2013a).

Barbiturates depress the central nervous system (CNS). Thiopental sodium, for example, causes cardiovascular depression and negative inotropy, resulting in hypotension, decreased CO, and peripheral vascular resistance. Barbiturates also cause respiratory depression, which puts the patient at risk for apnea, airway obstruction, and, at higher doses, loss of laryngeal reflexes; the latter effect puts the patient at risk for aspiration (Drain, 2013a). Other side effects may include headache, emergence agitation, prolonged somnolence, and nausea. Nursing considerations include monitoring for the prolonged effects of thiopental, which could persist for as long as 36 hours (Tembelopoulos, Carr, & Tressy-Murphy, 2012).

Etomidate is a hypnotic agent with no analgesic effects. It is considered the agent of choice in patients with cardiovascular instability. When this agent is used, it is less likely to cause hypotension. Heart rate, contractility, and CO remain stable, and negative inotropic effects are negligible with etomidate (Drain, 2013a). Some patients may develop postoperative nausea and vomiting (PONV), hiccoughs, involuntary tremors, or suppressed adrenal function following administration of etomidate (Drain, 2013a).

Propofol (Diprivan®) is a sedative that is primarily used as an induction agent. Compared with barbiturates, it causes less myocardial depression. Hypotension seen following propofol administration is felt to be related to arterial and venous dilation (Drain, 2013a). An infusion of propofol is generally initiated en route to the ICU and discontinued 10 to 15 minutes prior to ventilator weaning. The maintenance infusion rate is 50 to 150 mcg/kg/min. Propofol has a low incidence of postoperative side effects and is less likely to cause PONV than etomidate. It allows the patient to quickly regain consciousness with minimal residual CNS effects, allowing for early extubation. Because propofol has no analgesic properties, postoperative analgesics will be required (Drain, 2013a).

Benzodiazepines are used as adjuncts to induction agents prior to cardiac surgery. Midazolam (Versed®) may also be used postoperatively for sedation in the patient who remains intubated. This agent can cause respiratory depression and mild vasodilation, but it minimizes PONV (Drain, 2013a). Nursing considerations include monitoring of vital signs and oxygen saturation. If severe, respiratory depression may be reversed by administering flumazenil (Romazicon®). The initial dose of flumazenil may be administered as 0.2 mg intravenous (IV) doses over 15 sec. If the initial dose is not effective, additional 0.2-mg doses may be administered over 1 minute. Additional doses may be administered over 1 minute after waiting 45 sec to determine if the drug is effective. The maximum amount of flumazenil that may be administered is 1 mg (Frandsen & Pennington, 2014).

Inhalation Agents

Inhalation agents cause circulatory depression and hypotension as a result of vasodilation and decreased contractility (Drain, 2013b). They may be administered either alone or in combination with intravenous anesthetics.

Nursing considerations include monitoring for ventricular ectopy, fibrillation, and tachycardia, which generally manifest during the immediate postoperative period. Inhalation agents typically do not possess analgesic properties. They are eliminated through the lungs; the amount of time it takes depends on the patient's CO. Patients will require oxygen therapy and encouragement to cough and deep breathe (Drain, 2013b). Hemodynamic monitoring is essential given the sensitization to catecholamines associated with many of these inhalation agents.

Because some of the inhalation agents are fat soluble and are absorbed into adipose tissue, elimination and recovery times are longer when these agents are given. Further, patients with higher percentages of body fat will have a longer recovery time when administered fat-soluble inhalation agents. Prompt management of pain and PONV are other vital ICU nursing responsibilities at this time (Drain, 2013b).

Sevoflurane and halothane have depressant effects on the respiratory system. Additionally, smooth bronchial muscles and laryngeal and pharyngeal reflexes are blunted by these agents, placing the patient at risk for aspiration. Sevoflurane and halothane side effects may include decreased responsiveness to oxygenation and ventilation and elevated carbon dioxide levels. Halothane decreases mucociliary function for as long as 6 hours, which increases the patient's risk for atelectasis and pneumonia. Its cardiovascular effects include myocardial depression and peripheral vasodilation. Two benefits of halothane are the associated low incidence of PONV and its bronchodilator properties, making this agent useful in patients with pulmonary disease. Sevoflurane does not appear to irritate the respiratory system or to sensitize the heart to catecholamines, although it may cause hypotension by decreasing afterload (Hudson, Herold, & Hemmings, 2013).

Enflurane and isoflurane may cause laryngospasm, coughing, and breath holding. These side effects predispose the patient to noncardiogenic pulmonary edema. Attributes of isoflurane include that it is not associated with increased cardiac sensitization to catecholamines, stabilizes the cardiovascular system, and has the least related increase in cerebral blood flow (Bojar, 2011).

Enflurane has residual CNS depressant effects, which manifest during the postoperative period. Other effects include decreased blood pressure, stroke volume, and SVR, and increased heart rate; this medication also sensitizes the heart to catecholamines. Enflurane causes mild coronary vasodilation and puts the patient at increased risk for development of junctional rhythms (Bojar, 2011). A benefit of enflurane is the low associated incidence of PONV (Drain, 2013b). Nursing considerations include anticipation of delayed awakening and extubation.

Isoflurane augments the effects of nondepolarizing muscle relaxants. It is a coronary artery vasodilator that is associated with increased coronary perfusion. Isoflurane and halothane can cause postoperative shivering, with an associated increase in myocardial oxygen demand (Drain, 2013b).

Neuromuscular Blocking Agents

Neuromuscular blocking agents (NMBAs) are used as adjuncts to inhalation agents to provide relaxation of skeletal muscles, facilitate intubation, and decrease shivering (Drain, 2013c). These agents are classified as either depolarizing or nondepolarizing agents. Neuromuscular blocking agents that are commonly administered during cardiac surgery include rocuronium, vecuronium, and succinylcholine. Succinylcholine is an example of a depolarizing NMBA; rocuronium and vecuronium are examples of nondepolarizing agents. They are short- to medium-acting agents, respectively. Rocuronium, cisatracurium, rapacuronium, and vecuronium have no cardiovascular side effects and, therefore, are useful in cardiac surgery. These agents are eliminated by the hepatic system (as opposed to the renal system) (Drain, 2013c). As a

consequence, their effects will be prolonged in patients with severe liver disease.

Return paralysis can occur during the early postoperative period. The ICU nurse should observe for a descending trend in minute ventilation, which can be caused by inadequate reversal of the NMBA. Nondepolarizing agents are reversed with anticholinesterase drugs (e.g., neostigmine [Prostigmin®]). Depolarizing NMBAs cannot be pharmacologically reversed because they are metabolized by pseudocholinesterase, an endogenous enzyme.

It is essential that the ICU nurse realize that NMBAs have no amnestic or analgesic properties, nor do they cause a loss of consciousness. Analgesics must be administered to the postoperative cardiac surgery patient despite the patient's inability to quantify pain levels (Hudson et al., 2013). Medications to achieve decreased level of consciousness or amnesia must similarly be administered if those effects are desired in the postoperative cardiac surgery patient.

Opioids

Intravenous opioids are used as analgesics or as induction agents. When administered, these medications decrease the response and perception to pain. The most frequently used opioid in cardiac surgery is fentanyl. Nursing considerations include monitoring for bradycardia, which may be treated with atropine or glycopyrrolate (Robinul®). Postoperative nausea and vomiting is a common side effect of opioids and is of clinical concern. Typically protocols include an order for an antiemetic.

POSTOPERATIVE CARE

Hemodynamic Management

The primary goal of care for the cardiac surgery patient in the immediate postoperative period is optimization of hemodynamic status to help achieve a balance between oxygen supply and demand. This goal can best be accomplished by maintaining an adequate CO.

As described in Chapter 9, CO is affected by a patient's preload, afterload, and contractility. Preload refers to the heart's filling pressures, reflected as the amount of volume returning to the right and left sides of the heart. It is evaluated by measuring CVP and PAOP, respectively. Afterload refers to the amount of work the heart must do to eject blood. Typically, left-sided afterload (SVR) is evaluated most often. These two parameters can be evaluated and manipulated by the ICU nurse to optimize a patient's hemodynamic profile.

Causes of alterations in preload in the postoperative cardiac surgery patient include vasodilation from a systemic inflammatory response associated with CPB procedures, medications, loss of vasomotor tone, vasodilation from rewarming, bleeding, third spacing from increased capillary permeability, and increased urinary output from hypothermia. Further, compliance of the left ventricle is often decreased following cardiac surgery from post-ischemic injury and myocardial stunning (Silvestry, 2014). Volume repletion is indicated for patients with decreased preload. The decision of whether to use crystalloids or colloids for fluid resuscitation remains unresolved given the pros and cons of each option. If volume resuscitation alone is inadequate to maintain filling pressures and CO in a patient who has adequate pump function and vasodilation, consideration should be given to adding an infusion of a vasopressor (e.g., phenylephrine [Neosynephrine®], vasopressin, methylene blue) (Silvestry, 2014). Methylene blue is an inhibitor of nitric oxide, which is released in large quantities in patients following CPB. Nitric oxide produces profound vasodilation and vasoplegia (hypotension with normal or high CO, low CVP, low PAOP, and low peripheral vascular resistance) (Skuza et al., 2009). Methylene blue is not U.S. Food and Drug Administration (FDA)–approved for the indication but is frequently used in the treatment of vasodilatory shock or vasoplegic

syndrome in the immediate postoperative CPB period (Lenglet, Mach, & Montecucco, 2011). Chapter 12 discusses vasopressor therapy in more detail.

An increase in afterload may be related to postoperative hypertension, use of medications that cause vasoconstriction, hypothermia, pain, anxiety, hypovolemia, or postoperative pump failure. Infusion of a vasodilator (e.g., sodium nitroprusside [Nipride®], clevidipine [Cleviprex®], nitroglycerin [Tridil®], esmolol [Brevibloc®], or nicardipine [Cardene®]) is indicated for patients who are hypertensive or who have inadequate pump function but with individual-specific normal blood pressure (Bojar, 2011). Increased afterload may result in decreased stroke volume and cardiac output and increased myocardial oxygen demand (Silvestry, 2014). Vasodilator therapy is discussed in more detail in Chapter 12.

A decrease in afterload may be caused by vasodilation from the CPB-associated systemic inflammatory response, administration of medications that cause vasodilation, or fever (Silvestry, 2014).

Once a patient's preload and afterload have been optimized, if CO is inadequate, administration of an inotropic agent to augment contractility may be considered. Agents such as milrinone (Primacor®) or dobutamine (Dobutrex®) increase CO by augmenting contractility and decrease afterload by causing vasodilation (Silvestry, 2014). Chapter 12 discusses inotropic agents in more detail.

As described in Chapter 13, although acceptable postoperative hemodynamic values will vary with the patient's cardiac history, optimal hemodynamic parameters in a postoperative cardiac surgery patient include a cardiac index of more than 2 L/min/m^2, PAOP of approximately 15 mmHg, CVP less than 15 mmHg, mean arterial pressure (MAP) more than 65 mmHg, systolic blood pressure (SBP) in the range of 90–140 mmHg, and systemic vascular resistance index in the range of 1,400–2,800 dyne/sec/cm^{-5}/m^2 (Bojar, 2011).

Alterations in Heart Rate and Rhythm

Postoperative dysrhythmias can be anticipated in the postoperative cardiac surgery patient. The most common dysrhythmias are atrial in origin; ventricular dysrhythmias and bradycardic rhythms are possible as well. Dysrhythmias may or may not manifest in the initial postoperative period. If present, however, dysrhythmias may cause hemodynamic instability. If the patient has a clinically significant dysrhythmia, then pharmacologic control of rate, rhythm, or both, may be indicated. Management of alterations in heart rate and rhythm is discussed in detail in Chapter 15.

Postoperative Nausea and Vomiting

Postoperative nausea and vomiting is a common occurrence in the immediate postoperative period, primarily due to the medications administered intraoperatively. Postoperative nausea and vomiting increases the risk of pulmonary aspiration, disrupts surgical repairs secondary to retching, increases postoperative bleeding, and causes electrolyte disturbances (e.g., hypokalemia, hyponatremia, hypochloremia), dehydration, and esophageal rupture and tears (O'Brien, 2013). Postoperative nausea and vomiting can be minimized by assessing for risk factors (e.g., age, gender, history of PONV or motion sickness, and use of volatile anesthetics and opioids) in the preoperative phase and by implementing preventive strategies utilizing a multimodal approach (see **Table 8-2**).

Administering prophylactic antiemetics that affect different receptor sites in the brain has been shown to decrease the incidence of PONV. Medications that may be used to treat PONV include ondansetron (Zofran®), promethazine (Phenergan®), and prochlorperazine (Compazine®). If PONV is not relieved following two doses of antiemetics, it should be reported to the anesthesia provider (O'Brien, 2013). If it is not contraindicated or if the cause of PONV is hypotension,

Table 8-2   Multimodal Management of Postoperative Nausea and Vomiting
Dexamethasone
5-HT3 receptor antagonists
H1 blockers
Scopolamine patch
Droperidol
NK1 antagonists
Hydration
Pain and comfort management

Source: Data from O'Brien, D. (2013). Postanesthesia care complications. In J. Odom-Forren (Ed.), *Drain's perianesthesia nursing: A critical care approach* (6th ed., pp. 394–414). St. Louis, MO: Elsevier Saunders.

hydration may also be effective in reducing the occurrence of PONV (Glick, 2014). Patients who are vomiting should be positioned to prevent aspiration (O'Brien, 2013).

Thermoregulation (Hypothermia)

According to American Society of PeriAnesthesia Nursing (ASPAN, 2006) standards, postoperative nursing considerations include the identification of patients at risk for hypothermia and application of passive and active warming devices (e.g., bonnet, cotton blankets, socks, forced air warming device). Patients are considered hypothermic if they have a temperature of less than 96.8 °F (36 °C) (ASPAN, 2006). Others define postoperative hypothermia as a core temperature of less than 95 °F (36 °C) (Karalapillai et al., 2011). Factors affecting the development of hypothermia include patient age, health status, surgical procedure, exposed body areas, duration of anesthesia or surgery, ambient room temperature, prepping and irrigation solutions, administration of cool IV fluids, and peripheral vascular disease (O'Brien, 2013).

The postoperative cardiac surgery patient should be monitored consistently until normothermia is achieved. Adjusting ambient room temperature or warming oxygen may also be beneficial (Hooper et al., 2009).

Attaining and maintaining postoperative normothermia is vital because inadvertent postoperative hypothermia has been linked to adverse effects. Overall, postoperative patients admitted from the OR with a core temperature less than 36 °C have prolonged mechanical ventilation, shivering, and increasing oxygen consumption. Hemodynamic effects of hypothermia include increased SVR and greater likelihood of developing dysrhythmias, hypertension, tachycardia, decreased preload, impaired contractility, or coronary graft spasm (Karalapillai et al., 2011; Nearman, Klick, Eisenberg, & Pesa, 2014).

Hypothermia alters drug metabolism, causing delays in patients' emergence from anesthesia. It also causes a disruption of the coagulation pathway, increasing the need for blood transfusions. Hypothermia leads to delays in wound healing, which increases susceptibility to surgical site infections, and shivering, which increases myocardial oxygen demand and consumption (Nearman et al., 2014).

Postoperative Respiratory Management

In addition to managing a patient's hemodynamic status, respiratory management is another pivotal role of the ICU nurse in the immediate postoperative cardiac surgery period. Unless the patient was "fast-tracked" and extubated in the OR, short-term mechanical ventilation is employed until anesthetic agents have been eliminated. Early extubation should be a goal for all patients.

Weaning and extubation protocols vary among facilities. Nevertheless, these processes are generally based on adequate muscle strength, pulmonary function, and hemodynamic stability (Bojar, 2011; Cartwright & Andrews, 2013). As discussed in Chapter 11, extubation criteria typically include presence of a heart rate less than 140, respiratory rate less than 25, normothermia, and absence of ischemia and infusion of vasoactive agents. The patient should be alert and cooperative (i.e., able to respond to commands).

Presence of a cough and gag reflex is important because the patient must be able to maintain a patent airway following extubation. The patient must also demonstrate adequate muscle strength by sustaining a head lift for at least 5 sec. Other weaning criteria include ability to breathe spontaneously and adequately while maintaining adequate oxygen saturation and ABG values. Physiologic parameters that may be measured to assess potential readiness for extubation include a negative inspiratory force (NIF) of at least 20-25 cmH_2O, minute volume no greater than 10 L/min, and vital capacity 10-15 mL/kg (Bauman & Hyzy, 2014; Bojar, 2011). Typically, cardiac surgery patients are extubated within 12 hours after their arrival in the ICU from the OR (Badhwar et al., 2014).

Upon determination that the patient is ready for extubation, the patient's mouth should be suctioned and the tube-securing device removed. The cuff on the endotracheal tube is deflated with a syringe. The presence of an air leak must then be ascertained; such a leak may be either heard or felt. The patient is instructed to take a deep breath and cough, with the tube being removed toward the end of the cough. Supplemental humidified oxygen is applied (Bojar, 2011). Placement on low-flow oxygen such as nasal cannula is common practice.

Stir-up Regimen

Cardiac surgery patients require the "stir-up regimen" in the immediate postoperative period if they received an inhalation agent as part of their anesthesia because these agents cause respiratory depression and are eliminated with ventilation. The stir-up regimen is accomplished by elevating the head of the bed and encouraging deep breathing and coughing at regular intervals. This practice facilitates movement of the inhalation agent from an area of higher concentration (the patient's lungs) to an area of lower concentration (room air), which is how the agent will be eliminated (Godden, 2012).

Complications Related to Extubation

Complications following extubation are fairly uncommon but may include laryngospasm, noncardiogenic pulmonary edema, bronchospasm, hypoventilation, and hypoxia.

Laryngospasm and Noncardiogenic Pulmonary Edema

Laryngospasm is a partial or total obstruction of air flow into and out of the lungs owing to spasms of the vocal cords (Al Ghofaily, Simmons, Chen, & Liu, 2013). Causes include aspiration, suctioning, and histamine release associated with some medications. Signs of laryngospasm include "rocking" respirations, wheezing, stridor, dyspnea, use of accessory muscles, and tachypnea. The patient should be encouraged to cough, as this action may be effective in eradicating a partial obstruction (O'Brien, 2013).

Patients can have laryngospasm during extubation, which can trigger noncardiogenic pulmonary edema. Noncardiogenic pulmonary edema occurs following an acute airway obstruction, such as when the patient forcefully inspires against a closed glottis, thereby creating an increase in intrathoracic pressure and resulting in pulmonary edema (Al Ghofaily et al., 2013). Protein and fluid accumulate and extravasate into the alveoli without an associated increase in PAOP (Nearman et al., 2014). Symptoms of this condition, which typically have a rapid onset, include agitation, tachypnea, tachycardia, decreased oxygen saturation, and pink, frothy sputum. Crackles will be audible.

Prompt recognition and treatment of both laryngospasm and noncardiogenic pulmonary edema are crucial; indeed, the patient may require reintubation until these problems resolve. Treatment of laryngospasm generally involves positive-pressure breathing with a bag-valve-mask device with 100% oxygen and mandibular support. If these measures prove ineffective, succinylcholine can be administered intravenously. Lidocaine may be effective in preventing a laryngospasm.

Noncardiogenic pulmonary edema management involves maintenance of a patent airway, supplemental oxygen, and administration of a diuretic. Mechanical ventilation with PEEP may be required in severe cases (O'Brien, 2013). Chest radiograph may reveal findings consistent with pulmonary edema. Treatment of noncardiogenic pulmonary edema includes supplemental oxygen, respiratory support, and diuretics (O'Brien, 2013).

Bronchospasm

Bronchospasm can occur as a result of constriction of bronchial smooth muscles after extubation. It resolves quickly after airway irritants are eliminated. Symptoms include wheezing, dyspnea, and tachypnea. Treatment involves administration of a bronchodilator and humidified oxygen. In severe cases, muscle relaxants, lidocaine, epinephrine, or hydrocortisone may be administered to relax the airway (O'Brien, 2013).

Hypoventilation and Hypoxia

Hypoventilation is common in the immediate postoperative period. It may result from the anesthetic agents administered or the surgical procedure itself. Treatment entails eradicating the underlying cause. If the underlying cause is related to opioid administration, then treatment may include administration of naloxone (Narcan®) for patients with shallow or slow respirations. Institutional policy varies regarding use of opioid antagonists (O'Brien, 2013).

Hypoxemia is defined as an oxygen saturation less than 90%. Hypoxemia can have numerous undesired sequelae, including cardiac dysrhythmias and myocardial ischemia. Signs and symptoms may include cyanosis, agitation, somnolence, tachycardia, bradycardia, hypertension, and hypotension. Depending on the severity of the symptoms or hypoxemia, reintubation and mechanical ventilation may be required (O'Brien, 2013).

Inadequate reversal of NMBAs' effects can cause hypoventilation and hypoxia after extubation. Extubation of a patient who is partially paralyzed increases the individual's risk of developing postoperative complications. Residual respiratory muscle weakness can cause airway obstruction, hypoventilation, and an impaired response to hypoxia. Cardiac surgery patients are at increased risk if they receive a long-acting NMBA whose action is inadequately reversed with anticholinesterase agents. Re-paralysis can occur when an NMBA has a longer half-life than the reversal agents. If this problem occurs, the patient will demonstrate weak, shallow respirations and poor chest rise; anxiety and restlessness may become apparent as well. Treatment involves administration of additional doses of a reversal agent, respiratory support, and temporary reintubation until muscle strength is regained.

During weaning and extubation, opioids should be used judiciously. Opioids decrease respiratory effort, oxygen saturation, and respiratory rate and depth. Pain management is of concern; however, small doses of short-acting analgesics (e.g., dexmedetomidine [Precedex™]) may be recommended (Bojar, 2011). Complications that arise after extubation can be minimized by recognizing and treating respiratory emergencies and by adhering to weaning and extubation criteria (Bojar, 2011).

POTENTIAL POSTOPERATIVE COMPLICATIONS

The ICU nurse plays a pivotal role in preventing or promptly identifying and treating postoperative complications. Among the more common complications seen in the immediate postoperative period are hemodynamic compromise, respiratory insufficiency, neurologic issues, and hematological problems. Some complications are related to patient comorbidities; others are related to the surgical procedure itself. These complications and the associated ICU nursing responsibilities

are discussed in detail in Chapters 13 and 16. Potential complications related to effects of anesthesia are addressed in this section. One unique complication related to the surgical procedure is covered here as well.

Malignant Hyperthermia

Malignant hyperthermia (MH) is a genetic, life-threatening disorder that is triggered by certain anesthetic agents, depolarizing skeletal muscle relaxants, and stress. With this condition, a defect in the sarcoplasmic reticulum leads to a buildup of excess calcium in the mycoplasma. This results in sustained skeletal muscle contraction that is intense and prolonged, leading to a hypermetabolic state of heat production.

The onset of MH usually occurs during induction of anesthetic agents. Halothane, enflurane, isoflurane, desflurane, and succinylcholine are the most common triggering agents. The triggering of events is characterized by muscle rigidity of the jaw (masseter rigidity), tachypnea, tachycardia, elevated CO_2 level, cyanosis, respiratory and metabolic acidosis, elevated serum creatine phosphokinase (CPK), and hyperkalemia. Late signs include temperature elevation, bleeding from venipuncture sites, and rhabdomyolysis. Malignant hyperthermia typically manifests in the OR but it can develop within 24 hours postoperatively (O'Brien, 2013).

Treatment of MH includes discontinuance of triggering agents and immediate intravenous administration of dantrolene sodium (Dantrium®) 2.5 mg/kg (up to a maximum dose of 10 mg/kg). Dantrolene inhibits the release of calcium. Once the loading dose is administered, dantrolene is infused at a dose of 1 mg/kg every 4 hours for at least 48 hours (McAuley, 2012). Hyperventilation, administration of 100% oxygen, body surface area cooling, administration of sodium bicarbonate, maintenance of fluid and electrolyte balance, and treatment of associated conditions (e.g., hypertension, dysrhythmias) are also essential interventions in the setting of MH.

Lab data that may be obtained include ABG, serum electrolytes, liver enzymes, renal function studies, blood counts, and coagulation profile (Hooper, 2013; Kaplow, 2013; O'Brien, 2013). Effective management involves prompt recognition, guidance of the multidisciplinary team, and expert direction from the Malignant Hyperthermia Association of the United States (MHAUS).

Pseudocholinesterase Deficiency

Prolonged mechanical ventilation after cardiac surgery may be caused by a deficiency in pseudocholinesterase. A small percentage of patients lack this enzyme, which is responsible for metabolizing medications such as succinylcholine. Patients with pseudocholinesterase deficiency who receive these medications exhibit prolonged responses to these medications, can have sustained skeletal muscle paralysis, and remain apneic for as long as 48 hours after administration. Management involves emotional support and mechanical ventilation until the effects of the medication are completely eliminated (Kaplow, 2013).

Protamine Sulfate Allergic Reactions

Protamine sulfate is administered as a reversal agent for heparin. If it is given too rapidly,

severe hypotension and anaphylactic reactions may result. Consequently, caution should be used when administering protamine sulfate to patients who may be at increased risk of allergic reaction—specifically, individuals who have previously undergone procedures such as coronary angioplasty or CPB, diabetics who have been treated with protamine insulin, patients who are allergic to fish, and men who have had a vasectomy or are infertile and may have antibodies to protamine. Patients undergoing prolonged procedures involving repeated doses of protamine should be subject to careful monitoring of clotting parameters. A rebound bleeding effect may occur as long as 18 hours postoperatively (Bojar, 2011). Protamine sulfate reactions are discussed in more detail in Chapter 12.

SUMMARY

Although much progress has been made with respect to the postoperative care of the cardiac surgery patient, critical thinking and caring practices of the ICU nurse are primary determinants of positive outcomes. The initial hours following cardiac surgery are tenuous. The patient's preoperative status, the intraoperative course, and the effects of anesthesia all contribute to the complexity of the patient's profile.

CASE STUDY

A 72-year-old patient with a history of ST-segment elevation myocardial infarction (STEMI) involving the inferior wall, diabetes, hyperlipidemia, and mitral regurgitation underwent mitral valve repair. His intraoperative course was uneventful. He received succinylcholine and enflurane as part of his general anesthesia. He is admitted to the cardiovascular ICU postoperatively. His admitting ABG results are as follows: pH 7.20, pCO_2 46, pO_2 63, O_2 sat 90%, HCO_3 18. His initial vital signs are: BP 140/92, HR 112, RR 26.

Critical Thinking Questions

1. What is a plausible explanation for this patient's admitting vital signs and ABG results?
2. What are the patient's risk factors for developing this condition?
3. What interventions should the ICU nurse anticipate?

Answers to Critical Thinking Questions

1. This patient is manifesting signs and symptoms of malignant hyperthermia. He has tachycardia and tachypnea, and has a respiratory and metabolic acidosis on his ABG.

2. He received succinylcholine and enflurane during general anesthesia. Both of these agents are triggers for the development of malignant hyperthermia.

3. The nurse should obtain the malignant hyperthermia cart and anticipate reconstituting and administering dantrolene sodium. The patient should be hyperventilated with 100% oxygen (either from the ventilator or with bag-valve-tube). As the patient's temperature is likely elevated, cooling should begin. The patient should have electrolytes obtained (to monitor for hyperkalemia).

SELF-ASSESSMENT QUESTIONS

1. Initial management of hypertension immediately following cardiac surgery may entail use of which of the following?
   a. Beta blocker
   b. Calcium channel blocker
   c. Opioid
   d. Angiotensin-converting enzyme inhibitor

2. A postoperative cardiac surgery patient develops the following vital signs: BP 78/50, HR 118, CVP 18 mmHg, CO 3.2 L/minute. A low-voltage QRS complex is noted on the cardiac monitor. The drainage from the mediastinal chest tube has dramatically decreased in the past hour. Which of the following should the nurse suspect?
   a. Acute coronary syndrome
   b. Hypovolemia
   c. Cardiac tamponade
   d. Cardiogenic shock

3. A patient develops cardiac tamponade following cardiac surgery. Which of the following should the nurse initially anticipate?
   a. Administration of fluids
   b. Preparation for pericardiocentesis
   c. Titration of vasopressors
   d. Performing a 12-lead ECG

4. A cardiac surgery patient received etomidate while in the operating room. Which of the following should the ICU anticipate?
   a. Emergence delirium
   b. Decreased cardiac output
   c. Involuntary tremors
   d. Increased adrenal function

5. A cardiac surgery patient received isoflurane in the operating room. For which of the following should the nurse observe?
   a. Noncardiogenic pulmonary edema
   b. Increased sensitization
   c. Hypercarbia
   d. Laryngospasm

6. Patients who receive opioids in the operating room should be observed for which of the following?

a.

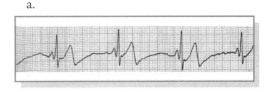

b.

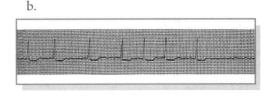

c.

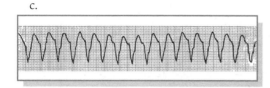

d.

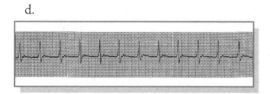

7. A cardiac surgery patient is admitted directly from the operating room. Initial temperature was 35.8 °C (96.4 °F). Which of the following should the nurse anticipate?
   a. SVR 900 dynes/sec/cm^{-5}
   b. BP 88/50
   c. CVP 9 mmHg
   d. HR 120

8. Which of the following is a potential effect of postoperative hypothermia?
   a. Decreased myocardial consumption
   b. Increased infection risk
   c. Increased clot formation
   d. Decreased need for transfusions

9. Post-extubation, a patient develops "rocking" respirations, tachypnea, stridor, and use of accessory muscles. The initial nursing intervention should be to:
   a. Prepare for reintubation
   b. Suction the oropharynx
   c. Encourage the patient to cough
   d. Administer a short-acting neuromuscular blocking agent

10. A patient received halothane as part of induction to anesthesia. Upon admission to the ICU, the patient has a temperature of 39 °C (102.2 °F). Which of the following should the ICU nurse perform initially?
   a. Begin cooling the patient
   b. Administer dantrolene sodium
   c. Hyperventilate with 100% oxygen
   d. Treat associated dysrhythmias

Answers to Self-Assessment Questions

1. c	6. a
2. c	7. d
3. a	8. b
4. c	9. c
5. a	10. c

Clinical Inquiry Box

Question: What are the experiences of patients who undergo cardiopulmonary bypass who develop postoperative abdominal complications?

Reference: Dong, G., Liu, C., Biao, X., Jing, H., Li, D., & Wu, H. (2012). Postoperative abdominal complications after cardiopulmonary bypass. *Journal of Cardiothoracic Surgery, 7,* 108. Retrieved from http://www.cardiothoracicsurgery.org/content/7/1/108

Objective: To determine the experiences of patients who undergo cardiopulmonary bypass who develop postoperative abdominal complications.

Method: Retrospective review of 2,349 consecutive patients.

Results: Of the 2,349 patients who underwent cardiopulmonary bypass, 33% developed gastrointestinal (GI) complications. These complications included paralytic ileus, GI hemorrhage, gastroduodenal ulcer perforation, acute cholecystitis, hepatic dysfunction, and ischemic bowel. There were five deaths. Risk factors for GI complications that were identified included history of peptic ulcer, advanced age, poor cardiac function, preoperative support with an intra-aortic balloon pump, prolonged CPB time, low cardiac output, and prolonged mechanical ventilation.

Conclusion: There was a low incidence of GI complications following CPB surgery but a higher mortality rate in those patients who experienced them. Early recognition and prompt intervention are pivotal for optimal patient outcomes.

REFERENCES

Al Ghofaily, L., Simmons, C., Chen, L., & Liu, R. (2013). Negative pressure pulmonary edema after laryngospasm: A revisit with a case report. *Journal of Anesthesia & Clinical Research, 3*(10), 252.

American Society of PeriAnesthesia Nurses. (2006). *Standards of perianesthesia nursing practice.* Cherry Hill, NJ: Author.

Aronson, S., Dyke, C. M., Levy, J. H., Cheung, A. T., Lumb, P. D., Avery, E. G., . . . Newman, M. F. (2011). Does perioperative systolic blood pressure variability predict mortality after cardiac surgery? An exploratory analysis of the ECLIPSE trials. *Anesthesia & Analgesia, 113*(1), 19–30.

Badhwar, V., Esper, S., Brooks, M., Mulukutla, S., Hardison, R., Mallios, D., . . . Subramaniam, K. (2014). Extubating in the operating room following adult cardiac surgery safely improves outcomes and lowers costs. *The Journal of Thoracic and Cardiovascular Surgery, 148*(6), 3103–3109.

Bauman, K., & Hyzy, R. (2014). *Extubation management.* Retrieved from http://www.uptodate.com/contents/extubation-management?source=machineLearning&search=extubation+cardiac+surgery&selectedTitle=1%7E150&sectionRank=2&anchor=H2#H2

Bojar, R. (2011). Cardiovascular management. In R. Bojar (Ed.), *Manual of perioperative care in adult cardiac surgery* (5th ed). Hoboken, NJ: Blackwell.

Cartwright, S., & Andrews, S. (2013). Perianesthesia nursing as a specialty. In J. Odom-Forren (Ed.), *Drain's perianesthesia nursing: A critical care approach* (6th ed., pp. 9–17). St. Louis, MO: Elsevier Saunders.

Drain, C. B. (2013a). Non-opioid intravenous anesthetics. In J. Odom-Forren (Ed.), *Drain's perianesthesia nursing: A critical care approach* (6th ed., pp. 265–277). St. Louis, MO: Elsevier Saunders.

Drain, C. B. (2013b). Inhalation agents. In J. Odom-Forren (Ed.), *Drain's perianesthesia nursing: A critical care approach* (6th ed., pp. 253–264). St. Louis, MO: Elsevier Saunders.

Drain, C. B. (2013c). Neuromuscular blocking agents. In J. Odom-Forren (Ed.), *Drain's perianesthesia nursing: A critical care approach* (6th ed., pp. 291–310). St. Louis, MO: Elsevier Saunders.

Faulk, S. A., Fleisher, L. A., Jones, S. B., & Nussmeier, N. A. (2014). Overview of anesthesia and anesthetic choices. Retrieved from http://www.uptodate.com/contents/overview-of-anesthesia-and-anesthetic-choices?source=machineLearning&search=anesthetic+agents&selectedTitle=1%7E150&sectionRank=1&anchor=H6#H28

Frandsen, G., & Pennington, S. S. (2014). Drug therapy with general anesthetics. In G. Frandsen & S. S. Pennington (Eds.), *Abrahms' clinical drug therapy: Rationales for nursing practice* (10th ed., pp. 915–933). Philadelphia, PA: Lippincott Williams & Wilkins.

Gil-Gomez, R., Blasco-Alonso, J., Reyes, J., Gonzalez-Correa, J., De La Cruz, J., & Milano, G. (2014). Post-operative systemic inflammatory response after cardiac surgery using extracorporeal circulation in children. *Experimental & Clinical Cardiology, 20*(6), 3906–3919.

Glick, D. (2014). *Overview of complications occurring in the post-anesthesia care unit.* Retrieved from http://www.uptodate.com/contents/overview-of-complications-occurring-in-the-post-anesthesia-care-unit?source=machineLearning&search=cardiac+surgery+care&selectedTitle=5%7E150&sectionRank=1&anchor=H1324456782#H1324456782

Go, A. S., Mozaffarian, D., Roger, V. L., Benjamin, E. J., Berry, J. D., Blaha, M. J., . . . Turner, M. B. (2014). Heart disease and stroke statistics—2014 update: A report from the American Heart Association. *Circulation, 129*(3), e28–e292.

Godden, B. (2012). Airway issues. In D. Stannard & D. Krenzischek (Eds.), *PeriAnesthesia nursing care: A bedside guide for safe recovery* (pp. 20–28). Burlington, MA: Jones & Bartlett Learning.

Gutsche, J. T., Erickson, L., Ghadimi, K., Augoustides, J. G., Dimartino, J., Szeto, W. Y., & Ochroch, E. A. (2014). Advancing extubation time for cardiac surgery patients using lean work design. *Journal of Cardiothoracic and Vascular Anesthesia, 8*(6), 1490–1496.

Hooper, V. D. (2013). Care of the patient with thermal imbalance. In J. Odom-Forren (Ed.), *Drain's perianesthesia nursing: A critical care approach* (6th ed., pp. 740–750). St. Louis, MO: Elsevier Saunders.

Hooper, V. D., Chard, R., Clifford, T., Fetzer, S., Fossum, S., Godden, B., . . . Ross, J. (2009). ASPAN's evidence-based clinical practice guideline for the promotion of perioperative normothermia. *Journal of PeriAnesthesia Nursing, 24*(5), 271–287.

Hudson, A. E., Herold, K. F., & Hemmings Jr., H. C. (2013). Pharmacology of inhaled anesthetics. In H. C. Hemmings, Jr. & T. D. Egan (Eds.), *Pharmacology and physiology for anesthesia: Foundations and clinical application* (pp. 159–179). Philadelphia, PA: Elsevier Saunders.

Kaplow, R. (2013). Safety of patients transferred from the operating room to the intensive care unit. *Critical Care Nurse, 33*(1), 68–70.

Karalapillai, D., Story, D., Hart, G. K., Bailey, M., Pilcher, D., Cooper, D. J., . . . Bellomo, R. (2011). Postoperative hypothermia and patient outcomes after elective cardiac surgery. *Anaesthesia, 66*(9), 780–784.

Landis, R. C., Murkin, J. M., Stump, D. A., Baker, R. A., Arrowsmith, J. E., De Somer, F., . . . Westaby, S. (2010). Consensus statement: Minimal criteria for reporting the systemic inflammatory response to cardiopulmonary bypass. *The Heart Surgery Forum, 13*(2), E116–E123.

Lenglet, S., Mach, F., & Montecucco, F. (2011). Methylene blue: Potential use of an antique molecule in vasoplegic syndrome during cardiac surgery. *Expert Review of Cardiovascular Therapy, 9*(12), 1519–1525.

McAuley, D. (2012). *Dantrolene-Dantrium®*. Retrieved from http://www.globalrph.com/dantrolene_dilution.htm

Morin, J. F., Mistry, B., Langlois, Y., Ma, F., Chamoun, P., & Holcroft, C. (2011). Fluid overload after coronary artery bypass grafting surgery increases the incidence of post-operative complications. *World Journal of Cardiovascular Surgery, 1*, 18.

Nearman, H., Klick, J. C., Eisenberg, P., & Pesa, N. (2014). Perioperative complications of cardiac surgery and postoperative care. *Critical Care Clinics, 30*(3), 527–555.

O'Brien, D. (2013). Postanesthesia care complications. In J. Odom-Forren (Ed.), *Drain's anesthesia nursing: A critical care approach* (6th ed., pp. 394–414). St. Louis, MO: Elsevier Saunders.

Reid, D., Collins, M., Rosalion, A., Newcomb, A., Yii, M., Nixon, I., . . . Dixon, B. (2011). Chest tube bleeding has a dose dependent relationship with hemodynamic features of cardiac tamponade and mortality following cardiac surgery. *American Journal of Respiratory and Critical Care Medicine, 183*, A3162.

Salhiyyah, K., Elsobky, S., Raja, S., Attia, R., Brazier, J., & Cooper, G. J. (2011). A clinical and economic evaluation of fast-track recovery after cardiac surgery. *The Heart Surgery Forum, 14*(6), E330–E334.

Sanders, J., Toor, I. S., Yurik, T. M., Keogh, B. E., Mythen, M., & Montgomery, H. E. (2011). Tissue oxygen saturation and outcome after cardiac surgery. *American Journal of Critical Care, 20*(2), 138–145.

Silvestry, F. E. (2014). *Postoperative complications among patients undergoing cardiac surgery.* Retrieved from http://www.uptodate.com/contents/postoperative-complications-among-patients-undergoing-cardiac-surgery?source=search_result&search=cardiac+surgery&selectedTitle=1%7E150

Skuza, K., Chmielniak, S., Dzluk, W., Kucewicz, E., Pawlak, S., & Knapik, P. (2009). Methylene blue therapy for vasoplegia after cardiac surgery. *Anaesthesiology Intensive Therapy, 341*(3), 129–132.

Tembelopoulos, K., Carr, J., & Tressy-Murphy, C. (2012). Emergence agitation: What it is and what we can do? *Journal of PeriAnesthesia Nursing, 27*(3), e24.

WEB RESOURCES

Dr. Bernadine Healy takes a tour of the hospital. The operating room is a virtual beehive during heart surgery and afterward in the intensive care unit: https://www.youtube.com/watch?v=9xx8PX77fOY

Cardiac tamponade: https://www.youtube.com/watch?v=C87TgEAMVOs

Postoperative Complications of Cardiac Surgery: https://www.youtube.com/watch?v=cUuFrd3iz88

Chapter 9

Hemodynamic Monitoring

Mary Zellinger

INTRODUCTION

Hemodynamic monitoring of the patient after cardiac surgery is a routine part of the immediate postoperative care. Data obtained during this period guide the clinician in initiating the optimal intervention to ensure a smooth recovery. Hemodynamics, or the study of the dynamics of blood circulation, can be assessed through both invasive and noninvasive mechanisms; the ultimate goal is to determine the adequacy of cardiac output (CO; the amount of blood ejected by the heart each minute). This chapter reviews the essentials of hemodynamic monitoring

in the patient who has undergone cardiac surgery. Both basic and newer technologies are discussed.

ESSENTIALS OF HEMODYNAMIC MONITORING

Monitoring assists in determining changes in fluid status and cardiac performance at the earliest possible time so that treatment fluctuations in three factors that affect cardiac output—preload, afterload, and contractility (see **Box 9-1**)—can be quickly addressed.

Box 9-1 Hemodynamic Monitoring Terms and Definitions

Preload: The volume of blood either in the right atrium or in the left ventricle at the end of diastole or the beginning of systole. Preload is quantified with central venous pressure (CVP) and pulmonary artery occlusive pressure (PAOP), respectively; these parameters reflect a patient's volume status. The end-diastolic volume (EDV) is related to the amount of stretch of the sarcomeres. Preload is a reflection of all of the elements that affect tension of the chamber wall at the end of filling (diastole).

Afterload: The amount of work the heart must do to eject blood; the impedance or resistance to ventricular contraction. Afterload reflects all of the elements that affect tension of the myocardial wall during systole.

Contractility: The ability of the myocardial muscle to shorten itself or the amount of strength produced by the myocardium when it ejects blood. It is influenced by neural factors and certain metabolic states (e.g., hypoxia, hypercarbia, or decrease in pH).

Cardiac output: The amount of blood ejected by the heart each minute.

Sources: Data from Dunn, J. M., & Heupler, F. (2013). Cardiac output. In S. Anwaruddin, J. M. Martin, J. C. Stephens, & A. T. Askari (Eds.), *Cardiovascular hemodynamics* (pp. 65–76). New York, NY: Springer; Sabe, M., & Heupler, F. (2013). Contractility. In S. Anwaruddin, J. M. Martin, J. C. Stephens, & A. T. Askari (Eds.), *Cardiovascular hemodynamics* (pp. 53–64). New York, NY: Springer;

Continued

Box 9-1   Hemodynamic Monitoring Terms and Definitions (*Continued*)

Vest. A. R., & Heupler, F. (2013a). Afterload. In S. Anwaruddin, J. M. Martin, J. C. Stephens, & A. T. Askari (Eds.), *Cardiovascular hemodynamics* (pp. 29–52). New York, NY: Springer; and Vest, A. R., & Heupler, F. (2013b). Preload. In S. Anwaruddin, J. M. Martin, J. C. Stephens, & A. T. Askari (Eds.), *Cardiovascular hemodynamics* (pp. 3–28). New York, NY: Springer.

New monitoring devices and techniques are introduced annually to the critical care arena, each of which has the goal of increasing accuracy and decreasing invasiveness of monitoring. It is imperative for the clinician to incorporate data from a variety of sources when assessing the hemodynamic picture so as not to rely on a single—and potentially misleading—parameter.

INITIAL POSTOPERATIVE ASSESSMENT

Following cardiac surgery, the intensive care unit (ICU) nurse will connect the patient to the bedside monitor upon receipt from the operating room (OR). The electrocardiogram (ECG) leads are connected to the bedside monitor from the transport monitor, and heart rate and rhythm are assessed. The pulse oximetry probe is connected to the finger, earlobe, or forehead. Pulse oximetry is a simple, noninvasive method of monitoring the percentage of hemoglobin that is saturated with oxygen. The target oxygen saturation (SpO_2) is 95% or greater in a patient without a history of chronic obstructive pulmonary disease (COPD).

Preparing Hemodynamic Equipment

After elevating the head of the bed (HOB), the transducers are leveled at the phlebostatic axis, which is located at the fourth intercostal space, midpoint of the anterior-posterior diameter (see Figure 7-7 in Chapter 7). The transducers are then zero-balanced, establishing atmospheric pressure as zero. Leveling at the phlebostatic axis is performed to eradicate the effects of hydrostatic forces on the hemodynamic pressures (American Association of Critical-Care Nurses, 2011). Cardiac pressures may be accurately obtained with the HOB elevated up to 60 degrees if the patient's legs are parallel to the floor (Rauen, Flynn, & Bridges, 2009). A square wave test is performed to ensure responsiveness (see **Box 9-2** and Figure 9-1). Proper setup

Box 9-2   Square Wave Test

A square wave test (also referred to as a fast flush or dynamic response test) is performed to assure that the waveforms that appear on the monitoring screen accurately reflect pulmonary artery pressures (American Association of Critical-Care Nurses [AACN], 2011). It is accomplished by pulling and releasing the pigtail or squeezing the button of the flush device so that the flow through the tubing is increased (from 3 mL/hr obtained with a pressure bag inflated to 300 mmHg). This causes a sudden rise in pressure in the system, such that a square wave is generated on the monitor oscilloscope. An acceptable response is the pressure waveform reverting to baseline within one to two oscillations. If the response is lacking in shape, amplitude, or time to return to baseline, the intensive care unit (ICU) nurse should troubleshoot the system until an acceptable response is achieved (Lockhart, 2007). If an underdamped or overdamped waveform is present, hemodynamic measurements will not be accurate. It is recommended that a square wave test (see **Figure 9-1**) be

Box 9-2   Square Wave Test (*Continued*)

performed when the system is being initially set up, at least once a shift, after opening the catheter system (e.g., for rezeroing, blood sampling, or changing tubing), and whenever the pressure waveform appears to be damped or distorted (AACN, 2011).

An overdamped waveform is sluggish and has an exaggerated or falsely widened and blunt tracing. It will cause the patient's systolic blood pressure (SBP) to be recorded as falsely low and the diastolic blood pressure (DBP) to be recorded as falsely high. Causes of an overdamped waveform include the presence of large bubbles in the system, loose connections, no or low fluid in the flush bag, low pressure of the flush solution pressure bag, or a kink in the catheter (AACN, 2011) (see **Figure 9-2**).

An underdamped waveform consists of an overresponse, which is seen as an exaggerated, narrow, artificially peaked tracing. In this case, the waveform overestimates the patient's SBP and underestimates the DBP. Causes of an underdamped waveform include the presence of small bubbles in the system, the pressure tubing being too long, or a defective transducer (AACN, 2011) (see **Figure 9-3**).

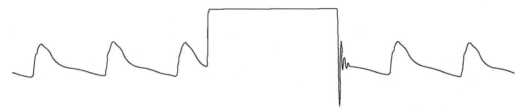

Figure 9-1 Square wave test.
Source: Illustrated by James R. Perron.

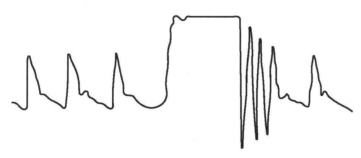

Figure 9-2 Overdamped waveform.
Source: Illustrated by James R. Perron.

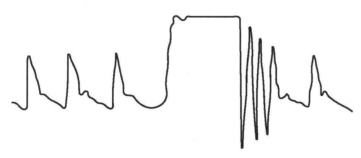

Figure 9-3 Underdamped waveform.
Source: Illustrated by James R. Perron.

and functioning of the monitoring system itself are essential to obtain accurate values, regardless of the specific parameter being measured. A number of variables—such as the number of stopcocks, the length of the tubing, the responsiveness of the tubing, and the presence of air bubbles—can influence the accuracy of the readings.

Vital Signs and Hemodynamic Assessment

An initial assessment of vital signs and hemodynamic parameters (see **Box 9-3**) is obtained, ensuring that the latter are assessed at end-expiration. Readings are obtained at this point in the respiratory cycle to eliminate the effects of changes in intrathoracic pressure that occur with breathing (Arora, Singh, Goudra, & Sinha, 2014). The frequency of obtaining subsequent sets of vital signs and hemodynamic parameters varies by facility and according to the patient's clinical status. It is imperative to obtain the patient's baseline and hemodynamic status from the OR during hand-off report, which includes the cardiac surgeon/resident, cardiac anesthesiologist,

---

Box 9-3   Hemodynamic Parameters and Normal Values

Parameters	Normal Values
Systolic and diastolic blood pressure	100–130/60–90 mmHg
Mean arterial pressure	70–105 mmHg
Right atrial pressure (central venous pressure)	0–8 mmHg
Right ventricular pressure	25–30/0–8 mmHg
Pulmonary artery pressure	15–30/6–12 mmHg
Pulmonary artery occlusive pressure	4–12 mmHg
Derived Hemodynamic Parameters	
Cardiac output/cardiac index	4–8 L/min / 2.5–4.2 L/min/m^2
Systemic vascular resistance	770–1,500 dynes/sec/cm^{-5}
Pulmonary vascular resistance	20–120 dynes/sec/cm^{-5}
Systemic vascular resistance index	1,680–2,580 dynes/sec/cm^{-5}
Pulmonary vascular resistance index	69–177 dynes/sec/cm^{-5}
Stroke volume/index	60–130 mL/beat / 30–65 mL/beat/m^2
Right ventricular stroke work	8–16 gm-m/beat
Right ventricular stroke work index	5–10 gm-m/m^2/beat
Left ventricular stroke work	58–104 gm-m/beat
Left ventricular stroke work index	50–62 gm-m/m^2/beat
Oxygenation Parameters	
Arterial oxygen saturation	95–100%
Mixed venous oxygen saturation	60–80%
Arterial oxygen content	17–20 mL/dL
Venous oxygen content	12–15 mL/dL
Oxygen delivery	900–1,150 mL/min
Oxygen consumption	200–290 mL/min
Oxygen extraction ratio	22–30%

Sources: Data from Blount, K. (2007). Hemodynamic monitoring. In R. Kaplow & S. R. Hardin (Eds.), *Critical care nursing: Synergy for optimal outcomes* (pp. 139–159). Sudbury, MA: Jones and Bartlett; and McCleaster, S., & Heuer, A. J. (2010). Review existing data in patient's record. In C. L. Scanlan, A. J. Heuer, & L. M. Sinopoli (Eds.), *Certified respiratory therapist's exam: Review guide* (pp. 43–60). Sudbury, MA: Jones and Bartlett.

Box 9-4   Postoperative Cardiac Surgery Initial Admission Responsibilities

Assessment of Chest Drainage System
- Connect chest drainage system to suction.
- Note and record the amount of drainage from the OR. Correlate these findings with the patient's baseline hemodynamic profile.

Assessment of Fluid Status
- Compare intraoperative intake and output with baseline hemodynamic profile and vital signs to help determine fluid volume status.

Diagnostics
- Obtain lab samples per protocol (e.g., electrolytes, arterial blood gas [ABG], complete blood count [CBC], coagulation profile) and other diagnostic procedures (e.g., 12-lead ECG) to check for potential intraoperative or postoperative ischemia, chest radiograph to verify endotracheal tube and central line placement and assess for presence/degree of pneumothorax or pulmonary congestion).

ICU medical provider, and bedside registered nurse (RN). Knowing the trends and status of the hemodynamics from the past several hours will help guide the management in the ICU.

Depending on unit-specific protocols and, perhaps, healthcare provider order, in addition to baseline hemodynamic values, CO/cardiac index (CI) may be measured. From CO/CI and invasive pressure data, several hemodynamic calculations can be performed, yielding valuable information about cardiac performance.

The ICU nurse will check the vasoactive drips and other fluids infusing to verify their type, infusion status, and dosages. The relationships among the amount of volume infused and lost in the OR, baseline postoperative vital signs, and hemodynamic status are assessed. Setting monitor alarm limits specific to the patient's baseline profile and ensuring these alarms are activated are crucial at this stage.

Patient Assessment

A complete baseline physical assessment is then completed. While the primary nurse is performing the baseline assessment, a number of concomitant essential activities related to the patient's hemodynamic status are performed. These activities are listed in **Box 9-4**.

A comprehensive head-to-toe assessment will enable the nurse to evaluate several indices to determine the overall adequacy of perfusion. A complete neurological assessment may prove challenging if the patient has not been reversed from general anesthesia or is receiving a continuous infusion of an anesthetic agent or sedation. Some hospital protocols require the anesthetic agent or sedation infusion be weaned and temporarily discontinued in the immediate postoperative period so that appropriate neurological function can be confirmed. The infusion can then be restarted until the ventilator weaning process begins. An awake and alert patient is one indicator of adequacy of CO. More often now, most hospital protocols encourage lighter sedation so that the patient is comfortable but arousable. If the patient is receiving a sedative, it is one that has little to no impact on respiratory effort so that continuous assessment for ventilator weaning is possible.

Extremity movement, warm skin, and palpable pulses indicate acceptable perfusion, unless obstructive peripheral vascular disease is present and limits perfusion to the distal extremities. Assessment of heart sounds provides additional information about cardiac function and any valve dysfunction. The presence of extra heart sounds, although normal in certain situations, warrants further investigation. An S3 or S4 heart sound may be a sign of decreased ventricular compliance. The presence or sudden absence of murmurs may indicate changes in native or prosthetic valve function. Placing the HOB between 30 and 45 degrees and observing for jugular vein distention will reinforce other findings of right-sided heart failure or fluid overload.

Breath sounds should be auscultated in all fields, noting any areas that are diminished or abnormal. Pulmonary congestion may be indicative of pulmonary dysfunction from the surgical process, be the effect of complications from mechanical ventilation, or occur as a result of cardiac dysfunction. In addition, transfusion-related acute lung injury (TRALI) from numerous intraoperative transfusions may develop.

Urinary output is another indication of adequacy of cardiac output, although it may sometimes misrepresent the adequacy of perfusion to the kidneys. Postoperatively, cardiac surgery patients should be evaluated for renal insufficiency if urinary output is less than 0.5 mL/kg/hr for 2 to 3 consecutive hours and serum creatinine levels are increasing (Kolh, 2009). Given that cardiac surgery patients may exhibit a relative diuresis of 200–400 mL/hr owing to the effects of hemodilution and osmotic agents sometimes administered during cardiopulmonary bypass (CPB) as well as elevated levels of atrial natriuretic peptide

(Walker & Butterworth, 2008), urinary output may not be indicative of perfusion for the first several hours after the surgery. Following the initial few hours postoperatively, urinary output should be at least 0.5 mL/kg/hr.

BLOOD PRESSURE MONITORING

In the immediate postoperative period, maintaining hemodynamic stability is the priority. Intra-arterial pressure monitoring provides for the direct measurement of arterial blood pressure, and in many clinical situations it is more accurate than the auscultatory measurement. Variables such as cuff size can influence indirect (noninvasive) pressure readings. Indirect pressure readings can underestimate actual systolic pressures by several mmHg in hypotensive patients (Veiga, Arcuri, Cloutier, & Santos, 2009). This difference occurs because of the Korotkoff sounds produced by blood flow. As blood flow diminishes, the sound becomes less audible, to the point that the faint early sounds may be missed. Indirect measurement of blood pressure, whether obtained manually or with a noninvasive automated pump, provides the best estimate of SBP but underestimates DBP when the patient is at rest (Jahangir, 2013).

Intra-arterial monitoring is indicated in situations when the patient's condition necessitates close hemodynamic observation. Patients who undergo mechanical manipulation of the heart as in cardiac surgery, those who receive drug therapy, and those in whom an intra-aortic balloon pump (IABP; discussed in Chapter 10) is used will all require frequent assessment of arterial pressure postoperatively. An intra-arterial line will also assist in assessing perfusion associated with dysrhythmias. When an intra-arterial catheter is in place in a peripheral artery, the SBP readings may be falsely elevated because of the amplitude of the waveform. However, mean arterial pressure (MAP) and DBP data are accurate (Schroeder, Barbesto, Bar-Yosef, & Mark, 2010).

Mean arterial pressure is the driving force for peripheral blood flow and the preferred pressure to be evaluated in unstable patients. On the monitor screen, it appears as a digital readout adjacent to the displayed blood pressure, usually in parentheses. Mean arterial pressure can also be calculated by the nurse using the formula given in **Box 9-5**. Mean arterial pressure readings do not change as the pressure waveform moves distally along the arterial tree. This pressure is measured electronically by first integrating the area under the arterial pressure waveform and then dividing by the duration of the cardiac cycle. Many clinical conditions may be reflected by changes in the arterial waveform.

Pulsus alternans (see **Figure 9-4**) is believed to be a sign of decreased myocardial contractility. A paradoxical pulse is an exaggeration of the normal variation in the pulse during the inspiratory phase of respiration, in which the pulse becomes weaker as the person inhales and stronger as the person exhales. Pulsus alternans is an indicator of the presence of severe ventricular systolic failure (Vidwan & Stouffer, 2009) and can be a sign of several conditions, including cardiac tamponade, which is a concern following cardiac surgery.

Complications associated with an intra-arterial catheter include ischemia or thrombosis of the affected extremity, infection, and bleeding. Prolonged hyperextension of the wrist can cause nerve conduction deficits. Close assessment for proper positioning and for signs of any complications related to indwelling intra-arterial catheters (e.g., presence of paresthesias, redness, extremity temperature and color) is an essential nursing responsibility and should be included in routine assessments (Clermont & Theodore, 2014). An armboard is frequently used to stabilize the catheter position because excessive movement may cause the catheter to perforate the intima of the artery.

CENTRAL VENOUS PRESSURE MONITORING

Because of the lack of supportive data on current use of pulmonary artery catheters (PACs), CVP catheters are being used more often in the cardiac surgical population. In one study, researchers compared low-risk patients undergoing coronary artery bypass grafting (CABG) with CVP with patients undergoing the same procedure with a PAC. Patients who had surgery with a PAC in place had higher weight gain and longer intubation time. Further, it is also speculated that the PAC may be associated with increased morbidity and resource utilization (Stewart, Psyhojos, Lahey,

---

Box 9-5   Mean Arterial Pressure Calculation

$$MAP = \frac{Systolic\ blood\ pressure + (Diastolic\ blood\ pressure \times 2)}{3}$$

For example, if the patient's blood pressure is 120/80, the MAP can be calculated as follows:

$$\frac{120 + (80 \times 2)}{3} = \frac{120 + 160}{3} \quad or \quad \frac{280}{3} = 93\ mmHg$$

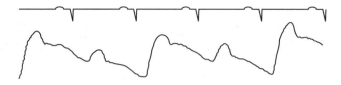

Figure 9-4   Pulsus alternans.

Source: Illustrated by James R. Perron.

Levitsky, & Campos, 1998). Circumstances in which a PAC may be used include patients with pulmonary hypertension, low CO, and predicted postoperative hemodynamic instability following cardiac surgery; it may also be used when assessing the hemodynamic response to therapies (Paunovic, 2013).

It can be anticipated that patients will manifest a decrease in blood and plasma volume within the first 24 hours following cardiac surgery. Patients who undergo CPB often will experience a systemic inflammatory response, which causes fluid to leak from the vessels to the interstitium. Vasodilation also occurs during rewarming and secondary to use of vasodilator therapy. Diuretic use in the postoperative period further contributes to hypovolemia (Roekaerts & Heijmans, 2012). Other etiologic factors for a decrease in plasma and blood volume include the patient's underlying cardiac disease, medications (preoperative, anesthesia, and vasoactive agents), procedure-induced hypothermia, rewarming, and bleeding. There is no reported agreement on which data should be used to guide fluid therapy in these patients. Filling pressures (i.e., CVP and PAOP) are often misleading as signs of optimal left ventricular (LV) filling, especially in patients with alterations in ventricular compliance (Boldt, 2005). In a landmark study, significant variations were reported in hemodynamic data following cardiac surgery. Because hemodynamic reference data had not been previously reported and great variability existed among the participants in this

study, it remains difficult to use hemodynamic data as the sole basis for treatment decisions. Indeed, using acceptable values to guide treatment may result in overtreatment of some patients (Sloth et al., 2008). Rather, correlating hemodynamic data with the patient's clinical presentation may be the most advantageous course of action.

Causes of elevated CVP readings may include hypervolemia, increased venous tone, right ventricular (RV) or LV dysfunction, valve disease (mitral, tricuspid), pulmonary hypertension, atrial fibrillation (AF), high pericardial pressures (such as seen in tamponade), high intrathoracic pressure (such as seen in pneumothorax or with positive-pressure ventilation), and high intra-abdominal pressure. A low CVP value is most often indicative of hypovolemia or a decrease in cardiac output (Roekaerts & Heijmans, 2012). Volume repletion with a crystalloid, colloid, blood, or blood product, along with identifying and treating the source of fluid loss, will resolve the problem. The most common sources of hypovolemia are overzealous diuresis, third spacing, and hemorrhage, but causes may also include diaphoresis and vasodilation. Central venous pressure readings are influenced by the relationships among intravascular volume status, ventricular compliance, and intrathoracic pressure. As a consequence, trending data and correlating them with the patient's clinical status is more likely to optimize the patient's hemodynamic status than evaluating and treating just one isolated numeric value.

To further help assure the accuracy of CVP readings, pressure waveforms are read at end-expiration. Reading the tracing at this point minimizes the influence of intrathoracic pressure on the values.

In addition to aligning the transducer to the phlebostatic axis and interpreting the waveforms at end-expiration, analysis of waveform morphology is essential when the nurse is collecting hemodynamic data. A typical CVP tracing consists of three waves and two descents. An "A" wave represents contraction of the right atrium and corresponds with the P wave on an ECG tracing. An "A" wave will not be seen in patients with tricuspid stenosis, RV hypertrophy, pulmonary hypertension, pulmonary stenosis, or AF. Giant "A" waves may be visible if the right atrium is attempting to eject blood into the RV through a closed tricuspid valve, as occurs in tricuspid stenosis (Chen & Pai, 2009). Pericardial constriction may be reflected by a prominent "A" wave.

A "C" wave is produced with bulging of the tricuspid valve into the right atrium at the start of ventricular systole. It corresponds with the start of the QRS complex on an ECG tracing (Chatterjee, 2007). A large "C" wave may be present in patients who have tricuspid regurgitation.

The "X descent" represents atrial relaxation and corresponding displacement of the tricuspid valve during ventricular systole (Chatterjee, 2007). Absence of the "X descent" may be present in patients who have tricuspid regurgitation.

A "V" wave represents filling of the right atrium with a closed tricuspid valve. It corresponds to the area immediately following the T wave on an ECG tracing. A giant "V" wave may be seen where an acute increase in pressure in the RV occurs (Foucha, 2009), as is seen in patients who have tricuspid regurgitation. Pericardial constriction may be reflected by a prominent "V" wave.

Finally, a "Y descent" represents opening of the tricuspid valve. At this time, blood is flowing from the right atrium (causing an associated decrease in right atrial pressure) into the RV (Chatterjee, 2007) (see **Figure 9-5**). An attenuated "Y descent" may be seen in tricuspid stenosis, reflecting obstruction to right atrial emptying.

The nurse must keep in mind that alterations in waveforms may result in inaccurate numeric displays and that analysis of the waveforms is essential to obtain accurate hemodynamic data.

Table 9-1 lists complications associated with use of a CVP catheter. Some of these complications are site dependent—for example, pneumothorax is associated with internal jugular or subclavian insertion sites but not external jugular or femoral site use.

The risk of vascular injuries may be reduced with use of real-time ultrasound imaging during catheter insertion. Infectious complications may be minimized when steps to prevent infection

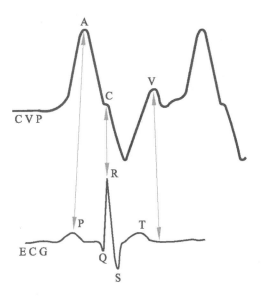

Figure 9-5 CVP waveform.

Source: Illustrated by James R. Perron.

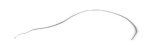

Table 9-1 Complications Associated with CVP Catheters
Pneumothorax (usually occurs during catheter placement)
Thrombus
Infection
Air embolism
Adjacent vessel perforation
Catheter shearing and embolization
Thrombophlebitis
Extravasation of fluid or medication into the mediastinum, pericardium, retroperitoneum, or pleural cavity
Hemothorax
Vascular injuries (e.g., local hematoma, arterial laceration, perforation of the superior vena cava, pericardial perforation)
Arterial puncture
Subpleural hematoma
Uncontrolled venous bleeding

Sources: Data from Gerhardt, M. A., & Skeehan, T. M. (2007). Monitoring the cardiac surgery patient. In F. A. Hensley, D. E. Martin, & G. P. Gravlee (Eds.), *A practical approach to cardiac anesthesia* (pp. 104–141). Philadelphia, PA: Lippincott Williams & Wilkins; Roe, E. J. (2012). *Central venous access via subclavian approach to the subclavian vein*. Retrieved from http://emedicine.medscape.com/article/80336-overview#a17; Young, M. P. (2014). *Complications of central venous catheters and their prevention*. Retrieved from http://www.uptodate.com/contents/complications-of-central-venous-catheters-and-their-prevention

are taken—and such steps should be part of every hospital's protocol. Preventive strategies include hand hygiene, maximal barrier precautions, chlorhexidine skin antisepsis, optimal catheter site selection, and use of antibiotic-impregnated catheters. These components are all part of the "call to order" that should be performed by the medical provider and RN prior to catheter insertion. A daily review of catheter necessity must be performed during change-of-shift report and during multidisciplinary rounds (American Society of Anesthesiologists, 2012).

Finally, staff should keep in mind that an excellent maneuver to reinforce or validate CVP findings is by performing the passive leg raise (PLR). The PLR is easily performed at the bedside by keeping the patient in the supine position and raising the patient's legs to 45 degrees for at least 1 minute. This action will draw blood from the venous compartments in the abdomen and lower limbs and allow the clinician to determine if the patient is volume depleted. It is easily reversible and may be performed quickly and at any time (Cavallaro et al., 2012) (see **Figure 9-6**).

MONITORING USING A PULMONARY ARTERY CATHETER

A PAC may be used to assess cardiac function, cardiac output/index, and intracardiac pressures (Paunovic, 2013). Achieving a cardiac index in the range of 2.5–4.2 L/min/m² is a goal for most postoperative cardiac surgery patients. Obtaining these hemodynamic data directly from the left ventricle would be ideal. Unfortunately, because of the potential for both damage to the LV wall and dysrhythmias, it is not possible to directly monitor these pressures on a continuous basis. Some indications for using a PAC may include patients undergoing CABG who have poor LV performance; those undergoing LV aneurysmectomy; those who recently had a myocardial infarction; those who have pulmonary hypertension, diastolic dysfunction, or acute ventricular septal rupture; or those having a LV assist device inserted (Kanchi, 2011).

A PAC may also be inserted following cardiac surgery if signs of RV failure are present.

Patient in semi-recumbent position

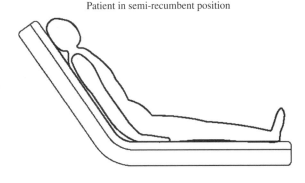

Patient supine with legs elevated to 45 degrees

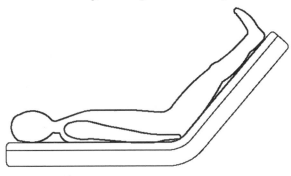

Figure 9-6   Passive leg raise.
Source: Illustrated by James R. Perron.

Ideally, capacity for continuous mixed venous oxygen saturation (SvO$_2$) is available. The catheter may help distinguish between pulmonary hypertension and RV ischemia so that appropriate therapy can be initiated. Other indications for pulmonary artery catheter insertion include unstable hemodynamic status, low cardiac output syndrome, or hypovolemia (Roekaerts & Heijmans, 2012).

A change in left atrial pressure is the earliest indicator of a change in LV preload if no obstruction to flow is present (e.g., mitral stenosis). The line may be used for direct vasoactive medication infusion when the drug administered may be deleterious if routed through the pulmonary system before reaching the left heart. However, because the possibility of tamponade with catheter removal and entry of air or catheter dislodgement exist while the catheter is in place, a left atrial pressure line is not a routine choice for most clinicians.

A PAC may be the next choice because it sits in the pulmonary artery and would provide an earlier indication of changes in the LV than a CVP line. With no obstruction to flow, pulmonary artery pressure (PAP) will indirectly reflect left atrial pressure and approximate value of LV end-diastolic pressure (LVEDP) (left-sided preload). Values obtained with a PAC include pulmonary artery systolic (PAS), pulmonary artery diastolic (PAD), pulmonary artery mean (PAM), and PAOP:

- The PAS reflects pressure measured from the tricuspid to the mitral valve and is a good overall indicator of PAP. Conditions such as COPD, acute respiratory distress syndrome, and pulmonary hypertension are likely to increase PAS pressure.

- The PAD reflects pressure in the area between the pulmonic and aortic valves. If there is no obstruction to blood flow, PAD is a good indicator of LV function.

- The pressure in the pulmonary artery is dynamic; it increases when blood is ejected from the right ventricle and then decreases until the next ejection of blood. The mean PAP is the continuous average of the pressure in the pulmonary artery during one complete cardiac cycle (from the start of ejection of blood to the next) (Costanzo, 2008).

- The PAOP, obtained by inflating the PAC balloon, reflects the pressure between the tip of the PAC and the aortic valve. Because it assesses less surface area, the PAOP is more reflective of LV function than is the PAD. In most circumstances, the PAOP is thought to closely equate to left atrial pressure and LVEDP or LV preload.

Fluid therapy and titration of vasoactive agents are based on these data. In some conditions, the PAOP is reported as greater than LVEDP—for example, in mitral valve disease, increased pulmonary vascular resistance, use of positive-pressure ventilation with associated increase in intrathoracic pressure, tachycardia, and COPD. In other conditions, the PAOP is reported as less than LVEDP—for example, in the presence of aortic regurgitation, a noncompliant left ventricle, or pulmonary embolism. There are data suggesting that during revascularization procedures, patients may have an elevated PAOP while having a low-volume status (Kassick, 2014).

Normally, the PAD is slightly higher than the PAOP, and the normal correlation is less than 5 mmHg (Kassick, 2014). To obtain the PAOP, the balloon must be inflated, which increases the potential risk of pulmonary artery rupture, pulmonary infarction, pulmonary thrombosis or embolism, and pulmonary artery hemorrhage. Obtaining PAOP readings may not be performed routinely but may be done if an acute change in the patient's clinical status or PAD occurs, or if no correlation between the PAD and PAOP exists. Unit-specific protocols for obtaining hemodynamic data should be followed.

When obtaining PAOP readings, balloon inflation time should be minimized. The balloon should be inflated slowly to avoid migration of the catheter into a smaller pulmonary artery or vessel rupture. The balloon should be left deflated at all other times (Weinhouse, 2013).

CARDIAC OUTPUT MEASUREMENT

The PAC also allows measurement of CO via thermodilution or the assumed Fick method. A bolus of either normal saline or D_5W is injected into the right atrium (proximal) port. The fluid mixes with the blood as it travels past the tricuspid valve, through the right ventricle, and into the pulmonary artery. The overall temperature of the mixed blood and injectate is measured by the thermistor (a temperature-sensing device) at the tip of the catheter. The amount of time it takes the cooler blood to pass the thermistor is used to calculate CO. The longer it takes for the cooler blood to pass, the lower the CO. An electronic display of the time–temperature curve and calculated numerical CO value are displayed on the monitor.

Several variables must be assessed to assure the accuracy of the CO displayed. Accuracy of CO results is essential because many of the hemodynamic calculations listed earlier and subsequent therapeutic modalities are based on accurate CO determination (Walsh et al., 2010). Intracardiac shunts produce shunting of cold injectate into the left heart, which decreases pulmonary artery cooling and lowers the peak of the time–temperature curve, as seen with a right-to-left shunt; this condition also results in an underestimation of CO. Tricuspid regurgitation causes underestimation of the CO, because the injectate will reflux back into the right atrium and prevent adequate mixing.

In patients with a left-to-right shunt, increased right heart volume dilutes the injectate, resulting in an overestimation of CO. Temperature of the injectate, injectate technique, minimal manipulation of the injectate-filled syringe, time between measurements, and lack of obstruction to a smooth injection must be confirmed and the patient's body position assessed to ensure accuracy of measurements. The monitor must be preset with the gauge of the PAC in place and the amount of injectate to be infused (5 mL or 10 mL). In addition, forward flow—so that adequate mixing occurs—is important (Walsh et al., 2010).

Dysrhythmias, such as AF, will prevent thorough mixing. Thus, the trend in CO values obtained is extremely important to monitor.

Continuous Cardiac Output

Potential causes of errors in obtaining intermittent measurements of CO have been discussed. Continuous cardiac output (CCO) catheters use a tracer that is not cool but warm; a 10-cm thermal filament is placed on the outside of the catheter at the level of the right ventricle. The filament warms the catheter every 30–60 sec, with low levels of heat energy being transferred to the blood that is adjacent to the filament. The same process is used to determine CO as with the intermittent injectate method. The only difference is that with this technology CO is calculated based on the amount of time it takes the warmed blood to pass the thermistor instead of cooled blood. The CO value is averaged over 3–6 minutes, and a numeric display of the calculated value appears on the monitor screen (Alhashemi, Cecconi, & Hofer, 2011).

Benefits of contour CO include avoidance of individual variations in the volume and speed of infusion of the tracer bolus, and the fact that CO is based on a time-weighted average versus a single instantaneous measurement. Drawbacks include the expense and delayed response time after changes in CO (Alhashemi et al., 2011). Light sedation and the initiation of early mobility are essential for any ICU patient to prevent delirium; therefore, frequent assessment of the need and potential ability to remove the PAC must be discussed at every opportunity. Although mobilization of a patient with a PAC is certainly possible without complications (Winkelman, 2011), logistically it is easier for the patient and staff without the burden of excessive monitoring lines.

Alternative Methods to Determine Cardiac Output

Even as the incorporation of goal-directed therapy using CO or similar parameters to guide intravenous fluid and inotropic therapy continues to increase, other less invasive options for monitoring CO are being adopted in many practices. Minimally invasive CO monitoring devices use one of four main principles to measure CO: pulse contour analysis, pulsed Doppler technology, applied Fick principle, and bioimpedance/bioreactance (Alhashemi et al., 2011). Technologies that are based on arterial pressure can provide CO determinations and measure other clinically important variables, such as stroke volume variation (SVV), pulse pressure variation (PPV), and systolic pressure variation (SPV). Clinical use of these parameters is emerging as a means for determining the patient's ability to respond to changes in fluid levels. Stroke volume variation occurs due to changes in intrathoracic pressure during spontaneous breathing; blood pressure decreases during inhalation and increases during exhalation. The opposite changes are observed when a patient is receiving positive-pressure ventilation.

Arterial Pulse Contour CCO

Arterial pulse contour CCO monitoring estimates CO based on pulse contour analysis; it is an indirect method based on analysis of the arterial pressure pulsation waveform. This technology relies on the concept that the contour of the arterial pressure waveform is proportional to stroke volume. The arterial pressure waveform is used to calculate CO, stroke volume variance, intrathoracic volumes, and extravascular lung water. These data are then used to predict response to fluid therapy (Marik, Monnet, & Teboul, 2011). The arterial waveform is typically recorded from an intra-arterial catheter, although noninvasive recordings have also been used. The efficacy of arterial pulse contour-based CO technology has been demonstrated in some patients who underwent CABG procedures (de Waal, Rex, Kruitwagen, Kalkman, & Buhre, 2008). Despite prior exclusion of well-known confounding factors, PPV has also been shown to be globally of poor clinical utility to predict fluid responsiveness, and digital pleth variability index is not discriminant for routine practice in the conventional cardiac surgery setting (Fischer et al., 2013).

Three of the currently available pulse contour CO systems use intra-arterial waveform analysis. The Pulse index Continuous Cardiac Output (PiCCO) system uses thermodilution for calibration and requires femoral or axillary arterial catheterization. It incorporates use of a catheter with a thermistor on the tip. The catheter records aortic pressure waveforms, and CO is then calculated using a formula based on the area under the systolic portion of the waveform (Grensemann, Wappler, & Sakka, 2013). Data from several studies have led some researchers to question the correlation between CO measurements obtained using this technology and the intermittent injectate method in hypothermic patients, including those undergoing CPB and patients with an upper-body warming device in use (Ostergaard, Nielsen, Rasmussen, & Berthelsen, 2006; Rocca, Costa, Pompei, Coccia, & Pietropaoli, 2002). The second pulse contour CO system available is LiDCO®, which uses lithium dilution for calibration and arterial pulse wave analysis from PulseCO®. The radial or brachial artery is used as the access site. With this technique, a small dose of intravenous lithium chloride is administered. Cardiac output is then determined by a dilution curve made by a lithium-sensitive electrode that is attached to the intra-arterial catheter (Drummond & Murphy, 2011).

FloTrac™/Vigileo™, the third method of pulse contour analysis, does not employ a calibration process to improve monitor precision but instead uses a formula or algorithm to continually update a constant that is used to determine CO (Compton, Zukunft, Hoffmann, Zidek, & Schaefer, 2008). The FloTrac sensor and Vigileo monitor together constitute the FloTrac system. As with the other pulse contour CO systems, SVV may be calculated. Data used to calculate SVV include the patient's blood pressure, age, gender, and body surface area. The patient's CO is determined from the stroke volume and heart rate. An accurate arterial pressure waveform is essential for accurate contour CO determination. Any factor that may alter the tracing (e.g., dysrhythmias, hypotension, equipment issues) may affect the results.

Data suggest that each of the three methods for pulse contour CO is comparable to using a PAC with the intermittent injectate method (Button et al., 2007).

Stroke Volume Variation

Stroke volume variation produces data on changes in preload that occur with mechanical ventilation. It is "the difference between the maximum and minimum stroke volume during one mechanical breath relative to the mean stroke volume" (Berkenstadt et al., 2005, p. 721). Stroke volume variation monitoring can provide data that suggest whether a patient's stroke volume will improve with volume repletion (Suehiro & Okutani, 2010).

There are conflicting data regarding the ability of SVV to predict response to fluid therapy. Some data suggest that SVV predicted preload responsiveness in cardiac surgery patients (Hofer, Senn, Weibel, & Zollinger, 2008). Conversely, other data reported that SVV did not predict an increase in CO or stroke volume in cardiac surgery patients (de Waal et al., 2008).

Possible explanations for the discrepancies in results include differences in tidal volumes used and differences in the cardiac stability of the two groups of patients (Pinsky, 2003).

Pulse Pressure Variation

Pulse pressure variation is "the difference between the maximum and minimum values of the arterial pulse pressure during one mechanical breath divided by the mean of the two values" (Berkenstadt et al., 2005, p. 721). Reports suggest that variations in PPV can accurately predict response to fluid therapy in patients with shock and in surgical procedures. Upon evaluating the Frank-Starling curve, an increase in preload is associated with a decrease in PPV; conversely, a decrease in preload is associated with an increase in PPV and contractility. It has been suggested that PPV is more accurate in predicting fluid response than CVP and PAOP, SPV, and SVV (Michard, Lopes, & Auler, 2007).

Systolic Pressure Variation

Systolic pressure variation is "the difference between the maximum and minimum systolic blood pressure during one mechanical breath" (Berkenstadt et al., 2005, p. 721). It can reportedly indicate decreases in CO from blood loss and predict a patient's response to volume repletion. This parameter is used to estimate circulating volume (Gouvêa & Gouvêa, 2005).

In a study of patients in the ICU who underwent CABG, researchers determined that PPV and SPV were both able to predict whether a patient would respond to volume repletion with an increase in CO. While PPV was demonstrated to be superior to SPV at predicting response to fluid therapy, the researchers concluded that both PPV and SPV were far superior to CVP and PAOP data (Marik, 2011).

Doppler Methods

Doppler-based methods use ultrasound and the Doppler effect to determine CO. When ultrasound waves strike moving objects, the waves are reflected back to their source at a different frequency, which is directly related to the velocity of the moving objects and the angle at which the ultrasound beam strikes these objects. Proper probe placement is essential when using these methods to monitor CO. Several different Doppler-based methods may be used to measure CO, each of which uses a slightly different site in the body for measuring blood flow. Data comparing ultrasound determination of CO with data from a PAC have conflicting results (Marik, 2013).

The esophageal Doppler technique is another method to measure blood flow velocity in the descending aorta by means of a Doppler transducer placed at the tip of a flexible probe. The probe is introduced into the esophagus of sedated, mechanically ventilated patients and then rotated so the transducer faces the descending aorta and a characteristic aortic velocity signal is obtained. The CO is calculated based on the diameter of the aorta (measured or estimated), the distribution of the CO to the descending aorta, and the measured flow velocity of blood in the aorta (Marik, 2013).

Electrical Bioimpedance

Electrical bioimpedance is a noninvasive method to determine CO. Using this technology, CO is measured based on changes in impedance that occur as blood is ejected from the left ventricle into the aorta and is calculated from changes in thoracic impedance. With this method, changes in thoracic blood volume during the cardiac cycle can be used to calculate CO. This technique is a successful method of monitoring CO because the algorithm eliminates the impedance due to body tissue and lung volume changes, instead using only the change in thoracic blood volume for CO determination. An alternative approach uses a specially designed endotracheal tube to measure electrical impedance changes in the ascending aorta (Fellahi & Fischer, 2013).

ASSESSMENT OF OXYGENATION PARAMETERS

Venous Oxygen Saturation

In addition to direct pressure measurements and CO assessment, other hemodynamic data may assess a patient's condition following cardiac surgery. Another type of PAC provides for continuous monitoring of SvO_2, which reveals the association between oxygen delivery (the amount of oxygen that is carried to the tissues each minute) and oxygen consumption (the amount of oxygen used by the tissues) or tissue oxygen balance (Teboul, Hamzaoui, & Monnet, 2011).

Mixed venous blood represents the amount of oxygen in the systemic circulation after the blood's passage through the tissues. Venous oxygen saturation data reflect tissue oxygenation and cardiopulmonary function and can be used to discover whether a patient is clinically deteriorating. Normal SvO_2 is in the range of 60% to 80%. Trends and changes in oxygen delivery, oxygen consumption, or tissue oxygenation may be identified by reviewing data related to venous oxygen saturation. These data can also be used to determine the efficacy of interventions implemented to optimize these variables as well as procedures performed by the ICU nurse while caring for a postoperative cardiac surgery patient (Groesdonk et al., 2009). With continuous digital readout of SvO_2 measurements, early recognition and prompt intervention to eradicate effects of poor tissue oxygenation can be implemented by the ICU nurse. Causes of changes in SvO_2 are many and include most variables affecting preload, afterload, and contractility. Although not specific to any one factor, any change in SvO_2 alerts the ICU nurse to quickly investigate.

Central Venous Oxygen Saturation

Catheters that allow for assessment of central venous oxygen saturation ($ScvO_2$) are being used in some cardiac surgical programs as the transition away from PACs continues. With this monitoring approach, a blood sample is obtained from a central venous catheter and is analyzed. A normal $ScvO_2$ is 70% or greater. If the value is less than 70%, it indicates that the tissues are extracting more oxygen than is normal and that the tissues do not perceive that their oxygen needs are being met; this is an indicator of a bad outcome (Goodrich, 2006; van Beest, Wietasch, Scheeren, Spronk, & Kuiper, 2011).

One of the newest noninvasive CO monitors is the Nexfin® monitor. Rather than a minimally invasive monitor, it is a completely noninvasive method of determining the patient's hemodynamic parameters, as the need for an invasive arterial catheter or a central line is obviated. The monitor is connected to the patient by wrapping an inflatable cuff around the middle phalanx of the finger. The pulsating finger artery is "clamped" to a constant volume by applying a varying counter pressure equivalent to the arterial pressure, resulting in a pressure waveform. The finger arterial pressure is then reconstructed into brachial arterial pressure waveform using a transfer function and a level correction based on a vast clinical database. The resulting brachial pressure waveform serves as the basis for determining continuous CO (Monnet et al., 2012). However, Nexfin does not provide consistent results at this time (Maass, Roekaerts, & Lancé, 2014).

Postoperative Hemodynamic Assessment

Some of the initial goals for patients in the immediate postoperative period following cardiac surgery include promoting satisfactory oxygen levels and ventilation, repleting intravascular volume, and augmenting perfusion by stabilizing blood pressure and CO (Roekaerts & Heijmans, 2012). The ICU nurse caring for a postoperative cardiac surgery patient must be aware of both normal and baseline parameter values so that any clinical deterioration or improvement in the patient may be promptly noted. Some patients, because of their comorbidities or their disease process (such as valve disease), may require higher filling pressures postoperatively to maintain an adequate cardiac output/index.

An adequate cardiac index in the range of 2.5–4.2 L/min/m^2 will be sustained by normalizing heart rate and stroke volume as soon as possible. Many variables may affect heart rate and rhythm in the postoperative period. The most common causes in the postoperative cardiac surgery patient include hypovolemia and pain, both of which should be addressed promptly. Despite sedation, the nurse should assess for other signs and symptoms that indicate the presence of pain. Pain assessment and management are discussed in detail in Chapter 14.

Dysrhythmias that may be seen in the postoperative period include AF, premature ventricular contractions, and ventricular tachycardia; the latter two dysrhythmias may occur due to electrolyte imbalance. All of the dysrhythmias may arise as a result of cardiac irritability from operative manipulation. Ventricular fibrillation, although rare, may also occur. The presence of any dysrhythmia may affect a patient's hemodynamic status and requires rapid intervention. The etiology and management of postoperative dysrhythmias are discussed in detail in Chapter 15.

After assessing heart rate, an adequate stroke volume should be ensured. Variables that influence stroke volume—preload, afterload, and contractility—often are affected in the intraoperative and postoperative periods. For example, preload may be decreased as the patient undergoes the rewarming process, which may lead to vasodilation. Bleeding from chest tubes or third spacing that results from the inflammatory process may also decrease preload, resulting in a decrease in CO. Postoperative bleeding is always a concern for the cardiac surgical patient. Blood loss will decrease the oxygen-carrying capacity to vital organs and tissues (Tsai, Hofmann, Cabrales, & Intaglietta, 2010). Logically, decreased circulating volume will decrease preload, stroke volume, and CO.

The causes of postoperative bleeding are many. For instance, the CPB circuit may cause platelet destruction as the blood circulates through it, in addition to decreasing levels of clotting factors. Inadequate hemostasis from incomplete heparin reversal or excessive protamine administration is another potential cause of altered hemostasis, as is a surgical bleed from a suture site.

If chest tube drainage exceeds 100 mL/hr for more than 3 hours, 200 mL/hr for 3 hours, or 300 mL in the first hour following surgery, the surgeon should be notified. Transfusion of blood or blood products may be ordered if the coagulation studies are outside of the normal range or if the patient's hematocrit level is low. If the patient is hypertensive, the blood pressure must be decreased to prevent stress on the suture sites, which may cause further bleeding. The patient may need to undergo surgical reexploration. Decreases in blood pressure, cardiac filling pressures, and urinary output are signs of hypovolemia that must be evaluated. Adjustments to volume administration are frequently necessary as well. Volume repletion is accomplished by administration of isotonic crystalloids (e.g., lactated Ringer's or normal saline) or colloids (e.g., albumin, blood, or blood products) as determined by the patient's hemodynamic status and lab results. Conversely, if preload indices are too high, holding further volume administration, diuretics, or vasodilators (e.g., nitroglycerin) may be indicated.

An increased afterload may result from severe LV dysfunction, hypovolemia, vasoconstriction, hypothermia, or increased catecholamine stimulation from the surgical procedure. Along with volume-related interventions and use of a warming blanket, arterial vasodilator administration may be beneficial in such cases. A decreased afterload may be the result of significant vasodilation from warming; this condition may be treated with administration of an agent that causes vasoconstriction.

Decreased contractility in the postoperative period may be the result of an increase or decrease in preload, an increase in afterload, or factors that affect myocardial contractility directly (e.g., ischemia, RV or LV failure, and aneurysms). Electrolyte imbalance and tamponade may also alter contractility. In such a scenario, preload and afterload are optimized while other interventions to treat the underlying cause are completed. If indicated, administration of positive inotropic agents is initiated. If further afterload reduction is needed after the use of vasodilators, an IABP is added. The IABP can increase CO by as much as 1 liter and may be necessary to support the patient through an acute event. Intra-aortic balloon pump therapy is discussed in detail in Chapter 10. The use of biventricular pacing has also been reported to improve contractility following bypass procedures (Wang et al., 2013).

If blood builds up inside the mediastinum, cardiac tamponade may occur, resulting in physical compression of the heart, limitation of diastolic filling time, and a decrease in CO. Cardiac tamponade and several other postoperative complications are discussed in detail in Chapter 13.

SUMMARY

The number of cardiac surgical patients with pulmonary artery catheters has decreased worldwide. Although little published evidence exists to associate use of patient monitoring with improved clinical outcomes, this lack of evidence does not necessarily equate to a lack of benefit. Thus, catheters will still be used, albeit with caution.

Intensive care unit nurses play a pivotal role in monitoring the postoperative hemodynamic status of patients following cardiac surgery. They must obtain accurate data, integrate those monitoring data with information gained by assessing the patient's clinical status, and use clinical judgment to select the best interventions to optimize the patient's status given the patient's current condition and past medical history. Having expertise helps to ensure that obtained parameters are not reflecting nonphysiologic events such as patient turning, artifact, and inaccurate leveling, and that values are assessed at end-expiration. The ICU nurse with high levels of critical judgment and clinical inquiry competencies will use accurate information and evidence-based guidelines to determine when activities can be clustered or when oxygen consumption is too high to do so.

By definition, the cardiac surgical patient always has underlying cardiac pathology that will have a major impact on postoperative recovery. Monitoring that incorporates a clinical evaluation, review of physiology, and expected responses relative to the type of cardiac surgery performed is essential. Invasive catheters may be used to augment—but not replace—monitoring for subtle changes. The expert ICU nurse validates signs and intervenes quickly. Each of these competencies is essential to achieve an optimal patient outcome following cardiac surgery.

CASE STUDY

A 72-year-old male patient, with a history of ST-segment elevation myocardial infarction (STEMI) and drug-eluting stent to the right coronary artery 3 years ago, is admitted to the ICU after on-pump cardiac surgery. Triple bypass was completed on the left anterior descending and circumflex arteries. At the time of admission to the ICU after surgery, the patient data were as follows: BP 98/52, MAP 74 mmHg, HR 110, PAS 22 mmHg, PAD 7 mmHg, PAOP 6 mmHg, CVP 2 mmHg, temperature 35.4 °C, CI 2.2 L/min/m^2; Hct 26%.

Critical Thinking Questions

1. What else should be part of this patient's initial admission assessment?
2. Which of the parameters given in the case study may indicate the patient's volume status?
3. What are two reasons why sinus tachycardia might occur in the immediate postoperative period?

Answers to Critical Thinking Questions

1. Following cardiac surgery, the ICU nurse will connect the patient to the bedside monitor upon receipt from the operating room. The ECG leads are connected to the bedside monitor from the transport monitor, and heart rate and rhythm are assessed. The pulse oximetry probe is connected to either the finger, earlobe, or forehead. Pulse oximetry is a simple, noninvasive method of monitoring the percentage of hemoglobin that is saturated with oxygen. The target SpO$_2$ is 95% or greater.
2. CVP and PAOP
3. Tachycardia may arise as a result of cardiac irritability from intraoperative manipulation, electrolyte imbalance, pain, anxiety, hypovolemia, or decreased cardiac output/index.

SELF-ASSESSMENT QUESTIONS

1. The nurse notices an overdamped waveform on the arterial line tracing. Which of the following should the nurse suspect?
   a. Small bubbles in the system
   b. Pressure tubing too long
   c. Defective transducer
   d. Low pressure in the flush bag

2. A cause of an underdamped waveform may include which of the following?
   a. Large bubbles in the system
   b. Loose connections
   c. Low pressure in the flush solution pressure bag
   d. Pressure tubing too long

3. Placement of the transducer below the phlebostatic axis will result in which of the following?
   a. Small air bubbles gathering in the pressure tubing
   b. Falsely elevated pressure readings
   c. Decreased perfusion to the area of insertion
   d. An overdamped waveform

4. Presence of pulsus alternans following cardiac surgery may indicate which of the following?
   a. Diastolic failure
   b. Loose connections of the pressure bag
   c. Increasing pleural effusion
   d. Decreased myocardial contractility

5. Which of the following hemodynamic parameters should the nurse anticipate in the first 24 hours after cardiac surgery?
   a. Systolic BP greater than 140 mmHg
   b. Pulmonary artery pressure 35/20
   c. Central venous pressure 1 mmHg
   d. Cardiac index 4 L/min/m²

6. Which of the following may cause an elevated CVP reading following cardiac surgery?
   a. Decreased pulmonary artery pressures
   b. Atrial fibrillation
   c. Pulmonic valve disease
   d. Pleural effusion

7. You are caring for a patient following cardiac surgery who is on mechanical ventilation. The patient has not been reversed. The following CVP tracing is seen on the monitor. What CVP reading should be documented?

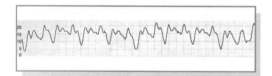

   a. 16 mmHg
   b. 3 mmHg

   c. 5 mmHg
   d. 12 mmHg

8. Which of the following is true about a V wave?
   a. It represents atrial relaxation.
   b. It corresponds with the QRS complex of the ECG tracing.
   c. It will not be seen in patients with pulmonary hypertension.
   d. If prominent, it may indicate pericardial constriction.

9. Pulmonary artery systolic pressure:
   a. represents left-sided preload
   b. is a good indicator of left ventricular function
   c. may be decreased in patients with acute respiratory distress syndrome
   d. reflects pressure measured from the tricuspid to mitral valve

10. When observing PAOP readings:
   a. Balloon inflation should not exceed 3 L.
   b. Balloon inflation should occur in 1 sec to avoid catheter migration.
   c. Values should be obtained hourly and compared to PAD values.
   d. The balloon should remain inflated for no more than 3 sec.

Answers to Self-Assessment Questions

1. d	6. b
2. d	7. d
3. b	8. d
4. d	9. d
5. c	10. d

Clinical Inquiry Box

Question: Are each of three methods to measure fluid responsiveness reliable?
Reference: Belloni, L., Pisano, A., Natale, A., Piccirillo, M. R., Piazza, A., Ismeno, G., . . . DeMartino, G. (2008). Assessment of fluid-responsiveness parameters for off-pump coronary artery bypass surgery: A comparison among LiDCO, transesophageal echocardiography (TEE), and pulmonary artery catheter. *Journal of Cardiothoracic and Vascular Anesthesia, 22*(2), 243–248.

Clinical Inquiry Box (*Continued*)

Objective: Determine the reliability of different methods to measure fluid responsiveness during cardiac surgery

Methods: A clinical, prospective non-blinded, non-randomized study was conducted in a community hospital. Central venous pressure and PAOP (from a PAC), LiDCO, and TEE parameters were measured before (t0) and after (t1) a fluid challenge was performed 20 minutes after induction of anesthesia, but before sternotomy and without inotropic infusion.

Results: Two groups of patients were identified following the fluid challenge—those who responded and those who did not respond. Mean PPV and mean SVV before the fluid challenge were significantly different between the two groups. No significant differences were shown in SPV, left ventricular end-diastolic area, or left ventricular end-diastolic volume. A statistically significant correlation was observed between the cardiac index following the fluid challenge and PPV, cardiac index following the fluid challenge and SVV (R = 0.809), and cardiac index following the fluid challenge and SPV. No correlation among cardiac index following the fluid challenge and central venous pressure, pulmonary capillary wedge pressure, or transesophageal echocardiography was found.

Conclusion: Responses to fluid therapy measured by LiDCO are highly sensitive for assessment of intravascular volume status during off-pump coronary artery bypass surgery. In contrast, even if static parameters by TEE reflect changes in ventricular diastolic volume, they were poor indicators of fluid responsiveness.

REFERENCES

Alhashemi, J. A., Cecconi, M., & Hofer, C. K. (2011). Cardiac output monitoring: An integrative perspective. *Critical Care, 15*(2), 214. Retrieved from http://ccforum.com/content/15/2/214

American Association of Critical-Care Nurses. (2011). *Pulmonary artery pressure measurement.* Retrieved from http://www.aacn.org/WD/Practice/Docs/PAP_Measurement_05-2004.pdf

American Society of Anesthesiologists. (2012). Practice guidelines for central venous access. *Anesthesiology, 116*(3), 539–573.

Arora, S., Singh, P. M., Goudra, B. G., & Sinha, A. C. (2014). Changing trends of hemodynamic monitoring in ICU—from invasive to non-invasive methods: Are we there yet? *International Journal of Critical Illness & Injury Science, 4*(2), 168–177.

Berkenstadt, H., Friedman, Z., Preisman, S., Keidan, I., Livingstone, D., & Perel, A. (2005). Pulse pressure and stroke volume variations during severe haemorrhage in ventilated dogs. *British Journal of Anaesthesia, 94*(6), 721–726.

Blount, K. (2007). Hemodynamic monitoring. In R. Kaplow & S. R. Hardin (Eds.), *Critical care nursing: Synergy for optimal outcomes* (pp. 139–159). Sudbury, MA: Jones and Bartlett.

Boldt, J. (2005). Volume therapy in cardiac surgery. *Annals of Cardiac Anaesthesia, 8*(2), 104–116.

Button, D., Weibel, L., Reuthebuch, O., Genoni, M., Zollinger, A., & Hofer, C. K. (2007). Clinical evaluation of FloTrac/Vigileo™ system and two established continuous cardiac output monitoring devices in patients undergoing cardiac surgery. *British Journal of Anaesthesia, 99*(3), 329–336.

Cavallaro, F., Sandroni, C., Marano, C., La Torre, G., Mannocci, A., De Waure, C., . . . Antonelli, M. (2012). Diagnostic accuracy of passive leg raising for prediction of fluid responsiveness in adults: Systematic review and meta-analysis of clinical studies. *Applied Physiology in Intensive Care Medicine, 36*(9), 225–233.

Chatterjee, K. (2007). Physical examination. In E. J. Topol, R. M. Califf, E. N. Prystowsky, J. D. Thomas, & P. D. Thompson (Eds.), *Textbook of cardiovascular medicine* (3rd ed., pp. 193–226). Philadelphia, PA: Lippincott Williams & Wilkins.

Chen, D., & Pai, P.-Y. (2009). Cannon a wave. *Circulation, 119*, e381–e383.

Clermont, G., & Theodore, A. C. (2014). *Arterial catheterization techniques for invasive monitoring.*

Retrieved from http://www.uptodate.com/contents/arterial-catheterization-techniques-for-invasive-monitoring

Compton, F. D., Zukunft, B., Hoffmann, C., Zidek, W., & Schaefer, J. H. (2008). Performance of a minimally invasive uncalibrated cardiac output monitoring system (FloTrac™/Vigileo™) in unstable haemodynamically unstable patients. *British Journal of Anaesthesia, 100*(4), 451–456.

Costanzo, L. S. (2008). Cardiovascular physiology. In L. S. Costanzo, *Physiology cases and problems* (3rd ed., pp. 47–56). Philadelphia, PA: Lippincott Williams & Wilkins.

de Waal, E. E. C., Rex, S., Kruitwagen, C. L. J. J., Kalkman, C. J., & Buhre, W. F. (2008). Stroke volume variation obtained with Flo-Trac/Vigileo™ fails to predict fluid responsiveness in coronary artery bypass graft patients. *British Journal of Anaesthesia, 100*(5), 725–726.

Drummond, K. E., & Murphy, E. (2011). Minimally invasive cardiac output monitors. *Continuing Education in Anaesthesia, Critical Care & Pain*, 11. Retrieved from http://ceaccp.oxfordjournals.org/content/early/2011/12/21/bjaceaccp.mkr044.full.pdf+html

Dunn, J. M., & Heupler, F. (2013). Cardiac output. In S. Anwaruddin, J. M. Martin, J. C. Stephens, & A. T. Askari (Eds.), *Cardiovascular hemodynamics* (pp. 65–76). New York, NY: Springer.

Fellahi, J.-L., & Fischer, M.-O. (2013). Electrical bioimpedance cardiography: An old technology with new hopes for the future. *Journal of Cardiothoracic and Vascular Anesthesia, 28*(3), 755–760.

Fischer, M., Pelissier, A., Bohadana, D., Gérard, J. L., Hanouz, J. L., & Fellahi, J. L. (2013). Prediction of responsiveness to an intravenous fluid challenge in patients after cardiac surgery with cardiopulmonary bypass: A comparison between arterial pulse pressure variation and digital plethysmographic variability index. *Journal of Cardiothoracic and Vascular Anesthesia, 27*(6), 1087–1093.

Foucha, B. K. (2009). The ABCs of A to V: Right atrial/left atrial (PCW) pressures. *Cath Lab Digest, 17*(5). Retrieved from http://www.cathlabdigest.com/articles/The-ABCs-A-V-Right-Atrial-Left-Atrial-PCW-Pressures

Gerhardt, M. A., & Skeehan, T. M. (2007). Monitoring the cardiac surgery patient. In F. A. Hensley, D. E. Martin, & G. P. Gravlee (Eds.), *A practical approach to cardiac anesthesia* (pp. 104–141). Philadelphia, PA: Lippincott Williams & Wilkins.

Goodrich, C. (2006). Continuous central venous oximetry monitoring. *Critical Care Nursing Clinics of North America, 18*(2), 203–209.

Gouvêa, G., & Gouvêa, F. G. (2005). Measurement of systolic pressure variation on a Datex AS/3 monitor. *Anesthesia & Analgesia, 100*(6), 1864.

Grensemann, J., Wappler, F., & Sakka, S. G. (2013). Erroneous continuous cardiac output by calibrated pulse contour analysis. *Journal of Clinical Monitoring and Computing, 27*(5), 567–568.

Groesdonk, H. V., Shpachenko, T., Hanke, H., Heinze, K. U., Berger, J., Schön, M., . . . Eleftheriadis, S. (2009). Continuous SvO$_2$ monitoring is reliable after on-pump cardiac surgery. *World Congress on Medical Physics and Biomedical Engineering, 25*(7), 634–637.

Hofer, C. K., Senn, A., Weibel, L., & Zollinger, A. (2008). Assessment of stroke volume variation for prediction of fluid responsiveness using the modified FloTrac™ and PiCCOplus™ system. *Critical Care, 12*(3). Retrieved from http://ccforum.com/content/12/3/r82

Jahangir, E. (2013). *Blood pressure assessment.* Retrieved from http://emedicine.medscape.com/article/1948157-overview

Kanchi, M. (2011). Do we need a pulmonary artery catheter in cardiac anesthesia?—An Indian perspective. *Annals of Cardiac Anaesthesia, 14*, 25–29.

Kassick, M. A. (2014). Clinical monitoring: Cardiovascular system. In J. J. Nagelhout & K. L. Plaus (Eds.), *Nurse anesthesia* (5th ed., pp. 292–312). St. Louis, MO: Elsevier Saunders.

Kolh, P. (2009). Renal insufficiency after cardiac surgery: A challenging clinical problem. *European Heart Journal, 30*(15), 1824–1827.

Lockhart, A. (2007). Cardiovascular care. In A. Lockhart (Ed.), *Best practices* (2nd ed., pp. 193–281). Philadelphia, PA: Lippincott Williams & Wilkins.

Maass, S. W., Roekaerts, P. M., & Lancé, M. D. (2014). Cardiac output measurement by bioimpedance and noninvasive pulse contour analysis compared with the continuous pulmonary artery thermodilution technique.

Journal of Cardiothoracic and Vascular Anesthesia 28(3), 534–539.

Marik, P. (2013). Noninvasive cardiac output monitors: A state-of the-art review. *Journal of Cardiothoracic and Vascular Anesthesia, 27*(1), 121–134.

Marik, P. E. (2011). Hemodynamic parameters to guide fluid therapy. *Transfusion Alternatives in Transfusion Medicine, 11*(3), 102–112. from http://www.medscape.com/viewarticle/741748_6

Marik, P. E., Monnet, X., & Teboul, J.-L. (2011). Hemodynamic parameters to guide fluid therapy. *Annals of Intensive Care,* 1. Retrieved from http://www.annalsofintensivecare.com/content/pdf/2110-5820-1-1.pdf

McCleaster, S., & Heuer, A. J. (2010). Review existing data in patient's record. In C. L. Scanlan, A. J. Heuer, & L. M. Sinopoli (Eds.), *Certified respiratory therapist exam: Review guide* (pp. 43–60). Sudbury, MA: Jones and Bartlett.

Michard, F., Lopes, M. R., & Auler, J.-O. (2007). Pulse pressure variation: Beyond fluid management of patients in shock. *Critical Care, 11*(3), 131.

Monnet, X., Picard, F., Lidzborski, E., Mesnil, M., Duranteau, J., Richard, C., . . . Teboul, J. L. (2012). The estimation of cardiac output by the Nexfin device is of poor reliability for tracking the effects of a fluid challenge. *Critical Care,* 16, R212.

Ostergaard, M., Nielsen, J., Rasmussen, J. P., & Berthelsen, P. G. (2006). Cardiac output-pulse contour analysis vs. pulmonary artery thermodilution. *Acta Anaesthesiologica Scandinavica, 50*(9), 1044–1049.

Paunovic, B. (2013). *Pulmonary artery catheterization.* Retrieved from http://emedicine.medscape.com/article/1824547-overview#a03

Pinsky, M. R. (2003). Probing the limits of arterial pulse contour analysis to predict preload responsiveness. *Anesthesia & Analgesia, 96*(5), 1245–1247.

Rauen, C., Flynn, M., & Bridges, E. (2009). Evidence-based practice habits: Transforming research into bedside practice. *Critical Care Nurse, 29*(2), 46–59.

Rocca, G. D., Costa, M. G., Pompei, L., Coccia, C., & Pietropaoli, P. (2002). Continuous and intermittent cardiac output measurement: Pulmonary artery catheter versus aortic transpulmonary technique. *British Journal of Anaesthesia, 88*(3), 350–356.

Roe, E. J. (2012). *Central venous access via subclavian approach to the subclavian vein.* Retrieved from http://emedicine.medscape.com/article/80336-overview#a17

Roekaerts, M. M. H. J., & Heijmans, J. H. (2012). *Early postoperative care after cardiac surgery, perioperative considerations in cardiac surgery.* Retrieved from http://www.intechopen.com/books/howtoreference/perioperative-considerations-in-cardiac-surgery/-early-postoperative-care-after-cardiac-surgery-

Sabe, M., & Heupler, F. (2013). Contractility. In S. Anwaruddin, J. M. Martin, J. C. Stephens, & A. T. Askari (Eds.), *Cardiovascular hemodynamics* (pp. 53–64). New York, NY: Springer.

Schroeder, R. A., Barbesto, A., Bar-Yosef, S., & Mark, J. B. (2010). Cardiovascular monitoring. In R. D. Miller, L. I. Eriksson, L. A. Fleisher, J. P. Wiener-Kronish, & W. L. Young (Eds.), *Miller's anesthesia* (7th ed., pp. 1267–1328). Philadelphia, PA: Elsevier.

Sloth, E., Lindskov, C., Lorentzen, A.-G., Nygaard, M., Kure, H. H., & Jakobsen, C-J. (2008). Cardiac surgery patients present considerable variation in pre-operative hemodynamic variables. *Acta Anaesthesiologica Scandinavica, 52*(7), 952–958.

Stewart, R. D., Psyhojos, T., Lahey, S. J., Levitsky, S., & Campos, C. T. (1998). Central venous catheter use in low-risk coronary artery bypass grafting. *Annals of Thoracic Surgery, 66*(4), 1306–1311.

Suehiro, K., & Okutani, R. (2010). Stroke volume variation as a predictor of fluid responsiveness in patients undergoing one-lung ventilation. *Journal of Cardiothoracic and Vascular Anesthesia, 24*(5), 772–775.

Teboul, J.-L., Hamzaoui, O., & Monnet, X. (2011). SvO_2 to monitor resuscitation of septic patients: Let's just understand the basic physiology. *Critical Care,* 15. Retrieved from http://ccforum.com/content/15/6/1005

Tsai, A. G., Hofmann, A., Cabrales, P., & Intaglietta, M. (2010). Perfusion vs. oxygen delivery in transfusion of "fresh" and "old" red blood cells: The experimental evidence. *Transfusion and Apheresis Science, 43*(1), 69–78.

van Beest, Wietasch, G., Scheeren, T., Spronk, P., & Kuiper, M. (2011). Clinical review: Use of venous oxygen saturations as a goal—A yet unfinished puzzle. *Critical Care, 15.* Retrieved from http://ccforum.com/content/pdf/cc10351.pdf

Veiga, E. V., Arcuri, E. A. M., Cloutier, L., & Santos, J. L. F. (2009). Blood pressure measurement: Arm circumference and cuff size availability. *Revista Latino-Americana de Enfermagem, 17*(4), Retrieved from http://www.scielo.br/scielo.php?script=sci_arttext&pid=S0104-11692009000400004

Vest, A. R., & Heupler, F. (2013a). Afterload. In S. Anwaruddin, J. M. Martin, J. C. Stephens, & A. T. Askari (Eds.), *Cardiovascular hemodynamics* (pp. 29–52). New York, NY: Springer.

Vest, A. R., & Heupler, F. (2013b). Preload. In S. Anwaruddin, J. M. Martin, J. C. Stephens, & A. T. Askari (Eds.), *Cardiovascular hemodynamics* (pp. 3–28). New York, NY: Springer.

Vidwan, P., & Stouffer, G. A. (2009). Biventricular pulsus alternans. *Cardiology Research and Practice, 2009,* Article ID 703793. Retrieved from http://www.hindawi.com/journals/crp/2009/703793/

Walker, S. G., & Butterworth, J. F. (2008). Endocrine, metabolic, and electrolyte responses. In G. P. Gravlee, R. F. Davis, A. H. Stammers, & R. M. Ungerleider (Eds.), *Cardiopulmonary bypass: Principles and practice* (3rd ed., pp. 282–310). Philadelphia, PA: Lippincott Williams & Wilkins.

Walsh, E., Adams, S., Chernipeski, J., Cloud, J., Gillies, E., Fox, R., . . . Ash, T. (2010). Iced vs room-temperature injectates for cardiac index measurement during hypothermia and normothermia. *American Journal of Critical Care, 19*(4), 365–372.

Wang, D. Y., Kelly, L. A., Richmond, M. E., Quinn, T. A., Cheng, B., Spotnitz, M. D., . . . Spotnitz, H. M. (2013). Feasibility of temporary biventricular pacing after off-pump coronary artery bypass grafting in patients with reduced left ventricular function. *Texas Heart Institute Journal, 40*(4), 403–409.

Weinhouse, G. L. (2013). *Pulmonary artery catheterization: Indications and complications.* Retrieved from http://www.uptodate.com/contents/pulmonary-artery-catheterization-indications-and-complications#H8

Winkelman, C. (2011). Ambulating with pulmonary artery or femoral catheters in place. *Critical Care Nurse, 31*(5), 70–73.

Young, M. P. (2014). *Complications of central venous catheters and their prevention.* Retrieved from http://www.uptodate.com/contents/complications-of-central-venous-catheters-and-their-prevention

WEB RESOURCES

NTI 2010 Hemodynamic Boot Camp: http://www.cardionursing.com/pdfs/Boot-Camp-Hemodynamic-Monitoring.pdf

Central Venous Pressure Monitoring: https://www.youtube.com/watch?v=JWf0NSQtWKs

Advanced Technology Swan-Ganz Catheter: Using Continuous SvO_2 and EDVI for Patient Management: https://www.youtube.com/watch?v=fGiZiZF9wDk

Chapter 10

Intra-aortic Balloon Pump

Barbara Hutton-Borghardt

INTRODUCTION

The intra-aortic balloon pump (IABP) is a mechanical device that is temporarily used to improve cardiac function. In many situations, the IABP is life-saving in its ability to stabilize patients as they await procedures such as heart transplant, coronary artery bypass grafting, or percutaneous coronary interventions (PCI) such as percutaneous transluminal coronary angioplasty/stent placement (Chen, Yin, Ling, & Krucoff, 2014; Hatch & Baklanov, 2014).

An IABP may be further indicated in the management of cardiogenic shock (Haddad & Robertson, 2013; Sharma, Lumley, & Perera, 2013). Medications such as vasodilators and inotropes are used initially to improve cardiac function. If they are not effective, the IABP may be used alone or with pharmacotherapy to assist left ventricular (LV) function

and improve cardiac output (CO) (Hatch & Baklanov, 2014).

Since its introduction in the late 1960s, IABP has become a widely used device in preoperative, intraoperative, and postoperative cardiac surgery patients (Parissis, Soo, & Al-Alao, 2012). In the United States, it is estimated that more than 70,000 IABP catheters are inserted annually (Rastan et al., 2010). A description of how an IABP improves cardiac function is provided in **Box 10-1**.

COMPONENTS OF AN IABP

The IABP consists of two main parts: (1) a double-lumen catheter with an inflatable balloon attached to the distal end and (2) a console that regulates the inflation and deflation of the balloon. One lumen of the balloon

---

Box 10-1   Goals of IABP Therapy

The IABP achieves its goals of stabilizing cardiac function by several mechanisms:

- It improves cardiac function (i.e., CO) by decreasing LV end-diastolic volume (preload) and by decreasing afterload.
- It improves myocardial oxygen supply by increasing blood flow to the coronary arteries.
- It decreases myocardial oxygen demand by decreasing LV wall tension.
- It stabilizes cardiac function in patients with dysrhythmias and myocardial ischemia.

Sources: Data from Elliot, D., Aitken, L., & Chaboyer, W. (2012). *ACCCN's critical care nursing* (2nd ed.). Chatswood, Australia: Elsevier Australia; and Krishna, M., & Zacharowski, K. (2009). Principles of intra-aortic balloon counterpulsation. *Continuing Education in Anaesthesia, Critical Care & Pain, 9*(1), 24–28.

catheter is attached to a pressure-transducer device that monitors the patient's arterial aortic pressure; the other lumen (with the balloon) is attached to a gas reservoir. The console allows for appropriate timing of balloon inflation and houses the helium) tanks. The tanks contain the helium gas that will be used to inflate the balloon during therapy. Additionally, the console has a monitor that displays the arterial waveforms, electrocardiogram (ECG), and balloon-pressure waveforms. Waveforms assist practitioners in determining whether the timing of balloon inflation/deflation is appropriate and allow for any necessary adjustments to be made (Goldich, 2014).

Physiology of Balloon Function

The IABP is timed to inflate and deflate in opposition to the cardiac cycle. The goal of inflation of the IABP balloon is to enhance perfusion. The balloon inflates at the beginning of diastole and deflates before ventricular systole, a process known as counterpulsation (Krishna & Zacharowski, 2009). To correlate the inflation and deflation to the ECG, the balloon begins to inflate in the middle of the T wave and to deflate before the end of the QRS complex (Hanlon-Pena & Quaal, 2011).

Inflation of the balloon at the beginning of diastole displaces blood upward toward the aortic root and augments the diastolic pressure between the balloon and the aortic origin. The increase in diastolic pressure, which is known as diastolic augmentation, forces blood back into the coronary arteries, which are normally perfused during diastole (Krishna & Zacharowski, 2009). Consequently, blood flow to the coronary arteries is increased, with a resultant improvement in myocardial oxygen supply. Intra-aortic balloon pump inflation further causes a decrease in heart rate and afterload and enhances LV function. Ischemia of the myocardial muscle

is diminished or relieved with the ensuing improved CO (Krishna & Zacharowski, 2009). During inflation, blood is also pushed forward to the periphery. In this way, blood flow is increased below the inflated balloon, which may enhance perfusion of the renal arteries and systemic blood vessels (Chen, 2010).

Deflation of the balloon immediately before systole occurs pulls blood forward away from the left ventricle, allowing for more complete emptying. This enhanced LV emptying decreases preload (or end-diastolic volume) and myocardial oxygen demand. The tension caused by the pressure of blood on the left ventricle as it ejects blood (afterload) is diminished as well, further decreasing myocardial oxygen demand and increasing CO and ejection fraction (EF). Systolic blood pressure is noted to be lower with the reduction in afterload (Castellucci, 2011).

Secondary effects of the IABP placement result from the improvement in cardiac function as well. Heart rate, pulmonary artery diastolic, and pulmonary artery occlusive pressures (PAOP) are decreased; mean arterial pressure (MAP), CO, and perfusion to vital organs such as the brain and kidneys are increased (Krishna & Zacharowski, 2009; Laham & Aroesty, 2013).

INDICATIONS FOR IABP THERAPY

The IABP is used in a variety of clinical situations but was initially used for patients in cardiogenic shock. Although still used for this purpose, the recently completed IAPB-SHOCK II trial, which studied the effect of the use of the IABP for 600 patients in cardiogenic shock after an acute myocardial infarction (AMI), did not demonstrate a significant improvement in the mortality rates of patients who received therapy with the IABP as compared with those who did not (Thiele et al., 2013). Cardiogenic shock is a complication in approximately 6% to

10% of patients with an AMI and carries a historically high mortality rate in the range of 50% to 80%. Early revascularization with angioplasty, fibrinolysis, or bypass surgery is initiated to improve mortality in such circumstances (Haddad & Robertson, 2013; Hochman & Reyentovich, 2014). In the case of the patient with cardiogenic shock, the IABP may be used to reduce myocardial ischemia and improve cardiac function, especially as the patient is prepared for a revascularization procedure (Parissis et al., 2012; Xiushui, 2014). In post-myocardial infarction (MI) patients, data suggest that persistent ischemia and reinfarction may also be prevented through use of an IABP (Chen et al., 2014; Parissis et al., 2012).

For patients with unstable angina who are receiving maximum medical therapy but who still experience chest pain/discomfort, the IABP has been successful in reducing or entirely eliminating symptoms. The patient's condition can be stabilized in preparation for surgery or revascularization procedure (Anderson et al., 2013; Parissis et al., 2012).

In post-MI patients, structural damage such as a ventriculoseptal defect (VSD) or mitral regurgitation may occur. The IABP can help hemodynamically stabilize these patients until surgical repair can be performed (Kettner, Sramko, Holek, Pirk, & Krautzner, 2013). With a VSD, there is an abnormal opening between the right ventricle and left ventricle. Because pressure is higher in the left ventricle than in the right ventricle, blood is shunted into the right ventricle, resulting in a lower CO and right ventricular failure. The decrease in afterload produced by the IABP decreases the right-to-left shunt (Testuz, Roffi, & Bonvini, 2013).

Mitral regurgitation in post-MI patients is often due to papillary muscle dysfunction or rupture. The papillary muscles, which are located in the mid- to lower ventricles, are connected to the valve leaflets by the string-like chordae tendineae. When LV systole

occurs, the papillary muscles contract and pull on the chordae. This action prevents the mitral valve leaflets from inverting. In the setting of papillary muscle dysfunction, the mitral valve becomes incompetent and regurgitant blood flow occurs. Blood is then forced back up into the left atrium during ventricular systole, increasing the pressure in that chamber. The increased left atrial pressure is transmitted into the pulmonary vasculature, causing pulmonary congestion and edema. Use of the IABP to decrease afterload can diminish this regurgitant blood flow, thereby relieving pulmonary congestion as the patient awaits surgical repair (Ihdayhid, Chopra, & Rankin, 2014).

The IABP may be essential to assist cardiac function in patients with end-stage cardiac disease or damage while they are awaiting transplant (i.e., as a bridge to transplant) (Parissis et al., 2012). The IABP may be used on a longer basis—as long as 6 months—in these instances. Its use may enable these patients to ambulate as they await transplant (Estep et al., 2013).

Refractory ventricular dysrhythmias may also be responsive to IABP therapy. Poor LV function, coupled with an increase in afterload and increased myocardial oxygen demand, will produce ventricular stretching. Ventricular stretching increases irritability, resulting in difficult-to-treat dysrhythmias. The use of the IABP improves coronary blood flow, thereby helping to reduce irritability. Additionally, because the IABP decreases preload and afterload, the ventricle will be less distended, which further decreases irritability and arrhythmogenicity (Ihdayhid et al., 2014).

It is often difficult to wean postoperative on-pump cardiac surgery patients from cardiopulmonary bypass (CPB) due to preexisting poor cardiac function and the effects of CPB itself (Krishna & Zacharowski, 2009). Placing patients on CPB involves stopping the heart, usually with the use of a cold electrolyte solution (cardioplegia), and inducing a controlled state of ischemia. In the postoperative period, the myocardial muscle is stunned and may need assistance to function effectively (Jones, 2010; Moon, 2012). The IABP stabilizes the hemodynamic profile of these cardiac surgery patients and allows them to be weaned more slowly with less risk of organ damage from a failing heart. Myocardial stunning is discussed in detail in Chapter 13.

Preoperative use of the IABP in patients who are considered at high risk for cardiac surgery has been shown to lower the postoperative mortality rate and shorten intensive care recovery (Hatch & Baklanov, 2014; Moon, 2012). High-risk patients include those with two of the following characteristics: poor LV function (EF less than 30%), unstable angina, left main coronary artery stenosis of greater than 70%, multi-vessel disease, cardiomyopathy, and hemodynamic instability (Hatch & Baklanov, 2014; Krishna & Zacharowski, 2009).

In a worldwide study known as the Benchmark Registry, the largest study to date, nearly 17,000 patients who had undergone IABP support were evaluated. The most common indications for initiating IABP therapy were to provide hemodynamic support during or after a cardiac catheterization procedure, cardiogenic shock, postoperative cardiac surgery in which CPB was used, preoperative cardiac support in high-risk patients, and unstable angina refractory to medical therapy (Ferguson et al., 2001).

CONTRAINDICATIONS TO IABP THERAPY

Contraindications to the use of the IABP are few and can be divided into absolute and relative contraindications. Absolute contraindications are those in which the patient should not receive IABP therapy; they include abdominal aortic aneurysm, aortic dissection, and aortic insufficiency (Haddad & Robertson, 2013). Relative contraindications

are those in which the potential risk of using the IABP must be weighed against the potential benefit; they include patients with peripheral vascular disease, coagulopathies or thrombocytopenia (Haddad & Robertson, 2013), terminal diseases, uncontrolled sepsis, and end-stage cardiomyopathies that are not suitable for transplant (Krishna & Zacharowski, 2009).

INSERTION OF AN IABP

Insertion of an IABP catheter may be performed at the bedside in the intensive care unit (ICU), in the catheterization lab, or in the operating room. Generally, institutional policy requires an informed consent to be signed and reviewed for completeness prior to insertion.

After preparation of the area and administration of a local anesthetic, the balloon catheter is inserted into either the right or left femoral artery. It is threaded up into the descending aorta so that the tip of the catheter is located 1 to 2 centimeters below the subclavian branch of the aortic arch and above the branches of the renal arteries (Haddad & Robertson, 2013; Hatch & Baklanov, 2014) (see **Figure 10-1**). In bridge-to-transplant patients, the catheter may be inserted in the axillary/subclavian fossa, with the distal end

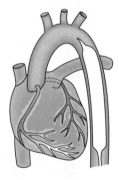

Figure 10-1   Inflated balloon catheter in descending aorta.
Source: Illustrated by James R. Perron.

being located above the renal arteries (Haddad & Robertson, 2013).

Traditionally, the balloon catheter is inserted through an introducer sheath, although many newer catheters are designed to be sheathless. The latter design results in a smaller diameter catheter in the femoral artery, decreasing the chance of ischemic complications to the lower extremity (Laham & Aroesty, 2013; Lewis, Ward, & Courtney, 2009).

The catheter may be inserted under fluoroscopy, which facilitates direct visualization—a key consideration in ensuring proper placement of the catheter. If fluoroscopy is not used, a radiograph film will be checked immediately following the procedure (Castellucci, 2011). When viewed, the tip of the catheter should be located at the second or third intercostal space. Proper positioning is essential because a catheter placed too high will obstruct blood flow to the subclavian artery, which supplies the head and upper extremities. A catheter placed too low can obstruct blood flow to the renal arteries (Goldich, 2014; Rastan et al., 2010).

After the catheter is secured in place, a sterile dressing is applied to the insertion site. The patient's ECG tracing is displayed on the console's monitor; review of the ECG is important to maintain proper triggering of the pump. The central lumen of the balloon catheter is attached to a pressure-monitoring device with continuous flush to monitor the arterial pressure waveform. The balloon lumen is attached to the gas reservoir of the IABP console. A heparin drip, which prevents thrombus formation on the catheter, is usually started after a bolus infusion. The goal is to maintain an activated partial thromboplastin time (aPTT) of 60–80 sec (Haddad & Robertson, 2013).

Upon its initial setup and every hour thereafter, the balloon will be inflated with a syringe, or by the autofill function on some consoles, with the appropriate volume of helium. Helium, which has replaced carbon dioxide (CO_2) on most pump systems, is beneficial, especially with faster heart rates, because it is lighter in density than CO_2 and can travel at a faster speed in and out of the balloon circuit. Balloon volume size varies from 25 or 34 mL for a smaller adult to 40 or 50 mL for a larger adult. Most balloons used are 40 mL in size (Haddad & Robertson, 2013; Krishna & Zacharowski, 2009).

TIMING

Correct timing of balloon inflation and deflation is imperative to achieve the optimal benefit (Hanlon-Pena & Quaal, 2011). Usually, the ECG is used to trigger the pump: The pump identifies the "R" wave to signify ventricular systole. Other triggers, such as an arterial pressure waveform or pacer spikes, may also be used (Lewis et al., 2009). If the designated trigger is not noted, the pump will not initiate inflation and deflation of the balloon. In such a case, the trigger must be restored or a different trigger selected for the pump to work.

The arterial waveform displayed on the console's monitor is used to identify whether the timing of inflation and deflation is accurate. Balloon inflation should start at the beginning of diastole; deflation occurs just before systole or at the onset of systole. Initially, the inflation frequency is set at 1:2 (every other beat assisted) so that the unassisted and assisted waveforms can be compared. Later, the frequency may be switched to 1:1 (every beat assisted) if the patient's status requires this timing. As the patient's condition improves, the frequency may be weaned to 1:2, 1:3, 1:4, or 1:8 before IABP therapy is discontinued, usually over 6 to 12 hours (Krishna & Zacharowski, 2009).

To confirm that the timing of inflation and deflation is correct, specific characteristics are observed on the arterial waveform. First, it is necessary to become familiar with the normal arterial waveform, noting the dicrotic notch (see **Figure 10-2**). Next, the arterial waveform of a patient receiving IABP therapy is

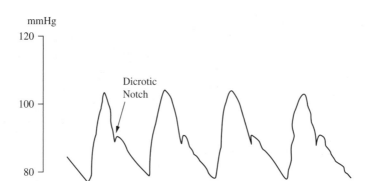

Figure 10-2   Normal arterial waveform.

Source: Illustrated by James R. Perron.

observed. The unassisted systole, the dicrotic notch signifying closure of the aortic valve, and the unassisted aortic end-diastolic pressure should be identified (see **Figure 10-3**). Following the dicrotic notch of an assisted beat will be diastolic augmentation. The dicrotic notch should form a distinct "V" shape between the unassisted systole and the augmented diastolic, indicating that pressure increased in the aortic root during balloon inflation. Following the augmented diastolic is the assisted end-diastolic pressure, which is lower than the unassisted diastolic pressure

because deflation of the balloon results in lower aortic pressure.

Balloon inflation is optimal when (1) a sharp "V" is noted at the dicrotic notch and (2) following the dicrotic notch, the augmented diastolic is as high as or higher than the previous systolic blood pressure. Balloon deflation is optimal when (1) the assisted end-diastolic pressure is lower, usually by 5 to 10 mmHg, than the unassisted aortic end-diastolic pressure and (2) the assisted systolic blood pressure is 5 to 10 mmHg lower than the unassisted systolic pressure (Krishna & Zacharowski, 2009).

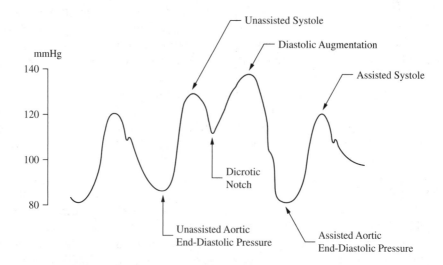

Figure 10-3   Arterial waveform of IABP patient, 1:2 counterpulsation.

Source: Illustrated by James R. Perron.

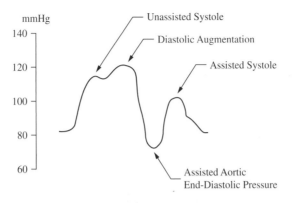

Figure 10-4 Arterial waveform with early balloon inflation.

Source: Illustrated by James R. Perron.

Timing Errors

Although most IABPs have automatic timing, it is essential that continuous monitoring be maintained. Often, manual adjustments to optimize timing are needed. With timing errors, not only are patients not receiving optimal benefit, but they may also suffer deleterious consequences, especially when inflation is not timed correctly (Lewis et al., 2009).

Timing errors occur when there is early or late inflation or early or late deflation of the balloon. With early balloon inflation, the balloon inflates before closure of the aortic valve. This action forces the valve to close early, resulting in aortic regurgitation and subsequent reduction in stroke volume, as well as increases in end-diastolic volume and myocardial oxygen demand (Haddad & Robertson, 2013). In such a case, the arterial waveform will lose its characteristic "'V" shape before diastolic augmentation (see **Figure 10-4**). With late inflation, the balloon inflates later than the appropriate time after closure of the aortic valve, with resultant lower augmented diastolic and coronary perfusion pressures. As a result, the IABP's key benefit—improving blood and oxygen supply to the coronary arteries—is lost or reduced. On the waveform, the peak of the augmented diastolic will be farther away from the dicrotic notch and will be lower, instead of higher, than the unassisted systolic (see **Figure 10-5**).

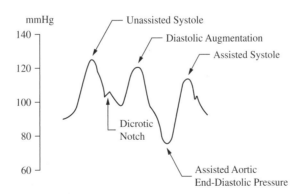

Figure 10-5 Arterial waveform with late balloon inflation.

Source: Illustrated by James R. Perron.

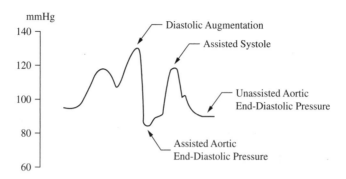

Figure 10-6   Arterial waveform with early balloon deflation.

Source: Illustrated by James R. Perron.

Normally, balloon deflation occurs just before the beginning of systole. If it occurs too far before the onset of systole (early balloon deflation), however, the patient's diastolic pressure will rise, leading to increases in afterload and myocardial oxygen demand. The arterial waveform reveals a sharp drop-off in the augmented diastolic curve, followed by a "U"-shaped curve before the next systolic upstroke (see **Figure 10-6**). When the balloon deflates later than the optimal time (late balloon deflation), its volume decreases as the aortic valve opens instead of before it opens. This results in the loss of the afterload reduction benefit; it may also increase afterload (and myocardial oxygen demand) as

the inflated balloon impedes the ejection of blood from the left ventricle. The waveform will reveal a widened augmented diastolic wave and a slow rise of the next assisted systole (Haddad & Robertson, 2013; Lewis et al., 2009) (see **Figure 10-7**).

Most IABP consoles have a display for the balloon pressure waveform. This waveform represents the pressure as gas is propelled in and out of the balloon catheter. Monitoring this waveform is beneficial as it will assist the ICU nurse in determining whether the balloon is functioning effectively (Castellucci, 2011) (see **Figure 10-8**). Caregivers may find it necessary to follow the specific manufacturer's directions for many settings on such

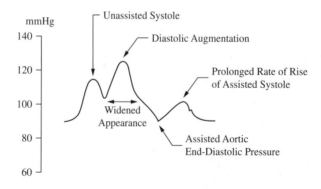

Figure 10-7   Arterial waveform with late balloon deflation.

Source: Illustrated by James R. Perron.

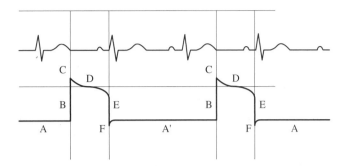

Figure 10-8   IABP waveform. A = balloon pressure baseline; B = rapid inflation; C = peak inflation artifact; D = balloon pressure plateau (balloon is completely inflated); E = rapid deflation; F = balloon deflation artifact; A′ = return to baseline (balloon completely deflated)

Source: Illustrated by James R. Perron.

devices because consoles offered by different companies may have unique properties.

Refer to **Box 10-2** for definitions related to IABP therapy.

COMPLICATIONS OF IABP THERAPY

Although the mortality rate directly associated with the use of the IABP is low, the rate of all complications is reported to be around 6.5%, with serious complications in about 2.1% (Moon et al., 2012; Parissis et al., 2012).

The most prevalent complications are vascular in nature, with the most common being lower-limb ischemia below the insertion site. Fortunately, catheter sizes are becoming smaller and many do not require a sheath for placement. Over the years, smaller catheter size and sheathless introducers have helped to

---

Box 10-2   IABP Therapy Waveform Definitions

Dicrotic notch: An area on the downstroke of the arterial waveform that results from the slight pressure increase created by closure of the aortic valve.

Diastolic augmentation: The increase in pressure in the aorta above the balloon catheter that results with balloon inflation during diastole. It increases perfusion in the coronary arteries and myocardial oxygen supply.

Unassisted aortic end-diastolic pressure: The pressure in the aorta at the end of diastole when counterpulsation via the balloon pump has not assisted that cardiac cycle.

Assisted aortic end-diastolic pressure: The pressure in the aorta at the end of diastole when counterpulsation has assisted the cardiac cycle. It is usually lower than the unassisted end-diastolic pressure.

Unassisted systole: The systolic aortic pressure when counterpulsation has not assisted the cycle.

Assisted systole: The systolic aortic pressure when counterpulsation has assisted the cardiac cycle. It is usually lower than the unassisted systole due to the action of balloon deflation.

Sources: Data from Goldich, G. (2014). Getting in sync with intra-aortic balloon pump therapy. *Nursing, 11*, 10–13; and Krishna, M., & Zacharowski, K. (2009). Principles of intra-aortic balloon counterpulsation. *Continuing Education in Anaesthesia, Critical Care & Pain, 9*(1), 24–28.

reduce complication rates (Laham & Aroesty, 2013; Lewis et al., 2009). Some patients, however, are more prone to limb ischemia. Especially vulnerable populations include the elderly, diabetics, females, obese patients, and individuals with peripheral vascular disease (Haddad & Robertson, 2013; Parissis, Soo, & Al-Alao, 2011). Limb ischemia can occur while the catheter is in place or within hours of its removal and is related to presence of a clot at the catheter site. Thrombectomy is usually required to treat this complication (Goldich, 2014).

Other vascular complications include bleeding or hemorrhage from the insertion site, perforation of the femoral artery, superficial or deep vein thrombosis, stroke, aortic dissection or perforation, and compartment syndrome (Moon, 2012; Parissis et al., 2011). Vascular complications can result in severe consequences, to the point that the patient may require an amputation, thrombectomy, blood transfusions, or vascular surgery.

Balloon-related complications can occur as well. Balloon rupture will result in the release of a helium bolus into the bloodstream because the gas will no longer be contained within the balloon circuit. Blood noted within the gas tubing, inability to maintain augmentation, and low pressure/gas alarms are indicators of possible balloon rupture. Balloon rupture is more likely to occur in patients with atherosclerosis, in whom the balloon will be inflating against rough calcium deposits in the aorta (Castellucci, 2011; Goldich, 2014).

Balloon migration within the aorta is also possible. If the balloon migrates upward, blood supply to the upper extremities and head may be compromised. If the balloon migrates downward, blood supply to the renal arteries and visceral arteries may be impaired (Rastan et al., 2010).

The ICU nurse should monitor for a variety of other complications when an IABP is used. Infection at the insertion site or in the systemic circulation may occur due to the presence of an indwelling catheter; red blood cell hemolysis and thrombocytopenia are possible due to the action of the balloon on blood components as they pass through the aorta (Haddad & Robertson, 2013; Lewis et al., 2009). Other complications include spinal cord ischemia, visceral ischemia, renal failure, and peripheral neuropathy (Laham & Aroesty, 2013).

WEANING FROM IABP THERAPY

The IABP is a temporary device that is usually discontinued postoperatively. Occasionally, some patients who are awaiting cardiac transplant may have it in place longer. Others may have IABP therapy discontinued intraoperatively if it was used to stabilize the patient's condition in the preoperative period. Unless complications occur, the IABP is removed after a period of weaning. Weaning will depend on the improvement in the patient's cardiac function and on a decrease in dependence on inotropes/vasoactive medications (Lewis et al., 2009; Moon, 2012). The ICU nurse, while monitoring the patient on an ongoing basis, is often the first to assess readiness for weaning. Although the orders for weaning will be instituted by a healthcare provider, the ICU nurse is responsible for determining the patient's tolerance to the weaning process. Some of the parameters that may suggest readiness for weaning are listed in **Box 10-3**.

Weaning from the IABP involves decreasing the frequency of assisted beats, decreasing the volume in the balloon over time, or both. Frequency weaning involves switching from 1:1 (every beat assisted by IABP) to 1:2 (every other beat assisted). Switching from a 1:1 to 1:2 ratio provides the most marked decrease in blood flow to the coronary arteries—more than switching from 1:2 to 1:3 or 1:4, or from 1:4 to 1:8 (Krishna & Zacharowski, 2009; Lewis et al., 2009). As a consequence,

Box 10-3   Parameters for IABP Weaning

- Stable hemodynamic parameters: Stable on low doses of vasoactive medications.
- No unstable dysrhythmias: Heart rate should be normal or near normal without dysrhythmias that compromise hemodynamic parameters.
- Low or normal serum lactate levels.
- Normal electrolyte levels.
- Acceptable hemoglobin/hematocrit levels.
- No chest pain/discomfort or dyspnea.
- No mental status changes indicative of poor cerebral perfusion.
- Urine output greater than 0.5 mL/kg/hr.

Source: Goldich, G. (2014). Getting in sync with intra-aortic balloon pump therapy. *Nursing, 11*, 10–13.

the patient who is weaned in this manner will require frequent monitoring, especially during the first stage of weaning.

Volume weaning involves gradually reducing the amount of gas in the balloon. Usually, the volume is lowered by 20% with each reduction. Because there is an increased risk of thrombus formation in the balloon folds, volume weaning is not recommended as readily as frequency weaning. Volume weaning, however, may be better tolerated by patients who do not tolerate frequency weaning (Lewis et al., 2009). Weaning is successful when the patient is able to remain hemodynamically stable with IABP therapy off.

Anticoagulation used during IABP therapy should be tapered and ultimately discontinued prior to catheter removal. Frequency of balloon inflation can be set to 1:8 while the heparin effect is allowed to wear off (Goldich, 2014).

Once the catheter is removed, pressure should be applied to the site for 30 to 45 minutes, followed by application of a sterile pressure bandage for 2 to 4 hours (Castellucci, 2011). After placement of the pressure bandage, the patient should be checked for bleeding every 30 minutes for 2 to 4 hours, then every 2 hours for 24 hours. Monitoring should confirm that a hematoma is not developing under the bandage because hematomas can be a significant source of blood loss. The

patient should be instructed to keep the head of the bed at 30 degrees or less, with no flexion of the hip for at least 8 hours following IABP catheter removal (Castellucci, 2011).

TROUBLESHOOTING THE IABP

With the IABP, as with any mechanical device, problems may occur that need to be addressed promptly. Often, it is best to refer to the manufacturer's troubleshooting guide because it contains a complete reference of problems likely to be encountered. A few of the most common problems are discussed here.

Low Diastolic Augmentation

Low diastolic augmentation is noted when the pressure in the aortic root (above the balloon) does not rise enough after balloon inflation to sufficiently perfuse the coronary arteries. Potential causes of low diastolic augmentation include incorrect balloon timing, dysrhythmias that result in low stroke volume, hypotension or low vascular resistance, balloon leak or rupture, incorrect balloon catheter placement or balloon migration, inappropriate balloon size, and balloon not fully opened.

If the balloon or balloon catheter is found to be faulty, it should be removed as soon as possible (within 30 minutes) to avoid thrombus development on an idle catheter (Moon, 2012). Most consoles have an alarm system that warns providers of a gas leak or a rapid loss of gas. Slow leaks may be the result of a hole in the balloon or a loose connection in the gas tubing. A rapid loss of gas, in contrast, is usually the result of balloon rupture or a disconnected gas circuit. In this scenario, the gas line should be clamped off immediately. If blood is noted in the balloon catheter or gas circuit, it is recommended that the pump be stopped immediately because the balloon or catheter has a leak. Continuing to pump will introduce gas into the bloodstream, producing an air embolus.

Faulty Trigger

On occasion, the ECG trigger may not function properly. Common causes of a faulty trigger include poor electrode placement, low ECG voltage, faulty electrode pads or cables, dysrhythmias, and other equipment's interference with the ECG signal (Chen, 2010; Moon, 2012). If the problem cannot be easily rectified, switching to the arterial pressure trigger will be necessary until the problem can be resolved.

Autofill Failure

The autofill feature on the IABP maintains the volume of gas within the balloon. Should this feature not function, an autofill alarm will sound. The cause of this problem could be an insufficient amount of gas in the tank or occlusion of the gas outlet. The amount of gas in the tank should be checked and the tank replaced as needed. Also, the provider should assess for and correct any kinks or leaks in the tubing and ensure that the valve on the tank is in the open position (Chen, 2010).

In the event of pump failure or if pumping needs to be stopped, the IABP balloon should be manually inflated with a syringe every 5 minutes. The syringe should be filled with a volume of gas that is 10 mL less than

balloon capacity to prevent thrombus formation (Castellucci, 2011).

Intensive care unit nurses caring for a patient receiving IABP therapy must be knowledgeable about the potential complications that can occur during catheter/balloon insertion and removal and during therapy. They must equally be aware of management strategies and preventive measures to implement to avoid or minimize associated morbidity. Patients receiving IABP therapy need to have continuous monitoring, and the nurse-to-patient ratio is encouraged to be 1:1. Often, these patients are critically ill and have complex problems related to their condition as well as the difficulties experienced by dependence, even for a few days, on highly specialized equipment. **Box 10-4** lists nursing interventions required by the patient who is receiving IABP therapy.

MONITORING FOR COMPLICATIONS OF IABP THERAPY

- *Limb ischemia.* Perform peripheral vascular checks, including checking pulses, capillary refill time, skin color, and temperature of lower extremities. After discontinuation of therapy, distal pulses should be checked every hour for 2 hours, then at least every 4 hours until the patient is discharged. Patients should be instructed to notify the nurse if they note any changes in circulation (Castellucci, 2011).

- *Bleeding at the insertion site.* Check the dressing and under the patient's thigh for bleeding every 2 hours. Check for hematoma development under dressing.

- *Anemia and thrombocytopenia.* Obtain a daily complete blood count (CBC). Transfuse platelets and red blood cells as indicated.

- *Infection.* Monitor for signs and symptoms of infection: greater than temperature

Box 10-4   Nursing Interventions for the Patient Receiving IABP Therapy

Pre-Insertion Interventions

- Perform a two-person identification verification and timeout to ensure the correct patient for the procedure.
- Provide as calm an environment as possible because the patient will likely be overwhelmed.
- Provide reassurance that the IABP therapy is temporary.
- Explain the procedure and the steps to help ensure safety (as time permits).
- Allow families to participate in discussions and to express concerns.
- Ascertain that consent is signed and complete if required.
- Obtain a 12-lead ECG; insert a urinary catheter.
- Assist with the insertion of invasive lines such as an arterial line and a pulmonary artery catheter.
- Obtain baseline hemodynamic readings: HR, RR, BP, MAP, PAP, PAOP, CVP, CO, or CI, SVR, and urine output.
- Obtain baseline blood work: ABG, mixed venous blood gas, chemistries with BUN/creatinine, CBC with platelets and differential, coagulation profile, and type and crossmatch.
- Perform a peripheral vascular assessment, including checking ankle-brachial index,* skin temperature, presence and strength of pulses, and capillary refill in lower extremities.
- Monitor for the presence of a left radial pulse. Inform the healthcare provider if the pulse is lost so that the catheter can be repositioned.

Post-Insertion Interventions

- Monitor and record hemodynamic measurements every 15 to 30 minutes until the patient is stable, then hourly and PRN.
- Obtain an ECG and chest radiograph daily and PRN.
- Titrate vasopressors/inotropic agents as required to desired hemodynamic parameters. Hemodynamic stability is essential to maintain optimal perfusion to the limb.
- Maintain IV fluid therapy as ordered to maintain an acceptable preload.
- Assess for pain/discomfort, anxiety, and mental status changes hourly.
- Document IABP settings hourly; include the assisted and unassisted pressures.
- Print and document the arterial waveform tracing every 12 hours and PRN with changes.
- Assess for presence and strength of distal pulses, indices of adequate limb perfusion, and sensorimotor function of both lower extremities every 15 minutes for 1 hour, then 30 minutes for 1 hour, and then hourly or according to unit protocol.
- Assess the ankle-brachial index every 4 hours.
- Monitor for the presence of a left radial pulse. Loss of pulse indicates that the catheter has migrated upward, is occluding the left subclavian artery, and requires repositioning.
- Maintain and titrate the heparin infusion to desired anticoagulation as ordered. Obtain coagulation studies 6 hours after dosage changes or follow the facility protocol.
- Obtain daily blood work: chemistries, CBC with platelets, coagulation profile, ABG, lactate level, and mixed venous blood gas.
- Monitor respiratory status: Assess breath sounds every 4 hours. Maintain oxygen, ventilator therapy, or both. Encourage coughing and deep breathing/incentive spirometry every 2 hours. Keep the head of bed at a 15- to 30-degree angle to prevent aspiration. Perform chest physiotherapy when the patient is logrolled.
- Maintain NPO or clear liquids as tolerated. If tolerated, maintain tube feedings via feeding tube. Check residual every 4 hours and notify the healthcare provider if it is greater than 200 mL.

(Continued)

Box 10-4   Nursing Interventions for the Patient Receiving IABP Therapy (*Continued*)

- Prevent skin breakdown related to immobility. Maintain the patient on bed rest, with sedation if needed. Encourage the patient not to flex the hip on affected side. Use a leg immobilizer if necessary. If tolerated, logroll the patient every 4 hours; perform meticulous skin care. Provide passive range-of-motion exercises for the lower extremity without a catheter and for upper extremities every 4 hours.

To check ankle-brachial index:

- With patient supine and at rest, apply blood pressure cuff around both ankles and arms.
- Inflate blood pressure cuffs above patient's normal SBP.
- Deflate blood pressure cuffs. Obtain blood pressure readings using a Doppler and record SBP measurements from the arms and ankles.
- Divide ankle systolic pressure by the highest arm pressure; this will yield an ABI value for each leg.

An index value of 0.9 to 1.3 is considered normal. Values greater than the normal range indicate the presence of some degree of peripheral vascular disease. Presence of mild, moderate, or severe peripheral vascular disease warrants reevaluation of vein selection for cardiac surgery.

ABG, arterial blood gas; ABI, ankle-brachial index; BP, blood pressure; BUN, blood urea nitrogen; CBC, complete blood count; CI, cardiac index; CO, cardiac output; CVP, central venous pressure; ECG, electrocardiogram; HR, heart rate; MAP, mean arterial pressure; PAOP, pulmonary artery occlusive pressure; PAP, pulmonary artery pressure; PRN, as needed; NPO, nothing by mouth; RR, respiratory rate; SBP, systolic blood pressure; SVR, systemic vascular resistance (afterload).

Sources: Castellucci, D. (2011). Intraaortic balloon pump management. In D. L. Weigand (Ed.), *AACN procedural manual for critical care* (6th ed., pp. 443-463). St. Louis, MO: Elsevier Saunders; Chen, M. (2010). Mechanical circulatory assist devices. In S. Woods, E. S. Froelicher, S. Motzer, & E. Bridges (Eds.), *Cardiac nursing* (6th ed., pp. 623-637). Philadelphia, PA: Wolters Kluwer Health/Lippincott Williams & Wilkins; and Goldich, G. (2014). Getting in sync with intra-aortic balloon pump therapy. *Nursing, 11*, 10-13.

101.8 °F, white blood cell count greater than 10,000 cells/mm³, chills, mental status changes. If infection is suspected, send specimens for peripheral blood, urine, and sputum cultures. Culture the IABP port as well. Change the insertion site dressing according to facility policy and examine the skin around site for redness, increased temperature, or purulent drainage. Institute antibiotics promptly as prescribed. Infection can occur at the insertion site or systemically, and the risk increases as the length of time the catheter is left in the patient increases (Chen, 2010).

- *Catheter migration.* Monitor the patient's pulses, skin color, and temperature; assess for altered sensation in the left upper extremity every 1–2 hours. Report urine output of less than 0.5 mL/kg/hr, increasing blood urea nitrogen (BUN)/

creatinine, or flank pain. Assess the patient for increased abdominal girth or discomfort with absent bowel sounds. Monitor the level of consciousness and evaluate the patient for unilateral neurologic impairment. Obtain a chest radiograph and anticipate repositioning or reinsertion of the catheter if migration is suspected (Laham & Aroesty, 2013).

- *Aortic dissection.* This complication occurs very rarely in IABP insertions. Assess the patient for abdominal, back, intrascapular, or shoulder pain, usually of sudden onset. The pain may be described as "tearing." Other symptoms include increased abdominal girth and absent or unequal peripheral pulses with concomitant decreased blood pressure and urine output. Obtain a computed tomography scan or magnetic resonance imaging if dissection is suspected. Treatment consists of prompt surgical repair (Juang, Braverman, & Eagle, 2008).

SUMMARY

Care of the patient receiving IABP therapy is complex and challenging. Patients require prompt intervention for problems and empathy for their critical illness. For the ICU nurse, additional instruction both in theory and in hands-on experience is required to be able to maintain and troubleshoot the complex IABP apparatus. Management of this device is accomplished while balancing evidence-based care that involves critical thinking and decision making, preventing and detecting complications, and providing emotional support to patients and families who are experiencing one of the most vulnerable times in their lives.

CASE STUDY

B. C. is a 57-year-old male with a known history of coronary artery disease, hyperlipidemia, and diabetes mellitus. He presented to the emergency department with shortness of breath and unrelieved chest pain. Upon ECG, an anterior wall ST-segment elevation MI (STEMI) was noted. B. C. underwent PCI with insertion of a drug-eluting stent. The procedure was uncomplicated. Post-procedure, B. C. was transferred to a cardiac step-down unit. One hour after admission, his vital signs were noted: BP 78/64, HR 144, RR 34, SpO_2 91%. Bibasilar crackles were auscultated. Following attempts to correct the hypotension with fluids and dopamine at 5 mcg/kg/min, he was transferred to the ICU. Dobutamine titrated up to 20 mcg/kg/min and a milrinone load followed by an infusion of 0.5 mcg/kg/minute did not completely resolve B. C.'s hemodynamic status. An IABP was placed in the descending aorta via the femoral artery. After 24 hours, B. C.'s condition improved. He ultimately was weaned from the IABP therapy and was transferred back to the cardiac step-down unit the next day. He will be followed by his cardiology team and it will be determined if he needs cardiac surgery in the future.

Critical Thinking Questions

1. What was the indication for IABP therapy for B. C.?
2. What nursing care should be provided to a patient receiving IABP therapy?
3. What criteria should be used to determine readiness to wean from IABP therapy?

Answers to Critical Thinking Questions

1. Cardiogenic shock; signs of decreased cardiac output that did not respond to other therapies.
2. After insertion, an occlusive sterile dressing should be applied and maintained. Other nursing care includes titration of the heparin infusion based on aPTT results, monitoring of the ECG to maintain proper triggering of the pump, confirming timing of inflation and deflation, and monitoring for complications of therapy.
3. Parameters that should be assessed to determine readiness to wean from IABP therapy include presence of stable hemodynamic parameters, no unstable dysrhythmias, normal or below normal serum lactate level, normal electrolyte and CBC results, no chest pain or discomfort, no dyspnea, no mental status changes, and urinary output at least 0.5 mL/kg/hour.

SELF-ASSESSMENT QUESTIONS

1. Intra-aortic balloon pump inflation should correspond with which part of the ECG?
   a. On the R wave
   b. Middle of the T wave
   c. Just before the P wave
   d. In the PR interval

2. Intra-aortic balloon pump deflation should correspond with which part of the ECG?
   a. Before end of the T wave
   b. At the beginning of the P wave
   c. Before the end of the QRS
   d. In the middle of the PR interval

3. Intra-aortic balloon pump inflation causes which of the following?

	HR	SVR	LV function
a.	increased	increased	decreased
b.	decreased	increased	decreased
c.	increased	decreased	increased
d.	decreased	decreased	increased

4. Deflation of the intra-aortic balloon pump balloon results in which of the following?
   a. Increased blood flow to the coronary arteries
   b. Increased myocardial oxygen delivery
   c. Decreased heart rate
   d. Decreased preload

5. Inflation of the intra-aortic balloon pump balloon results in which of the following?
   a. Decreased myocardial oxygen demand
   b. Decreased heart rate
   c. Increased ejection fraction
   d. Decreased systolic blood pressure

6. Patients with which of the following rhythms may benefit from intra-aortic balloon pump therapy?

a.

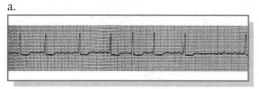

b.

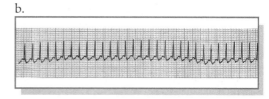

c.

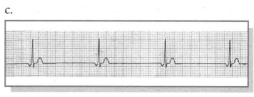

d.

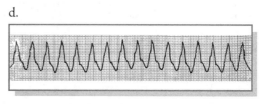

7. Which of the following is an absolute contraindication for intra-aortic balloon pump therapy?
   a. Peripheral vascular disease
   b. Thrombocytopenia
   c. End-stage cardiomyopathy
   d. Aortic insufficiency

8. Early balloon inflation results in which of the following?
   a. Aortic regurgitation
   b. Decreased PAOP
   c. Decreased myocardial oxygen demand
   d. Mitral regurgitation

9. Early intra-aortic balloon pump deflation will result in which of the following?
   a. Increased diastolic blood pressure
   b. Decreased afterload
   c. Decreased myocardial oxygen demand
   d. Increased coronary artery perfusion

10. You are caring for a patient with an intra-aortic balloon pump in place and note blood within the gas tubing. Which of the following should the nurse suspect?
    a. Red blood cell hemolysis
    b. Balloon migration
    c. Thrombocytopenia
    d. Balloon rupture

Answers to Self-Assessment Questions

1. b	4. d	7. d	9. a
2. c	5. b	8. a	10. d
3. d	6. d		

Clinical Inquiry Box

Question: Is there a difference in morbidity and mortality data between patients who receive IABP therapy before or after cardiac surgery?

Reference: Dhaliwal, A. S., Chu, D., Huh, J., Ghadir, M., Sansgiry, S., Atluri, P., . . . Bakaeen, F. G. (2009). Prognostic impact of intra-aortic balloon pump insertion before versus after cardiac surgical intervention in a veteran population. *American Journal of Surgery, 198*(5), 628–632.

Objective: To determine if there is difference in morbidity and mortality data between patients who receive IABP therapy before or after cardiac surgery.

Method: Retrospective data analysis.

Results: The patients who received IABP therapy after cardiac surgery had higher morbidity (71% versus 42%) and mortality rates (43% versus 14%) than the patients who received IABP therapy before cardiac surgery. Survival rates at 1 year (50% versus 83%) and 3 years (46% versus 80%) were lower in the patients who received IABP therapy after surgery as compared to those who received IABP therapy before surgery.

Conclusion: Patients who receive IABP therapy following cardiac surgery may have worse outcomes as compared to those who receive IABP therapy before cardiac surgery.

REFERENCES

Anderson, J. L., Adams, C. D., Antman, E. M., Bridges, C. R., Califf, R. M., Casey, Jr., D. E., . . . Wright, S. (2013). 2012 ACCF/AHA focus update incorporated into the ACCF/AHA 2007 guidelines for the management of patients with UA/Non-ST elevation MI: A report of the American College of Cardiology Foundation/American Heart Association Task Force on Practice Guidelines. *Journal of the American College of Cardiology, 61*(23), e179–e347.

Castellucci, D. (2011). Intraaortic balloon pump management. In D. L. Weigand (Ed.), *AACN procedural manual for critical care* (6th ed., pp. 443–463). St. Louis, MO: Elsevier Saunders.

Chen, M. (2010). Mechanical circulatory assist devices. In S. Woods, E. S. Froelicher, S. Motzer, & E. Bridges (Eds.), *Cardiac nursing* (6th ed., pp. 623–637). Philadelphia, PA: Wolters Kluwer Health/Lippincott Williams & Wilkins.

Chen, S., Yin, Y., Ling, Z., & Krucoff, M. W. (2014). Short and long term effect of adjunctive intra-aortic balloon pump use for patients undergoing high risk reperfusion therapy: A meta-analysis of 10 international randomised trials. *Heart (British Cardiac Society), 100*(4), 303–310.

Elliot, D., Aitken, L., & Chaboyer, W. (2012). *ACCCN's critical care nursing* (2nd ed.). Chatswood, Australia: Elsevier Australia.

Estep, J. D., Cordero-Reyes, A. M., Bhimaraj, A., Trachtenberg, B., Khalil, N., Loebe, M., . . . Torre-Amione, G. (2013). Percutaneous placement of intra-aortic balloon pump in left axillary/subclavian position provides safe, ambulatory, long-term support as a bridge to heart transplant. *JACC Heart Failure, 1*(5), 382–388.

Ferguson, J. J., Cohen, M., Freedman, R. J., Stone, G. W., Miller, M., Joseph, D. L., & Ohman, E. M. (2001). The current practice of intra-aortic balloon counterpulsation: Results from the Benchmark Registry. *Journal of the American College of Cardiology, 38*(5), 1456–1462.

Goldich, G. (2014). Getting in sync with intra-aortic balloon pump therapy. *Nursing*, 11, 10–13.

Haddad, E. V., & Robertson, C. H. (2013). *Intra-aortic balloon counterpulsation.* Retrieved from http://emedicine.medscape.com/article/1847715-overview

Hanlon-Pena, P. M., & Quaal, S. J. (2011). Intra-aortic balloon pump timing: Review of evidence supporting current practice. *American Journal of Critical Care*, 20, 323–334.

Hatch, J., & Baklanov, D. (2014). Percutaneous hemodynamic support in PCI. *Current Treatment Options in Cardiovascular Medicine*, 16(4), 293.

Hochman, J. S., & Reyentovich, A. (2014). *Prognosis and treatment of cardiogenic shock complicating acute myocardial infarction.* Retrieved from http://www.uptodate.com/contents/prognosis-and-treatment-of-cardiogenic-shock-complicating-acute-myocardial-infarction

Ihdayhid, A. R., Chopra, S., & Rankin, J. (2014). Intra-aortic balloon pump: Indications, efficacy, guidelines and future directions. *Current Opinion in Cardiology*, 29, 285–292.

Jones, B. (2010). Postoperative complications of cardiac surgery and nursing interventions. In S. Hardin & R. Kaplow (Eds.), *Cardiac surgery essentials* (pp. 257–286). Sudbury, MA: Jones and Bartlett.

Juang, D., Braverman, A. C., & Eagle, K. (2008). Aortic dissection. *Circulation*, 118, e507–e510.

Kettner, J., Sramko, M., Holek, M., Pirk, J., & Krautzner, J. (2013). Utility of intra-aortic balloon pump support for ventricular septal rupture and acute mitral regurgitation complicating acute myocardial infarction. *American Journal of Cardiology*, 112, 1709–1713.

Krishna, M., & Zacharowski, K. (2009). Principles of intra-aortic balloon counterpulsation. *Continuing Education in Anaesthesia, Critical care & Pain*, 9(1), 24–28.

Laham, R. J., & Aroesty, J. M. (2013). *Intraaortic balloon counterpulsation.* Retrieved from http://www.uptodate.com/contents/intraaortic-balloon-pump-counterpulsation

Lewis, P. A., Ward, D. A., & Courtney, M. D. (2009). The intra-aortic balloon pump in heart failure management: Implications for nursing practice. *Australian Critical Care*, 22(3), 125–131.

Moon, C. (2012). Preoperative intra-aortic balloon pumping in high-risk cardiac surgery patients.

Dimensions of Critical Care Nursing, 31(4), 223–227.

Parissis, H., Soo, A., & Al-Alao, B. (2011). Intra aortic balloon pump: Literature review of risk factors related to complications of the intra aortic balloon pump. *Journal of Cardiothoracic Surgery*, 6, 147. Retrieved from http://www.cardiothoracicsurgery.org/content/6/1/147

Parissis, H., Soo, A., & Al-Alao, B. (2012). Intra-aortic balloon pump (IABP): From the old trends and studies to the current "extended" indications of its use. *Journal of Cardiothoracic Surgery*, 7, 128. Retrieved from http://www.cardiothoracicsurgery.org/content/7/1/128

Rastan, A. J., Tillman, E., Subramanian, S., Lehmkuhl, L., Funkat, A. K., Leontyev, S., . . . Mohr, F. W. (2010). Visceral arterial compromise during intra-aortic balloon counterpulsation therapy. *Circulation*, 122(Suppl. 1), S92–S99.

Sharma, S., Lumley, M., & Perera, D. (2013). Intra-aortic balloon pump use in high-risk percutaneous coronary intervention. *Current Opinion in Cardiology*, 28, 671–675.

Testuz, A., Roffi, M., & Bonvini, R. F. (2013). Left-to-right shunt reduction with intra-aortic balloon pump in postmyocardial infarction ventricular septal defect. *Catheterization and Cardiovascular Interventions*, 81, 727–731.

Thiele, H., Zeymer, U., Neumann, F. J., Ferenc, M., Olbrich, H. G., Hausleiter, J., . . . Schuler, G. (2013). Intra-aortic balloon counterpulsation in acute myocardial infarction complicated by cardiogenic shock (IABP-SHOCK II): Final 12 month results of a randomised, open-label trial. *Lancet*, 382, 1638–1645.

Xiushui, R. (2014). *Cardiogenic shock.* Retrieved from http://emedicine.medscape.com/article/152191

WEB RESOURCES

Intra-aortic balloon pump information: http://www.cprworks.com/IABP.html

Intra-aortic balloon pump: https://www.youtube.com/watch?v=o11fhdVOYWA

Timing and triggering of the intra-aortic balloon pump: https://www.youtube.com/watch?v=Ff-1YXaUBO0

Ankle Brachial Index: https://www.youtube.com/watch?v=KnJDrmfIXGw

Chapter 11

Mechanical Ventilation After Cardiac Surgery

Mary Jane Bowles

INTRODUCTION

Mechanical ventilation may be essential in the postoperative management of patients undergoing cardiac surgery and cardiopulmonary bypass (CPB). Prior to the 1990s, patients were mechanically ventilated until the morning after surgery before weaning was attempted. In more recent decades, the need for cost containment has resulted in "fast-tracking" patients by implementing early weaning protocols and reversible sedation. By utilizing appropriate anesthetic techniques and postoperative management, the cardiac surgery patient may be extubated within 6 hours without complications, thus leading to better patient outcomes. The reported benefits of earlier extubation include improved preload, decreased hemodynamic compromise, early discharge from the intensive care unit (ICU), early ambulation, prevention of potential complications of prolonged intubation, and decreased neurologic compromise (in elderly patients). Early extubation protocols have also shown a decrease in morbidity associated with both cardiac and respiratory complications (Akhtar & Hamid, 2009; Schadler et al., 2012).

The majority of patients are extubated within 24 hours following coronary artery bypass grafting (CABG) procedures. However, prolonged mechanical ventilation may occur in as many as 22.7% of cardiac surgery patients (Piotto et al., 2012). In one study, 48% of patients were still receiving mechanical ventilation on day 10 after surgery (Trouillet et al., 2009).

The Society of Thoracic Surgeons (STS; 2014) was formed to provide the highest quality patient care through education, research, and advocacy in chest surgery. The Virginia Cardiac Surgery Quality Initiative (VCSQI), a subgroup of STS, identified in 2007 the timely extubation of patients and reduction in rates of prolonged ventilation as a priority to improve outcomes. In the VCSQI review, the ability to achieve early extubation included the use of less sedation and shorter-acting muscle relaxants. Some institutions utilized Bispectral Index Monitoring as part of the cardiac anesthesia protocol, extubations while still maintained on the intra-aortic balloon pump (IABP), moderate hypothermia intraoperatively with more aggressive rewarming postoperatively, standard protocol orders, and transparency regarding results of extubation times (VCSQI, 2014).

Nurses in the ICU who are caring for patients in the immediate postoperative period following cardiac surgery must have an understanding of the pathophysiology of the lungs, use of mechanical ventilation, weaning protocols, and ability to interpret the clinical significance of diagnostic tests such as arterial blood gases (ABGs) and radiographic findings. They must be able to identify complications of patients on mechanical ventilation and implement measures to prevent morbidities associated with therapy so optimal patient outcomes can be attained.

PREDICTORS OF PROLONGED MECHANICAL VENTILATION

Several factors have been identified as predictors of the need for prolonged mechanical ventilation following cardiac surgery. These include older age, chronic renal failure, chronic obstructive pulmonary disease (COPD), CABG associated with other procedures, and aortic cross-clamping time (Piotto et al., 2012); aortic aneurysm surgery, emergency surgery, valve procedures, and preoperative stroke (Knapik, Ciesla, Borowik, Czempik, & Knapik, 2011); admission to the ICU on IABP therapy, and redo procedure within 24 hours of admission to the ICU because of bleeding (Zante, Kubik, & Reichenspurner, 2010); older age and longer surgical time (Giakoumidakis et al., 2011); age 70 years and above, left ventricular ejection fraction (LVEF) 30% or less, preexisting respiratory disease, preexisting renal failure, emergent surgery, redo surgery, and preoperative use of inotropes (Faritous, Aghdaie, Yazdanian, Azarfarin, & Dabbagh, 2011); higher than New York Heart Association (NYHA) class II, requiring renal dialysis, age, decreased respiratory function, and obesity (body mass index greater than 35 kg/m^2) (Salah et al., 2012); age 65 years and older, chronic renal failure, COPD, redo surgery, emergent surgery, NYHA class higher than II, LVEF 30% or less, need for transfusion of four or more units of packed red blood cells or fresh frozen plasma during surgery, and CPB time more than 77 minutes (Cislaghi, Conderni, & Corona, 2009).

Anesthesia and Postoperative Complications

General anesthesia is used for pain control, muscle relaxation, and amnesia effect during cardiac surgery. A combination of medications are utilized: inhalation, intravenous, and sometimes epidural agents; these agents all have effect on the patient related to duration, mechanism of action, and side effects and will impact duration of ventilation and extubation.

A higher mortality rate is also associated with patients who require prolonged ventilation (Akhtar & Hamid, 2009). Data suggest that patients who undergo cardiac surgery who have prolonged ventilator time postoperatively have lower probability of being discharged from the ICU to a general unit, from a general unit to a rehabilitation unit, or have higher in-hospital mortality rates (Cislaghi et al., 2009). Similarly, postoperative cardiac surgery patients who developed pneumonia also had a higher mortality rate (Ibañez et al., 2014).

Delays Related to Bypass Complications

Several clinical conditions, when present, are likely to result in failure of ventilator weaning. When these conditions are compounded with complications associated with CPB, ventilation time may be prolonged due to a decrease in surfactant production, potential for pulmonary microemboli, and interstitial fluid accumulation in the lungs. Furthermore, red blood cell damage in the pump circuit may potentially occur, decreasing the number of oxygen-carrying capacity cells (Khalpey, Ganim, & Rawn, 2008).

Complications of Prolonged Ventilation

Prolonged use of mechanical ventilation is not without risk. In one study, patients who required prolonged ventilation (more than 72 hours) were more likely to experience sepsis, endocarditis, gastrointestinal bleeding, stroke, renal failure, or deep sternal wound infection (Durham & Gold, 2008).

PATHOPHYSIOLOGY OF THE LUNGS

The main function of the respiratory system is to transport air into the lungs so that oxygen can enter the body and carbon dioxide (CO_2) can be eliminated. Air enters the nose or mouth and moves through the trachea into the bronchi and then into each lung. Once air is in the lungs, gas exchange occurs in the approximately 300 million alveoli. Oxygen and carbon dioxide can cross between the lung capillaries and the alveolar spaces, allowing gas exchange to occur. The nasal passages and bronchi warm and moisten the air before it enters the alveoli as a method of preventing damage to delicate alveolar structures.

The mechanism of breathing involves the diaphragm and the intercostal muscles. During normal breathing, inspiration is an active process and expiration is a passive process. Inspiration involves contraction of the diaphragm and the intercostal muscles to allow for the movement of air into the respiratory tract. The diaphragm and intercostal muscles then relax during expiration.

The respiratory center, which is located in the medulla oblongata (the lower part of the brain stem), receives neural, chemical, and hormonal signals that can control the rate and depth of movements of the diaphragm and other respiratory muscles. An increase in carbon dioxide or a decrease in oxygenation, for example, will increase the rate or depth of breathing. Injury, medications, and disease processes can affect the respiratory center's ability to respond to changes in carbon dioxide or oxygen, resulting in respiratory compromise. The use of mechanical ventilation may be needed in these circumstances.

The autonomic nervous system is also involved in breathing. The parasympathetic nervous system may stimulate bronchoconstriction, whereas stimulation of the sympathetic nervous system may cause bronchodilation.

ASSESSMENT OF READINESS FOR WEANING

While many postoperative cardiac surgery patients are extubated prior to their admission to the ICU and many others remain on mechanical ventilation for only a few hours after surgery, all intubated patients should be evaluated for their readiness for weaning. Data suggest that it may be safe to extubate patients 2 hours following cardiac surgery (Parmer, Clarke, Lau, Porter, & Allsager, 2014). Despite the relatively short amount of time during which patients are intubated postoperatively, it has been reported that more than 22% of patients experience difficulty with weaning. A number of criteria have been suggested for the ICU nurse to use to determine patient readiness, including the patient's ability to cough adequately, presence of minimal secretions, pulmonary mechanics, and cardiovascular reserve (Kulkami & Agarwal, 2008). In addition, hemodynamic stability, bleeding control, normothermia, and ability to follow commands must be assessed when deciding if a patient is ready for extubation (Dirks & Waters, 2014).

General Physiologic and Hemodynamic Stability

The patient's overall condition should be assessed because a number of conditions may potentially influence the success of weaning from mechanical ventilation. Presence of excessive bleeding or an electrolyte imbalance may affect the patient's ability to oxygenate or eliminate carbon dioxide (Dirks & Waters, 2014). Similarly, if the patient is not hemodynamically stable—a common finding in the postoperative cardiac surgery patient—success with weaning may be impaired. The ICU nurse should assess vital signs and hemodynamic parameters, and evaluate the patient for presence of dysrhythmias, tachycardia, bradycardia, weak peripheral pulses, and signs of heart failure (e.g., increase in pulmonary artery occlusive pressure or decrease in cardiac output or mixed venous saturation) (Dirks & Waters, 2014).

A number of clinical conditions have been found to influence the ability to wean by affecting either the capacity of or the demand on the respiratory system. In addition to hemodynamic instability and electrolyte imbalances, administration of morphine causes delays in weaning from mechanical ventilation (Parmer et al., 2014). Patient factors that should be optimized prior to extubation include cardiovascular, respiratory, metabolic/temperature, and neuromuscular factors (Popat et al., 2012). Electrolyte imbalances can decrease muscle contractility and, therefore, may influence success with weaning. Specifically, phosphorus, calcium, magnesium, and potassium deficits should be corrected prior to attempting to wean the patient from mechanical ventilation (Eskandar & Apostolakos, 2007).

A patient's mental status should be adequate enough to allow for maintenance of a patent airway and the ability to cooperate with coughing and deep breathing to prevent post-extubation respiratory compromise and complications (Eskandar & Apostolakos, 2007).

Mechanical weaning parameters are, in general, insufficient at predicting weaning success because they do not take into account cardiac reserves. Therefore, it is necessary for nursing personnel to understand cardiovascular response to mechanical ventilator weaning. Porhomayon, Papadakos, and Nader (2012) reported serum B-type natriuretic peptide (BNP) and N-terminal pro B-type natriuretic peptide (NT-proBNP) appear to signify patients with heart failure during the weaning process. Ischemic heart disease, valvular heart disease, or systolic or diastolic dysfunction can be part of the cause of cardiac load increase and weaning failure. The extra demand on cardiac load during spontaneous breathing trials (SBTs) may become apparent when transferring patient from positive to spontaneous ventilation. In these situations, diuretic therapy may be considered for excessive preload, and weaning to noninvasive positive-pressure ventilation may be beneficial (Porhomayon et al., 2012; Schadler et al., 2012). However, BNP levels are increased in multiple disorders, such as sepsis unrelated to cardiac disease, and needs further research in the usefulness as an indicator of weaning in cardiac surgery (Aydogan et al., 2013).

Pulmonary Mechanics

Evaluation of certain parameters is suggested to evaluate patient readiness to wean—namely, vital capacity, minute ventilation (or volume), respiratory rate, oxygenation, tidal volume, intact airway protection, and negative inspiratory pressure (or force) (Coleman, 2012):

- Vital capacity is the amount of air that can be exhaled forcibly following a full inspiration (Des Jardins, 2013).

- Minute ventilation is the volume of gas exchange (inhaled and exhaled) in 1 minute. It is measured by multiplying respiratory rate and tidal volume (Des Jardins, 2013).

- Respiratory rate is the number of breaths taken by a patient in a minute.

- Tidal volume refers to the amount of air inhaled by the patient during a normal breath (versus a forced inhalation) (Des Jardins, 2013). If tidal volume is too low, it is surmised that the patient will develop atelectasis or pneumonia post-extubation.

- Negative inspiratory pressure refers to the amount of negative pressure that the patient generates during a forced inspiration when working against an obstruction to flow (Des Jardins, 2013). It is a reflection of the patient's ability to take a deep breath and generate a cough that is strong enough to clear secretions.

The ICU nurse should be mindful that these physiologic weaning parameters are not perfect predictors of a patient's success with extubation. Rather, when assessed in combination with the other criteria discussed in this section, these data will provide some insight into the patient's condition and possible tolerance to breathing without mechanical support.

Assessment of readiness to wean has been studied extensively utilizing the Burns Weaning Assessment Program (BWAP). The BWAP consists of a 26-factor bedside checklist; the BWAP score is derived by simply dividing the number of factors scored as yes by 26. Not all BWAP factors are significantly associated with weaning success but are predictive of weaning success (Burns et al., 2012). When studied in a variety of units, including cardiovascular, the BWAP scores of less than 50 were weaned successfully 74% of the time. However, the patients with BWAP scores of 50 or more were weaned successfully 96% of the time. After 3 consecutive days of mechanical ventilation, several conditions complicate and delay weaning (Burns et al., 2012).

Respiratory Physiologic Issues

Infrequently, a postoperative patient may require prolonged ventilator support for more than several days. Failure to wean has two primary causes: failure of gas exchange at the alveolar level and failure to ventilate adequately.

Atelectasis

One of the most common reasons for deficiency in gas exchange in the postoperative cardiac surgery patient is atelectasis. Atelectasis affects as many as 70% of cardiac surgery patients. It is the most common respiratory complication following cardiac surgery. Etiologic factors identified include preoperative risks such as smoking, chronic bronchitis, obesity, cardiogenic pulmonary edema, and lungs not being perfused during CPB (Al-Qubati, Damag, & Noman, 2013). Pain from median sternotomy or thoracotomy incisions inhibits deep breathing efforts, which can result in atelectasis and pneumonia (Silvestry, 2014). Aggressive pulmonary toileting and pain management are needed post-extubation to prevent further respiratory compromise. Atelectasis is discussed in more detail in Chapter 13.

Left Ventricular Failure

Persistent left ventricular failure after cardiac surgery causes an increase in hydrostatic pressure, with resultant fluid extravasation into alveoli. Interstitial fluid in the alveoli inhibits oxygen transfer and increases shunting. Consideration of baseline cardiac reserve may be an important factor in the selection of an appropriate mode of spontaneous ventilation following controlled mechanical ventilation (Porhomayon et al., 2012).

Pleural Effusion

Postoperative cardiac surgery patients may also develop a pleural effusion, usually on the left side. Although the specific etiology of this condition is not known, contributing factors are thought to include volume overload, hypoalbuminemia, inflammation of the pericardium and pleura (postpericardiotomy syndrome), atelectasis, pneumonia, and pulmonary embolism (Khalpey et al., 2008). Development of a pleural effusion may lead to hypoxia, thereby affecting the success of weaning from mechanical ventilation.

A small pleural effusion is common in the early postoperative course following CABG procedures. It occurs with less frequency in patients who have undergone mitral or aortic valve replacement surgery, and typically occurs more commonly on the left side than on the right side. Effusions may necessitate thoracentesis or occasionally placement of a chest tube. Pleural effusions can present with different symptoms depending on the size of the effusion. Typically, the ICU nurse can expect to percuss dullness or decreased resonance and to auscultate diminished or inaudible breath sounds or a pleural friction rub. Pleural effusions rarely result in an increased mortality rate or increased length of stay (Heffner, 2013). This complication is discussed in more detail in Chapter 13.

Phrenic Nerve Injury

Another potential cause of weaning failure is phrenic nerve injury. This can result from cold cardioplegia or mechanical stretching during cardiac surgery. It can also result from harvesting procedures for internal thoracic artery grafts (Kamangar, 2013), dissection of the internal thoracic artery (Bojar, 2011), or from the use of cold slush (topical hypothermia solution) (Aguirre et al., 2013). The reported incidence of phrenic nerve injury during cardiac surgery is up to 60% (Aguirre et al., 2013).

Phrenic nerve injury may be associated with either unilateral or bilateral paralysis; the former is more common. It is more common to occur on the left side than the right (Aguirre et al., 2013). Patients with unilateral involvement typically do not experience respiratory symptoms and will be successfully extubated. It is noted that patients with COPD may experience shortness of breath and may require reintubation. Patients with bilateral involvement typically have tachypnea, paradoxical abdominal breathing, and hypercarbia during weaning attempts (Aguirre et al., 2013; Bojar, 2011).

Arterial Blood Gas

Another method of evaluating the effectiveness of breathing and determining readiness for weaning from mechanical ventilation following cardiac surgery is by obtaining an ABG. An ABG provides data with which to evaluate the patient's condition and the need for potential intervention; specifically, it includes pH, PaO_2, SaO_2, $PaCO_2$, and HCO_3 levels. Accurate interpretation will assist in determining the patient's acid–base balance and any required interventions. **Table 11-1** lists normal values for an ABG.

Acid–Base Disorders

The pH is a measurement of acidity and alkalinity of the blood. If a patient has an acidic pH, a decrease in myocardial contractility, vascular response to catecholamines, and response to effects and actions of certain medications may result. An alkalotic pH may result in interference with tissue oxygenation, normal neurologic functioning, and normal muscular functioning.

RESPIRATORY ACIDOSIS

The definition of respiratory acidosis is a pH of less than 7.35 with a $PaCO_2$ greater than 45 mmHg. It is important to treat a respiratory

Table 11-1　Components and Normal Values of Arterial Blood Gas	
ABG Component	**Normal Value**
pH	7.35–7.45
PaO_2	80–100 mmHg
$PaCO_2$	35–45 mmHg
HCO_3	22–26 mEq/L
SaO_2	94–100%
Base excess	–2 to +2 (A negative base excess indicates a base deficit in the blood.)

acidosis, because its presence increases the minute ventilation required to normalize pH (Eskandar & Apostolakos, 2007). **Table 11-2** lists common causes of respiratory acidosis in the postoperative cardiac surgery patient.

Signs and symptoms of respiratory acidosis are respiratory, neurologic, and cardiovascular in nature. Respiratory symptoms may include dyspnea, respiratory distress, and shallow respirations. Headache, restlessness, combativeness, hallucinations, and confusion are neurologic symptoms. If CO_2 levels continue to increase, symptoms can progress to agitation or delirium, somnolence, stuporousness, constricted pupils, drowsiness, seizures, and coma. Cyanosis may be present if the acidosis is accompanied by hypoxemia. Superficial blood vessels may become dilated and papilledema may be noted on retinal examination (Byrd, 2014a). Treatment for respiratory acidosis entails treating the underlying cause of hypoventilation and increasing ventilation.

RESPIRATORY ALKALOSIS

Respiratory alkalosis is defined as a pH greater than 7.45 with a $PaCO_2$ less than 35 mmHg. Conditions that cause hyperventilation can result in respiratory alkalosis. **Table 11-3** lists common causes of respiratory alkalosis in the postoperative cardiac surgery patient.

Respiratory alkalosis is associated with both nervous and cardiac system sequelae. Lightheadedness, dizziness, agitation, numbness or tingling of the extremities, laryngospasm, confusion, and blurred vision are common neurologic symptoms. Cardiac symptoms may include chest pain, ischemic changes on electrocardiogram (ECG), peripheral vasoconstriction, dysrhythmias, and palpitations. The patient often experiences dry mouth, diaphoresis, muscle twitching, weakness, and tetanic spasms of the arms and legs; some patients may also develop seizures (Edgren, 2008).

Treatment of respiratory alkalosis focuses on eradicating the underlying cause. The patient must be monitored for respiratory muscle fatigue and acute respiratory failure. If these situations occur, temporary reinstitution of mechanical ventilation may be indicated.

Table 11-2   Causes of Respiratory Acidosis

Impaired Respiratory Muscle Function Related to:

- Neuromuscular blocking agents

Pulmonary Disorders

- Atelectasis
- Pneumonia
- Pneumothorax
- Pulmonary edema
- Pulmonary embolism

Increased CO_2 Production

- Shivering
- Sepsis

Hypoventilation Secondary to:

- Pain
- Sternal incision
- Residual anesthesia
- Awakening with inadequate analgesia and impaired respiratory mechanics
- Opioid side effects

User Error

- Inappropriate ventilator settings
- Hypoventilation during transfer from the operating room

Sources: Data from Akhtar, M. I., & Hamid, M. (2009). Success and failure of fast track extubation in cardiac surgery patients of tertiary care hospital: One year audit. *Journal of the Pakistan Medical Association, 59,* 154–156; and Gerhardt, M. A. (2007). Postoperative care of the cardiac surgical patient. In F. A. Hensley, D. E. Martin, & G. P. Gravlee (Eds.), *A practical approach to cardiac anesthesia* (pp. 261–288). Philadelphia, PA: Lippincott Williams & Wilkins.

Table 11-3   Causes of Respiratory Alkalosis
Hypoventilation Secondary to:
• Anxiety or fear
• Pain or generalized discomfort
Increased Oxygen Demand
• Fever
• Sepsis
Pulmonary Disorders
• Pneumonia
• Pulmonary edema
• Pneumothorax/hemothorax
• Aspiration
• Asthma
• Emphysema
• Chronic bronchitis
Medications
• Respiratory stimulants
• Catecholamines
• Nicotine
User Error
• Inappropriate ventilator settings
• Hyperventilation during transfer from operating room
Sources: Data from Byrd, R. P. (2014b). *Respiratory alkalosis*. Retrieved from http://emedicine.medscape.com/article/301680-clinical#a0218; and Gerhardt, M. A. (2007). Postoperative care of the cardiac surgical patient. In F. A. Hensley, D. E. Martin, & G. P. Gravlee (Eds.), *A practical approach to cardiac anesthesia* (pp. 261–288). Philadelphia, PA: Lippincott Williams & Wilkins.

Table 11-4   Causes of Metabolic Acidosis
Hemodynamics
• Decreased cardiac output
• Inadequate systemic perfusion
• Decreased cardiac function
• Decreased peripheral perfusion
• Hypotension
• Hypovolemia
• Vasoconstriction from hypothermia
Physiologic Conditions (increasing acids)
• Sepsis
• Low cardiac output
• Tissue hypoperfusion
• Impaired renal perfusion
• Low filling pressures
• Renal failure
• Regional ischemia
• Diabetic ketoacidosis
• Anaerobic metabolism
Medication
• Metformin (Glucophage®)
Sources: Gerhardt, M. A. (2007). Postoperative care of the cardiac surgical patient. In F. A. Hensley, D. E. Martin, & G. P. Gravlee (Eds.), *A practical approach to cardiac anesthesia* (pp. 261–288). Philadelphia, PA: Lippincott Williams & Wilkins; and Lemmer, J. H. & Vlahakes, G. J. (2010). *Handbook of patient care in cardiac surgery* (7th ed., pp. 81–135). Philadelphia, PA: Lippincott Williams & Wilkins.

METABOLIC ACIDOSIS

Metabolic acidosis is defined as a bicarbonate level less than 22 mEq/L and a pH less than 7.35. **Table 11-4** lists possible causes of metabolic acidosis in the postoperative cardiac surgery patient.

Metabolic acidosis symptoms arise in relation to the neurologic, cardiovascular, gastrointestinal, and respiratory systems. Fatigue, dyspnea on exertion, nausea and vomiting, deep respirations, use of accessory muscles, tachycardia, and hypotension are possible (Seifter, 2011). Kussmaul respirations occur when the body attempts to maintain a normal pH by blowing off CO_2. Laboratory findings may include hyperkalemia, hyperphosphatemia, hyperuricemia, and hypocalcemia (Seifter, 2011). The ICU nurse should attempt to identify the underlying cause of the metabolic acidosis. Hypoxia of any tissues will produce metabolic acids from anaerobic metabolism even if the PaO_2 is normal. The only way to treat acidosis is to restore tissue perfusion, thereby preventing further hypoxemia and hypoxia from developing. If renal failure is the etiology of the metabolic acidosis, the ICU nurse should attempt to attain and maintain normovolemia, administer diuretics based on the patient's hemodynamic profile, and possibly support the patient during dialysis or hemofiltration. Treatment may also entail administration of sodium bicarbonate (depending on the severity of the acidosis or pH level) (Thomas, 2013a).

METABOLIC ALKALOSIS

Metabolic alkalosis is defined as a bicarbonate level greater than 26 mEq/L with a pH greater than 7.45. **Table 11-5** lists conditions that may cause a metabolic alkalosis in the postoperative cardiac surgery patient.

Metabolic alkalosis symptoms are primarily associated with the neurologic and musculoskeletal systems. Weakness, myalgia, polyuria, and cardiac dysrhythmias may be expected. The patient also may develop hypoventilation, which can manifest with feeling jittery, perioral tingling, and muscle spasms (Thomas, 2013b). Electrolyte imbalances associated with metabolic alkalosis include hypokalemia, hypocalcemia, hypomagnesemia, and hypophosphatemia (Thomas, 2013b).

Treatment of metabolic alkalosis can be difficult. Acetazolamide (Diamox®) is commonly given after cardiac surgery when excess diuretics have been administered. It may take hours to days to resolve the alkalosis. Acetazolamide blocks the action of carbonic anhydrase, thereby promoting renal excretion of sodium, potassium, phosphorus, bicarbonate, and water (Thomas, 2013b). Renal excretion of potassium and phosphorus may be excessive with acetazolamide therapy, however. In severe cases (pH $\geq$ 7.55), intravenous administration of hydrochloric acid may be necessary. It may also be considered in patients who cannot receive sodium chloride or potassium chloride because of fluid overload or acute kidney injury. Administration of hydrochloric acid may also be indicated for patients who require rapid correction of this metabolic imbalance (Thomas, 2013b).

Administration of ammonium chloride may be considered in severe cases of metabolic alkalosis. Ammonium chloride converts in the liver to ammonia and hydrochloric acid. Release of hydrochloric acid may help to correct the metabolic alkalosis (Thomas, 2013b).

Supplementation with potassium may be part of the treatment plan for patients with a metabolic alkalosis. This is typically done in patients who have a metabolic alkalosis due to hypokalemia (Thomas, 2013b).

Table 11-5   Causes of Metabolic Alkalosis
Loss of Acids • Nasogastric suctioning • Excessive administration of diuretics without adequate potassium and chloride repletion • Hypochloremia **Hypokalemia** **Massive Transfusion (from citrate)** Source: Data from Lemmer, J. H. & Vlahakes, G. J. (2010). *Handbook of patient care in cardiac surgery* (7th ed., pp. 81–135). Philadelphia, PA: Lippincott Williams & Wilkins.

Intrapulmonary Shunt

Intrapulmonary shunt (IPS) is the percentage of cardiac output that does not participate in gas exchange. This blood passes through the lungs but is not exposed to ventilated alveoli, so gas exchange does not take place; as a consequence, the blood leaves the lungs in a desaturated state. Intrapulmonary shunt can occur as a result of a number of conditions (e.g., collapsed or fluid-filled alveoli) and is a major cause of hypoxemia in the ICU. A frequent cause of

IPS following cardiac surgery is atelectasis (Samantaray & Hemanth, 2011). A normal shunt is in the range of approximately 2% to 5%. Some patients, however, may have a shunt as high as 40% or 50% (e.g., patients with acute respiratory distress syndrome). Because the desaturated blood has not been exposed to ventilated alveoli, increasing oxygen delivery will not correct the resultant hypoxia. Instead, correction of the underlying pathology is necessary to resolve this condition.

A-a Gradient

In addition to assessing acid–base balance, another assessment criterion that may be used to determine patient readiness to wean from mechanical ventilation is calculation of the Alveolar-arterial oxygen gradient (A-a gradient), a method of measuring IPS. This calculation determines the difference between the percentage of alveolar oxygen entering the alveoli and the percentage of oxygen diffusing into the arterial blood. The result of this calculation will aid the clinician in assessing for the presence of dysfunction in oxygenation as well as the degree of IPS (Theodore, 2013). The higher the A-a gradient, the more severe the problem with oxygen reaching the blood. If the shunt is too extensive, the patient is not ready for weaning from mechanical ventilation.

Hypoventilation during cardiac surgery results in atelectasis, increasing A-a gradient. As the alveoli re-expand postoperatively, the A-a gradient normalizes (300 mmHg), revealing the patient's readiness for weaning.

The formula for calculating an A-a gradient is complex. Fortunately, Internet sources offer calculator programs to facilitate the process. In one such calculator, the ICU nurse would need to insert the local barometric pressure P_B (which is preset at 760 mmHg), PaO_2 and $PaCO_2$ data from the ABG, and the patient's FiO_2 level, and then click the "Calculate Aa Gradient" button for the result to appear (McAuley, 1993–2014).

PaO_2/FiO_2 Ratio

A suggested alternative to the A-a gradient that is easy to calculate and considered a reliable indicator of gas exchange is the PaO_2/FiO_2 (P/F) ratio (Markou, Myrianthefs, & Baltopoulos, 2004). This ratio is an index of oxygenation that is commonly used by clinicians because of its ease in calculation. A PaO_2/FiO_2 ratio of less than 200 is associated with a significant shunt. Criticisms of the PaO_2/FiO_2 ratio include the fact that it is affected by changes in $PaCO_2$ and SvO_2, it is reportedly not equally sensitive across the entire range of FiO_2, and it cannot provide information about the functional status of the lungs based on interventions to augment oxygenation (e.g., positive end-expiratory pressure [PEEP], lateral or prone positioning) (Slutsky, 2014).

$PaO_2/(FiO_2 \times Mean\ P_{aw})$

Another oxygenation index, $PaO_2/(FiO_2 \times mean\ P_{aw})$, where P_{aw} is mean airway pressure, takes into account the effects of PEEP. In a study of cardiac surgery patients, data suggested that $PaO_2/(FiO_2 \times mean\ P_{aw})$ measurements may be more reliable than other oxygenation measurements in reflecting intrapulmonary shunt (El-Khatib & Jamaleddine, 2004).

POSTOPERATIVE MECHANICAL VENTILATION

Prolonged mechanical ventilation following cardiac surgery is associated with increased ICU and hospital lengths of stay, resource use and costs, and poorer physiologic outcomes (Natarajan, Patil, Lesley, & Ninan, 2006). Results of "fast-track" programs have shown that postoperative intubation can be safely limited in cardiac surgery patients. In one study, older age and LVEF less than 35% were revealed as predictors of failure of the fast-track program (Haanschoten et al., 2012).

If not extubated in the operating room, the patient is placed on mechanical ventilation upon arrival to the ICU. The mode of ventilation and settings used will depend on the patient's clinical status. Cardiac surgical patients have multiple risk factors for postoperative respiratory dysfunction. Because patients are at risk for surgery-related complications (e.g., hemodynamic instability, temperature dysregulation, blood loss from the mediastinum) for the first 2-6 hours postoperatively, it is suggested that extubation occurs after that period of time. It is further recommended that the extubation process be based on a protocol (Roekaerts & Heijmans, 2012).

Initial Postoperative Ventilator Settings

For patients who remain on mechanical ventilation in the postoperative period, the settings used should be based on a plan intended to optimize gas exchange, decrease work of breathing, and minimize complications associated with positive-pressure ventilation (Chikwe, Beddow, & Glenville, 2006). **Table 11-6** shows the initial ventilator settings.

Patient Monitoring

When the patient is admitted to the ICU, the nurse should auscultate breath sounds to

Table 11-6	Initial Postoperative Ventilator Settings
Mode	IMV, Assist Control, Pressure Support Ventilation, or Pressure Control
FiO_2	Range = 0.4–1.0. Depends on the patient's ABG results and SpO_2 measurements. It is modified to the lowest level while maintaining SpO_2 levels at least 92% or what is reasonable according to the patient's baseline and past medical history.
Tidal volume	8–12 mL/kg ideal body weight. Tidal volume may be increased to decrease carbon dioxide levels, and vice versa. Tidal volume may also be adjusted to maintain pH within appropriate limits for the patient and to achieve a minute ventilation of 100 mL/kg/min. It may also be adjusted to maintain peak inspiratory pressure less than 35 cmH_2O.
Rate	8–10 breaths/minute. Respiratory rate may be increased to decrease carbon dioxide levels and to achieve a minute ventilation of 100 mL/kg/min.
Minute volume	100–120 mL/kg/min. Minute volume may be increased by increasing the rate, the tidal volume, or both to decrease carbon dioxide levels.
PEEP	3–10 cmH_2O. PEEP levels may be increased to improve oxygenation.
Pressure support	5–8 cmH_2O.
Inspiratory:expiratory (I:E) ratio	1:2–1:3. If a patient has difficulty with oxygenation, the ratio may be changed to either 1:1 or 2:1 (inverse I:E ratio).
Inspiratory flow rate	30–60 L/min.

ABG, arterial blood gas; IMV, intermittent mandatory ventilation; PEEP, positive end-expiratory pressure.

Sources: Data from Bojar, R. M. (2011). Post-ICU care and other complications. In R. M. Bojar (Ed.), *Manual of perioperative care in adult cardiac surgery* (pp. 641–726). Hoboken, NJ: Blackwell; Herlihy, J. P., Koch, S. M., Jackson, R., & Nora, H. (2006). Course of weaning from prolonged mechanical ventilation after cardiac surgery. *Texas Heart Institute Journal, 33*(2), 122–129; Khalpey, Z. I., Ganim, R. B., & Rawn, J. D. (2008). Postoperative care of cardiac surgery patients. In L. H. Cohn (Ed.), *Cardiac surgery in the adult* (pp. 465–486). New York, NY: McGraw-Hill; Lytle, F. T., & Brown, D. R. (2008). Appropriate ventilatory settings for thoracic surgery: Intraoperative and postoperative. *Seminars in Cardiothoracic and Vascular Anesthesia, 12*(2), 97–108; and Samantaray, A., & Hemanth, N. (2011). Comparison of two ventilation modes in post-cardiac surgical patients. *Saudi Journal of Anaesthesia, 5*(2), 173–178.

confirm good bilateral air entry and absence of bronchospasm. The postoperative cardiac surgery patient will be monitored with pulse oximetry and potentially with waveform capnometry (end-tidal carbon dioxide [$ETCO_2$]) (Bojar, 2011). These noninvasive monitoring devices provide the ICU nurse with continuous estimates of the patient's oxygenation and ventilation status, respectively, and will likely expedite the weaning process. For capnography, an infrared gas analyzer is placed in the exhalation port of the ventilator or closest to the endotracheal tube. The normal $ETCO_2$ is 2–6 mmHg less than the $PaCO_2$.

WEANING CRITERIA

Anesthesia traditionally utilizes short-acting anesthetic agents so that the patient will wake up quickly. The ICU nurse assesses the patient for readiness to wean on an ongoing basis.

Initiating the weaning process commences when the patient is hemodynamically stable, normothermic, and adequately resuscitated; does not have any clinically significant dysrhythmias; is draining less than 100 mL/hr from the chest tube; is not shivering; and is on minimal vasoactive support. The patient must be awake, oriented, able to cooperate with instructions, and triggering the ventilator by taking spontaneous breaths (Bojar, 2011; Roekaerts & Heijmans, 2012).

The patient should also demonstrate adequate muscle strength as demonstrated by either a strong hand grasp or a sustained head lift for 5 sec (Lytle & Brown, 2008). A chest radiograph should be reviewed prior to extubation to ascertain the presence of any indicators that the patient might not tolerate extubation. Lab values (e.g., electrolytes, lactate level) should be within normal ranges. The ABG results should be at or close to the patient's baseline or normalized.

The patient should be normothermic before weaning is attempted because shivering causes an increase in carbon dioxide production. Shivering following hypothermic CPB causes a twofold to threefold increase in oxygen consumption (Scaravilli, Bonacina, & Citerio, 2012) as well as carbon dioxide production and increased peripheral vascular resistance (Royster, Thomas, & Davis, 2008).

Weaning from Mechanical Ventilation

Optimal management of mechanical ventilation and weaning requires dynamic and collaborative decision making among nursing, respiratory therapists, and healthcare providers to minimize complication and avoid delays in liberation from the ventilator. Weaning may be accomplished in several different ways, depending on the mode of ventilation and the patient's condition. The first goal is to wean the patient as tolerated while maintaining a SpO_2 > 92–94% on FiO_2 .40 and PEEP 5 cmH_2O. If the patient is receiving pressure support, as the patient's respiratory effort increases, pressure support levels can be gradually titrated down (Khalpey et al., 2008).

Once physiologic parameters have been met, the amount of support the patient receives from the ventilator is gradually decreased or else the patient typically undergoes a spontaneous breathing trial. Data suggest more successful weaning and extubation with SBTs (Robertson et al., 2008). An alternative to an SBT for weaning is to gradually and incrementally decrease the amount of support from pressure support ventilation or the intermittent mandatory ventilation (IMV) rate. Data are conflicting regarding whether earlier weaning occurs with SBTs versus pressure support ventilation or use of IMV; however, in a recent study, researchers report no differences (Lourenço, Franco, Bassetto, & Rodrigues, 2013). Older data suggest that patients who were weaned with SBTs were successfully extubated two to three times earlier than patients who were weaned with either of the alternative methods (Esteban et al., 1995). Regardless of the method used, once the patient has satisfactory ABG results and has demonstrated the ability to breathe independently without signs of distress, extubation can be considered. In addition to assessment of pulmonary mechanics, if the patient is able to maintain a patent airway and manage secretions and the criteria in **Box 11-1** are met, the patient is considered ready to be extubated.

The ICU nurse plays a pivotal role in assessing tolerance to weaning. Signs and symptoms that would indicate poor tolerance to weaning include a respiratory rate of 35 or greater; SpO_2 less than 90%; heart rate greater than 140; systolic or diastolic blood pressure higher than 180 or 90 mmHg, respectively; and presence of agitation, diaphoresis, or anxiety (Khalpey et al., 2008). Further, if the patient has an inadequate minute volume, tidal volume, episodes of apnea lasting more than 25 sec, mental status changes, a decrease in SpO_2 to less than 92%, or $ETCO_2$ greater than 55 mmHg, the trial is stopped, the patient is restored to the prior ventilator settings, and an ABG is obtained. It has been recommended that spontaneous breathing trials be attempted hourly until weaning is successful (Lytle & Brown, 2008).

When ABG results are obtained and are within the appropriate range, collaboration with the healthcare provider regarding extubation is indicated. If the ABG results are not acceptable, the patient should be placed back on the previous support settings and reassessed in 30 minutes to an hour (Lytle & Brown, 2008).

Researchers have compared intubation times using SmartCare™, a knowledge-based system for automated weaning with conventional healthcare provider–controlled weaning after off-pump coronary artery bypass. No complications or increase in reintubations occurred with this computer-driven weaning system, and SmartCare reduced

Box 11-1   Readiness for Extubation Criteria

NIP –25 cmH$_2$O

RR < 25 bpm

HR < 140

Minute volume (VE) 10 L/min

Vital capacity (VC) 10–15 mL/kg

Rapid Shallow Breathing Index (RSBI) f/V_T

Cardiac status:
- No signs of ischemia
- Not receiving vasopressor therapy or low-dose inotropic agents

Neurologic status:
- Alert
- Able to respond to commands
- Cough and gag reflex
- Able to protect airway and clear secretions
- Able to sustain a head lift for at least 5 sec

NIP, negative inspiratory pressure; RR, respiratory rate.

Sources: Data from BouAki, I., Bou-Khalil, P., Kanazi, G., Ayoub, C., & El-Khatib, M. (2012). Weaning from mechanical ventilation. *Thoracic Anesthesia, 25*(1), 42–47; and Khalpey, Z. I., Ganim, R. B., & Rawn, J. D. (2008). Postoperative care of cardiac surgery patients. In L. H. Cohn (Ed.), *Cardiac surgery in the adult* (pp. 465–486). New York, NY: McGraw-Hill.

the duration of mechanical ventilation (Kataoka et al., 2007). More recent data suggest that an automated ventilation method was safe in patients who were hemodynamically stable following cardiac surgery (Lellouche, Bouchard, Simard, L'Her, & Wysocki, 2013). Another study evaluated the Siemens Servo 300A ventilator, which has an automode function allowing for automated weaning from mechanical ventilation. Data suggest that the automode decreased ventilation time by 2 hours, decreased peak airway pressure during spontaneous ventilation, and improved patients' cardiac index (Hendrix, Kaiser, Yusen, & Merk, 2006).

Weaning from Prolonged Ventilation

In long-term weaning, the physiologic or rapid, shallow breathing index is a reliable predictive indicator of failure to wean and extubation. The physiologic index is determined by assessing the minute frequency of spontaneous ventilation (f) and dividing this value by the tidal volume (V_T) in liters. When this index is high, it reflects a clinical picture of a patient with rapid, shallow breathing. When f/V_T is less than 105, 78% of patients can be weaned and extubated successfully. When f/V_T is greater than 105, 95% of patients cannot be weaned and extubated successfully (Teixeira et al., 2008).

A study investigating the temporal pattern of weaning from mechanical ventilation for patients undergoing prolonged mechanical ventilation after cardiac surgery found a specific temporal pattern. Data analysis suggested that a turn in weaning success was improvement of pulmonary mechanics rather than improvement in gas exchange or respiratory load (Herlihy et al., 2006).

Collaborative decision making for ventilation and weaning was influenced by nurse-to-patient ratio and presence of a protocol. If there was not a collaboration of disciplines, this delayed adaptation of ventilator to changes in physiologic parameters and delayed recognition of weaning and extubation readiness, leading to prolongation of ventilation (Rose et al., 2011).

POST-EXTUBATION CARE

Prior to extubation with the cuff of the endotracheal tube deflated and then upon extubation, the patient is assessed for a patent airway and absence of laryngeal edema. The ICU nurse should ask the patient to speak a few words. Once extubated, the patient should be placed on a humidified face mask set to deliver an FiO_2 10% greater than what was received when on mechanical ventilation. The FiO_2 level may be titrated down according to SpO_2 values, which should initially be maintained above the range of 97% to 98%. After the initial post-extubation period, FiO_2 can be titrated to maintain SpO_2 at least 95% for the first 2 to 3 days. After that point, a nasal cannula can be used to maintain SpO_2 at least 90% (Salenger, Gammie, & Vander Salm, 2003).

Extubation failure in postoperative cardiac surgery patients has a reported overall incidence of up to 47% (Kulkami & Agarwal, 2008). Identified risk factors of extubation failure include older age, severity of illness upon admission to the ICU, prolonged ventilation before attempting extubation, and use of continuous sedation. Reasons for extubation failure include upper airway obstruction, impaired ability to clear secretions, respiratory failure, hypoxemia, hypercarbia, cardiac failure, neurological impairment, and insecure airway (Kulkami & Agarwal, 2008). Renal failure, IABP requirement, longer surgical time, and longer time on bypass have also been implicated (Khalpey et al., 2008).

Trouillet and colleagues (2009) studied patients still mechanically ventilated after day 3 post-cardiac surgery. Several factors were associated with successful weaning odds: urine output 500 mL/24 hours or greater, platelet count 100 g/L or greater, patients without inotropic support with epinephrine/ norepinephrine, Glasgow coma score of 15, arterial bicarbonate 20 mmol/L or greater, and absence of lung injury.

Post-extubation, the ICU nurse should initially observe for laryngospasm for as long as 1 hour and stridor for as long as 24 hours; both conditions may result in the need for reintubation. Prophylactic administration of dexamethasone has been shown to be effective in decreasing the incidence of post-extubation stridor in patients who are at risk for developing laryngeal edema (Lee, Peng, & Wu, 2007).

After cardiac surgery, many patients will have decreased breath sounds secondary to lower lobe atelectasis (Khalpey et al., 2008). For this reason, the ICU nurse must frequently evaluate the patient in terms of work of breathing, respiratory rate, use of accessory muscles, and expiratory phase of breathing. Nursing care must include encouraging mobility, use of incentive spirometry, bronchial hygiene, and frequent auscultation of breath sounds. Chest physiotherapy will promote lung expansion, mobilize secretions, encourage coughing, and prevent the side effect of retained secretions, which might otherwise cause atelectasis and potentially pneumonia (Westerdahl & Olsén, 2011).

One of the sequelae of bypass procedures is activation of the inflammatory response, which can cause marked pulmonary dysfunction (Khalpey et al., 2008). A variety of interventions are being studied for their potential to mitigate the deleterious effects of bypass procedures that can cause delays in weaning from mechanical ventilation. These interventions include use of a leukocyte filtration to reduce the effects of CPB, intraoperative use of heparin-bonded circuits designed to prevent complement activation and subsequent increase in neutrophil activation, and use of antioxidants and anti-inflammatory drugs with the serine protease inhibitor activity of aprotinin in combination with leuko-cyte-reduction filters. The last combination has been shown to improve post-bypass lung performance by reducing inflammatory response and its sequelae (Zakkar, Taylor, & Hornik, 2008).

SUMMARY

Caring for patients following cardiac surgery is often challenging. While many patients are admitted to the ICU having already been extubated, others require management with mechanical ventilation for either a short or prolonged period of time. Mechanical ventilation is suggested to be associated with—and may even cause—lung damage and many other complications.

Prolonged use of mechanical ventilation is correlated with an increased mortality rate. The cardiac surgery ICU nurse must continuously assess the post-cardiac surgery patient for tolerance to therapy, prevent complications associated with mechanical ventilation, minimize the effects of the patient's comorbidities and the procedure-associated complications, and assess the patient's readiness for and tolerance of weaning from mechanical ventilation. Although the majority of patients are quickly weaned from mechanical ventilation and extubated, extubation failure must be minimized or recognized promptly. Identifying patients at risk for prolonged mechanical ventilation following cardiac surgery based on preoperative assessment variables may assist to mitigate complications postoperatively. Using high levels of clinical judgment and caring practices will affect the ICU nurse's ability to optimize outcomes of the postoperative cardiac surgery patient.

CASE STUDY

A 72-year-old obese male had a 3-month history of progressive typical angina pain. He had a stent placed in the left anterior descending artery 24 months prior to the current admission. His history includes hyperlipidemia, hypertension, COPD, and insulin-dependent diabetes. The patient is being treated with 325 mg aspirin daily, atorvastatin (Lipitor®), insulin, and an angiotensin-converting enzyme (ACE) inhibitor.

The patient presented with substernal pain and "heaviness" in his chest. Upon admission, the 12-lead ECG revealed ST-segment elevation in leads II, III, and aVF, and elevation in V5 and V6 with additional ST-segment depression in V3 and V4. The patient reported his chest pain to be 8 out of 10; he was treated with sublingual nitroglycerin, which decreased the pain to 6 out of 10. Initial electrolytes and complete blood count were within normal limits although troponin I was elevated and HbA1c was 7.5%. Cardiac catheterization revealed the following:

- Severe triple-vessel coronary artery disease.
- The right coronary artery had 90% dominant obstruction.
- The circumflex had 80% obstruction.
- The left anterior descending (LAD) coronary artery with previous stent was 70% obstructed.
- The aortic and mitral valves were normal without significant stenosis or regurgitation.

The patient was scheduled for CABG. The left internal thoracic artery was used to bypass the LAD, and the saphenous vein was used to bypass the remaining blockages. The intraoperative course was uneventful, and the patient was admitted to the ICU postoperatively.

Critical Thinking Questions

1. For which post-extubation complications should the ICU nurse assess on this patient?
2. Which pulmonary interventions will be necessary to facilitate respiratory functioning in this patient?
3. What are possible pulmonary complications from cardiac surgery?

Answers to Critical Thinking Questions

1. In the post-extubation patient, the nurse should initially observe for laryngospasm for as long as 1 hour and stridor for as long as 24 hours; either of these complications may result in the need for reintubation. After cardiac surgery, the patient would be expected to have decreased breath sounds secondary to lower lobe atelectasis, particularly in the left lower lobe. The patient will need frequent assessment in terms of work of breathing, respiratory rate, use of accessory muscles, and the expiratory phase of breathing, which can indicate compromised pulmonary function.

2. Nursing care must include mobility and bronchial hygiene, and frequent auscultation of breath sounds. Bronchial hygiene will promote lung expansion, mobilize secretions, and prevent retention of secretions that cause atelectasis and potentially pneumonia. This care should include pulmonary toileting of effective coughing and incentive spirometry. Incentive spirometry has only limited effectiveness, however, because many patients are unable to cooperate adequately to use it correctly. Care for this patient should include early mobility beginning with dangling at bedside upon extubation and walking on postoperative day 1.

3. Potential pulmonary complications include phrenic nerve injury, atelectasis, pleural effusions, and air leak syndrome.

SELF-ASSESSMENT QUESTIONS

1. Respiratory acidosis would be indicated by:
   a. pH less than 7.35
   b. pCO_2 less than 45
   c. HCO_3 more than 26
   d. pH more than 7.45

2. A postoperative patient is evaluated for extubation in the intensive care unit. Which of the following findings regarding respiratory mechanics meets extubation criteria?
   a. Vital capacity: 8 mL/kg
   b. Negative inspiratory pressure: − 23 cmH_2O
   c. Spontaneous respiratory rate: 28 breaths/min
   d. Tidal volume: 6 mL/kg

3. The most common cause of respiratory acidosis in the extubated cardiac surgery patient is:
   a. Hyperglycemia
   b. Hypoventilation
   c. Acute lung injury
   d. Electrolyte imbalance

4. The postoperative cardiac surgery patient has been in the ICU for 1 hour. The patient has a core temperature of 34.9°C, cardiac index of 2.5 L/min/m², chest tube drainage of 50–75 mL/hr, serum glucose of 240 mg/dL, and MAP of 65 mmHg. What would prohibit extubation at this time?
   a. Chest tube drainage of 50–75 mL/hr
   b. Serum glucose of 240 mg/dL
   c. One hour post arrival in the ICU
   d. Temperature of 34.9°C

5. A 70-kg open heart surgery patient with acute respiratory failure is being mechanically ventilated on the following settings: FiO_2 of 0.40, rate 6 breaths/min, tidal volume 600 mL. Arterial blood gas results obtained on these settings are: pH 7.26, $PaCO_2$ 55, PaO_2 66, and HCO_3 27. What ventilator adjustments would you make based on the ABG?
   a. Increase the I:E ratio
   b. Decrease the tidal volume
   c. Increase the rate
   d. Decrease the FiO_2

6. Which of the following best defines hypoventilation in your post–open heart patient indicating weaning failure with current assessment?
   a. RR less than 10 breaths/min
   b. PaO_2 greater than 75
   c. Arterial pH of 7.37
   d. $PaCO_2$ of 52

7. An ABG sample obtained on postoperative day 1 after cardiac surgery, on room air, is as follows: pH 7.17, $PaCO_2$ 82, PaO_2 37, HCO_3 28. The ABG indicates:
   a. Respiratory acidosis with severe hypoxemia
   b. Combined respiratory and metabolic acidosis
   c. Respiratory acidosis with mild hypoxemia
   d. Metabolic acidosis with respiratory compensation

8. The cause of the previous ABG in the cardiac surgery patient is probably due to:
   a. Low cardiac index
   b. Hypoventilation
   c. Hemoglobin of 7.5 g/dL
   d. Cardiac dysrhythmias

9. Which of the following signs are an indication that your postoperative patient has developed a tension pneumothorax?
   a. Distended neck veins, absent breath sounds on the affected side, hypotension
   b. Flat neck veins, wheezing on the affected side, hypertension
   c. Flat neck veins, absent breath sounds on the affected side, hypertension
   d. Equal breath sounds, + 3 – 4 pulses, hypotensive

10. Which of the following would be the most appropriate initial treatment for your cardiac surgery patient with COPD, in respiratory distress, and O_2 saturation of 85% 2 hours after extubation?

   a. Chest x-ray, blood cultures, and antibiotics

   b. O_2 via nasal cannula at 2 L/min and bronchodilators

   c. Immediate intubation and mechanical ventilation

   d. 100% non-rebreather mask and bronchodilators

Answers to Self-Assessment Questions

1. a
2. d
3. b
4. d
5. c

6. d
7. a
8. b
9. a
10. c

Clinical Inquiry Box

Question: What are the predictors of postoperative prolonged ventilation following cardiac surgery?

Reference: Knapik, P., Ciesla, D., Borowik, D., Czempik, P., & Knapik, T. (2011). Prolonged ventilation post cardiac surgery—tips and pitfalls of the prediction game. *Journal of Cardiothoracic Surgery, 6*, 158. Retrieved from http://www.cardiothoracicsurgery.org/content/6/1/158

Objective: To compare two ICU-developed prediction models for prolonged ventilator requirements following cardiac surgery.

Methods: Retrospective review of two patient cohorts in two subsequent 18-month periods.

Results: The percentage of patients who required prolonged ventilation decreased from 5.7% to 2.4% following changes in techniques for postoperative ventilation. Preoperative and procedure-related variables were identified: abdominal aneurysm surgery, emergent surgery, combined procedures, valve procedures, preoperative renal dysfunction, and preoperative stroke.

Conclusion: Prediction models for postoperative ventilation need to be updated on a regular basis based on changes in patient demographics, surgical techniques, and anesthetic methods.

REFERENCES

Aguirre, V. J., Sinha, P., Zimmet, A., Lee, G. A., Kwa, L., & Rosenfeldt, F. (2013). Phrenic nerve injury during cardiac surgery: Mechanisms, management and prevention. *Heart Lung and Circulation, 22*(11), 895–902.

Akhtar, M. I., & Hamid, M. (2009). Success and failure of fast track extubation in cardiac surgery patients of tertiary care hospital: One year audit. *Journal of the Pakistan Medical Association, 59*, 154–156.

Al-Qubati, F. A. A., Damag, A., & Noman, T. (2013). Incidence and outcome of pulmonary complications after open cardiac surgery, Thowra Hospital, cardiac center, Sana'a Yemen. *The Egyptian Journal of Chest Diseases and Tuberculosis, 62*(4), 775–780.

Aydogan, M., Balta, S., Kucuk, U., Demirkol, S., Unlu, M., & Gumus, S. (2013). Future studies should consider multiple predisposing conditions in predicting weaning failure from mechanical ventilation in patients after cardiac surgery. *Clinics, 68*(5), 725. Retrieved from http://www.ncbi.nlm.nih.gov/pmc/articles/PMC3654291/

Bojar, R. M. (2011). Post-ICU care and other complications. In R. M. Bojar (Ed.), *Manual of perioperative care in adult cardiac surgery* (pp. 641–726). Hoboken, NJ: Blackwell.

BouAki, I., Bou-Khalil, P., Kanazi, G., Ayoub, C., & El-Khatib, M. (2012). Weaning from mechanical ventilation. *Thoracic Anesthesia, 25*(1), 42–47.

Burns, S. M., Fisher, C., Tribble, S. S., Lewis, R., Merrel, R., Conaway, M., & Beck, T. P. (2012). The relationship of 26 clinical factors to weaning outcome. *American Journal of Critical Care, 12*(21), 52–59.

Byrd, R. P. (2014a). *Respiratory acidosis clinical presentation.* Retrieved from http://emedicine.medscape.com/article/301574-clinical#aw2aab6b3b3

Byrd, R. P. (2014b). *Respiratory alkalosis clinical presentation.* Retrieved from http://emedicine.medscape.com/article/301680-clinical#a0218

Chikwe, J., Beddow, E., & Glenville, B. (2006). Cardiac intensive care. In J. Chikwe, E. Beddow, & B. Glenville, *Cardiothoracic surgery* (pp. 127–250). New York, NY: Oxford University Press.

Cislaghi, F., Conderni, A. M., & Corona, A. (2009). Predictors of prolonged mechanical ventilation in a cohort of 5123 cardiac surgical patients. *European Journal of Anaesthesiology, 26*(5), 396–403.

Coleman, M. (2012). Post-op ventilation of the surgical patient. In L. F. Chu & A. J. Fuller (Eds.), *Manual of clinical anesthesiology.* Philadelphia, PA: Lippincott Williams & Wilkins.

Des Jardins, T. (2013). Pulmonary function measurements. In T. Des Jardins (Ed.), *Cardiopulmonary anatomy and physiology* (pp. 145–160). Clifton Park, NY: Delmar.

Dirks, J., & Waters, J. (2014). Cardiovascular therapeutic management. In L. D. Urden, K. M. Stacy, & M. E. Lough (Eds.), *Critical care nursing: Diagnosis and management* (7th ed., pp. 412–466). St. Louis, MO: Elsevier Mosby.

Durham, S. J., & Gold, J. P. (2008). Late complications of cardiac surgery. In L. H. Cohn (Ed.), *Cardiac surgery in the adult* (pp. 535–548). New York, NY: McGraw-Hill.

Edgren, A. R. (2008). Respiratory alkalosis. *Encyclopedia of medicine.* Retrieved from http://www.encyclopedia.com/doc/1G2-3451601396.html

El-Khatib, M. F., & Jamaleddine, G. W. (2004). A new oxygenation index for reflecting intrapulmonary shunting in patients undergoing open-heart surgery. *Chest, 125*(2), 592–596.

Eskandar, N., & Apostolakos, M. J. (2007). Weaning from mechanical ventilation. *Critical Care Clinics, 23*(2), 263–274.

Esteban, A., Fruto, F., Tobin, M. J., Alia, I., Solsona, J. F., Valverdu, V., . . . Blanco, J. (1995). A comparison of four methods of weaning patients from mechanical ventilation. *New England Journal of Medicine, 332*(6), 345–350.

Faritous, Z. S., Aghdaie, N., Yazdanian, F., Azarfarin, R., & Dabbagh, A. (2011). Perioperative risk factors for prolonged mechanical ventilation and tracheostomy in women undergoing coronary artery bypass graft with cardiopulmonary bypass. *Saudi Journal of Anaesthesia, 5*(2), 167–169.

Gerhardt, M. A. (2007). Postoperative care of the cardiac surgical patient. In F. A. Hensley, D. E. Martin, & G. P. Gravlee (Eds.), *A practical approach to cardiac anesthesia* (pp. 261–288). Philadelphia, PA: Lippincott Williams & Wilkins.

Giakoumidakis, K., Eltheni, R., Rokalaki, H., Galanis, P., Nenekidis, I., & Fildissis, G. (2011). Preoperative and intraoperative risk factors for prolonged mechanical ventilation among cardiac surgery patients. *Health Science Journal, 5*(4), 297–305.

Haanschoten, M. C., van Straten, A. H. M., ter Woorst, J. F., Stepaniak, P. S., van der Meer, A.-D., van Zundert, A. A. J., . . . Hamad, M. A. S. (2012). Fast-track practice in cardiac surgery: Results and predictors of outcome. *Interactive Cardiovascular and Thoracic Surgery, 17.* Retrieved from http://icvts.oxfordjournals.org/content/early/2012/09/05/icvts.ivs393.long

Heffner, J. E. (2013). *Pleural effusions following cardiac surgery.* Retrieved from http://www.utdol.com/online/content/topic.do?topicKey=pleurdis/8523&selectedTitle=1~150&source=search_result

Hendrix, H., Kaiser, M. E., Yusen, R. D., & Merk, J. (2006). A randomized trial of automated versus conventional protocol-driven weaning from mechanical ventilation following coronary artery bypass surgery. *European Journal of Cardio-Thoracic Surgery, 29*(6), 957–963.

Herlihy, J. P., Koch, S. M., Jackson, R., & Nora, H. (2006). Course of weaning from prolonged mechanical ventilation after cardiac surgery. *Texas Heart Institute Journal, 33*(2), 122–129.

Ibañez, J., Riera, M., Amezaga, R., Herrero, J., Colomar, A., Campillo-Artero, C., . . . Bonnin, O. (2014). Long-term mortality after pneumonia in cardiac surgery patients. A propensity-matched analysis. *Journal of Intensive Care Medicine, 10.* Retrieved from http://jic.sagepub.com/content/early/2014/02/26/0885066614523918.abstract

Kamangar, N. (2013). *Diaphragmatic paralysis follow-up.* Retrieved from http://emedicine.medscape.com/article/298200-followup

Kataoka, G., Murai, N., Kodera, K., Sasaki, A., Asano, R., Ikeda, M., . . . Takeuchi, Y. (2007). Clinical experience with Smart Care after off-pump coronary artery bypass for early extubation. *Journal of Artificial Organs, 10*(4), 218–222.

Khalpey, Z. I., Ganim, R. B., & Rawn, J. D. (2008). Postoperative care of cardiac surgery patients. In L. H. Cohn (Ed.), *Cardiac surgery in the adult* (pp. 465–486). New York, NY: McGraw-Hill.

Knapik, P., Ciesla, D., Borowik, D., Czempik, P., & Knapik, T. (2011). Prolonged ventilation post cardiac surgery—tips and pitfalls of the prediction game. *Journal of Cardiothoracic Surgery, 6,* 158. Retrieved from http://www.cardiothoracicsurgery.org/content/6/1/158

Kulkami, A. P., & Agarwal, V. (2008). Extubation failure in intensive care unit: Predictors and management. *Indian Journal of Critical Care Medicine, 12*(1), 1–9.

Lee, C.-H., Peng, M.-J., & Wu, C.-L. (2007). Dexamethasone to prevent postextubation airway obstruction in adults: A prospective, randomized, double-blind, placebo controlled study. *Critical Care, 11*(4), R72.

Lellouche, F., Bouchard, P., Simard, S., L'Her, E., & Wysocki, M. (2013). Evaluation of fully automated ventilation: A randomized controlled study in post-cardiac surgery patients. *Intensive Care Medicine, 39,* 463–471.

Lemmer, J. H., & Vlahakes, G. J. (2010). *Handbook of patient care in cardiac surgery* (7th ed., pp. 81–135). Philadelphia, PA: Lippincott Williams & Wilkins.

Lourenço, I. S., Franco, A. M., Bassetto, S., & Rodrigues, A. J. (2013). Pressure support-ventilation versus spontaneous breathing with "T-Tube" for interrupting the ventilation after cardiac operations. *Revista Brasileira de Cirurgia Cardiovascular, 28*(4). Retrieved from http://www.scielo.br/scielo.php?pid=S0102-76382013000400008&script=sci_arttext

Lytle, F. T., & Brown, D. R. (2008). Appropriate ventilatory settings for thoracic surgery: Intraoperative and postoperative. *Seminars in Cardiothoracic and Vascular Anesthesia, 12*(2), 97–108.

Markou, N. K., Myrianthefs, P. M., & Baltopoulos, G. J. (2004). Advancements in respiratory management, part 2. *Critical Care Nursing Quarterly, 27*(4), 353–379.

McAuley, D. (1993–2014). *Aa gradient.* Retrieved from http://www.globalrph.com/aagrad.htm

Natarajan, K., Patil, S., Lesley, N., & Ninan, B. (2006). Predictors of prolonged mechanical ventilation after on-pump coronary artery bypass grafting. *Annals of Cardiac Anaesthesia, 9*(1), 31–36.

Parmer, J., Clarke, J., Lau, G., Porter, R., & Allsager, C. (2014). Delays in extubation following elective adult cardiac surgery. *Critical Care, 18*(Suppl. 1). Retrieved from http://ccforum.com/content/18/S1/P185

Piotto, R. F., Ferreira, F. B., Colósimo, F. C., de Silva, G. S., de Sousa, A. G., & Braile, D. M. (2012). Independent predictors of prolonged mechanical ventilation after coronary artery bypass surgery. *Revista Brasileira de Cirurgia Cardiovascular, 27*(4). Retrieved from http://www.scielo.br/scielo.php?pid=S0102-76382012000400009&script=sci_arttext&tlng=en

Popat, M., Mitchell, V., Dravid, R., Patel, A., Swampillai, C., & Higgs, A. (2012). Difficult Airway Society guidelines for the management of tracheal extubation. *Anaesthesia, 67,* 318–340.

Porhomayon, J., Papadakos, P., & Nader, N. D. (2012). Failed weaning from mechanical ventilation and cardiac dysfunction. *Critical Care Research and Practice, 2012.* Retrieved from http://www.hindawi.com/journals/ccrp/2012/173527

Robertson, T. E., Sona, C., Schallom, L., Buckles, M., Cracchiolo, L., Schuerer, D., . . . Buchman, T. G. (2008). Improved extubation rates and earlier liberation from mechanical ventilation with implementation of a daily spontaneous-breathing trial protocol. *Journal of the American College of Surgeons, 206*(3), 489–495.

Roekaerts, M. M. H. J., & Heijmans, J. H. (2012). *Early postoperative care after cardiac surgery, perioperative considerations in cardiac surgery.* Retrieved from http://www.intechopen .com/books/howtoreference/perioperative-considerations-in-cardiac-surgery/-early-postoperative-care-after-cardiac-surgery-

Rose, L., Blackwood, B., Egerod, I., Haugdahl, H., Hofhuis, J., Isfort, M., . . . Schultz, M. (2011). Decisional responsibility for mechanical ventilation and weaning: An international survey. *Critical Care, 15,* R295. Retrieved from http: //ccforum.com.content/15/6/R295

Royster, R. L., Thomas, S. J., & Davis, R. F. (2008). Termination of cardiopulmonary bypass. In G. L. Gravlee, R. F. Davis, A. H. Stammers, & R. M. Ungerleider (Eds.), *Cardiopulmonary bypass: Principles and practice* (3rd ed., pp. 614–631). Philadelphia, PA: Lippincott Williams & Wilkins.

Salah, H. Z., Shaw, M., Al-Rawi, O., Yates, J., Pullan, M., Chalmers, J. A. C., & Fabri, B. M. (2012). Outcomes and predictors of prolonged ventilation in patients undergoing elective coronary surgery. *Interactive Cardiovascular and Thoracic Surgery.* Retrieved from http://icvts.oxford-journals.org/content/early/2012/04/11/icvts. ivs076.full

Salenger, R., Gammie, J. S., & Vander Salm, T. J. (2003). Postoperative care of cardiac surgical patients. In L. H. Cohn & L. H. Edmunds (Eds.), *Cardiac surgery in the adult* (pp. 439–469). New York, NY: McGraw-Hill.

Samantaray, A., & Hemanth, N. (2011). Comparison of two ventilation modes in post-cardiac surgical patients. *Saudi Journal of Anaesthesia, 5*(2), 173–178.

Scaravilli, V., Bonacina, D., & Citerio, G. (2012). Rewarming: Facts and myths from the systemic perspective. *Critical Care, 16*(Suppl. 2). Retrieved from http://ccforum.com/content/16/S2/A25

Schadler, D., Engel, C., Elke, G., Pulletz, S., Haake, N., Frerichs, I., . . . Weiler, N. (2012). Automatic control of pressure support for ventilator weaning in surgical intensive care patients. *American Journal of Respiratory and Critical Care Medicine, 185*(6), 637–644.

Seifter, J. (2011). Acid-base disorders. In L. Goldman & A. I. Schafer (Eds.), *Goldman's Cecil medicine* (24th ed.). Philadelphia, PA: Elsevier Saunders.

Silvestry, F. E. (2014). *Overview of the postoperative management of patients undergoing cardiac surgery.* Retrieved from http://www.utdol.com/online/ content/topic.do?topicKey=cc_medi/22438& selectedTitle=12~150&source=search_result

Slutsky, A. S. (2014). *Optimizing gas exchange in mechanically ventilated patients with acute respiratory failure.* Retrieved from http://www.med-scape.org/viewarticle/443575

Society of Thoracic Surgeons. (2014). *About STS.* Retrieved from http://www.sts.org/about-sts

Teixeira, C., Zimermann Teixeira, P. J., Höhër, J. A., de Leon, P. P., Brodt, S. F., & da Siva Moreira, J. (2008). Serial measurements of f/VT can predict extubation failure in patients with f/ VT < or = 105. *Journal of Critical Care, 23*(4), 572–576.

Theodore, A. C. (2013). *Oxygenation and mechanisms of hypoxemia.* Retrieved from http://www .uptodate.com/contents/oxygenation-and-mechanisms-of-hypoxemia

Thomas, C. P. (2013a). *Metabolic acidosis.* Retrieved from http://emedicine.medscape.com/article /242975-overview

Thomas, C. P. (2013b). *Metabolic alkalosis.* Retrieved from http://emedicine.medscape.com/article /243160-overview

Trouillet, J., Combes, A., Vaissier, E., Luyt, C., Ouattara, A., Pavie, A., . . . Chastre, J. (2009). Prolonged mechanical ventilation after cardiac surgery: Outcomes and predictors. *The Journal of Thoracic and Cardiovascular Surgery, 138,* 948–953.

Virginia Cardiac Surgery Quality Initiative. (2014). *The Virginia Cardiac Surgery Quality Initiative.* Retrieved from http://www.vcsqi.org/ about_us.php

Westerdahl, E., & Olsén, M. F. (2011). Chest physiotherapy and breathing exercises for cardiac surgery patients in Sweden—a national survey of practice. *Monaldi Archives for Chest Disease, 75*(2), 112–119.

Zakkar, M., Taylor, K., & Hornick, P. I. (2008). Immune system and inflammatory responses. In G. L. Gravlee, R. F. Davis, A. H. Stammers, & R. M. Ungerleider (Eds.), *Cardiopulmonary bypass: Principles and practice* (3rd ed., pp. 321–337). Philadelphia, PA: Lippincott Williams & Wilkins.

Zante, B., Kubik, M., & Reichenspurner, H. (2010). Predictors of prolonged ventilation after cardiac surgery. *The Thoracic and Cardiovascular Surgeon, 58*, 45. Retrieved from https://www.thieme-connect.com/products/ejournals/abstract/10.1055/s-0029-1246815

WEB RESOURCES

Respiratory assessment: http://www.youtube.com/watch?v=IepL5u5lAtE

Mechanical ventilation tutorial: http://www.ccmtutorials.com/rs/mv/

Patient education guides on mechanical ventilation: http://patients.thoracic.org/information-series/en/resources/mechanical-ventilation.pdf

Ventilator case studies: http://www.ventworld.com/education/casestudies.asp

Chapter 12

Pharmacologic Support Following Cardiac Surgery

April Miller Quidley and Roberta Kaplow

INTRODUCTION

Hemodynamic compromise, dysrhythmias, and coagulopathy following cardiac surgery are common therapeutic challenges. The etiology of these complications may be the patient's underlying cardiac disease, postoperative filling pressures, decreased ventricular compliance, loss of vasomotor tone, increased capillary permeability, increased urinary output, inflammatory response to cardiopulmonary bypass (CPB), poor myocardial protection during aortic cross-clamping, pulmonary edema, cardiac tamponade, or ventricular dysfunction. Even though the surgery has been completed, there may not be an immediate improvement in contractility in some patients (Sidebotham & Gillham, 2007).

In the care of the postoperative cardiac surgery patient, the intensive care unit (ICU) nurse must be aware of the intricate balance between physiologic data and the medications utilized to treat and prevent complications. This chapter discusses several medications used in the immediate postoperative setting, including their mechanism of action, therapeutic uses, and side effects. In addition, nurse precautions that are utilized in the delivery of care are described. Many of the medications profiled in this chapter have a number of mechanisms of action and indications. Because of the potential for interaction of some of these medications and their sometimes burdensome side effect profiles,

the ICU nurse needs a high level of clinical judgment to help optimize the patient's outcome.

AGENTS USED TO MANAGE POSTOPERATIVE HYPERTENSION

Hypertension is common following postoperative cardiac surgery and is frequently linked to vasoconstriction and decreased sensitivity of baroreceptors. The vasoconstriction may be linked to induced hypothermia during CPB (Silvestry, 2014). Development of hypertension, vasoconstriction, or both may be due to decreased oxygen levels or inflammatory responses to CPB (Silvestry, 2014). Hypertension leads to increased afterload with resultant metabolic acidosis, increased systemic vascular resistance (SVR), decreased cardiac output (CO), decreased stroke volume (SV), tissue hypoxia of skeletal muscles, and increased myocardial oxygen consumption (Silvestry, 2014). From previous studies of anesthesia and postoperative complications, potential causes of increased afterload include hypothermia, hypovolemia, hypercarbia, inadequate rewarming, volume overload, cardiogenic shock, pain, and anxiety. The latter two causes arise as a result of increased sympathetic nervous system stimulation. Hypertension must be managed after cardiac surgery because extreme vasoconstriction places patients at risk of developing life-threatening hypertension and decreased CO. Controlling hypertension is also important after cardiac surgery to reduce

bleeding from surgical sites and enhance CO. Refer to **Table 12-1** for a summary of medications used to treat hypertension following cardiac surgery.

Table 12-1   Antihypertensive Agents Used in Postoperative Cardiac Surgery Patients and Hemodynamic Effects

Agent	Dose	Mechanism of Action	Hemodynamic Effects
Vasodilators			
Nitroglycerin (Tridil®, Nitronal®)	3–10 mcg/min; titrated in 5-mcg increments every 3–5 minutes.	Venous and arterial vasodilation (dose dependent). Increases coronary blood flow, dilates coronary arteries.	Decreases preload and afterload (dose dependent). Decreases PAP, CVP, SVR, PVR, myocardial oxygen consumption.
Nitroprusside (Nitropress®, Nipride®)	0.25–0.5 mcg/kg/min; titrated in 0.5 mcg/kg/min increments every 10 minutes up to 10 mcg/kg/min.	Smooth muscle relaxant; arterial vasodilation. Generates nitric oxide.	Decreases SVR and PVR; increases venous capacitance, decreases coronary vascular resistance.
Nicardipine (Cardene®)	Infusion at 5 mg/hr. Dose may be slowly increased by 2.5 mg/hr to a maximum of 15 mg/hr. May reduce by 3 mg/hr once goal blood pressure is reached.	Blocks flow of calcium. Acts directly on arterioles. Also been shown to dilate the coronary vasculature.	Peripheral vascular and coronary vasodilation and lower blood pressure.
Clevidipine (Cleviprex®)	1–2 mg/hr via continuous infusion. Dose may be doubled in 90 sec intervals. Once blood pressure begins to approach goal, incremental dosing should be every 5–10 min and be less than double the dose. A maximum initial dose is 16 mg/hr. Total 24-hr dosing should not exceed 21 mg/hr.	Blocks calcium channels. Smooth muscle relaxant and arterial vasodilator.	Decreases MAP and SVR.

Table 12-1   Antihypertensive Agents Used in Postoperative Cardiac Surgery Patients and Hemodynamic Effects (*Continued*)

Fenoldopam mesylate (Corlopam®)	Initial dose of 0.03–0.1 mcg/kg/min. Titration in increments of 0.05–0.1 mcg/kg/min every 5–15 min, to maximum of 1.6 mcg/kg/min, to achieve desired blood pressure. Should not be used for more than 48 hrs.	Selective dopamine-1-receptor agonist and moderately binds to alpha$_2$ receptors.	Vasodilator; increases renal blood flow; decreases SVR and PVR and enhances cardiac output.
Beta Blockers			
Esmolol (Brevibloc®)	Loading dose: 500–1,000 mcg/kg IV bolus over 1 minute. Maintenance dose: 50 mcg/kg/min titrated in 50 mcg/kg/min increments every 4 minutes to a maximum dose of 300 mcg/kg/min.	Cardioselective beta-adrenergic receptor blocker. Inhibits effects at beta$_1$ receptors. Inhibits beta$_2$ receptors at higher doses.	Decreases heart rate, blood pressure, contractility, and cardiac output.
Labetalol (Normodyne®, Trandate®)	10–20 mg IV push over 2 minutes. Additional 10–20 mg doses every 10 min up to a maximum of 300 mg in 24 hours may be given. Infusion dosing: Initial rate 2 mg/min to a maximum cumulative dose of 300 mg.	Non-cardioselective adrenergic blocking agent. Exerts inhibitory effects on beta$_1$, beta$_2$, and alpha$_1$ receptors.	
ACE Inhibitors			
Enalaprilat (Vasotec®)	0.625–1.25 mg, infused over 5 min every 6 hrs. Additional doses, up to a maximum of 5 mg every 6 hrs, may be administered.	Prevents conversion of angiotensin I to angiotensin II (a potent vasoconstrictor) by inhibiting ACE in the pulmonary and systemic vascular endothelium.	Vasodilation; decreases SVR.

(Continued)

Table 12-1   Antihypertensive Agents Used in Postoperative Cardiac Surgery Patients and Hemodynamic Effects (*Continued*)

ARBs

No specific ARB recommendations noted in literature and no commercially available IV ARB agents	Dosage is drug dependent.	Blocks production of angiotensin II from sources of angiotensin II other than the liver (i.e., blood vessels, in the adrenals, and within all other tissues).	The adrenal-related blockage results in a decrease in aldosterone levels, thereby leading to increased excretion of sodium and water from kidneys.

Calcium Channel Blockers

Nicardipine (Cardene®)	Start 5 mg/hr IV. Increase by 2.5 mg/hr every 5–15 min.	Inhibits calcium ion influx into vascular smooth muscle and myocardium.	Decrease in coronary resistance and SVR.
Clevidipine (Cleviprex®)	1–2 mg/hr via continuous infusion. Dose may be doubled in 90 sec intervals. Once blood pressure begins to approach goal, incremental dosing should be every 5–10 min and be less than double the dose. A maximum initial dose is 16 mg/hr. Total 24-hr dosing should not exceed 21 mg/hr.	Smooth muscle relaxant and arterial vasodilator.	Decreases MAP and SVR.

Selective Dopamine-1-Receptor Agonist

Fenoldopam Mesylate (Corlopam®)	Start 0.025–0.3 mcg/kg/min IV. Titrate by 0.05–0.1 mcg/kg/min.	Stimulates dopamine D_1-like and alpha$_2$ adrenergic receptors.	Increases heart rate; decreases mean, systolic, and diastolic arterial blood pressure.

Notes: ACE, angiotensin-converting enzyme; ARB, angiotensin receptor blocker; CVP, central venous pressure; IV, intravenous; MAP, mean arterial pressure; PAP, pulmonary artery pressure; PVR, pulmonary vascular resistance; SVR, systemic vascular resistance.

Sources: Data from Rhoney, D., & Peacock, W. (2009). Intravenous therapy for hypertensive emergencies. *American Journal of Health-System Pharmacy, 66*(15), 1343–1352; Katz, E. A. (2007). Pharmacologic management of the postoperative cardiac surgery patient. *Critical Care Nursing Clinics of North America, 19*(4), 487–496; Singla, N., Warltier, D. C., Ghandi, S. D., Lumb, P. D., Sladen, R. N., Aronson, S., . . . Corwin, H. L. (2008). Treatment of acute postoperative hypertension in cardiac surgery patients: An efficacy study of clevidipine assessing its postoperative antihypertensive effect in cardiac surgery-2 (ESCAPE-2), a randomized, double-blind, placebo-controlled trial. *Anesthesia & Analgesia, 107*(1), 59–67.; Soto-Ruiz, K. M., Peacock, W. F., & Varon, J. (2010). Perioperative hypertension: Diagnosis and treatment. *Netherlands Journal of Critical Care, 15*(3), 143–148.

Vasodilators

Vasodilators are the agents of choice to decrease hypertension in the immediate postoperative cardiac surgery patient. Nitroprusside is the agent of choice (Silvestry, 2014). Vasodilators are utilized to control hypertension, reduce afterload by decreasing vasoconstriction, and prevent angina pectoris, myocardial infarction (MI), and heart failure, all of which could occur in the postoperative cardiac surgery patient. These agents may also be used in postoperative cardiac surgery patients who have normal blood pressure despite poor pump function (Silvestry, 2014). Agents may dilate either the arterial or venous system, or both. The most commonly used vasodilators in this patient population are nitroglycerin (Tridil®), nitroprusside (Nipride®), nicardipine (Cardene®), clevidipine (Cleviprex®), and fenoldopam mesylate (Corlopam®).

Care must be taken to correct hypovolemia in hypertensive patients prior to administering a vasodilator. Abrupt, life-threatening hypotension may develop when vasodilators are used and there is an inadequate volume to fill the vasculature. The ICU nurse should always be prepared to administer a rapid fluid bolus when starting any vasodilator, should hypotension occur. As with all vasoactive agents, use of the smallest dose necessary to accomplish the desired effect is recommended. The risk of side effects escalates with higher infusion rates.

Nitroglycerin

MECHANISM OF ACTION

Nitroglycerin (NTG) has many uses in postoperative cardiac surgery patients. It decreases preload and, in higher doses, afterload. Patients with high preload benefit because NTG lowers pulmonary artery pressure (PAP) and central venous pressure (CVP) via its vasodilatory action. Nitroglycerin also decreases SVR and pulmonary vascular resistance (PVR)

(Lemmer & Vlahakes, 2010a). Whenever myocardial ischemia is suspected postoperatively, NTG may be ordered because of its ability to dilate the coronary arteries and increase coronary blood flow. This agent also decreases pulmonary congestion and myocardial oxygen consumption (Clark, Harvey, Finkel, Ray, & Whalen, 2012a).

In addition to treating hypertension, decreasing preload or afterload, and treating myocardial ischemia, NTG is also used in some centers on a short-term basis (12–48 hours) to prevent spasm of internal thoracic arteries in the postoperative period.

DOSAGE

Infusion rates for NTG may be set as low as 5–10 mcg/min. The rate is titrated in 5-mcg increments until a mean arterial pressure (MAP) goal has been attained. Titration to effect can occur as often as every 5–10 minutes owing to the short half-life of NTG. This agent has an immediate onset of action and the drug effects last 30 minutes (Alexander, 2014).

SIDE EFFECTS

One potential side effect of NTG is hypoxia—a condition caused by the drug's inhibition of pulmonary arterial vasoconstriction, which in turn increases blood flow through poorly oxygenated lung areas (Katz, 2007). Other side effects that are often reported with NTG administration include lightheadedness, headache, hypotension, reflex tachycardia, dizziness, and flushing of the face and neck. Tachyphylaxis (decrease in response to the drug) occurs within 6 hours of initiation of therapy (Alexander, 2014). Although rare, methemoglobinemia has been reported as being associated with intravenous (IV) administration of NTG (Singla et al., 2008).

NURSING IMPLICATIONS

Abrupt discontinuation of NTG can cause coronary vasospasm. For this reason, close monitoring of rhythm, blood pressure, and hemodynamic parameters is warranted when the infusion is stopped. The drug dosage used depends on the desired effect, the patient's blood pressure, and hemodynamics, bearing in mind that increasing coronary blood flow may improve cardiac function. The advantages of NTG are its ease of titration and short half-life.

Nitroprusside (Nitropress®)

MECHANISM OF ACTION

Nitroprusside is a smooth muscle relaxant that is used to control hypertension and reduce afterload (SVR and PVR). A powerful arterial vasodilator, it lowers blood pressure by generating nitric oxide. Nitroprusside also increases venous capacitance and decreases coronary vascular resistance (Clark, Harvey, Finkel, Ray, & Whalen, 2012b).

DOSAGE

For afterload reduction, initial doses as low as 0.3–0.5 mcg/kg/min should be used and slowly titrated (every 10 minutes) up to 10 mcg/kg/min to maintain the blood pressure within specified goals. Nitroprusside has an immediate onset of action (the peak effect occurs in 2 minutes), and its effects dissipate rapidly (within 3 minutes) when the infusion is discontinued (Clark et al., 2012b). It rapidly reduces blood pressure and is converted in the body to cyanide and then to thiocyanate. Its adverse effects can be attributed mainly to excessive hypotension and excessive cyanide accumulation; thiocyanate toxicity may also occur. To avoid cyanide toxicity, its use should be limited to low doses (< 2 mcg/kg/min) for less than 72 hours, and use at the maximum dose (10 mcg/kg/min) should not occur for more than 10 minutes. Thiocyanate toxicity can also occur, especially in patients with renal impairment who receive infusions for more than 72 hours (Singla et al., 2008).

SIDE EFFECTS

Administration of nitroprusside may produce reflex tachycardia, hypotension, and renal dysfunction. Rarely, patients may develop a decreased platelet count or hypothyroidism (thiocyanate impairs iodine transport). Owing to its dilation of the pulmonary arterioles, nitroprusside can decrease arterial oxygen content and cause—or worsen—any existing ventilation/perfusion mismatch, leading to hypoxia. Methemoglobinemia may also occur, which will decrease the blood's oxygen-carrying capacity. It typically occurs when nitroprusside infuses for more than 16 hours (Aschenbrenner & Venable, 2009). Cerebral vasodilation with resultant increased intracranial pressure may occur, and it should be avoided in patients with suspected stroke or head injury. Nitroprusside may also inhibit platelet function, cause hypothyroidism, bradycardia or tachycardia, electrocardiogram (ECG) changes, and decrease renal and cerebral blood flow (Aschenbrenner & Venable, 2009).

An excessive amount of cyanide in the plasma (more than 80 ng/mL) following nitroprusside administration—as a consequence of overdosage or depletion of endogenous thiosulfate (which converts cyanide to thiocyanate)—may result in nausea, malaise, headache, vertigo, dizziness, disorientation, confusion, psychosis, weakness, muscle spasm, shortness of breath, or generalized seizures (Leybell, 2014). Metabolic acidosis may be the first sign of cyanide toxicity. Cyanide poisoning occurs when the infusion rate of the drug exceeds the excretion rate of cyanide (Aschenbrenner & Venable, 2009). Early symptoms of cyanide toxicity can include tachypnea/hyperpnea, hypertension, confusion, headache, and/or nausea. Thiocyanate levels should be monitored daily; excess amounts can be removed with dialysis.

NURSING IMPLICATIONS

Nitroprusside can cause sudden, life-threatening hypotension if its use is not closely monitored. Care should be taken not to flush or initiate new medications in lines that contain nitroprusside because doing so can result in abrupt hypotension. When nitroprusside is discontinued, the line should be aspirated and then flushed to avoid this possibility.

Like NTG, nitroprusside can cause pulmonary vasodilation with shunting of blood to atelectatic areas of the lung, resulting in hypoxia and a need for higher oxygen delivery. This effect is usually seen immediately and can be dose dependent. If it occurs, another therapy may be chosen. Increasing positive end-expiratory pressure is helpful in resolving atelectasis.

Beta Adrenergic Antagonists

Depending on the etiology of hypertension, beta adrenergic antagonists (also called beta blockers) may be effective. The net effects of beta blockers are a decrease in heart rate, blood pressure, and CO. Beta blockers are discussed in detail later in this chapter.

Esmolol (Brevibloc®)

MECHANISM OF ACTION
Esmolol is an ultra-short-acting, cardioselective, beta-adrenergic receptor blocker. It inhibits the effects of beta$_1$ receptors. At higher doses, this agent inhibits beta$_2$ receptors located in bronchial musculature and blood vessels (Che, Schreiber, & Rafey, 2009).

INDICATIONS
Esmolol is indicated for intraoperative and postoperative hypertension, management of acute MI, and management of intraoperative and postoperative tachydysrhythmias. It is also used in the management of hypertension in patients with aortic dissection (Mancini, 2014).

DOSAGE
For postoperative hypertension, the dose of esmolol is 500 mcg/kg, given as an IV bolus administered over 1 minute. This bolus should be followed by a maintenance dose of 50 mcg/kg/min given over 4 minutes. If

additional dosing is required after 5 minutes, the same loading dose followed by 100 mcg/kg/min may be infused over 4 minutes. This titration may continue by increasing the maintenance dose in 50 mcg/kg/min increments until the desired therapeutic endpoint or a maintenance dosage of 300 mcg/kg/min is reached. Because esmolol has a short half-life, it is a practical choice for treating patients with a labile blood pressure (Mancini, 2014).

SIDE EFFECTS
Side effects commonly associated with esmolol include bradycardia, chest pain, hypotension, confusion, headache, dizziness, agitation, dyspnea, wheezing, fatigue, constipation, and nausea and vomiting. Serious, but less common side effects include seizures, bronchospasm, and pulmonary edema. Anemia may prolong the half-life of esmolol. Esmolol should not be used in patients with acute heart failure, bradycardia, heart block (greater than first degree), or bronchospasm (Gupta, Gupta, & Khoynezhad, 2009; Mancini, 2014).

NURSING IMPLICATIONS
Logically, any patient who requires an agent that causes beta-receptor stimulation should not receive beta-blocker therapy. Esmolol is contraindicated in patients with cardiogenic shock, hemodynamic compromise, second- or third-degree heart block, first-degree heart block (if the PR interval is greater than 0.24 sec), or severe sinus bradycardia. Caution should be exercised when this agent is administered to patients with heart failure, bronchospastic disease, atrial fibrillation (AF) with associated hypotension, diabetes, renal impairment, or hyperthyroidism (Minczak, 2014). Because esmolol may require large volumes of fluid for its administration, thought should be given as to whether it is the appropriate drug for patients who may not be able to tolerate this excessive fluid intake.

The ICU nurse should monitor heart rate, blood pressure, and for signs of heart failure in patients receiving esmolol. Similarly, patients with diabetes should have their blood glucose monitored on a regular basis because esmolol my mask symptoms of hypoglycemia. Sudden withdrawal of therapy should be avoided because it can cause myocardial ischemia and hyperdynamic circulation (Butterworth, 2013).

Labetalol (Normodyne®, Trandate®)

MECHANISM OF ACTION

Labetalol is a nonselective, adrenergic blocking agent that exerts inhibitory effects on $beta_1$, $beta_2$, and $alpha_1$ receptors.

INDICATIONS

Labetalol is used on an off-label basis for postoperative hypertension. Data suggest it is effective when used on postoperative vascular surgery patients and in patients with aortic dissection (Upadhye & Schiff, 2012).

DOSAGE

For postoperative hypertension, patients receive 10 mg intravenously over 2 minutes. If additional doses are needed, 10–20 mg may be given every 10 minutes, up to a maximum dose of 300 mg in a 24-hour period (Butterworth, 2013). A continuous infusion starting at 2 mg/min may be used, with the same maximum cumulative 300 mg dose in 24 hours.

SIDE EFFECTS

When labetalol is given for on-label conditions, serious side effects have included bronchospasm, hyperkalemia, and ventricular dysrhythmias. Commonly experienced side effects include bradycardias, edema, postural hypotension, diaphoresis, increased liver enzymes (less common), dizziness, paresthesias, elevated renal function tests, dyspnea, wheezing, and fatigue (Prometheus, 2013).

NURSING IMPLICATIONS

Like esmolol, labetalol is contraindicated in patients with cardiogenic shock, second- or third-degree heart block, or severe sinus bradycardia. It is also contraindicated in patients with bronchial asthma or chronic obstructive pulmonary disease. Caution should be exercised when labetalol is administered to patients with heart failure, bronchospastic disease, diabetes, heart failure, ischemic heart disease, liver disease, peripheral vascular disease (PVD), or hyperthyroidism. Monitoring by the ICU nurse should include heart rate, blood pressure, and signs of heart failure. Similarly, patients with diabetes should have their serum glucose monitored on a regular basis due to the potential masking of the signs and symptoms of hypoglycemia. Sudden withdrawal of therapy should be avoided (Butterworth, 2013). As with esmolol, any patient who requires an agent that causes beta-receptor stimulation should not receive beta-blocker therapy.

Angiotensin-Converting Enzyme Inhibitors

Enalaprilat (Vasotec®)

HEMODYNAMIC EFFECTS

Angiotensin-converting enzyme (ACE) inhibitors act on the renin–angiotensin–aldosterone system (RAAS). Specifically, they prevent the conversion of angiotensin I to angiotensin II by inhibiting ACE in the pulmonary and systemic vascular endothelium (Alexander, 2014). Because angiotensin II is a potent vasoconstrictor, inhibition results in vasodilation. Additionally, these agents prevent the production of aldosterone, which blocks the reabsorption of sodium in the kidneys. These agents cause a decrease in SVR and typically have little effect on heart rate. With the dosage described in this section, patients should experience improvements in both blood pressure and CO (Hillis et al., 2011).

INDICATIONS

Angiotensin-converting enzyme inhibitors may be administered early after cardiac surgery to patients with mild left ventricular (LV) dysfunction, even in the face of moderate renal impairment (Hillis et al., 2011). Enalaprilat is the only ACE inhibitor available in an IV dosage form.

DOSAGE

The initial dose of enalaprilat is 0.625–1.25 mg, infused over 5 minutes. Additional doses, up to a maximum of 5 mg every 6 hours, may be administered.

SIDE EFFECTS

The most common side effects with enalaprilat are cough, hyperkalemia, and renal failure. The cough is thought to occur due to the accumulation of bradykinin in the lung and vasculature (Aronson, 2009). While benign, it should be treated by discontinuation of enalaprilat rather than with antitussive agents. Hyperkalemia occurs when aldosterone is inhibited secondary to the inhibition of angiotensin II. Enalaprilat should be avoided in patients with bilateral renal artery stenosis because a decrease in glomerular filtration rate (GFR) may occur. If acute kidney injury should occur, enalaprilat should be discontinued (Kaplan, 2014). Angioedema with potential airway compromise is a rare side effect. The ICU nurse should observe the patient for facial swelling or reported airway swelling. Neutropenia can be a rare but serious complication. Patients may also rarely report dysgeusia (altered sense of taste) or blurred vision. The ICU nurse should observe for signs of onset of these complications and anticipate possible discontinuation of the medication if they occur.

NURSING IMPLICATIONS

For patients who have a history of renal insufficiency and who are receiving enalaprilat, nurses should monitor serum creatinine levels (Kaplan, 2014). Meticulous monitoring of the patient's hemodynamic profile and hourly measurement of urinary output may help avoid the development of renal failure sometimes associated with ACE inhibitors.

Angiotensin Receptor Blockers

Angiotensin receptor blockers (ARBs) influence the RAAS by blocking production of angiotensin II from sources of angiotensin II other than the liver. The blocking of angiotensin receptors occurs on blood vessels, in the adrenals, and within all other tissues. The adrenal-related blockage results in a decrease in aldosterone levels, thereby leading to increased excretion of sodium and water from the kidneys. Common ARBs include oral losartan (Cozaar®), valsartan (Diovan®), and candesartan (Atacand®). There are no parenteral dosage forms.

Angiotensin receptor blockers cause less cough than ACE inhibitors, but otherwise have similar side effects. They are utilized predominately for hypertension management and require blood pressure monitoring after their initiation. Both ACE inhibitors and ARBs are contraindicated in patients with bilateral renal artery stenosis.

Calcium Channel Blockers

Nicardipine (Cardene®)

HEMODYNAMIC EFFECTS

Nicardipine blocks the flow of calcium on vascular smooth muscle. It acts directly on arterioles to cause peripheral vascular and coronary vasodilation and lower blood pressure. It has little effect on contractility or atrioventricular (AV) node conduction. Nicardipine has also been shown to dilate the coronary vasculature (Bush, 2010). Administration did not affect ventricular preload or afterload or CO despite significant decreases in blood pressure (Bush, 2010).

INDICATIONS

Nicardipine is indicated for the treatment of hypertension, including in the postoperative period (Bush, 2010).

DOSAGE

Therapy is initiated at an infusion rate of 5 mg/hr. The dose may be slowly increased by 2.5 mg/hr to a maximum of 15 mg/hr. Once the blood pressure endpoint is reached, a maintenance infusion may be run at 3 mg/hr (Cannon et al., 2013).

SIDE EFFECTS

The most common side effects of nicardipine are headache, hypotension, nausea, vomiting, peripheral edema, headache, dizziness, and tachycardia. Serious adverse events that have been reported include angina and myocardial ischemia or infarction. Severe bradycardia has also been reported (Aronson, 2009).

NURSING IMPLICATIONS

Because of nicardipine's potential to cause negative inotropic effects, especially in patients with heart failure, portal hypertension, or significant LV dysfunction, caution should be exercised when administering this agent with a beta blocker. Close blood pressure and heart rate monitoring are required during therapy. Nicardipine is contraindicated in patients with advanced aortic stenosis because diastolic pressure and afterload reduction may worsen rather than improve myocardial oxygen balance (Walker, 2013). Nicardipine is prepared as a dilute solution, and patients requiring large doses for extended periods may receive too much fluid.

Clevidipine (Cleviprex®)

HEMODYNAMIC EFFECTS

Clevidipine is an ultra-short-acting intravenous calcium channel blocker. It functions as both a smooth muscle relaxant and an arterial vasodilator. This agent causes a decrease in MAP and SVR, but it does not reduce filling pressures (Deeks, Keating, & Keam, 2009).

INDICATIONS

Clevidipine is used to treat postoperative hypertension without impairing cardiac function. In one study of postoperative cardiac surgery patients, treatment with this calcium channel blocker was effective in 91.8% of patients (Singla et al., 2008).

DOSAGE

The initial dose of clevidipine is 1–2 mg/hr via continuous infusion. The dose may be doubled in 90-second intervals. Once the patient's blood pressure begins to approach the goal, less rapid dose titration (every 5–10 minutes) should occur. A maximum initial dose of 16 mg/hr is recommended, and a therapeutic effect is achieved for most patients at infusion rates of 4–6 mg/hr. The total 24-hour dosing should not exceed an average of 21 mg/hr (or 1,000 mL total) because of lipid load restrictions (Bojar, 2011).

SIDE EFFECTS

Reported side effects of clevidipine include headache, sinus tachycardia, hypotension, nausea, vomiting, and dizziness (Singla et al., 2008). Other side effects that have been reported include AF and acute renal failure. Although rare, cardiac arrest, MI, hypotension, and reflex tachycardia have occurred with use of this agent (Ndefo, Erowele, Ebiasah, & Green, 2010).

NURSING IMPLICATIONS

Administration of clevidipine is contraindicated in patients with an allergy to soy or egg products or with alterations in lipid metabolism (e.g., hyperlipidemia) due to its formulation in a lipid vehicle. Because of the phospholipid vehicle, it is recommended that the intravenous tubing be changed every 4 hours. Clevidipine is also contraindicated in patients with severe aortic stenosis, because it may reduce myocardial oxygen delivery secondary to afterload reduction. Caution should be exercised when administering clevidipine concomitantly with a beta blocker. Heart failure symptoms may be exacerbated due to this agent's negative inotropic effects. Patients may develop hypotension and reflex tachycardia when rapid titration takes place in an effort to increase the dosage. Rebound hypertension may develop following extended infusions of clevidipine (Ndefo et al., 2010).

When a patient is receiving clevidipine, the ICU nurse should continuously monitor heart rate and blood pressure during the infusion and until vital signs become stable. Blood pressure monitoring should continue for a minimum of 8 hours following discontinuation of clevidipine if the patient is not converted to another antihypertensive agent. Patients should also be monitored for exacerbation of heart failure symptoms (de Araujo, Fagundes, Leite, & Fonseca, 2010).

Selective Dopamine-1-Receptor Agonists

Fenoldopam Mesylate (Corlopam®)

HEMODYNAMIC EFFECTS

Fenoldopam mesylate is a dopamine-1-receptor agonist. The dopamine-1 (D_1) receptors are located in the coronary, mesenteric, and renal vasculature; when stimulated, they cause vasodilation (Levy, Tanaka, & Bailey, 2008). Fenoldopam also moderately binds to alpha$_2$ receptors, which results in lowered SVR and PVR and enhanced CO. This agent has rapid action as a vasodilator and increases renal blood flow (Ranucci et al., 2010).

INDICATIONS

Fenoldopam is indicated for the short-term treatment of severe hypertension, including during the perioperative period (Ranucci et al., 2010). It is believed to be especially useful in patients with renal insufficiency when it is administered in the prescribed dose range. Due to stimulation of dopamine-1 receptors in the kidneys, fenoldopam causes an increase in GFR, renal blood flow, and sodium excretion (Ranucci et al., 2010).

DOSAGE

The initial dose of fenoldopam is 0.01–1.6 mcg/kg/min. Titration can occur in increments of 0.05–0.1 mcg/kg/min every 5–15 minutes, to a maximum of 1.6 mcg/kg/min, to achieve the desired blood pressure. The doses must be administered as a continuous infusion; no bolus doses should be given. Fenoldopam should not be used for more than 48 hours. Fenoldopam may be discontinued progressively or rapidly once the desired effect has been achieved (Gahart & Nazareno, 2013).

SIDE EFFECTS

Possible adverse effects of fenoldopam include hypotension, dose-related tachyarrhythmias, flushing, nausea, vomiting, dizziness, headache, angina, cardiac dysrhythmias, heart failure, MI, hypokalemia (to less than 3 mEq/L), and serum creatinine elevation (Tse, Lip, & Coats, 2011).

NURSING IMPLICATIONS

Caution should be used when fenoldopam is administered to patients who are concomitantly receiving beta blockers or in patients with hypokalemia, hypotension, liver disease, tachycardia, or glaucoma (increased intraocular pressure may result). During administration of this agent, the ICU nurse should monitor blood pressure, heart rate, and serum electrolytes, particularly potassium.

AGENTS USED TO MANAGE POSTOPERATIVE LOW CARDIAC OUTPUT AND HYPOTENSION

Some degree of myocardial depression, low CO, and hypotension are common in the immediate postoperative period following cardiac surgery. These conditions can be related to preexisting cardiac disease, inflammation related to CPB, post-ischemic dysfunction, or reperfusion injury (Kouchoukos, Blackstone, Hanley, & Kirklin, 2013).

Low CO following CPB procedures is primarily due to LV dysfunction. This LV dysfunction may occur secondary to cardioplegic arrest, decreased preload, loss of vasomotor tone, intraoperative blood loss, increased capillary permeability, increased urinary output from hypothermia, dysrhythmias, or intraoperative MI (Apostolakis, Baikoussis, Parissis, Siminelakis, & Papadopoulos, 2009). Low cardiac output syndrome (LCOS), which may occur in postoperative cardiac surgery patients, is a decrease in CO secondary to a brief episode of myocardial dysfunction.

Contributing factors to postoperative hypotension include hypovolemia, vasodilation (relative hypovolemia), anemia, pneumothorax, hemothorax, cardiac tamponade, electrolyte imbalance, hemorrhage, metabolic alterations, and dysrhythmias.

Effective treatment of low CO and hypotension depends on quickly identifying the causes and initiating the appropriate treatment. Detrimental complications can occur even with brief periods of hypotension, so aggressive and prompt intervention is warranted.

When low CO or hypotension is accompanied by low CVP and pulmonary artery occlusive pressure (PAOP), volume resuscitation is needed to correct hypovolemia. A combination of crystalloids, colloids, and blood products may be used for this purpose. An in-depth discussion of volume resuscitation appears in Chapter 17.

If hypotension persists after volume resuscitation, it may be secondary to significant vasodilation. In this scenario, adrenergic agonists or vasopressors may be required to normalize blood pressure if the patient has normal pump function and remains unresponsive to volume repletion alone. It is best to begin pharmacologic intervention once the patient has adequate filling pressures and acid–base and electrolyte balance has been achieved (Silvestry, 2014).

Many cardiac surgery patients require vasopressor and inotropic support. In these patients, volume repletion, administration of vasodilators, pacing, or any combination of these may not be adequate (Silvestry, 2014). Typically, patients who improve with inotropic support are those with a cardiac index (CI) less than 2 L/min/m² who have optimal heart rate, cardiac rhythm, filling pressures, afterload, and absence of tamponade (Khalpey, Schmitto, & Rawn, 2012).

Adrenergic Agonists

Adrenergic agonists are used to normalize blood pressure when all known causative factors are corrected but hypotension persists. Any patient receiving an adrenergic agonist should be continuously assessed for hypovolemia, which may occur even after adequate volume repletion. Adrenergic agonists are often referred to as sympathomimetics, reflecting their ability to activate adrenergic receptors by direct receptor binding, promotion of norepinephrine (NE) release, blockade of NE reuptake, and inhibition of NE inactivation.

Adrenergic agonists are classified as either catecholamines or non-catecholamines. Catecholamines include epinephrine (Adrenaline®), norepinephrine (Levophed®), dopamine (Intropin®), and dobutamine (Dobutrex®). An example of a non-catecholamine is phenylephrine (Neosynephrine®).

Adrenergic agonists are notable for their specificity, with the various agents acting on alpha$_1$, alpha$_2$, beta$_1$, beta$_2$, or a combination of these receptors (see **Table 12-2**). The precise ability of a drug to selectively activate certain receptors to the exclusion of others is dose dependent. Clinical activation of alpha$_1$ receptors results in vasoconstriction. Activation of alpha$_2$ receptors inhibits NE release and often has central effects. When beta$_1$ receptors are activated, patients experience a positive inotropic effect (increased force of contraction) and increased blood pressure, heart rate, CO, and impulse conduction through the AV node. Activation of beta$_2$ receptors can also have positive inotropic (increase in contractility) and chronotropic (increase in heart rate) effects on the heart

Table 12-2 Adrenergic Receptors and Effects When Stimulated	
Adrenergic Receptor Type	**Effects When Stimulated**
β_1	Increased heart rate, blood pressure, contractility (increased inotropic effect), cardiac output, conduction velocity, and automaticity
β_2	Bronchodilation
α_1	Vasoconstriction
α_2	Vasodilation by inhibition of central norepinephrine release
Dopamine$_1$ (D$_1$), post-synaptic	Direct vasodilation
D$_2$, pre-synaptic	Vasodilation by inhibition of norepinephrine release
Vasopressin (V$_1$) (on vascular smooth muscle)	Increased peripheral vascular resistance and vasoconstriction of capillaries and arterioles

Sources: Data from Fawzy, A., & Pool, J. L. (n.d.). *Part I: The physiology and function of the alpha-adrenergic nervous system.* Retrieved from http://www.medscape.org/viewarticle/440787; Klabunde, R. C. (2011). *Cardiovascular physiology concepts* (2nd ed.). Philadelphia, PA: Lippincott Williams & Wilkins.

and cause peripheral vasodilation (especially in skeletal and muscle vasculature). When beta$_2$ receptors in the lung are stimulated, bronchodilation occurs.

Stimulation of dopamine-1 (D$_1$, post-synaptic) receptors, by contrast, causes direct vasodilation. Stimulation of dopamine-2 (D$_2$, pre-synaptic) receptors causes vasodilation by inhibiting the release of NE (Klabunde, 2011).

Use of adrenergic agonists is typically initiated in the operating room (OR) during cardiac surgery, and patients can often be weaned from their agents rapidly after recovery from anesthesia. These drugs are titrated so as to maintain blood pressure within the ordered parameters—typically a MAP of more than 65 mmHg or a systolic blood pressure (SBP) of at least 90 mmHg. Higher pressures may be required to perfuse organs when patients have a history of extreme hypertension, carotid artery disease, PVD, or renal dysfunction (Khalpey et al., 2012).

All adrenergic agonists cause vasoconstriction such that significant tissue damage can occur if extravasation of these agents into the subcutaneous tissue occurs. Decreased blood flow to tissue as a result of vasoconstriction may lead to tissue death. Immediate treatment with an appropriate agent should be utilized promptly after extravasation of adrenergic agonists is suspected or identified. These agents should be given ideally via a central line to limit the risk of extravasation.

Six adrenergic agonists are typically used after cardiac surgery: phenylephrine, norepinephrine, epinephrine, vasopressin (antidiuretic hormone), dopamine, and dobutamine. These medications are used to elevate blood pressure for patients in hypotensive states.

Phenylephrine Hydrochloride (Neosynephrine®)

HEMODYNAMIC EFFECTS AND INDICATIONS

Phenylephrine is a vasoconstrictor that is often used after cardiac surgery to manage mild to moderate hypotension and to increase SVR when hypotension coexists (Bojar, 2011).

It causes vasoconstriction by activating alpha$_1$ receptors on vascular smooth muscle; no other adrenergic receptors are stimulated. The vasoconstrictor effects lead to an increase in SVR. Phenylephrine is also valuable in patients with a high CI who are profoundly vasodilated. A decrease in CO is seen with use of this agent, and either an increase or a decrease in heart rate may be seen (Murfin, 2011).

DOSAGE

Phenylephrine should be started at a dose relative to the clinical situation. Effects are often seen immediately. The dose range is 0.05–1.5 mcg/kg/min (Bojar, 2011). Patients may become refractory after several hours of phenylephrine infusing; a change to norepinephrine may be required.

SIDE EFFECTS

Because of its vasoconstrictor activity, phenylephrine causes hypoperfusion to tissues and end organs, which can lead to visceral and renal ischemia. It also causes an increase in myocardial oxygen consumption and may exacerbate metabolic acidosis. Other reported side effects include hypertension, MI, tachyarrhythmias, ventricular dysrhythmias, and pulmonary edema. Care should be taken when administering phenylephrine or any other alpha agonist to patients who have undergone revascularization procedures with arterial grafts; spasm may occur (Bojar, 2011).

NURSING IMPLICATIONS

The patient should receive adequate volume resuscitation prior to receiving phenylephrine or receiving a significantly increased dose of this agent. Phenylephrine is contraindicated for use in patients with severe hypertension and tachycardia. Caution should be exercised when administering this drug to patients with bronchial asthma, diabetes, or hypertension. Heart rate and blood pressure should be monitored, preferably continuously.

Norepinephrine Bitartrate (Levophed®)

HEMODYNAMIC EFFECTS AND INDICATIONS

Norepinephrine is a powerful vasopressor and adrenergic agonist that stimulates alpha$_1$ and beta$_1$ receptors, causing vasoconstriction, increased inotropic effects, and cardiac stimulation. A small amount of beta$_2$-receptor stimulation occurs as well. Norepinephrine is classified as a vasopressor and an inotrope (Bojar, 2011). It is typically used in profound hypotension when volume repletion is inadequate; it can also be administered concomitantly with fluid resuscitation if the patient's blood pressure and CO are significantly impaired (Bojar, 2011).

INDICATIONS

Norepinephrine is indicated when patients have slightly low blood pressure due to low SVR. If CI is less than 2 L/min/m^2, another inotrope should be administered with norepinephrine (Bojar, 2011).

DOSAGE

Norepinephrine is used in the dose range of 2–20 mcg/min or 0.01–3 mcg/kg/min and titrated so as to reach the desired response, usually a MAP of at least 70 mmHg (Bojar, 2011). This dose will likely produce decreased peripheral and visceral blood flow, which may lead to development of a metabolic acidosis.

SIDE EFFECTS

The most clinically significant side effects experienced by the postoperative cardiac surgery patient receiving norepinephrine are an increase in myocardial workload and oxygen consumption. End-organ damage (e.g., damage to the kidneys and mesentery) may also occur secondary to alpha$_1$-receptor stimulation (Katz, 2007). Norepinephrine exacerbates hyperglycemia and metabolic acidosis, with acidosis occurring secondary to an increase in lactate production (Bojar, 2011).

NURSING IMPLICATIONS

High doses and long-term use of norepinephrine cause decreased perfusion to the skin and can lead to tissue necrosis and limb loss. Patients should be assessed regularly for cyanosis, decreased capillary refill time, and diminished peripheral pulses, all of which are signs of decreased perfusion (Bojar, 2011). They should receive adequate volume resuscitation prior to receiving this therapy or receiving a significantly increased dose of norepinephrine.

Epinephrine (Adrenalin®)

HEMODYNAMIC EFFECTS AND INDICATIONS

Epinephrine stimulates $alpha_1$, $beta_1$, and $beta_2$ receptors (Bojar, 2011). It may be used after cardiac surgery as an inotrope to improve cardiac function and enhance SV, as an adrenergic agonist and vasopressor for refractory hypotension, or as a positive chronotropic agent to increase heart rate in bradycardia (Bojar, 2011). Epinephrine is also useful in the cardiac arrest situation owing to its ability to enhance automaticity (Sinz, Navarro, & Soderberg, 2010).

DOSAGE

Epinephrine's effects on different adrenergic receptors vary with the dosage used. At low doses (less than 0.02 mcg/kg/min), epinephrine causes stimulation of $beta_2$ receptors with resultant mild peripheral vasodilation and relaxation of the bronchial smooth muscle. At higher doses (0.008–0.06 mcg/kg/min), $beta_1$ stimulation results in an increased blood pressure, CO, and contractility. At doses of 0.5–4.0 mcg/kg/min, positive chronotropic effects are noted. At the highest dosage (more than 2 mcg/kg/min), $alpha_1$-receptor stimulation causes vasoconstriction, which results in an increase in SVR. The blood pressure effects of epinephrine vary in postoperative cardiac surgery patients. In particular, patients who are post-CPB demonstrate inconsistent hemodynamic responses to epinephrine administration. Variable responses in CO, heart rate, and MAP have been reported (Bojar, 2011).

SIDE EFFECTS

When higher doses of epinephrine are administered, patients may develop atrial or ventricular ectopy and tachyarrhythmias owing to $beta_1$-receptor stimulation. The higher the dose, the more likely that atrial or ventricular ectopy and tachyarrhythmias will be seen (Royal Flying Doctor Service, 2013).

Epinephrine can raise the serum glucose levels so profoundly that insulin drips should be anticipated. Higher than normal doses of insulin may be required to maintain adequate glycemic control. The hyperglycemia is attributable to increased gluconeogenesis and the stress response to catecholamine administration (Rosas, Giocoechea-Turcott, Ortiz, Salazar, & Palma, 2012). Hyperglycemia typically occurs in patients who receive epinephrine within the first 6–8 postoperative hours and usually disappears within a few hours after epinephrine is discontinued (Rosas et al., 2012).

Patients receiving low doses of epinephrine may also develop metabolic acidosis; low serum bicarbonate levels (typically between 17 and 21 mEq/L). This metabolic acidosis may occur secondary to the inadequate metabolism and lactate buildup that occurs in response to $beta_1$ stimulation. It is not related to hypoperfusion, as patients' cardiac performance is acceptable when the acidosis develops. Cardiac output and mixed venous saturation levels also remain within acceptable parameters (Bojar, 2011). As with hyperglycemia, metabolic acidosis typically occurs in patients who receive epinephrine within the first 6–8 postoperative hours and usually disappears within a few hours of epinephrine's discontinuation (Bojar, 2011).

NURSING IMPLICATIONS

While on epinephrine, the patient must be monitored closely for tachycardia and signs of myocardial ischemia—administration of this agent will increase PVR, SVR, lactate, and myocardial oxygen consumption. Adequate oxygenation should be maintained and the patient monitored for signs of ischemia, given that epinephrine increases myocardial oxygen demand. The ICU nurse should be prepared to quickly wean the patient from insulin if the epinephrine drip is reduced or discontinued. Hyperglycemia usually resolves within a few hours (6 or fewer) after the epinephrine infusion is discontinued.

While increasing blood pressure and CO/CI are goals of therapy, vasodilators may be necessary to control elevated blood pressure when epinephrine must be used at high doses to maintain CO. Similarly, when epinephrine is infused at higher doses, alpha$_1$ stimulation causes an increase in myocardial workload, SVR, and PAOP (Bojar, 2011).

Vasopressin (Pitressin®)

Cardiopulmonary bypass frequently causes the release of vasopressin, an antidiuretic hormone, which may contribute to post-bypass vasoconstriction. Data indicate that vasopressin levels may diminish as hypotension continues. This finding suggests that the body may have a limited supply of vasopressin that is depleted following the initial hypotensive episode (Levy et al., 2008).

HEMODYNAMIC EFFECTS AND INDICATIONS
Vasopressin is used to treat vasodilatory shock following CPB procedures in patients with profound hypotension (MAP less than 70 mmHg) despite fluid resuscitation, afterload reduction, inotropic therapy, and norepinephrine administration. Postoperative CPB patients who have protracted hypotension can demonstrate poor vascular smooth-muscle response to catecholamines. Vasopressin, when administered in high doses, promotes contraction of vascular smooth muscle, which in turn causes vasoconstriction of the capillaries and small arterioles and can increase

MAP (Yimin, Xiaoyu, Yuping, Weiyan, & Ning, 2013). It is also believed that some patients have low vasopressin concentrations, such that exogenous administration may improve these patients' clinical status (Yimin et al., 2013). The postoperative cardiac surgery patients with vasodilatory shock who benefit most from vasopressin are those with a deficiency, often manifested by reduced response to high doses of other vasopressors. Those with a low ejection fraction (EF) who take chronic ACE inhibitors may also benefit (Thoma, 2013).

Vasopressin stimulates V$_1$ receptors on vascular smooth muscle, which causes an increase in peripheral vascular resistance and vasoconstriction of capillaries and arterioles. Vasopressin may improve LV function, which would result in an increase in CO and coronary blood flow (Yimin et al., 2013). Vasopressin increases secretion of corticotropin, a hormone produced by the anterior pituitary gland that stimulates the adrenal cortex. The adrenal cortex produces cortisol, a major hormone responsible for blood pressure regulation.

Vasopressin also has indications in cardiac arrest situations as an early substitute for epinephrine in patients with ventricular fibrillation (VF), pulseless ventricular tachycardia, or asystole (Sinz et al., 2010).

DOSAGE
The dosage of vasopressin needed to achieve vasoconstrictor effects is 0.01–0.1 unit/min by continuous IV infusion (Bojar, 2011; Yimin et al., 2013).

SIDE EFFECTS
Side effects of vasopressin are rare but include end-organ damage from vasoconstriction, leading to hypoperfusion, hyponatremia, and increased SVR. All of these effects occur secondary to the drug's vasoconstrictive effects. Patients may also develop nausea, abdominal cramping, bronchoconstriction, water intoxication with resultant hyponatremia, and

decreased myocardial oxygen delivery secondary to constriction of the coronary arteries (Klabunde, 2011).

NURSING IMPLICATIONS

Extreme caution should be used in patients with coronary artery disease who are receiving vasopressin because of the potential for extreme vasoconstriction associated with this agent. The ICU nurse should monitor for a number of adverse effects in the postoperative cardiac surgery patient, including decreased CO, chest pain, myocardial ischemia, ventricular dysrhythmias, bronchoconstriction, metabolic acidosis, tremors, gastrointestinal infarction, abdominal cramping, and water intoxication (Klabunde, 2011).

Dopamine (Intropin®) and Dobutamine (Dobutrex®)

The use of dopamine and dobutamine is required in many postoperative cardiac surgery patients even when careful attention is paid to intraoperative myocardial protection. Prolonged surgery, myocardial edema, advanced age, reperfusion injuries, and poor preoperative cardiac function are all factors that put the patient at higher risk for low CO postoperatively. Both dopamine and dobutamine cause an increase in CO and heart rate (Alexander, 2014).

Before these agents are administered, CO/CI should be high enough to sustain end-organ perfusion and deliver adequate amounts of oxygen to tissues. This criterion should be judged subjectively for each patient based on adequate urine output, normal capillary refill time, appropriate mentation, adequate blood pressure, warm skin temperature, and lack of acidosis. Objectively, CI should be more than 2 L/min/m^2 before use of dopamine and dobutamine is considered; normal CI in the nondiseased heart is in the range of 2.5–4.5 L/min/m^2. When preload has been optimized and SV remains low, poor contractility is the likely etiology and inotropes are

indicated. Adding inotropes will increase the amount of contractile force and result in an improved SV and CO/CI.

Dopamine

HEMODYNAMIC EFFECTS AND INDICATIONS

Like epinephrine, dopamine's effects on different adrenergic receptors vary with dosage. Dopamine stimulates dopaminergic, alpha$_1$, beta$_1$, and beta$_2$ receptors, resulting in either vasoconstriction or positive inotropic and chronotropic effects (Lemmer & Vhahakes, 2010b). Stimulation of beta$_2$ receptors is less than that seen with the other adrenergic agents. Dopamine is used to increase blood pressure, CO, and perfusion through the renal vasculature. At higher doses, this drug has vasopressor properties, as it stimulates the release of endogenous NE. Dopamine also stimulates D$_1$ and D$_2$ receptors when administered in doses less than 8 mcg/kg/min (Lemmer & Vlahakes, 2010b).

Some data suggest that dopamine administration to post-cardiac surgery patients results in an increase in renal oxygenation secondary to vasodilation. No increase in GFR, sodium reabsorption, or renal oxygen consumption were reported (Redfors, Bragadottir, Sellgren, Sward, & Rickstein, 2010).

DOSAGE

Renal vasodilation occurs due to stimulation of dopaminergic receptors in the kidneys at doses of 0.5–3.0 mcg/kg/min. At an infusion rate of 4–10 mcg/kg/min, beta$_1$ stimulation is seen. Positive inotropic and chronotropic effects lead to an increase in heart rate, blood pressure, contractility, and CO. At doses exceeding 10 mcg/kg/min, alpha$_1$ stimulation occurs, along with associated vasoconstriction and increased SVR. Dopamine's effect on renal perfusion in terms of long-term outcomes remains controversial (Silvestry, 2014). This agent should be started at a low dose and doses titrated upward slowly to achieve the desired effect.

SIDE EFFECTS

Common side effects of dopamine include chest pain, hypertension, palpitations, tachyarrhythmias, headache, anxiety, dyspnea, oliguria, nausea, and vomiting. Serious side effects include ectopic beats (including ventricular dysrhythmias), widening QRS complex, and gangrenous disorder (Lemmer & Vlahakes, 2010b).

NURSING IMPLICATIONS

Systolic pressures are often elevated with dopamine use, making it a poor choice in patients with pulmonary hypertension. Dopamine is also contraindicated in patients with tachyarrhythmias. As with other inotropes, caution should be exercised when administering this agent to patients with angina, hypovolemia, or ventricular dysrhythmias.

Like epinephrine, dopamine causes vasoconstriction, such that significant tissue damage can result if extravasation into the subcutaneous tissue occurs. Decreased blood flow to tissue from vasoconstriction may lead to tissue sloughing and death. Immediate infiltration with phentolamine (Regitine®) to the ischemic area should be implemented promptly after extravasation of adrenergic agonists is suspected or identified.

Dobutamine

HEMODYNAMIC EFFECTS AND INDICATIONS

Dobutamine is a synthetic catecholamine and positive inotrope that acts primarily as a beta$_1$ agonist. It causes an increase in CO/CI, while lowering SVR and increasing heart rate (Lemmer & Vlahakes, 2010b). It achieves these effects by increasing contractility and causing peripheral vasodilation (Khalpey et al., 2012). Dobutamine causes minimal amounts of alpha$_1$-receptor stimulation and a small amount of beta$_2$-receptor stimulation (Lemmer & Vlahakes, 2010b). This agent is useful when patients have low CO with high SVR or PVR and cannot tolerate vasodilators to decrease afterload. Dobutamine administration also results in enhanced coronary blood flow and decreased LV preload and afterload—more so than is noted with dopamine (Carmona et al., 2010). Following cardiac surgery, vasodilation is frequently present with LCOS. Dobutamine is the drug of choice in this situation (Hajjir, Fukushima, Osawa, Almeida, & Galas, 2011).

Patients with high pulmonary pressures, including those who have undergone mitral valve replacement, with or without a history of pulmonary hypertension, and with low heart rates may benefit more from dobutamine than from dopamine. This preference arises because dobutamine administration is associated with a decrease in PAP, LV stroke work index, CI, PAOP, and SVR (Carmona et al., 2010).

DOSAGE

The onset of action of dobutamine is rapid, and it is rapidly cleared (2–3 minutes) when discontinued, allowing for rapid titration of the drug. The dose is 2–20 mcg/kg/min, and doses as high as 40 mcg/kg/min have been reported (Yancy et al., 2013).

SIDE EFFECTS

While administering dobutamine, the ICU nurse should observe for hypotension, ventricular dysrhythmias, nausea, palpitations, shortness of breath, and myocardial ischemia (Aronson, 2009). Other reported side effects include angina, dyspnea, tachyarrhythmias (increase in heart rate 5–15 beats/minute), hypertension (increase in SBP 1–20 mmHg), and headache (Aronson, 2009). Of note, dobutamine is less likely to cause dysrhythmias than other positive inotropic agents. As with other catecholamines, mild hypokalemia may develop.

NURSING IMPLICATIONS

Like other agents in this category, dobutamine should not be given to hypovolemic patients. Monitoring of blood pressure, heart rate, PAP, PAOP, CVP, CO, SVR, and urinary output should be performed on an ongoing basis to determine the drug's efficacy and the patient's tolerance of therapy. Evaluation of the patient's ECG and electrolyte status should also be performed on a regular basis.

Phosphodiesterase Inhibitors

Another category of medications that may be used to treat low CO after cardiac surgery comprises the phosphodiesterase (PDE) inhibitors. Two direct phosphodiesterase inhibitors—inamrinone (formerly amrinone, Inocor®) and milrinone (Primacor®)—are especially well known agents. Inamrinone is no longer commercially available in the United States.

Milrinone
HEMODYNAMIC EFFECTS AND INDICATIONS
Milrinone is a positive inotrope with vasodilator properties. Its administration will cause a decrease in SVR and PVR, making it an ideal agent for patients with right ventricular (RV) failure. Milrinone also decreases coronary vascular resistance and, therefore, has a highly favorable effect on myocardial oxygen consumption (Yancy et al., 2013).

Milrinone enhances CO by directly inhibiting phosphodiesterase from metabolizing cyclic adenosine monophosphate (AMP) in myocardial cells. An increase in cyclic AMP causes an increase in the amount of calcium that moves into cells through the ion channels, thereby resulting in a more forceful contraction (inotropic effect).

Milrinone also produces venous and arterial vasodilation, and decreases SVR, PVR, and LV preload (PAOP), while minimally affecting myocardial oxygen demand (Bojar, 2011). All of these actions contribute to an improvement in CO/CI. The drug has little effect on heart rate, however (Bojar, 2011). It also produces vasodilation in vascular smooth muscle by decreasing intracellular calcium concentration. This effect causes relaxation of the vasculature and ventricles, thereby increasing SV and CO/CI and lowering afterload. In addition, milrinone promotes myocardial relaxation and improves coronary and mesenteric blood flow (Bangash, Kong, & Pearse, 2012).

Milrinone is indicated for the management of ventricular failure in the postoperative cardiac surgery patient (Katz, 2007). Because of its vasodilator properties, it is a valuable option in the management of patients with pulmonary vasoconstriction and RV dysfunction (Bangash et al., 2012).

DOSAGE
A loading dose of 50 mcg/kg of milrinone may be given over 10 minutes but is no longer recommended by heart failure guidelines. It should be administered via continuous infusion at a rate of 0.375–0.75 mcg/kg/min (Yancy et al., 2013). Milrinone has a rapid onset of action, and a half-life of 2–3 hours following titration or discontinuation (Gorodeski et al., 2009). The half-life is longer than that for dobutamine, making milrinone more challenging to titrate (Gorodeski et al., 2009).

SIDE EFFECTS
Ventricular tachycardia or supraventricular tachycardia (SVT) may occur when milrinone is given, owing to the drug's proarrhythmic properties. Hypotension should be anticipated related to the vasodilatory properties of milrinone (Yancy et al., 2013).

NURSING IMPLICATIONS
Patients receiving milrinone may require concomitant administration of an adrenergic agonist to counteract the profound vasodilation that occurs (Bojar, 2011). Aggressive replacement of potassium and magnesium are recommended as well, because the dysrhythmias are more likely to occur when an electrolyte imbalance is present. Patients receiving milrinone should also be observed for hypotension during therapy. Patient improvement may be reflected by increased CO, decreased PAOP, and favorable changes in clinical indices. See **Table 12-3** and **Box 12-1** for a summary of medications used to treat LCOS and hypotension following cardiac surgery.

Table 12-3   Select Agents Used to Manage Postoperative Low Cardiac Output and Hypotension and Hemodynamic Effects

Agent	Dose	Mechanism of Action	Hemodynamic Effects
Adrenergic Agonists			
Epinephrine (Adrenaline®)	0.008–0.06 mcg/kg/ min by continuous IV infusion	Stimulation of β_1 receptors	Increased contractility and stroke volume, and cardiac stimulation
	0.5–4.0 mcg/min by continuous IV infusion		Increased heart rate
	Less than 0.02 mcg/kg/ min by continuous IV infusion	Stimulation of β_2 receptors	Vasodilation and relaxation of the bronchial smooth muscle
	Greater than 2 mcg/min by continuous IV infusion	Stimulation of α_1 receptors	Vasoconstriction; increased SVR
Norepinephrine (Levophed®)	2–20 mcg/min or 0.01–3 mcg/kg/min by continuous IV infusion	Stimulation of α_1 receptors	Vasoconstriction; increased SVR; decreased cardiac output; increase or decrease in heart rate
		Stimulation of β_1 receptors	Increased inotropic effects and cardiac stimulation
Dopamine (Intropin®)	0.5–3.0 mcg/kg/min	Stimulation of dopaminergic receptors	Renal vasodilation
	4–10 mcg/kg/min by continuous IV infusion	Stimulation of β_1 receptors	Increased heart rate, blood pressure, contractility, and cardiac output
	Greater than 10 mcg/kg/ min	Stimulation of α_1 receptors	Vasoconstriction; increased SVR
	Less than 8 mcg/kg/min by continuous IV infusion	Stimulation of D_1 and D_2 receptors	Vasodilation
Dobutamine (Dobutrex®)	2–20 mcg/kg/min by continuous IV infusion	Stimulation of β_1 receptors (increased contractility) and peripheral vasodilation	Increased CO/CI, and heart rate; decreased SVR and PAOP (more so than dopamine), PAP, left ventricular stroke work index, enhanced coronary blood flow
		Minimal amounts of α_1 stimulation	Vasoconstriction

Table 12-3   Select Agents Used to Manage Postoperative Low Cardiac Output and Hypotension and Hemodynamic Effects (*Continued*)

		Small amount of β_2 receptor stimulation	Relaxation of the bronchial smooth muscle
Phenylephrine (Neosynephrine®)	100–200 mcg/min OR 0.4–9.1 mcg/kg/min by continuous IV infusion	Activation of α_1 receptors	Vasoconstriction; increased SVR; decreased CO; increase or decrease in heart rate
Vasopressin (antidiuretic hormone)	0.01–0.1 unit/min by continuous IV infusion	Stimulates V1 receptors	Contraction of vascular smooth muscle, which causes vasoconstriction of the capillaries and small arterioles and can increase mean arterial pressure
Phosphodiesterase (PDE) Inhibitors			
Inamrinone (Inocor®)	Loading dose: 0.75 mg/kg administered over 2–3 min Maintenance: 10–30 mcg/kg/min by continuous infusion Additional loading doses at 0.75 mg/kg may be administered. Total daily dose should not exceed 10 mg/kg/day.	PDE inhibitor; venous and arterial vasodilation; vasodilation in vascular smooth muscle by decreasing intracellular calcium concentration.	Increased CO/CI and SV; decreased SVR, PVR, and PAOP; promotes myocardial relaxation and improves coronary skeletal muscle, and mesenteric blood flow
Milrinone (Primacor®)	Maintenance dose: 0.125–0.75 mcg/kg/min by continuous infusion	PDE inhibitor; positive inotrope and vasodilator	Increased CO/CI and SV; decreased SVR, PVR, and PAOP; promotes myocardial relaxation and improves coronary skeletal muscle, and mesenteric blood flow
Other agent			
Methylene blue (Urolene Blue®)	1–2 mg/kg, administered as a slow IV push	Inhibitor of nitric oxide	Vasodilation

CO/CI, cardiac output/cardiac index; IV, intravenous; PAOP, pulmonary artery occlusive pressure; PAP, pulmonary artery pressure; PDE, phosphodiesterase; PVR, pulmonary vascular resistance; SV, stroke volume; SVR, systemic vascular resistance.

Sources: Data from Alexander, E. (2014). Pharmacology. In S. Burns (Ed.), *AACN essentials of progressive care nursing* (3rd ed., pp. 151–180). New York, NY: McGraw-Hill; Bojar, R. (2011). Cardiovascular management. In R. Bojar (Ed.), *Manual of perioperative care in adult cardiac surgery* (5th ed., pp. 437–580). Hoboken, NJ: Blackwell; McAuley, D. (2014a). *Vasopressors and inotropes*. Retrieved from http://www.globalrph.com/icu-agents.htm; Yancy, C. W., Jessup, M., Bozkurt, B., Butler, J., Casey Jr., D. E., Drazner, M. A., . . . Wilkoff, B. L. (2013). ACCF/AHA guideline for the management of heart failure: A report of the American College of Cardiology Foundation/American Heart Association Task Force on Practice Guidelines. *Circulation, 128*(16), e240–e327.

Box 12-1   Vasoactive Agents Used to Manage Postoperative Low Cardiac Output and Hypotension and Hemodynamic Effects

Agent	MAP	PAP	PAOP	CO/CI	SVR	PVR
Epinephrine	+	+/–	+/–	+	+/–	+/–
Norepinephrine	++	++	++	+	++	++
Dopamine	+/–	+/–	+/–	+	+/–	+/–
Dobutamine	+/–	–	–	+	–	–
Phenylephrine	++	~	+	~	++	++
Vasopressin	++	–	~	~	++	–/~
Inamrinone	–	–	–	+	–	–
Milrinone	–	–	–	+	–	–
Methylene blue	+	+	~	~	+	+

CI, cardiac index; CO, cardiac output; MAP, mean arterial pressure; PAOP, pulmonary artery occlusive pressure; PAP, pulmonary artery pressure; PVR, pulmonary vascular resistance; SVR, systemic vascular resistance.

+, increase; –, decrease; ~, no change

Sources: Data from Alexander, E. (2014). Pharmacology. In S. Burns (Ed.), *AACN essentials of progressive care nursing* (3rd ed., pp. 151–180). New York, NY: McGraw-Hill; Bojar, R. (2011). Cardiovascular management. In R. Bojar (Ed.), *Manual of perioperative care in adult cardiac surgery* (5th ed., 437–580); Hoboken, NJ: Blackwell; McAuley (2014a) Vasopressors and inotropes. Retrieved from http://www.globalrph.com/icu-agents.htm

Other Agents Used to Control Postoperative Hypotension

Methylene Blue (Urolene Blue®)

HEMODYNAMIC EFFECTS AND INDICATIONS
Methylene blue is an inhibitor of nitric oxide, which is released in large quantities in patients following CPB. Nitric oxide produces profound vasodilation and vasoplegia (hypotension with normal or high CO, low CVP, low PAOP, and low peripheral vascular resistance) (Skuza et al., 2009). Methylene blue is not U.S. Food and Drug Administration (FDA) approved for the indication but is frequently used in the treatment of vasodilatory shock or vasoplegia syndrome in the immediate postoperative CPB period (Lenglet, Mach, & Montecucco, 2011).

DOSAGE
The dosage of methylene blue is most commonly 2 mg/kg over 20–30 minutes with doses in the range of 0.5–3 mg/kg reported (Lenglet et al., 2011).

SIDE EFFECTS
The two main side effects of methylene blue administration are hypertension and a brief period of factitious low oxygen saturation on pulse oximetry (Lenglet et al., 2011). Other reported side effects include hypertension, hypotension, abdominal pain, dizziness, headache, confusion, nausea, vomiting, and diarrhea. Serious adverse events reported include cardiac dysrhythmias, malignant hyperthermia, and methemoglobinemia (Lenglet et al., 2011).

NURSING IMPLICATIONS
Following administration of methylene blue, the ICU nurse should observe for hypertension, urine discoloration, and transiently low oxygen saturation on pulse oximetry. The (false) decreased oxygenation saturation on pulse oximetry is short lived, lasting less than 10 minutes and results from interference with light absorption (Katz, 2007). If the patient's oxygen saturation is in question during this time, evaluation with an arterial

blood gas should be performed (Hariharan, Sood, Choudhery, Garg, & Haur, 2011). The ICU nurse should anticipate immediate increases in SVR and MAP and the need to significantly lower the infusion rate of norepinephrine. The ICU nurse should also monitor methemoglobin levels, complete blood count results, and blood pressure during administration of methylene blue. Caution should be exercised when this agent is administered to patients with renal impairment or G6PD deficiency (Lenglet et al., 2011).

Dexamethasone (Decadron®)

Despite supportive data, and possibly because the data are inconsistent (Murphy, Whitlock, Gutsche, & Augoustides, 2013), the routine use of steroids remains controversial in cardiac surgery patients. Their mechanism of action and the pathophysiologic changes that occur during cardiac surgery, which can result in adrenal insufficiency, have been cited as justifications for their administration in this scenario.

Any postoperative cardiac surgery patient exhibiting protracted vasodilatory shock should be suspected of having adrenal insufficiency. In cardiac surgery patients with physiologic stress, a low or normal cortisol level can be assumed to be associated with adrenal insufficiency (Krüger & Ludman, 2014). Cortisol plays a vital role in regulating blood pressure by increasing the sensitivity of the vasculature to endogenous epinephrine and norepinephrine. In the absence of normal cortisol levels, widespread vasodilation occurs secondary to the effects of pro-inflammatory mediators.

MECHANISM OF ACTION

Steroids decrease inflammation by suppressing neutrophil migration, decreasing production of pro-inflammatory mediators, and reversing the increase in capillary permeability. In patients with adrenal insufficiency, their mineralocorticoid effects can promote sodium and water retention (Merck Manual, 2014).

INDICATIONS

Corticosteroids are used in cardiac surgery cases involving persistent postoperative hemodynamic instability associated with a CPB-induced inflammatory response. They are additionally used in patients with known preoperative adrenal insufficiency (e.g., those on preoperative chronic steroid therapy).

Hydrocortisone (Solu-Cortef®)

INDICATIONS

Hydrocortisone is used in cases involving postoperative hemodynamic instability associated with a CPB-induced inflammatory response.

DOSAGE

The dosage of hydrocortisone is based on the indication. For acute adrenal insufficiency, the recommended dose is an initial 100 mg IV bolus, then 200–300 mg/day. Common doses including 100 mg every 8 hours or 50 mg every 6 hours. Alternatively, the total daily dose may be administered as a continuous infusion. Doses should be gradually tapered down over 3–7 days depending on patient response (Merck Manual, 2014). In patients receiving chronic preoperative steroids, patients should be tapered to their preoperative regimen.

SIDE EFFECTS

Side effects that are reported as being related to administration of hydrocortisone include insomnia, hyperglycemia, and delirium. Potentially serious adverse events include, but are not limited to, hypertension, edema, headache, seizure, mood swings, bruising, hypokalemia, Cushing's syndrome, sodium and water retention, abdominal distention, stress ulcer, and immunosuppression (Merck Manual, 2014).

NURSING IMPLICATIONS

Withdrawal and discontinuation of hydrocortisone should be done slowly, with gradual tapering of the dose (Merck Manual, 2014).

AGENTS USED TO PREVENT OR CONTROL POSTOPERATIVE DYSRHYTHMIAS

As discussed in Chapter 15, postoperative dysrhythmias are common in cardiac surgery patients. Several potential etiologic factors have been identified, including preexisting cardiac conditions (e.g., pericarditis); infarction, ischemia, or enlargement; respiratory complications; electrolyte imbalance (e.g., hypokalemia, hyperkalemia, hypomagnesemia); surgical trauma (intraoperative injury to the atrium, inadequate cardioprotection during CPB); hypothermia; hyperadrenergic state; acid–base imbalance; anxiety; and pain (Maesen, Nijs, Maessen, Allessie, & Schotten, 2012; Peretto, Durante, Limite, & Cianflone, 2014). Prior to intervening with pharmacotherapy, any underlying causes should be treated. Atrial and ventricular dysrhythmias, including bradyarrhythmias and tachyarrhythmias, may be experienced by cardiac surgery patients.

The most common antiarrhythmic medications used in the immediate postoperative phase are categorized as Class I, II, III, or IV agents. Class I agents are sodium channel blockers and include quinidine (Quinaglute®), procainamide (Pronestyl®), disopyramide (Norpace®), lidocaine (Xylocaine®), propafenone (Rythmol®), and flecainide (Tambocor®). Class II agents are beta blockers and include metoprolol (Lopressor®, Toprol®) and carvedilol (Coreg®). Class III agents delay repolarization and include amiodarone (Cordarone®) and ibutilide (Corvert®). Class IV agents include the calcium channel blockers diltiazem (Cardizem®) and verapamil (Calan®) (see **Box 12-2**). The agents used most often for postoperative cardiac surgery patients are discussed here and are summarized in **Table 12-4**.

Box 12-2   Categories of Antiarrhythmic Therapy

Category	Mechanism of Action
Class I	Sodium channel blockers
Class II	Beta blockers
Class III	Delays repolarization; prolongs action potential by affecting potassium channels
Class IV	Calcium channel blockers

Agents Used to Manage Atrial Dysrhythmias

As noted in Chapter 15, AF is a common dysrhythmia that may occur in postoperative cardiac surgery patients. Its peak onset is 2–4 days following surgery (Helgadottir, Sigurdsson, Ingvarsdottir, Arnar, & Gudbjartsson, 2012; Peretto et al., 2014), with a small percentage of patients developing AF after 6 days (Maesen et al., 2012). Given that most patients remain in the ICU for 24 hours or less, AF may not appear until after the patient leaves the ICU.

A wide array of medications is used to treat atrial dysrhythmias after cardiac surgery. The particular medication selected will depend on the drug's mechanism of action, the suspected cause of the dysrhythmia, and the drug's side effect profile.

Prior to initiating treatment of AF, three criteria are considered. First, determination is made as to whether the patient is hemodynamically stable or unstable with the presence of AF. The ICU nurse can identify the presence of hemodynamic compromise by assessing for hypotension, altered mental status, presence of chest pain, shortness of breath, poor peripheral perfusion, decreased urinary output, signs of impaired CO, or increased preload (Khalpey et al., 2012).

Table 12-4   Agents Used to Manage Postoperative Dysrhythmias

Dysrhythmia	Agent	Dose	Mechanism of Action
Atrial Fibrillation	Metoprolol	**PO:** Initial dose of 25–50 mg, followed by additional doses of 25 mg until heart rate is less than 100 beats/min. **IV:** 5–15 mg (usually 5 mg) over 2.5 minutes. Additional doses may be given at 7.5-minute intervals.	Class II, cardioselective beta blocker
	Carvedilol	**PO:** 6.25 mg BID or 3.125 mg BID in patients with heart failure. Titrated to a maximum dose of 25 mg PO BID.	Class II, non-selective beta blocker, alpha blocker
	Amiodarone	**IV:** 150 mg given over 10–15 minutes, followed by a 24-hour infusion given at a rate of 1 mg/min for the first 6 hours and at a rate of 0.5 mg/min for the next 18 hours, if required.	Class III but possesses properties in all four categories of agents. Blocks potassium channels, which prolongs the duration of the action potential and decreases membrane excitability. Slows heart rate by depressing SA node. Increases refractoriness of AV node. Decreases impulse conduction by indirectly blocking sodium channels, and blocking beta adrenergic receptors. Increases atrial and ventricular refractoriness. Inhibits alpha-adrenergic receptors.
	Ibutilide	**IV:** For patients who weigh ≥ 60 kg: 1 mg over 10 min. For patients who weigh < 60 kg: 0.01 mg/kg over 10 min. A second dose of equal strength may be administered over 10 min if conversion does not take place with initial dose.	Class III antiarrhythmic
	Diltiazem	**IV:** Initial bolus: 0.25 mg/kg over 5–10 min. Subsequent bolus: 0.35 mg/kg over 5–10 min after 15 minutes if needed.	Class IV. Blocks calcium ion influx during depolarization of cardiac and vascular smooth muscle.

(Continued)

Table 12-4   Agents Used to Manage Postoperative Dysrhythmias (*Continued*)

		Maintenance infusion: 5–15 mg/hr.	Decreases vascular resistance and causes relaxation of the vascular smooth muscle, resulting in a decrease in blood pressure. Negative inotropic effect.
	Digoxin	**IV or PO**: Total loading dose: 0.5–1 mg, given as ½ total dose initially, then ¼ total dose given at intervals of 6–8 hours in 2 follow-up doses. **PO maintenance dose**: 0.125–0.375 mg daily. **IV maintenance dose**: 0.125–0.25 mg daily.	May control ventricular rate. Slows conduction at the AV node and increases refractory period. Positive inotrope.
	Adenosine	**IV Initial dose**: 6 mg rapid IV push followed by 20 mL normal saline. **Subsequent IV doses**: 12 mg IV push followed by 20 mL normal saline. Two subsequent doses may be given.	Transient depression of LV function. Slows SA node impulse formation. Slows conduction through the AV node. Can interrupt reentry pathways through the AV node. Coronary vasodilation.
Ventricular Dysrhythmias	Amiodarone	**VF, pulseless VT initial bolus**: 300 mg IV push. A maximum of 2.2 g may be given in 24 hrs. **Continuous infusion**: 1 mg/min for the first 6 hrs and at a rate of 0.5 mg/min for the next 18 hrs, if required.	See description in AF.
	Lidocaine	**VF, pulseless VT initial bolus**: 1–1.5 mg/kg. **Subsequent bolus doses**: 0.5–0.75 mg/kg every 5–10 min. **Continuous infusion**: 1–4 mg/min. Maximum dose is 3 mg/kg in 24 hrs.	Class I antiarrhythmic agent.
	Sotalol	**PO**: 80 mg BID. If necessary, may increase dose to 240–320 mg/day.	Classes II and III; non-cardioselective beta blocker

AF, atrial fibrillation; AV, atrioventricular; BID, two times per day; CPB, cardiopulmonary bypass; IV, intravenous; PO, by mouth; LV, left ventricular; VF, ventricular fibrillation; VT, ventricular tachycardia.

Sources: Data from Alexander, E. (2014). Pharmacology. In S. Burns (Ed.), *AACN essentials of progressive care nursing* (3rd ed., pp. 151–180). New York, NY: McGraw-Hill; Bojar, R. (2011). Cardiovascular management. In R. Bojar (Ed.), *Manual of perioperative care in adult cardiac surgery* (5th ed., 437–580). Hoboken, NJ: Blackwell; Sinz, E., Navarro, K., & Soderberg, E. S. (Eds.). (2010). *Advanced cardiovascular life support provider manual*. Dallas, TX: American Heart Association.

Next, precipitating factors should be identified. These conditions may include ischemia, increased sympathetic tone, electrolyte or acid–base imbalance, or pulmonary disorders (Khalpey et al., 2012).

Lastly, the goal of therapy needs to be decided. Therapy can be aimed at restoring normal sinus rhythm (rhythm control) or at controlling the rate of AF (rate control). The ultimate goal is hemodynamic stability (Helgadottir et al., 2012; Maesen et al., 2012; Peretto et al., 2014). Agents that may be used to control rate include beta blockers or calcium channel blockers. Refer to Chapter 15 for details on each of the agents used to control postoperative cardiac surgery dysrhythmias.

Agents to Treat Electrolyte Imbalances

Correcting electrolyte imbalances is paramount in preventing and correcting all dysrhythmias. The goal of treatment is to lower the heart rate, thereby reducing the workload on the heart and promoting conversion back to sinus rhythm as soon as possible. As described in Chapter 17, numerous factors related to cardiac surgery put the patient at risk for developing postoperative acid–base and electrolyte disturbances. These factors include anesthesia, induced hypothermia, physiologic effects of CPB techniques, shock resulting in acute kidney injury, cardioplegia, rapid fluid and electrolyte shifts across fluid compartments following CPB, stress associated with surgery, intraoperative volume repletion, hemodilution, and the rewarming process that follows hypothermia (Khalpey et al., 2012). An in-depth discussion of the management of the common electrolyte imbalances experienced by postoperative cardiac surgery patients appears in Chapter 17.

OTHER AGENTS THAT MAY BE REQUIRED IN POSTOPERATIVE CARDIAC SURGERY PATIENTS

Naloxone (Narcan®)

Mechanism of Action

Naloxone is an opioid antagonist that effectively blocks the effects of opioids that have been administered. It has the greatest affinity for the mu receptor but competes for the mu, kappa, and sigma opiate receptor sites in the central nervous system (Butterworth, Mackey, & Wasnick, 2013).

Indications

Naloxone may be used in patients with hypoventilation following opioid analgesic administration.

Dosage

For reversal of opioid-induced respiratory depression, the dose is 0.4–2 mg IV. It may be repeated every 2–3 minutes as needed until the desired effect is achieved (Butterworth et al., 2013).

Side Effects

Side effects associated with naloxone are rare but include cardiac dysrhythmias, tachycardia, hypertension, hypotension, VF, pulmonary edema, and hepatotoxicity (Butterworth et al., 2013). Additionally, in patients with opioid dependence, it can precipitate acute withdrawal symptoms.

Nursing Implications

Care should be taken to closely monitor for continued hypoventilation because naloxone's duration is much shorter than many opioids. The dose should be titrated to patient effect. The ICU nurse should monitor blood pressure, heart rate, and respiratory rate following administration of naloxone. In addition, a decline in opioid medication effects, including worsening pain and possible withdrawal symptoms, should be anticipated.

PROPHYLACTIC ANTIBIOTICS

Patients who undergo CPB are at an increased risk of postoperative infection if they do not receive prophylactic antibiotic therapy. Administration of prophylactic antibiotics preoperatively and continuing for 24 hours postoperatively significantly decreases postoperative infection rates. The incidence of endotoxemia following CPB has been reported as high as 100% (Klein, Briet, Nisenbaum, Romaschin, & Mazar, 2011).

Cardiopulmonary bypass causes a number of physiologic consequences that suggest that stopping antibiotics may not be advisable. Specifically, CPB compromises humeral immunologic defenses, decreases phagocytosis, and activates white blood cells. Further, the length of the procedure puts the patient at increased risk for infection (Edwards, Engelman, Houck, Shahian, & Bridges, 2006).

Antibiotic selection is area and facility specific, typically based on the institutional biograms that are reported. However, first-generation cephalosporins, such as cefazolin, are generally recommended both preoperatively and for 24 hours postoperatively (Alexander, Solomkin, & Edwards, 2011).

AGENTS USED TO CONTROL POSTOPERATIVE BLEEDING

As discussed further in Chapter 13, the incidence of excessive postoperative bleeding (defined as loss of more than 500 mL of blood in the first postoperative hour) following cardiac surgery is reported to average up to 9.1%; the actual incidence is procedure dependent (Kubota et al., 2011). Postoperative bleeding may be surgical in origin, related to coagulation system dysfunction from exposure to CPB circuitry, or attributable to inadequate heparin reversal at the end of CPB (Ferraris et al., 2011). Depending on the etiology of the bleeding, pharmacologic intervention may be warranted.

Protamine Sulfate

Mechanism of Action

Protamine sulfate acts as a reversal agent for heparin that when combined with heparin forms an inactive salt. It can also partially reverse the activity of low-molecular-weight heparin, such as enoxaparin (Lovenox®) or dalteparin (Fragmin®) (van Veen et al., 2011).

Indications

In the intraoperative period, protamine sulfate is routinely given to reverse the effects of heparin administered during CPB. Postoperatively, protamine sulfate is indicated for patients with a postoperative coagulopathy due to inadequate heparin reversal (Schaub, Thomas, Fridh, & Schött, 2013).

Dosage

There are conflicting opinions about how to dose protamine. One way is based on the amount of heparin that needs to be reversed. In this case, the dosage is 1–1.5 mg of protamine sulfate for every 100 units of heparin that need to be reversed, up to a maximum dose of 50 mg. This dose should be administered no faster than 5 mg/min. The other method is based on heparin levels; it has been suggested that this method results in less postoperative bleeding (Lutjen & Arndt, 2012; O'Carroll-Kuehn & Meeran, 2007; Wang, Ma, & Zheng, 2013). Heparin is neutralized within 5 minutes of administration and the effect lasts for 2 hours (Katz, 2007).

Side Effects

Side effects of protamine sulfate administration include hypotension, wheezing, pulmonary artery hypertension (from pulmonary vasoconstriction secondary to a non-immunologic reaction), bradycardia, flushing, decreased myocardial contractility, cardiac arrest from VF, urticaria, angioedema, platelet dysfunction, and noncardiogenic pulmonary edema (Schaub et al., 2013).

A protamine reaction may manifest in any of several ways. If this medication is administered too quickly, a histamine reaction can occur. Hypotension develops as a result of histamine release, with resultant decreases in SVR and PVR. These effects can be reversed with administration of an alpha-receptor agonist.

A Type I reaction is either an anaphylactic or anaphylactoid reaction with associated hypotension, tachycardia, bronchospasm, flushing, and pulmonary edema. This reaction is often related to immunoglobulin E (IgE), causing release of histamine, leukotrienes, and kinins. The release of these substances results in capillary leak, hypotension, and pulmonary edema. Type I reactions may occur within the first 10–20 minutes (or more) following administration of protamine.

Protamine can also cause catastrophic pulmonary vasoconstriction, with associated increases in PAP, hypotension (secondary to peripheral vasodilation), left atrial depression, RV dilation, and myocardial depression. This kind of reaction is hypothesized to result from activation of various mediators of the inflammatory response. Complement activation leads to leukocyte aggregation, which causes pulmonary edema; the arachidonic acid pathway stimulates production of thromboxane, which causes constriction of pulmonary vasculature. The latter effect subsides in approximately 10 minutes (Nel & Eren, 2011).

Nursing Implications

Patients with allergies to fish have a high risk of the anaphylactoid type of protamine reaction because protamine sulfate is made of a protein found in fish sperm. In addition, caution should be used when administering protamine to men who are infertile or who have undergone a vasectomy, because antiprotamine antibodies may be present in these individuals (Bakchoul et al., 2013). There is also a 30- to 50-fold increased risk of protamine reaction in patients who take NPH insulin (Nel & Eren, 2011).

While a protamine reaction is more likely to occur in the OR, administration of protamine also may take place in the ICU if the patient experiences inadequate heparin reversal. If a protamine reaction occurs, in addition to administration of an alpha-receptor agonist to increase SVR, management strategies that may be implemented include administration of the following therapies: 500 mg IV calcium chloride to increase SVR and promote contractility, an inotropic agent (e.g., low-dose epinephrine, dobutamine, inamrinone, milrinone) to decrease PVR, a vasodilator (e.g., nitroglycerin, nitric oxide) to decrease preload and PVR, aminophylline to manage wheezing, and heparin to reverse a protamine reaction (Nel & Eren, 2011).

Desmopressin (DDAVP®)

Mechanism of Action

For patients with CPB-induced platelet dysfunction, desmopressin stimulates the release of von Willebrand factor, which increases levels of endogenous factor VIII, factor XII, prostacyclin, and tissue plasminogen activator, thereby decreasing bleeding time and activated partial thromboplastin time (Özgönenel, Rajpurkar, & Lusher, 2007).

Indications

Desmopressin may be used in patients with platelet dysfunction and bleeding secondary to CPB, and for prophylaxis of bleeding in patients with uremia (Ferraris et al., 2011).

Dosage

In cardiac surgery patients, a dose of 0.3 mcg/kg IV over 30 minutes is used. It is typically administered as a single dose, but dose may be repeated one additional time (Ferraris et al., 2011). Use should be limited to two doses total because of the lack of effect after two doses secondary to depletion of endogenous von Willebrand factor.

Side Effects

Desmopressin may cause hyponatremia, headache, or dizziness. While rare, thrombosis, including MI and cerebrovascular thrombosis, can occur (Özgönenel et al., 2007).

Nursing Implications

The ICU nurse should observe for improvement in bleeding including chest tube output, hemoglobin/hematocrit, and platelet counts. Urine output and serum sodium levels should also be monitored (Chapman, Blount, Davis, & Hooker, 2011).

Recombinant Activated Factor VII (NovoSeven®RT)

Mechanism of Action

Recombinant activated factor VII activates the extrinsic pathway of the coagulation system. This action stimulates the generation of thrombin and leads to a subsequently rapid correction of the patient's prothrombin time. Factor VII also expedites platelet activation and ultimate fibrin clot formation (Chapman et al., 2011).

Indications

As described further in Chapter 13, recombinant activated factor VII may prove helpful in achieving hemostasis in cardiac surgery patients with intractable bleeding (Ferraris et al., 2011). Factor VII is sometimes used following cardiac surgery in patients with coagulopathies who have already received standard therapies with blood and product

replacement (Ferraris et al., 2011). It should be used with extreme caution because it carries a thrombotic risk that could be detrimental to patients immediately following bypass grafting. In fact, some data suggest that because of an increased risk of stroke, factor VIIa is not recommended for routine use in cardiac surgery patients (Ponschab et al., 2011). In one study, patients who received factor VIIa had a two-fold increase in cryoprecipitate, fresh frozen plasma, packed red blood cells, and platelets. No statistically significant difference in venous thrombotic events, renal failure, or mortality were reported. However, there was a significantly higher reoperation rate for bleeding, increased incidence of pneumonia, ventilator hours, ICU hours, and rebleeding (Chapman et al., 2011).

Dosage

A wide range of activated factor VIIa doses has been used in the cardiac surgery population, with doses ranging from 40–80 mcg/kg, and 50 mcg/kg being a common dose (Gill et al., 2009). The smallest effective dose should be used due to thrombotic risk (Ferraris et al., 2011).

Side Effects

Serious adverse effects that have been reported with recombinant activated factor VII use include SVT and thrombotic events—including MI, arterial thromboembolism, bleeding, coagulopathies, venous thromboembolism, cerebral artery occlusion, cerebral ischemia, acute renal failure, and pulmonary embolism (Novo Nordisk A/S, 2014).

Nursing Implications

The ICU nurse must carefully observe for and anticipate thromboembolic complications when the patient receives recombinant activated factor VII (Chapman et al., 2011). Monitoring of coagulation profile results (i.e., prothrombin time, activated partial thromboplastin time, platelets, and international normalized ratio) and assessing for decreased postoperative bleeding are steps that should be taken to determine the efficacy of this treatment. Caution should be exercised when administering recombinant activated factor VII to patients with advanced atherosclerotic disease, coagulopathies, or septicemia because of the increased risk of thrombotic events associated with use of this medication.

Epsilon-Aminocaproic Acid (Amicar®)

Mechanism of Action

Epsilon-aminocaproic acid is an anti-fibrinolytic agent. It works by preventing plasminogen from binding to fibrin, thereby stopping the activation of plasmin and preventing clot breakdown (Network for the Advancement of Patient Blood Management, Haemostasis and Thrombosis, n.d.).

Indications

Aminocaproic acid is indicated for patients with postoperative bleeding that occurs secondary to fibrinolysis. It may be used to treat excessive bleeding following CPB, to decrease chest tube output, minimize blood transfusion requirements, and for fibrinolysis prophylaxis (Ferraris et al., 2011; Ortmann, Besser, & Klein, 2013).

Dosage

For prevention of bleeding, the dose of aminocaproic acid is 75–150 mg/kg over 20–30 minutes followed by 10–15 mg/kg/hr intraoperatively (Gravlee & Spiess, 2008). For postoperative bleeding, additional bolus doses of 100 mg/kg IV can be given.

Side Effects

Side effects of aminocaproic acid include thrombocytopenia, agranulocytosis, leukopenia, coagulation disorders, dysrhythmias, pulmonary embolism, decreased vision, seizures, delirium, dizziness, headache, malaise, hallucinations, intracranial hypertension, muscle weakness, elevated creatine phosphokinase, stroke, and abdominal pain (Martin et al., 2011; Ortmann et al., 2013). Reported serious adverse events include bradyarrhythmias, hypotension, renal failure, and rhabdomyolysis (Gravlee & Spiess, 2008).

Nursing Implications

Administration of aminocaproic acid is contraindicated in patients with disseminated intravascular coagulopathy. This medication should be used with caution in patients with cardiac, hepatic, or renal insufficiency. A definitive diagnosis of primary fibrinolysis must be made before administering aminocaproic acid.

Aminocaproic acid should not be administered rapidly. The ICU nurse should monitor the patient's complete blood count and coagulation profile prior to and after therapy. Evaluation for bradycardia, hypotension, dyspnea, and renal function tests should be conducted as well (Gravlee & Spiess, 2008). The ICU nurse should observe the patient for signs and symptoms of thrombosis, including pulmonary embolism or stroke, and arrange for appropriate testing as needed.

Other Coagulation Factors

In addition to fresh frozen plasma, factor eight inhibitor bypassing activity (FEIBA) and prothrombin complex concentrate (PCC) (Bebulin®, Profilnine®, Kcentra®) formulations have been used in "off-label" capacity in patients following cardiac surgery who have excessive bleeding. Prothrombin complex concentrate (human), as the name connotes, is a concentrate of coagulation factors that is derived from humans. Depending on the manufacturer, the product contains either three (factors II, IX, and X) or four factors (factors II, VII, IX, and X). It may also contain protein C and protein S, which are natural coagulation inhibitors. Most preparations contain a small amount of heparin (Seller & Peng, 2013). Further studies are needed on the use of these agents for cardiac surgery patients.

Mechanisms of Action

Factor eight inhibitor bypassing activity is a pro-coagulant (Maeda et al., 2013). Prothrombin complex concentrate increases plasma levels of factor IX and other factors in the concentrate to temporarily correct a coagulation defect caused by deficiency in these clotting factors (Medscape, 2014).

Indications

Factor eight inhibitor bypassing activity is used for hemophilia A (those with factor VIII deficiency). It has been used "off-label" in patients following cardiac surgery with CPB who have life-threatening coagulopathies or excessive bleeding (Rao et al., 2014; Song et al., 2014). Factor eight inhibitor bypassing activity is contraindicated in patients who underwent cardiac surgery under CPB and those procedures involving extracorporeal membrane oxygenation because of the high risk of thrombotic events, including a clotted hemothorax and distal extremity ischemia in one patient each (Balsam, Timek, & Pelletier, 2008).

Prothrombin complex concentrate is approved for use in patients with hemophilia B (those with factor IX deficiency) to prevent or control bleeding episodes. One formulation, Kcentra PCC, is indicated for adult patients with need for reversal of acute major

bleeding related to acquired factor deficiency induced by vitamin K antagonist (e.g., warfarin [Coumadin®]) therapy (McAuley, 2014b). Prothrombin complex concentrate is also used "off-label" to control excessive bleeding after CPB (Arnékian et al., 2012).

Dosage

Factor eight inhibitor bypassing activity is dosed based on body weight and is administered intravenously either with a syringe or with an infusion. Prothrombin complex concentrate is administered by intravenous infusion. The dose is based on different criteria, based on product. For example, Kcentra dosage is individualized based on the patient's current pre-dose international normalized ratio (INR) and body weight (McAuley, 2014b). Other product dosage is based on the number of factor IX international units (IU) required and is based on body weight. Dosage may also be based on the amount of postoperative bleeding (i.e., whether major bleeding exists or not). A 1% increase in Factor IX (0.01 IU)/IU administered/kg can be expected.

Side Effects

Factor eight inhibitor bypassing activity side effects include thrombotic events and myocardial infarction. In one study, there were three deaths—two from multiple organ failure and one from respiratory failure (Balsam et al., 2008). The most common side effects reported for PCC include disseminated intravascular coagulation, myocardial infarction, and thrombosis. The most serious adverse reactions of Kcentra were venous thromboembolic events (VTEs) (e.g., ischemic stroke, pulmonary embolism, deep vein thrombosis). There is a black box warning on Kcentra literature addressing VTEs. Common side effects of this agent include headache, nausea/

vomiting, hypotension, dizziness, urticaria, fever, chills, and anemia (McAuley, 2014b).

Nursing Implications

Because many of the PPC formulations contain heparin, their use is contraindicated in patients with heparin-induced thrombocytopenia. Other contraindications are product specific. The nurse should refer to the package insert or other facility-specific reference to obtain contraindications. Patient education should include the risk of blood-borne pathogens and Creutzfeldt-Jakob disease because this product is derived from humans; no cases have been reported to date. The nurse should also monitor for a hypersensitivity reaction (HSR), as this complication is a possibility. If an HSR occurs, the infusion should be stopped and facility-specific protocol for an HSR should be followed. Monitoring for intravascular clotting (e.g., disseminated intravascular coagulation) is essential. Upon suspicion of a thrombotic event, the infusion should be stopped and the patient should be evaluated.

SUMMARY

Patients who undergo cardiac surgery may develop several alterations in their hemodynamic profile and their cardiac rate and rhythm in the immediate postoperative period. Alterations in preload, afterload, and CO may be treated with a variety of agents, each of which has its own side effect profile. An understanding of the pharmacologic agents used in the immediate postoperative period is essential. Part of the role of the ICU nurse is to stay current with data regarding pharmacologic agents used in the management of postoperative cardiac surgery patients. Implementation of recommendations published in updates and Black Box Warnings issued by the FDA are essential to help ensure patient safety and optimal patient outcomes (see **Table 12-5**). The ICU nurse must be vigilant in managing the complexities associated with administration of these agents and use clinical judgment to help ensure optimal patient outcomes.

Table 12-5 Black Box Warnings Issued by the FDA	
Agent	**Black Box Warning**
Nitroprusside (Nipride®)	Medication must be diluted. Frequent blood pressure monitoring required due to hypotension. Cyanide toxicity can occur; therefore, monitoring of acid–base balance and venous oxygen concentration is needed.
Norepinephrine (Levophed®), dopamine Intropin®	Infiltration requires the use of phentolamine mesylate (Regitine®) as soon as possible to treat extravasation.
Phenylephrine (Neosynephrine®)	The complete contents of the package insert should be reviewed prior to prescribing.

Source: Data from U.S. Food and Drug Administration.

CASE STUDY

A 78-year-old patient has a history of class III angina, hypertension, ejection fraction 35%, and positive stress test with 3-vessel disease including proximal left anterior descending stenosis. The patient underwent on-pump coronary artery bypass grafting. The patient remains intubated and on mechanical ventilation. He developed postoperative hypertension and was placed on a nitroprusside infusion that was titrated to effect. After 24 hours, the blood pressure was improving and the nitroprusside infusion was discontinued. Arterial blood gas (ABG) results following the infusion being discontinued were as follows: pH 7.18, pCO_2 30, pO_2 70, HCO_3 15, base deficit 12. His color is usual for ethnicity.

Critical Thinking Questions

1. What is the etiology of this patient's ABG results?
2. Is his clinical picture consistent with his ABG results?
3. What treatment should be implemented?

Answers to Critical Thinking Questions

1. This patient developed cyanide toxicity from the nitroprusside infusion. He was at risk because of the length of time on the infusion as well as from being on CPB (hemolysis increases the risk of cyanide toxicity).

2. His clinical condition is consistent with his ABG results. Despite the metabolic acidosis, because of the cyanide toxicity, cells cannot utilize oxygen. Oxygen saturation levels remain high despite cellular hypoxia.

3. Increase the FiO_2 on the ventilator to 1.00, administer sodium bicarbonate because the pH is below 7.20, administer sodium thiosulfate 150–200 mg/kg over 15 minutes to facilitate removal of the cyanide, and consider insertion of a pulmonary artery catheter to measure mixed venous oxygen saturation.

SELF-ASSESSMENT QUESTIONS

1. Which of the following sets of hemodynamic parameters should the nurse anticipate as a result of hypertension following cardiac surgery?

SVR (dynes/sec/cm^{-5})	CI (L/min/m^2)	MvO$_2$
a. 2,900	2	85%
b. 1,200	5	55%
c. 1,000	1.8	50%
d. 3,000	4.5	90%

2. Which of the following ABG results should the nurse anticipate as a result of hypertension following cardiac surgery?

	pH	pCO$_2$	HCO$_3$
a.	7.28	35	19
b.	7.31	48	27
c.	7.48	45	29
d.	7.51	29	21

3. Which of the following sets of parameters indicates that a patient is at risk for increased afterload following cardiac surgery?

	CVP (mmHg)	pCO$_2$	Temp (°C/°F)
a.	1	50	35/95
b.	3	35	36/96.8
c.	8	33	37/98.6
d.	12	55	38/100.4

4. Which of the following should the nurse anticipate being used initially to manage hypertension in the immediate postoperative cardiac surgery patient?
   a. Nicardipine (Cardene®)
   b. Esmolol (Brevibloc®)
   c. Losartan (Cozaar®)
   d. Nitroprusside (Nipride®)

5. Which of the following sets of hemodynamic parameters indicates a patient will improve with inotropic support for the management of hypotension following cardiac surgery?

	CI (L/min/m²)	HR	SVR (dynes/sec/cm⁻⁵)
a.	1.8	90	1,400
b.	1.6	110	3,000
c.	3.0	80	1,100
d.	3.6	120	2,900

6. Which of the following sets of lab data should the nurse anticipate when caring for a patient on a norepinephrine infusion following cardiac surgery?

	Glucose	Lactate
a.	Elevated	Elevated
b.	Elevated	Decreased
c.	Decreased	Elevated
d.	Decreased	Decreased

7. Which of the following ABG results should the nurse anticipate when caring for a patient on an epinephrine infusion following cardiac surgery?

	pH	pCO_2	HCO_3
a.	7.30	50	26
b.	7.48	45	28
c.	7.50	30	22
d.	7.29	35	17

8. Your patient has undergone a mitral valve replacement and has postoperative hypotension and decreased cardiac output. Which of the following agents is preferred?
   a. Dopamine (Intropin®)
   b. Epinephrine (Adrenalin®)
   c. Dobutamine (Dobutrex®)
   d. Norepinephrine (Levophed®)

9. Your patient is receiving a milrinone (Primacor®) infusion following cardiac surgery. For which of the following should the nurse observe?
   a.

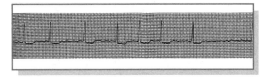

   b.

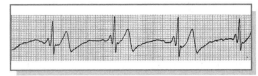

   c.

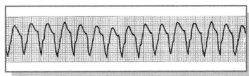

   d.

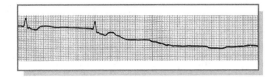

10. Your patient has protracted vasodilatory shock following cardiopulmonary bypass and is receiving dexamethasone (Decadron®). For which of the following should the nurse observe?
    a.

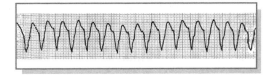

    b.

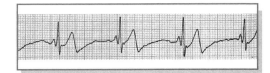

c.

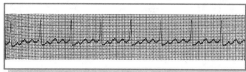

d.

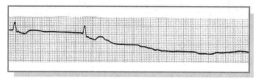

Answers to Self-Assessment Questions

1. a		6. a
2. a		7. d
3. a		8. c
4. a		9. c
5. a		10. b

Clinical Inquiry Box

Question: Is there a difference between dobutamine and levosimendan with regard to hepatic perfusion in patients with low cardiac output state after on-pump cardiac surgery?

Reference: Alvarez, J., Baluja, A., Selas, S., Oteru, P., Rial, M., Veira, S., . . . Rodriguez, J. (2013). A comparison of dobutamine and levosimendan on hepatic blood flow in patients with low cardiac output state after cardiac surgery. A randomized controlled study. *Anesthesia & Intensive Care, 41,* 719–727.

Objective: To determine if one inotrope over another is superior in improving hepatic perfusion with low cardiac output state following on-pump cardiac surgery.

Method: Randomized controlled trial of 25 patients. Patients either received levosimendan 12 mcg/kg over 15 minutes followed by an infusion of 0.2 mcg/kg/min for 24 hours or a dobutamine infusion at 7.5 mcg/kg/min for 24 hours.

Results: Systemic and hepatic hemodynamic parameters at 24 and 48 hours were better with levosimendan than dobutamine. The patients who received dobutamine had a cardiac index of 2.5 L/min/m² and a portal vein flow of 614 mL/min. Patients who received levosimendan had a cardiac index of 3.02 L/min/m² and a portal vein flow of 723 mL/min. Improvement in portal vein flow was greater in levosimendan than dobutamine at 48 hours (41% vs. 11% increment from baseline). There was a significant decrease in hepatic resistance following levosimendan but not dobutamine (a reduction of 6.5% vs. 0%).

Conclusion: Levosimendan is considered a selective liver vasodilator and can improve hepatic blood flow through the hepatic artery and portal venous system. Dobutamine can improve portal venous blood flow without vasodilation of the hepatic artery.

Note: Levosimendan, a positive inotrope and phosphodiesterase inhibitor, was granted fast-track status for Phase III clinical trials in the United States in early 2014. It is currently available in Europe.

REFERENCES

Alexander, E. (2014). Pharmacology. In S. Burns (Ed.), *AACN essentials of progressive care nursing* (3rd ed., pp. 151–180). New York, NY: McGraw-Hill.

Alexander, J. W., Solomkin, J. S., & Edwards, M. J. (2011). Updated recommendations for control of surgical site infections. *Annals of Surgery, 253*(6), 1082–1093.

Apostolakis, E. E., Baikoussis, N. G., Parissis, H., Siminelakis, S. N., & Papadopoulos, G. S. (2009). Left ventricular diastolic dysfunction of the cardiac surgery patient: A point of view for the cardiac surgeon and cardio-anesthesiologist. *Journal of Cardiovascular Surgery, 4,* 67. doi: 10.1186/1749-8090-4-67

Arnékian, V., Camous, J., Fattal, S., Rézaiguia-Delclaux, S., Nottin, R., & Stéphan, F. (2012). Use of prothrombin complex concentrate for excessive bleeding after cardiac surgery. *Interactive Cardiovascular and Thoracic Surgery, 15*(3), 382–389.

Aronson, J. K. (2009). Drugs used to treat hypertension, heart failure, and angina pectoris. In J. K. Aronson (Ed.), *Meyler's side effects of cardiovascular drugs* (pp. 1–196). Amsterdam, The Netherlands: Elsevier.

Aschenbrenner, D. S., & Venable, S. J. (2009). Drugs affecting blood pressure. In D. S. Aschenbrenner & S. J. Venable (Eds.), *Drug therapy in nursing* (3rd ed., pp. 493–534). Philadelphia, PA: Lippincott Williams & Wilkins.

Bakchoul, T., Zöllner, H., Amiral, J., Panzar, S., Selleng, S., Kohlmann, T., . . . Greinacher, A. (2013). Anti-protamine-heparin antibodies: Incidence, clinical reference and pathogenesis. *Blood, 121*(15). Retrieved from http://www.bloodjournal.org/content/121/15/2821?550-checked=true

Balsam, L. B., Timek, T. A., & Pelletier, M. P. (2008). Factor eight inhibitor bypassing activity (FEIBA) for refractory bleeding in cardiac surgery: Review of clinical outcomes. *Journal of Cardiac Surgery, 23*(6), 614–621.

Bangash, M. W., Kong, M.-L., & Pearse, R. M. (2012). Use of inotropes and vasopressor agents in critically ill patients. *British Journal of Pharmacology, 165*(7), 2015–2033.

Bojar, R. (2011). Cardiovascular management. In R. Bojar (Ed.), *Manual of perioperative care in adult cardiac surgery* (5th ed., 437–580). Hoboken, NJ: Blackwell.

Bush, T. G. (2010). Angina pectoris, myocardial infarction. In T. G. Bush (Ed.), *Clinically oriented pharmacology* (pp. 125–134). Retrieved from https://books.google.com/books?id=PaOhT_4zBL8C&printsec=frontcover&dq=Clinically+oriented+pharmacology&hl=en&sa=X&ei=WyiqVLjiIMegNsypgrgK&ved=0CB8Q6AEwAA#v=onepage&q=Clinically%20oriented%20pharmacology&f=false

Butterworth, J. F. (2013). Cardiovascular drugs. In J. F. Butterworth, F. A. Hansley, D. E., Jr., Martin, & G. P. Gravlee (Eds.), *A practical guide to cardiac anesthesia* (5th ed., pp. 23–88). Philadelphia, PA: Lippincott Williams & Wilkins.

Butterworth, J. F., Mackey, D. C., & Wasnick, J. D. (2013). Adjuncts to anesthesia. In J. F. Butterworth, D. C. Mackey, & J. D. Wasnick (Eds.), *Morgan & Mikhail's clinical anesthesiology* (5th ed., pp. 277–294). Philadelphia, PA: Lippincott Williams & Wilkins.

Cannon, C. M., Levy, P., Baumann, B. M., Borczuk, P., Chandra, A., Cline, D. M., . . . Peacock, W. F. (2013). Intravenous nicardipine and labetalol use in hypertensive patients with signs or symptoms suggestive of end-organ damage in the emergency department: A subgroup analysis of the CLUE trial. *British Medical Journal, 3*(3), ii.

Carmona, M. J. C., Martins, L. M., Vane, M. F., Longo, B. A., Doredes, L. S., & Malbouisson, L. M. S. (2010). Comparison of the effects of dobutamine and milrinone on hemodynamic parameters and oxygen supply in patients undergoing cardiac surgery with low cardiac output after anesthetic induction. *Revista Brasileira de Anesthesiologia, 60*(3), 237–246.

Chapman, A. J., Blount, A. L., Davis, A. T., & Hooker, R. L. (2011). Recombinant factor VIIa (NovoSeven RT) use in high-risk cardiac surgery. *European Journal of Cardio-Thoracic Surgery, 6,* 1314–1319.

Che, Q., Schreiber, M. J., & Rafey, M. A. (2009). Beta-blockers for hypertension: Are they going out of style? *Cleveland Clinical Journal of Medicine, 76*(9), 533–542.

Clark, M. A., Harvey, R. A., Finkel, R., Ray, J. A., & Whalen, K. (2012a). Anti-anginal drugs. In M. A. Clark, R. A. Harvey, R. Finkel, J. A. Ray, & K. Whalen (Eds.), *Pharmacology* (5th ed., pp. 224–226). Philadelphia, PA: Lippincott Williams & Wilkins.

Clark, M. A., Harvey, R. A., Finkel, R., Ray, J. A., & Whalen, K. (2012b). Antihypertensives. In M. A. Clark, R. A. Harvey, R. Finkel, J. A. Ray, & K. Whalen (Eds.), *Pharmacology* (5th ed., pp. 227–242). Philadelphia, PA: Lippincott Williams & Wilkins.

de Araujo, H. B. N., Fagundes, A. A. P., Leite, L. R., & Fonseca, G. T. (2010). Clevidipine for hypertensive emergency. *Revista Brasileira de Terapia Intensiva, 22*(1), 92–95.

Deeks, E. D., Keating, G. M., & Keam, S. J. (2009). Clevidipine: A review of its use in the management of acute hypertension. *American Medical Journal, 9*(2), 117–134.

Edwards, F. H., Engelman, R. M., Houck, P., Shahian, D. M., & Bridges, C. R. (2006). The

Society of Thoracic Surgeons Practice Guideline Series: Antibiotic prophylaxis in cardiac surgery, Part II: Antibiotic choice. *Annals of Thoracic Surgery, 81*, 397–404.

Fawzy, A., & Pool, J. L. (n.d.). *Part I: The physiology and function of the alpha-adrenergic nervous system.* Retrieved from http://www.medscape.org/viewarticle/440787

Ferraris, V. A., Brown, J. R., Despotis, G. J., Hammon, J. W., Reece, T. B., Saha, S. P., . . . Clough, E. R. (2011). 2011 Update to the Society of Thoracic Surgeons and the Society of Cardiovascular Anesthesiologists Blood Conservation Clinical Practice Guidelines. *Annals of Thoracic Surgery, 91*, 944–982.

Gahart, B. L., & Nazareno, A. R. (2013). *2013 intravenous medications: Patient handbook for nurses and health professionals* (29th ed., p. 504). St. Louis, MO: Elsevier Mosby.

Gill, R., Herbertson, M., Vuylsteke, A., Olsen, P. S., von Heymann, C., Mythen, M., . . . Schmidt, M. (2009). Safety and efficacy of recombinant activated factor VII: A randomized placebo-controlled trial in the setting of bleeding after cardiac surgery. *Circulation, 120*, 21–27.

Gorodeski, E. Z., Chu, E. C., Reese, J. R., Shishehbor, M. H., Hsich, E., & Starling, R. C. (2009). Prognosis on chronic dobutamine or milrinone infusions for Stage D heart failure. *Circulation, 2*, 320–324.

Gravlee, G. P., & Spiess, B. (2008). Pharmacologic prophylaxis for post-cardiopulmonary bypass bleeding. In G. P. Gravlee, R. F. Davis, A. H. Stammers, & R. M. Ungerleider (Eds.), *Cardiopulmonary bypass: Principles and practice* (3rd ed, pp. 522–542). Philadelphia, PA: Lippincott Williams & Wilkins.

Gupta, P. K., Gupta, H., & Khoynezhad, A. (2009). Hypertensive emergency in aortic dissection and thoracic aortic aneurysm—A review of management. *Pharmaceuticals, 2*, 66–76.

Hajjir, L. A., Fukushima, J. T., Osawa, E., Almeida, J. P., & Galas, F. R. B. G. (2011). Dobutamine administration in patients after cardiac surgery: Beneficial or harmful? *Critical Care, 15*, 444. Retrieved from http://ccforum.com/content/15/5/444

Hariharan, U., Sood, R., Choudhery, A., Garg, R., & Kaur, J. (2011). Oxygen desaturation following methylene blue injection: Not always spurious. *Saudi Journal of Anaesthesia, 5*(1), 113–114.

Helgadottir, S., Sigurdsson, M. I., Ingvarsdottir, I. L., Arnar, D. O., & Gudbjartsson, T. (2012). Atrial fibrillation following cardiac surgery: Risk analysis and long-term survival. *Journal of Cardiovascular Surgery, 7*(87), 1749–1753.

Hillis, D. L., Smith, P. K., Anderson, J. L., Bittl, J. A., Bridges, C. R., Byrne, J. G., . . . Winniford, M. D. (2011). 2011 ACCF/AHA guideline for coronary artery bypass graft surgery: A report of the American College of Cardiology Foundation/American Heart Association Task Force on practice guidelines. *Journal of the American College of Cardiology, 58*(24), 2584–2614.

Kaplan, N. M. (2014). *Major side effects of angiotensin-converting enzyme inhibitors and angiotensin II receptor blockers.* Retrieved from http://www.uptodate.com/contents/major-side-effects-of-angiotensin-converting-enzyme-inhibitors-and-angiotensin-ii-receptor-blockers

Katz, E. A. (2007). Pharmacologic management of the postoperative cardiac surgery patient. *Critical Care Nursing Clinics of North America, 19*(4), 487–496.

Khalpey, Z. I., Schmitto, J. D., & Rawn, J. D. (2012). Postoperative care of cardiac surgery patients. In L. H. Cohn (Ed.), *Cardiac surgery in the adult* (4th ed.). Retrieved from http://accesssurgery.mhmedical.com/content.aspx?bookid=476&Sectionid=39679028

Klabunde, R. C. (2011). Adrenergic and cholinergic receptors in the heart. *Cardiovascular physiology concepts* (2nd ed.). Philadelphia, PA: Lippincott Williams & Wilkins.

Klein, D. J., Briet, F., Nisenbaum, R., Romaschin, A. D., & Mazar, D. M. (2011). Endotoxemia related to cardiopulmonary bypass is associated with risk of infection after cardiac surgery: A prospective observational study. *Critical Care, 15*(1). Retrieved from http://ccforum.com/content/15/1/R69

Kouchoukos, N. T., Blackstone, E. H., Hanley, F. L., & Kirklin, J. K. (2013). Postoperative care. In N. T. Kouchoukos, E. H. Blackstone, F. L. Hanley, & J. K. Kirklin (Eds.), *Kirklin/Barratt-Boyes cardiac surgery* (4th ed., pp. 133–162). Philadelphia, PA: Elsevier.

Krüger, W., & Ludman, A. J. (2014). Shock. In W. Krüger & A. J. Ludman (Eds.), *Core knowledge in critical care medicine* (pp. 159–272). London: Springer.

Kubota, H., Miyata, H., Motomura, N., Ono, M., Takamoto, S., Haril, K., . . . Kyo, S. (2011). Deep sternal wound infection after cardiac surgery. *Journal of Cardiothoracic Surgery, 8*, 132. Retrieved from http://www.cardiothoracicsurgery.org/content/8/1/132

Lemmer, J. H., & Vlahakes, G. J. (2010a). Postoperative management. In J. H. Lemmer & G. J. Vlahakes (Eds.), *Handbook of patient care in cardiac surgery* (7th ed., pp. 81–135). Philadelphia, PA: Lippincott Williams & Wilkins.

Lemmer, J. H., & Vlahakes, G. J. (2010b). Postoperative complications involving the heart and lungs. In J. H. Lemmer & G. J. Vlahakes (Eds.), *Handbook of patient care in cardiac surgery* (7th ed., pp. 136–194). Philadelphia, PA: Lippincott Williams & Wilkins.

Lenglet, S., Mach, F., & Montecucco, F. (2011). Methylene blue: Potential use of an antique molecule in vasoplegic syndrome during cardiac surgery. *Expert Review of Cardiovascular Therapy, 9*(12), 1519–1525.

Levy, J. H., Tanaka, K. A., & Bailey, J. M. (2008). Cardiac surgical pharmacology. In L. H. Cohn (Ed.), *Cardiac surgery in the adult* (pp. 77–110). New York, NY: McGraw-Hill.

Leybell, I. (2014). *Cyanide toxicity*. Retrieved from http://emedicine.medscape.com/article/814287-clinical

Lutjen, D. L., & Arndt, K. L. (2012). Methylene blue to treat vasoplegia due to a severe protamine reaction: A case report. *American Association of Nurse Anesthetists Journal, 80*(3), 170–173.

Maeda, K., Asija, R., Hollander, S., Williams, G., Yeh, J., Rosenthal, D., . . . Reinhartz, O. (2013). Low dose factor eight inhibitor bypassing activity (FEIBA) for incessant bleeding in pediatric patients on mechanical circulatory support (MCS). *Journal of Heart and Lung Transplantation, 32*(4), S290.

Maesen, B., Nijs, J., Maessen, J., Allessie, M., & Schotten, U. (2012). Post-operative atrial fibrillation: A maze of mechanisms. *Eurospace, 14*(2), 159–174.

Mancini, M. C. (2014). *Aortic dissection medicine*. Retrieved from http://emedicine.medscape.com/article/2062452-medication #2

Martin, K., Knorr, J., Breuer, T., Gertler, R., Macquill, M., Lange, R., . . . Wiesner, G. (2011). Seizures after open heart surgery. Comparison of Σ-aminocaproic acid and tranexamic acid. *Journal of Cardiovascular and Vascular Anesthesia, 25*(1), 20–25.

McAuley, D. (2014a). *Vasopressors and inotropes*. Retrieved from http://www.globalrph.com/icu-agents.htm

McAuley, D. (2014b). *Kcentra prothrombin complex concentrate (Human)*. Retrieved from http://globalrph.com/drug_Kcentra.htm

Medscape. (2014). *Factor IX complex (Rx)*. Retrieved from http://reference.medscape.com/drug/bebulin-vh-profilnine-sd-factor-ix-complex-999858

Merck Manual. (2014). *Corticosteroids*. Retrieved from http://www.merckmanuals.com/vet/pharmacology/anti-inflammatory_agents/corticosteroids.html

Minczak, B. M. (2014). Cardiac procedures. In J. R. Roberts & J. R. Hedges (Eds.), *Clinical procedures in emergency medicine* (6th ed., pp. 213–227). Philadelphia, PA: Elsevier Saunders.

Murfin, D. (2011). Phenylephrine: In and out. *South African Journal of Anaesthesia & Analgesia, 12*(2), 200–201.

Murphy, G. S., Whitlock, R. P., Gutsche, J. T., & Augoustides, J. G. T. (2013). Steroids for adult cardiac surgery with cardiopulmonary bypass: Update on dose and key randomized trials. *Journal of Cardiothoracic and Vascular Anesthesia, 27*(5), 1053–1059.

Ndefo, U. A., Erowele, G. I., Ebiasah, R., & Green, W. (2010). Clevidipine: A new intravenous option for the management of acute hypertension. *American Journal of Public Health, 67*(5), 351–360.

Nel, L., & Eren, E. (2011). Perioperative anaphylaxis. *British Journal of Clinical Pharmacology, 71*(5), 647–658.

Network for the Advancement of Patient Blood Management, Haemostasis and Thrombosis. (n.d.). *Antifibrinolytics in open-heart surgery*. Retrieved from http://www.nataonline.com/np/419/antifibrinolytics-cardiac-surgery

Novo Nordisk A/S. (2014). *NovoSeven® RT*. Retrieved from http://www.novo-pi.com/novosevenrt.pdf

O'Carroll-Kuehn, B. U., & Meeran, H. (2007). Management of coagulation during cardiopulmonary bypass. *Continuing Education in Anaesthesia, Critical Care & Pain, 7*(6), 195–198.

Ortmann, E., Besser, M. W., & Klein, A. A. (2013). Antifibrinolytic agents in current anesthesia practice. *British Journal of Anaesthesia, 111*(4), 549–563.

Özgönenel, B., Rajpurkar, M., & Lusher, J. M. (2007). How do you treat bleeding disorders with desmopressin? *Postgraduate Medical Journal, 83*(97), 159–163.

Peretto, G., Durante, A., Limite, L. R., & Cianflone, D. (2014). Postoperative arrhythmias after cardiac surgery: Incidence, risk factors, and therapeutic management. *Cardiology Research and Practice, 2014,* 1–15.

Ponschab, M., Landoni, G., Biondi-Zoccai, G., Bignami, E., Frati, E., Nicolotti, D., . . . Zangrillio, A. (2011). Recombinant activated factor VII increases stroke in cardiac surgery: A meta-analysis. *Journal of Cardiothoracic and Vascular Anesthesia, 25*(5), 809–810.

Prometheus. (2013). *Trandate® (labetalol hydrochloride) product information.* Retrieved from http://www.prometheuslabs.com/Resources/PI/TrandateTab.pdf

Ranucci, M., DeBenedetti, D., Bianchini, C., Castelvecchio, S., Ballotta, A., Frigiola, A., . . . Menicanti, L. (2010). Effects of fenoldopam infusion in complex cardiac surgical operations: A prospective, randomized, double-blind, placebo-controlled study. *Minerva Anestesiologica, 76*(4), 249–259.

Rao, V. K., Lobato, R. L., Bartlett, B., Klanjac, M., Mora-Mangano, C. T., Soran, P. D., . . . van der Starre, P. J. (2014). Factor VIII inhibitor bypass activity and recombinant activated factor VII in cardiac surgery. *Journal of Cardiothoracic and Vascular Anesthesia, 28*(5), 1221–1226.

Redfors, B., Bragadottir, G., Sellgren, J., Sward, K., & Rickstein, S. (2010). Dopamine increases renal oxygenation: A clinical study in post-cardiac surgery patients. *Acta Anaesthesiologica Scandinavica, 54,* 183–190.

Rhoney, D., & Peacock, W. (2009). Intravenous therapy for hypertensive emergencies. *American Journal of Health-System Pharmacy, 66*(15), 1343–1352.

Rosas, M. M., Giocoechea-Turcott, E. W., Ortiz, P. L., Salazar, A., & Palma, B. A. (2012). Glycemic control in cardiac surgery. In C. Narin (Ed.), *Perioperative considerations in cardiac surgery.* Retrieved from http://cdn.intechopen.com/pdfs-wm/30207.pdf

Royal Flying Doctor Service. (2013). *Clinical manual. Part 2. Drug infusion guidelines* (p. 1). Retrieved from http://www.flyingdoctor.org.au/IgnitionSuite/uploads/docs/Part%202%20-%20Drug%20Infusion%20Guidelines%20June%202008%20Cover%20Bookmarked.pdf

Schaub, C., Thomas, O. D., Fridh, A., & Schött, U. (2013). Protamine dosage effects on complement activation and sonoclot coagulation analysis after cardiac surgery. *Herbert Open Access Journals, 1.* Retrieved from http://www.hoajonline.com/cardiovascsyst/2052-4358/1/1

Seller, A., & Peng, Y. G. (2013). Drug innovation update: Prothrombin complex concentrate use during cardiac surgery. *SCA Bulletin, 12*(7). Retrieved from http://www.scahq.org/sca3/newsletters/2013dec/drug-innovation-update.html

Sidebotham, D., & Gillham, M. (2007). Hemodynamic instability and resuscitation. In D. Sidebotham, A. McKee, M. Gillham, & J. Levy (Eds.), *Cardiothoracic critical care* (pp. 295–315). Philadelphia, PA: Butterworth-Heinemann.

Silvestry, F. E. (2014). *Postoperative complications among patients undergoing cardiac surgery.* Retrieved from http://www.uptodate.com/contents/postoperative-complications-among-patients-undergoing-cardiac-surgery

Singla, N., Warltier, D. C., Ghandi, S. D., Lumb, P. D., Sladen, R. N., Aronson, S., . . . Corwin, H. L. (2008). Treatment of acute postoperative hypertension in cardiac surgery patients: An efficacy study of clevidipine assessing its postoperative antihypertensive effect in cardiac surgery-2 (ESCAPE-2), a randomized, double-blind, placebo-controlled trial. *Anesthesia & Analgesia, 107*(1), 59–67.

Sinz, E., Navarro, K., & Soderberg, E. S. (Eds.). (2010). *Advanced cardiovascular life support provider manual.* Dallas, TX: American Heart Association.

Skuza, K., Chmielniak, S., Dzluk, W., Kucewicz, E., Pawlak, S., & Knapik, P. (2009). Methylene blue therapy for vasoplegia after cardiac surgery. *Anaesthesiology Intensive Therapy, 341*(3), 129–132.

Song, H. K., Tibayan, F. A., Kahl, E. A., Sera, V. A., Slater, M. S., Deloughery, T. G., . . . Scanlan, M. M. (2014). Safety and efficacy of prothrombin complex concentrates for the treatment of coagulopathy after cardiac surgery. *Journal of Thoracic and Cardiovascular Surgery, 147*(3), 1036–1040.

Soto-Ruiz, K. M., Peacock, W. F., & Varon, J. (2010). Perioperative hypertension: Diagnosis and treatment. *Netherlands Journal of Critical Care, 15*(3), 143–148.

Thoma, A. (2013). Pathophysiology and management of angiotensin-converting enzyme inhibitor-associated refractory hypotension during the perioperative period. *American Association of Nurse Anesthetists Journal, 81*(2), 133–140.

Tse, H.-F., Lip, G. Y., & Coats, A. J. S. (2011). Hypertension. In H.-F. Tse, G. Y. Lip, & A. J. S. Coats (Eds.), *Oxford desk reference: Cardiology* (p. 137). New York, NY: Oxford University Press.

Upadhye, S., & Schiff, K. (2012). Acute aortic dissection in the emergency department: Diagnostic challenges and evidence-based management. *Emergency Medical Clinics of North America, 30*(2), 307–327.

Van Veen, J. J., Maclean, R. M., Hampton, K. K., Laidlaw, S., Kitchen, S., Toth, P., . . . Makris, M. (2011). Protamine reversal of low molecular weight heparin: Clinically effective? *Blood Coagulation & Fibrinolysis, 12*(7), 565–570.

Walker, K. (2013). Aortic cross-clamp: Cardiovascular complications. In R. K. Modak (Ed.), *Anesthesiology key words review* (p. 59). Philadelphia, PA: Lippincott Williams & Wilkins.

Wang, J., Ma, H. P., & Zheng, H. (2013). Blood loss after cardiopulmonary bypass: Standard versus titrated protamine: A meta-analysis. *The Netherlands Journal of Medicine, 71*(3), 123–127.

Yancy, C. W., Jessup, M., Bozkurt, B., Butler, J., Casey, D. E., Jr., Drazner, M. A., . . . Wilkoff, B. L.; American College of Cardiology Foundation/American Heart Association Task Force on Practice Guidelines. (2013). ACCF/AHA guideline for the management of heart failure: A report of the American College of Cardiology Foundation/American Heart Association Task Force on Practice Guidelines. *Circulation, 128*(16), e240–e327.

Yimin, H., Xiaoyu, L., Yuping, H., Weiyan, L., & Ning, L. (2013). The effect of vasopressin on the hemodynamics in CABG patients. *Journal of Cardiothoracic Surgery, 16*(8), 49.

WEB RESOURCES

U.S. Food and Drug Administration: http://www.fda.gov/

Safety-related drug labeling changes: http://www.fda.gov/medwatch/safety.htm

FDA Safety News (recalls and safety alerts and preventing medical errors): http://www.accessdata.fda.gov/scripts/cdrh/cfdocs/psn/index.cfm

Adverse event reporting system (case reports): http://www.fda.gov/cder/aers/extract.htm

Herbal drug and supplement information: http://www.nlm.nih.gov/medlineplus/druginformation.html

Scientific Review of Alternative Medicine: http://www.sram.org/

Clinical drug trials (lists studies by drug intervention): http://www.clinicaltrials.gov

Chapter 13

Postoperative Complications of Cardiac Surgery and Nursing Interventions

Tamara S. Goda and Roberta Kaplow

INTRODUCTION

Coronary artery bypass grafting (CABG) and valve replacement procedures are among the most frequently performed surgical procedures, with more than 2 million operations being performed worldwide; more than 600,000 procedures are performed in the United States alone (Mao et al., 2013). Patients who are candidates for cardiac surgery often present with a number of comorbidities. Some of these comorbidities are directly related to the need for surgery, whereas others are attributable to advanced age and other noncardiac conditions. An extensive presurgical evaluation should always be performed, as discussed in Chapter 4. From these data and a thorough assessment of the patient's condition, management of the patient's complex problems may take place before, during, and following cardiac surgery.

Despite the trend toward cardiac surgery being performed on older persons and those with more complex health issues, the 30-day mortality associated with cardiac surgical procedures continues to decline. The overall mortality rate is now reported to be 1% to 5%. Patients having elective cardiac surgery who were considered to be low risk averaged a mortality rate of 1% (Silvestry, 2014). An important focus for the patient undergoing cardiac surgery is an assessment of cardiac risk. Calculation of risk potential

affords patients and their families insight into the risk of complications and possible mortality of the surgical procedure. It also heightens the healthcare team's awareness of the high-risk patient for whom more aggressive therapy may be warranted and alerts caregivers to the potential for postoperative complications. This chapter describes the most common postoperative complications associated with cardiac surgery and the intensive care unit (ICU) nursing management of these complications.

Once a patient has been deemed an acceptable candidate for cardiac surgery, a comprehensive preoperative evaluation must occur. The patient's history and presence of noncardiac comorbidities must be fully assessed to determine what, if any, perioperative complications should be factored into the patient's recovery. Additionally, numerous cardiac surgery risk models are available that can provide a patient with specific risk assessment, allowing for calculation and prediction of perioperative morbidity and mortality (Bojar, 2011). **Table 13-1** lists the most common risk factors that have been shown to have predictive value when determining postoperative complications and higher rates of mortality.

Complications of cardiac surgery have negative and variable effects on patient outcomes. Postoperative complications may occur secondary to patient comorbidities, and the

Table 13-1   Risk Factors for Postoperative Complications
Older age (older than 65 years)
BSA
Emergent need for procedure (vs. urgent need)
Reoperations
Recent smoking
Preexisting preoperative comorbidities: renal dysfunction (dialysis-dependent), COPD, diabetes, cerebrovascular disease, peripheral vascular disease, heart failure, acute myocardial infarction, pulmonary hypertension, hypertension, immunosuppressive therapy
CABG/valve surgery
Low ejection fraction
Pulmonary dysfunction
Preoperative presence of intra-aortic balloon pump
Cardiogenic shock
New-onset atrial fibrillation
Anemia

BSA, body surface area; CABG, coronary artery bypass grafting; COPD, chronic obstructive pulmonary disease.

Sources: Data from Bojar, R. (2011). *Manual of perioperative care in adult cardiac surgery* (5th ed.). Hoboken, NJ: Blackwell; Ji, Q., Mei, Y., Wang, X., Feng, J., Cai, J., & Ding, W. (2013). Risk factors for pulmonary complications following cardiac surgery with cardiopulmonary bypass. *International Journal of Medical Sciences, 10*(11), 1578–1583; Ji, Z., Mei, Y., Wang, X., Feng, J., Cai, J., Xie, S., . . . Hu, D. (2008). Study on the risk factors of postoperative hypoxemia in patients undergoing coronary artery bypass grafting. *Circulation, 72*(18), 1975–1980.

complexity of the surgical procedure, the use of cardiopulmonary bypass (CPB), or both. However, advances in surgical techniques and technology, improved understanding of CPB, and the creation of highly specialized critical care teams have positively influenced both postoperative management and outcomes. Perhaps the greatest advances have been related to the evolution of minimally invasive surgical procedures, allowing operations to be offered to older persons, and those patients with multiple comorbidities who might previously not have been considered surgical candidates. Additionally, postoperative care rendered in the ICU in terms of early extubation protocols, decreased utilization of blood products, and strict glycemic control has been directly correlated with lower morbidity and mortality rates (Bojar, 2011).

Despite these improvements, a few complications continue to be associated with a mortality rate of 50% or greater. The deleterious side effects of CPB, circulatory arrest, hypothermia, and aortic cross-clamping can cause a number of physiologic abnormalities in major organs in the perioperative period. Most notably, the loss of pulsatile blood flow while on CPB results in decreased perfusion pressure. Therefore, many organ systems—the brain, gut, and kidneys—can suffer damage when the surgical procedure and CPB time are protracted. Knowledge and early identification of potential postoperative complications are essential to successful patient management and outcomes following cardiac surgery.

CARDIAC COMPLICATIONS

Adequate cardiac function is the most important factor associated with recovery from cardiac surgery. Perioperatively, patients with poor cardiac function and low cardiac output (CO) have a higher mortality risk. Hence, the ICU nurse plays a vital role in identifying and treating a low CO state and preventing subsequent complications.

Hemodynamic compromise in the cardiac surgery patient is challenging to manage because the status of such patients tends to be labile in the immediate postoperative period. The etiology of hemodynamic compromise is multifactorial. It may be caused by the patient's underlying cardiac function, volume status, dysrhythmias, decreased ventricular compliance, loss of vasomotor tone, increased capillary permeability, postoperative bleeding, poor myocardial protection during aortic cross-clamping, or a systemic inflammatory response to CPB. Data suggest that a release of inflammatory mediators occurs in patients who undergo cardiac surgery, further contributing to these individuals' postoperative hemodynamic instability. Secretion of prostaglandins and other proinflammatory mediators (cytokines) stimulates release of nitric oxide, leading to profound vasodilation (Rodrigues, Evora, & Evora, 2014). Nitric oxide causes resistance to vasopressors by preventing vessels of some patients from vasoconstricting.

Perhaps the factor that influences cardiac performance most in the immediate postoperative period is the underlying preoperative cardiac pathology. Even though surgery has been performed, the patient will not experience an immediate improvement in contractility; inadequate inotropy is not uncommon after cardiac surgery (Silvestry, 2014). When decreased ventricular function is present, compensatory mechanisms such as sympathetic nervous system (SNS) stimulation and endogenous catecholamine production cause an increase in heart rate, contractility, and vasoconstriction. In turn, both preload and afterload increase (Guarracino, Baldassarri, & Pinsky, 2013). Initially, these compensatory factors will improve CO and blood pressure, albeit usually at the cost of increasing myocardial oxygen consumption, which can exacerbate myocardial ischemia. The compensatory mechanisms are temporary, however; when they are exhausted, poor tissue perfusion will ensue. Initial signs of poor tissue perfusion include tachycardia, diminished peripheral pulses, delayed capillary refill time, decreased urinary output, hypotension, and (possibly) metabolic acidosis (Wilson, 2012).

The primary objective of postoperative management of the cardiac surgery patient is attainment of an adequate CO. Optimal hemodynamic parameters in a postoperative cardiac surgery patient include a cardiac index (CI) of 2.2–4.4 L/min/m^2, pulmonary artery occlusive pressure (PAOP) 10–15 mmHg, central venous pressure (CVP) less than 15 mmHg, mean arterial pressure (MAP) 60–90 mmHg, systolic blood pressure in the range of 90–100 mmHg, and systemic vascular resistance (SVR) in the range of 1,400–2,800 dynes/sec/cm^{-5} (Silvestry, 2014). The patient should also have warm, well-perfused extremities and urine output at least 0.5 mL/kg/hr.

Low Cardiac Output Syndrome

To help ensure oxygen delivery, CO (the amount of blood ejected by the heart each minute) must be adequate. A related parameter to CO is CI, the amount of blood ejected by the heart each minute in relation to a patient's body surface area. Adequate tissue perfusion is dependent on satisfactory CO. Cardiac output and index are functions of stroke volume (SV), the amount of blood ejected by the heart with each beat), and heart rate. Stroke volume depends on myocardial contractility, preload (the amount of volume returning to the right or left side of the heart), and afterload (the amount of work the heart has to do to eject blood (Sherwood, 2012).

Low cardiac output syndrome (LCOS) is often seen after cardiac surgery and is associated with increased morbidity and mortality. Low cardiac output states are seen most commonly in patients with advanced age, left ventricular (LV) dysfunction, combined CABG/valve procedures, extended cross-clamping and CPB times, mitral valve procedures, and chronic kidney disease (Bojar, 2011). Low cardiac output syndrome can be defined as CI less than 2 L/min/m^2, elevated left-sided filling pressures (pulmonary artery diastolic pressure [PAD] > 20 mmHg) and an SVR exceeding 1,500 dynes/sec/cm^{-5}, and/or the need for administration of an inotropic infusion for more than 30 minutes or intra-aortic balloon pump (IABP) therapy (Bojar, 2011). Postoperative cardiac surgery patients may develop LCOS transiently within the first 6–8 hours due to myocardial ischemia and reperfusion injury following cardioplegic arrest; however, this usually returns to normal within 24 hours (Bojar, 2011).

The ICU nurse must monitor for signs and symptoms of impaired CO. Assessment of the patient with LCOS reveals decreased MAP, tachycardia, cool extremities and decreased or weak peripheral pulses, oliguria or anuria, and distended neck veins (Bojar, 2011).

Hemodynamic monitoring reveals mixed venous oxygen saturation (SvO_2) levels lower than normal in the setting of LCOS. Venous oxygen saturation is the percentage of hemoglobin saturated with oxygen in the pulmonary artery after blood has circulated systemically and oxygen has been extracted based on cellular need. Normal SvO_2 values are in the range of 70% to 75%. If the SvO_2 is less than 70%, it indicates that cells are sensing hypoperfusion or an increased metabolic rate and are extracting more oxygen from hemoglobin. Venous oxygen saturation monitoring provides data on the balance between oxygen supply and demand. Lab data that will help support a diagnosis of low CO include a metabolic acidosis or increasing base deficit on arterial blood gas and an elevated serum lactate level (Kraut & Madias, 2010).

Management of the patient with low CO depends on the underlying cause, hemodynamic profile, and patient assessment findings. Use of fluids, vasopressors, and inotropic agents will vary based on whether the patient has low preload or whether the SVR is elevated or low (Silvestry, 2014). If inotropic support is required, the chosen drug's efficacy must be carefully monitored because inotropic agents increase myocardial workload and metabolic rate. Epinephrine, norepinephrine (Levophed®), dopamine (Intropin®), or dobutamine (Dobutrex®) may be administered if contractility (ejection fraction, or EF) is below the expected values for the patient. These agents may have decreased efficacy in patients with chronic systolic dysfunction due to down regulation of beta receptors. Use of a phosphodiesterase inhibitor (e.g., milrinone [Primacor®]) may be a more effective means to augment contractility in this group of patients. Phosphodiesterase inhibitors augment myocardial contractility and coronary blood flow, and decrease SVR. These will result in increased CO and decreased preload and afterload of the left ventricle with minimal increase in myocardial oxygen demand (Silvestry, 2014). If vasodilation is the cause of the LCOS, administration of a vasoconstrictor (e.g., phenylephrine [Neosynephrine®]), norepinephrine, or vasopressin) is warranted (Silvestry, 2014).

If afterload is elevated, administration of nitroprusside (Nipride®), dobutamine, or IABP therapy may be indicated (Silvestry, 2014). Regardless of the cause of low CO, the primary goal of management will focus on decreasing metabolic demand. Interventions such as preventing hyperthermia, administering sedation and analgesia, decreasing work of breathing with mechanical ventilation, and preventing or treating tachycardia, dysrhythmias, and electrolyte and acid–base imbalances may need to be considered.

Preload Issues

Preload refers to the amount of volume returning to the right or left heart at the end of filling (diastole). It may be assessed by CVP and PAOP, which are the filling pressures of the right and left heart, respectively. Pulmonary artery occlusive pressure is a reflection of left ventricular end-diastolic pressure (LVEDP), from which estimates of LV end-diastolic volume can be made (Silvestry, 2014). The majority of patients are admitted to the ICU from the operating room (OR) with alterations in preload despite having a positive fluid balance.

The volume, however, is not in the intravascular space; instead, much of the fluid is located in the interstitium or other third space (e.g., pleural cavity).

Adequate preload is essential to maintain a satisfactory CO and tissue perfusion. Decreased preload in the immediate postoperative cardiac surgery patient can result from several factors, including excessive fluid output from diuresis or hypothermia, vasodilation during rewarming, inadequate intraoperative fluid resuscitation, intraoperative or postoperative bleeding, loss of vasomotor tone, infusion of vasodilator agents, decreased LV compliance, or capillary leak leading to third spacing of fluid. Further, after cardiac surgery, compliance of the left ventricle is typically decreased, which causes diastolic dysfunction. A higher LVEDP will be required during this time to maintain preload (Silvestry, 2014).

The type and amount of fluid resuscitation required will be based on the patient's history, cardiac function, amount and type of fluid lost, and hematocrit level. If the patient experiences excessive postoperative bleeding, transfusion of blood and blood products should be initiated while the source of the blood loss is being determined. The hemoglobin requirement should be determined by the patient's cardiac and hemodynamic status, age, and other clinical issues pertinent to the situation (Ferraris et al., 2011). Coagulation factors such as fresh frozen plasma and cryoprecipitate may also need to be given to correct coagulopathies usually caused by CPB.

If bleeding is not present, bolus administration of isotonic crystalloids (e.g., 0.9% normal saline, lactated Ringer's solution) or colloid (e.g., 5% albumin) may be used to optimize preload, usually to a PAOP of 18–20 mmHg. Administration of inotropic agents is not recommended for patients with decreased preload; intravascular volume repletion is required (Silvestry, 2014). Patients with a history of ventricular hypertrophy or diastolic dysfunction usually require a higher preload (Klabunde, 2013). Volume requirements may decrease after the patient has been removed from positive-pressure ventilation, as this change is often associated with an increase in venous return owing to the decrease in intrathoracic pressure (Levitov & Marik, 2011). Vasodilation is reported as the major contributor to a decrease in preload in the initial postoperative period; therefore volume repletion is typically required (Silvestry, 2014).

A therapeutic endpoint for volume resuscitation may be the MAP. The goal of a MAP in the range of 60–90 mmHg is suggested. Tachycardia is not believed to be an appropriate indicator of adequacy of preload, given the many preoperative and intraoperative factors that can affect the correlation between heart rate and hypovolemia. Ongoing monitoring of the patient's hemodynamic profile must take place concomitantly with volume repletion. Care must be taken not to overstretch the ventricle with excessive volume because an impaired CO may ensue (Beebe & Myers, 2011).

Cardiac Dysrhythmias

Dysrhythmias are a common complication following cardiac surgery. Additionally, they are a major source of morbidity and mortality, exposing patients to both extra days in the hospital and high-risk medications. As discussed in Chapter 15, atrial dysrhythmias are the most commonly encountered rhythm abnormalities encountered in the postoperative CABG patient. The overall incidence of atrial dysrhythmias is reported as high as 60%. A higher incidence is reported in patients who undergo valve surgery than CABG (Helgadottir, Sigurdsson, Ingvarsdottir, Arnar, & Gudbjartsson, 2012; Maesen, Nijs, Maessen, Allessie, & Schotten, 2012; Shen et al., 2011). The incidence of development of atrial dysrhythmias is reported to be 29% to 44% in patients undergoing CABG alone (Maesen et al., 2012;

Table 13-2   Common Causes of Dysrhythmias Following Cardiac Surgery

Patient-Related Factors

Age

Preexisting heart disease

Extracardiac morbidities—obesity, COPD, and stroke

Surgery-Related Factors

Tissue trauma and inflammation

Hemodynamic stress

Poor intraoperative myocardial protection/ ischemic injury

Pulmonary complications—hypoxia/ hypercapnia, ET tube misplacement, and pneumothorax

Electrolyte disturbances

Medications

Fever, pain, and anxiety

Hypothermia

COPD, chronic obstructive pulmonary disease; ET, endotracheal tube.

Sources: Data from Bojar, R. (2011). *Manual of perioperative care in adult cardiac surgery* (5th ed.). Hoboken, NJ: Blackwell; and Peretto, G., Durante, A., Limite, L., & Cianflone, D. (2014). Postoperative arrhythmias after cardiac surgery: Incidence, risk factors and therapeutic management. *Cardiology Research and Practice, 2014*, 615987. Retrieved from http://dx.doi.org/10.1155/2014/615987

Helgadottir et al., 2012; Nair, 2010; Shen et al., 2011), as high as 40% in patients undergoing valve replacements (Nair, 2010), and 50% to 64% following CABG and valve surgery combined (Helgadottir et al., 2012; Nair, 2010). Many factors have been implicated in the development of postoperative dysrhythmias (**Table 13-2**). Postoperative dysrhythmias are discussed in detail in Chapter 15.

Dysrhythmias can compromise CO when they interfere with diastolic filling. If a disturbance in heart rhythm is present, prompt identification and close assessment of the patient are essential. Assessment of the patient with cardiac dysrhythmias following cardiac surgery requires evaluation of the rhythm and its effects on systemic perfusion, as well as evaluation of precipitating factors. Treatment is based on whether the goal of therapy is to control the rate or to convert the rhythm. Postoperative dysrhythmias are discussed in detail in Chapter 15; the pharmacologic management of dysrhythmias is discussed in Chapters 12 and 15.

Diastolic Dysfunction

Diastolic dysfunction is characterized by reduced ventricular compliance and can be exacerbated by myocardial ischemia or edema from reperfusion injury (Bojar, 2011). Diastolic dysfunction commonly occurs following aortic valve replacement and is largely due to the LV hypertrophy that results from standing aortic stenosis. A second very common cause of postoperative diastolic dysfunction is poor intraoperative myocardial protection. The hemodynamic picture is one of elevated PAOP and low CO, EF greater than in preoperative setting, and small left ventricle (Alsaddique, Royse, Fouda, & Royse, 2012). If the left ventricle becomes stiff during filling (diastole), it may not be able to fill completely. As a result, fluid may back up to the lungs, and heart failure may ensue.

Treatment of diastolic dysfunction includes volume administration to maximize preload and administration of vasodilators. Patients with diastolic dysfunction from decreased LV compliance will require a higher PAOP to maintain adequate preload than do patients with a reduced preload from the other etiologies listed earlier. Because the ventricle has decreased compliance in this case, the PAOP may be elevated despite the need for additional preload (Alsaddique et al., 2012). Infusion of an inotropic agent should be administered at low doses if the patient's

EF is low to normal. A combination of dobutamine and norepinephrine may be effective. Monitoring for tachycardia is essential when using these agents because an increased heart rate will decrease ventricular filling time, which can result in decreased SV and CO. Milrinone, a phosphodiesterase inhibitor, causes vasodilation and may improve EF. If a vasodilator is used, it is important not to exceed baseline levels of dilation. Administration of a vasoconstrictor may be required in diastolic dysfunction after cardiac surgery if the patient is vasodilated from the inflammatory response common after these procedures. In this case, the goal is to normalize vascular resistance, but not elevate it. Calcium channel blockers may be helpful if the diastolic dysfunction is related to idiopathic cardiomyopathies (Alsaddique et al., 2012).

Right Ventricular Failure

Although most low-output states following cardiac surgery are attributable to LV failure, low CO can also be the result of right ventricular (RV) failure. Right ventricular failure after cardiac surgery is a significant cause of postoperative morbidity and mortality. The incidence is dependent on the procedure performed: 0.1% after cardiotomy, 2% to 3% after heart transplant, and 20% to 30% in patients who required an LV assist device (Haddad, Couture, Tousignant, & Denault, 2009). Etiology of RV dysfunction may include myocardial ischemia, infarction from right coronary artery disease, pulmonary hypertension of any cause, or any combination of these (Bojar, 2011). Preexisting conditions such as severe lung disease, including obstructive sleep apnea, aortic or mitral valve disease, tricuspid regurgitation, primary pulmonary hypertension, or RV hypertrophy, may commonly be associated with pulmonary hypertension and contribute to the development of postoperative RV failure (Bojar, 2011). Inadequate function of the right ventricle leads to decreased

filling of the left ventricle, reduced LV output, and poor systemic perfusion. The right ventricle then becomes distended, with RV failure being the ultimate outcome. Right ventricular failure can also occur following a heart transplant (Vlahakes, 2012). The diagnosis of RV failure is based on the presence of elevated CVP and low PAOP and CO (Khalpey, Ganim, & Rawn, 2008).

Management of RV failure includes optimizing preload, ensuring atrioventricular (AV) conduction, reducing RV afterload (pulmonary vascular resistance, or PVR), improving RV contractility, and maintaining systemic blood pressure (Bojar, 2011). Volume repletion is essential to optimize left heart function; care must be taken, however, to avoid overdistention of the right ventricle—the goal being a CVP of 18–20 mmHg (Khalpey et al., 2008). Inotropic support may be required; the key is to use medications that provide ventricular support without increasing PVR. Milrinone is commonly used in the treatment of RV failure because this agent improves RV contractility, resulting in vasodilation and reduced pulmonary artery pressures. Systemic hypotension may ultimately ensue, requiring an alpha agent to support SVR, which may in turn increase PVR (Bojar, 2011).

In the case of severe RV failure, pulmonary vasodilators should also be administered. Inhaled nitric oxide, nesiritide, or prostaglandin and prostacyclin analog infusions all may be beneficial in reducing pulmonary artery pressures and PVR and improving RV function when severe pulmonary hypertension occurs after cardiac surgical procedures (Bojar, 2011; Haddad et al., 2009).

Decreased Myocardial Contractility

Contractility is the shortening of myocardial fibers during systole (ventricular emptying) and the force produced by the myocardium to eject blood. It is evaluated with EF by echocardiography (Silvestry, 2014).

Cardiac contractility may be impaired postoperatively due to cross-clamping of the aorta without adequate myocardial protection, ischemia, decreased coronary blood flow, cardiac tamponade, myocardial infarction (MI), or coronary graft vasospasm or thrombosis (Silvestry, 2014). Other implicating factors include hypoxia, acidosis, electrolyte imbalance, narcotics, anesthesia, transient ischemic/reperfusion injury, impaired preoperative function (EF less than 35%), inadequate intraoperative myocardial protection, duration and extent of postoperative hypothermia, CPB time (especially if longer than 120 minutes), tamponade, valve function, or myocardial ischemia or infarction (Kouchoukos, Blackstone, Hanley, & Kirklin, 2013).

Left ventricular function/contractility may be reduced following cardiac surgery. It reaches its lowest point 24 hours after surgery and gradually returns to baseline within a week (Cool, Thomas, Nolan, & Parr, 2014). Decreased contractility may require inotropic support with vasoactive medications to support cardiac function. Both inotropic and vasodilator support with medications such as dobutamine, dopamine, milrinone, and epinephrine, used alone or in combination, may prove effective in improving cardiac contractility. No data support the use of inotropes to improve patient outcomes following cardiac surgery, nor do any data support use of one inotrope over another (Cool et al., 2014). Epinephrine, however, is associated with the development of temporary but significant hyperglycemia, metabolic acidosis, and increased serum lactate when used in the initial 6–8 postoperative hours. These effects usually resolve in 12 hours (Rosas, Giocoechea-Turcott, Ortiz, Salazar, & Palma, 2012).

In addition to titrating medications according to the patient's hemodynamic profile, the ICU nurse must monitor for signs and symptoms of inadequate perfusion related to the impaired contractility. Evaluation of CI,

hypotension, mottling, end-organ dysfunction (e.g., inadequate urinary output), and presence of a metabolic acidosis is vital. Urinary output may be increased in the initial postoperative period, however, so it is considered a less reliable indicator of poor perfusion.

Myocardial Stunning and Hibernation

Cardiovascular research has led to the identification of two important phenomena: myocardial stunning and myocardial hibernation.

Myocardial stunning is a period of impaired contractility following temporary ischemia, in which the dysfunction persists despite return of blood flow. Myocardial stunning may occur after CPB, and postoperative cardiac dysfunction (i.e., decreased ventricular function) is often attributed to its effects (Kouchoukos et al., 2013).

Hibernating myocardium is a condition of impaired LV function when the patient is at rest; it reflects a chronic reduction in blood flow. Heart function can be partially or totally normalized by improving blood flow or decreasing oxygen demand (Shavelle, 2014). Myocardial hibernation is considered a compensatory or protective mechanism to safeguard the capacity and integrity of the myocardium during times of decreased blood flow (Shavelle, 2014).

Increased Systemic Vascular Resistance (Afterload)

As with preload, right- and left-sided afterload can be evaluated to help determine cardiac performance. Right-sided afterload is reflected by PVR; left-sided afterload is reflected by SVR. Most of the discussion in this section refers to left-sided afterload.

Afterload is determined by intraventricular systolic pressure and the thickness of the ventricular wall. The latter factor is minimally affected with cardiac surgery. Systolic blood pressure will have the greatest effect on afterload and, therefore, SV and myocardial oxygen demand. By decreasing afterload, CO will improve (Silvestry, 2014).

Increased SVR is also often a compensatory result of the SNS response to low CO. Increased SVR may be poorly tolerated in a patient with already poor myocardial function.

Hypertension is a well-known complication of patients who undergo cardiac surgery (Singla et al., 2008) and is often associated with vasoconstriction related to hypothermia during CPB (Silvestry, 2014). Development of hypertension, vasoconstriction, or both may be related to decreased oxygen levels in the muscle with concomitant metabolic acidosis or inflammatory responses to CPB (Silvestry, 2014). Other potential causes of increased afterload include hypothermia, hypovolemia, hypercarbia, inadequate rewarming, volume overload, cardiogenic shock, pain, and anxiety. The latter two etiologies result from increased SNS stimulation. If vasoconstriction is extreme, the patient is at risk of developing life-threatening hypertension and decreased CO (Silvestry, 2014).

Treatment of increased afterload may entail administration of vasodilator therapy with medications such as sodium nitroprusside, nitroglycerin (Tridil®), or milrinone. Sodium nitroprusside is the treatment of choice (Silvestry, 2014). Given that vasodilators cause a decrease in preload, concomitant administration of fluids may be required to maintain adequate intravascular volume during their use. As the potential for abrupt hypotension exists when nitroprusside is administered, frequent blood pressure monitoring is essential, especially during rewarming (Silvestry, 2014). In severe cases of LV failure, IABP counterpulsation may be used to reduce afterload. Intra-aortic balloon pump therapy is discussed in detail in Chapter 10.

Decreased Systemic Vascular Resistance

While an increase in afterload is common following cardiac surgery, some patients develop a decreased SVR postoperatively. This condition, which is also referred to as vasodilatory shock, is associated with a CO that is either normal or increased (Silvestry, 2014). The incidence of vasodilatory shock is reported to range from 5% to 8%. Patients who are at higher risk for the development of a decreased SVR are those who have a low EF (less than 35%) and those with end-stage heart failure requiring assist device insertion. Vasodilatory shock also may be caused by an inflammatory response to CPB. Its treatment entails administration of a vasoconstrictor agent such as phenylephrine or norepinephrine. If patients do not respond to this therapy, vasopressin administration may be attempted. Finally, methylene blue administration may be considered because this agent inhibits nitric oxide production (Silvestry, 2014).

Mechanical Issues

A number of mechanical issues can contribute to the development of hemodynamic compromise in the postoperative cardiac surgery patient. These complications include cardiac tamponade, coronary artery or radial artery graft spasm, acute graft closure, prosthetic valve regurgitation, pneumothorax (PTX), and hemothorax (Silvestry, 2014).

Cardiac Tamponade

During cardiac surgery, the pericardial sac is excised to gain access to the epicardial surface of the heart. At the end of the procedure, the pericardial sac remains open, leaving a communication between the heart and the mediastinum. Excessive bleeding in the perioperative period may lead to the potential accumulation of blood and fluid in the mediastinal space. Such an accumulation may lead to compression of the atria, restriction of venous return to the heart, and reduced ventricular filling, resulting in a decrease or cessation of preload, causing a precipitous fall in CO (Floerchinger et al., 2013). Cardiac tamponade is most often the result of persistent mediastinal bleeding that is not adequately being evacuated by chest tubes.

Cardiac tamponade is one of several potential complications that may result in ventricular dysfunction (Silvestry, 2014). Diagnosis may be difficult because hypotension, tachycardia, and elevated filling pressures are common scenarios in most immediate postoperative cardiac surgery patients. In addition, some of the other characteristic symptoms of cardiac tamponade (e.g., muffled heart sounds, pulsus paradoxus, and neck vein distention) are not helpful in the cardiac surgery patient. While the patient may experience equalization of intracardiac pressures (CVP equal with PAOP or PAD), other signs and symptoms will likely suggest the presence of cardiac tamponade prior to this manifestation (Yarlagadda, 2014). Heightened awareness for tamponade should be present when the patient develops the signs and symptoms listed in **Table 13-3**.

Continuous hypotension that does not respond to fluid administration and the use of inotropic support with the presence of signs and symptoms listed in Table 13-3 requires prompt intervention with a bedside echocardiogram to differentiate between ventricular dysfunction and cardiac tamponade (Bojar, 2011). The patient may need to return to the OR for clot evacuation, bleeding site repair, or both. When an echocardiogram is not feasible or there is impending cardiac arrest, emergency mediastinal exploration is warranted for accurate diagnosis (Čanádyová, Zmeko, & Mikráček, 2012). **Box 13-1** lists the steps undertaken in an emergency resternotomy.

Coronary Vasospasm

A frequently unrecognized cause of sudden cardiovascular collapse in the early postoperative period is coronary artery/graft vasospasm. This complication usually presents itself as acute hypotension, ST-segment elevation in multiple leads, and low CO. All types of coronary grafts are implicated in the development of coronary vasospasm—saphenous vein grafts, arterial conduits, and normal cardiac vessels alike (Neto, Neto, Simões, & Stolf, 2010). In addition, vasoconstriction of an arterial conduit may occur; patients

Table 13-3　Signs and Symptoms of Cardiac Tamponade
Sudden decrease or cessation of significant mediastinal bleeding
Persistent low cardiac output state with hypotension
Narrowing pulse pressure
Inappropriately fluctuating MAP
Increased central venous pressure or equalization of intracardiac pressures: RA = PAOP = LA pressures
An increasing requirement for inotropic or vasopressor medications
Chest radiograph findings of an enlarged cardiac silhouette or widened mediastinum
ECG changes including decreased voltage QRS complex, a compensatory tachycardia, dysrhythmias, or pulseless electrical activity
Sudden oliguria
Altered mental status
Dyspnea
Diaphoresis
Cyanosis or pallor
Anxiety, restlessness, or both

ECG, electrocardiogram; MAP, mean arterial pressure; RA, right atrial; PAOP, pulmonary artery occlusive pressure; LA, left atrial.

Sources: Data from Bojar, R. (2011). *Manual of perioperative care in adult cardiac surgery* (5th ed.). Hoboken, NJ: Blackwell; Schiavone, W. A. (2013). Cardiac tamponade: 12 pearls. *Cleveland Clinic Journal of Medicine, 80*(2), 109–116; Yarlagadda, C. (2014). *Cardiac tamponade: Clinical presentation.* Retrieved from http://emedicine.medscape.com/article/152083-overview

Box 13-1   Emergency Resternotomy Procedures

1. Alert the surgeon and operating team.
2. Obtain an emergency open chest tray.
3. Obtain an electrocautery device, and apply the ground pads to the patient's skin to prevent a Bovie burn.
4. Set up sterile suction.
5. Obtain personal protective equipment, sterile gowns, antiseptic solution, and drapes.
6. Remove the dressing.
7. Cleanse skin with chlorhexidine solution.
8. Place sterile towels and drapes on the patient's skin.
9. Assist the surgeon by supplying scalpel and wire cutters.
10. Open the incision down to the sternum with the scalpel.
11. Cut the sternal wires with the wire cutters.
12. Place the sternal retractor to expose the heart, carefully locating the existing coronary artery bypass grafts.
13. Assist with controlling bleeding and suctioning, if needed.
14. Assist in irrigation of mediastinum with warm saline or antibiotics.
15. Assist in closing the sternum.
16. Apply a dressing to the incision, securing the epicardial pacer wires and chest tube sites.
17. Assess the patient's cardiovascular and hemodynamic status every 15 minutes until stable.
18. Monitor coagulation and hematology laboratory studies as needed.
19. Monitor chest tube drainage.

who received a radial artery graft are routinely given a prophylactic "cocktail," which includes a vasodilator, such as nitroglycerin, and a calcium channel blocker (Bojar, 2011). Vasospasm usually resolves on its own; however, treatment is aimed primarily at supportive care to maintain hemodynamic stability.

Myocardial Ischemia and Infarction

Myocardial ischemia, whether transient or leading to MI, may occur after cardiac surgery. Causative factors leading to perioperative myocardial ischemia include poor myocardial protection during CBP (e.g., insufficient cardioplegia, incomplete revascularization, coronary vasospasm, or coronary artery or intracoronary embolism). Other risk factors that have been identified include age over 70 years, female gender, acute kidney injury (AKI), diabetes, peripheral artery disease, emergency or redo surgery, left ventricular ejection fraction (LVEF) less than 35%, cardiogenic shock, or preoperative MI (Al-Attar, 2011). Myocardial infarction may also occur in the early postoperative period related to acute closure of a bypass graft. Patients may be started on aspirin, clopidogrel, or both within the initial few postoperative hours to reduce prevalence of MI. The incidence of postoperative MI has been reported to range from 2% to 15% for all cardiac surgery procedures (Al-Attar, 2011); however, the range is only 4% to 5% for patients who have undergone CABG specifically (Silvestry, 2014). It is typically due to poor perfusion of the more proximal coronary arteries after bypass grafting (Al-Attar, 2011).

The diagnosis of perioperative MI can be determined by electrocardiogram (ECG) changes (e.g., the presence of Q waves or ST elevation), evidence of new wall motion abnormalities, and the presence of elevated cardiac markers (troponin I or creatine kinase [CK-MB]). Significant ST elevation on a postoperative ECG may indicate acute graft closure; other suspect ECG findings include new bundle branch block, ventricular dysrhythmias, or complete heart block (Bojar, 2011; Lim et al., 2011). Troponin I is a myocardial protein that is a very sensitive and specific marker for myocardial damage. However, troponin elevation is common in the immediate postoperative period following cardiac surgery. The troponin elevation varies among surgical procedures. In fact, troponin concentrations may be present upon admission to the ICU. Higher levels are reported following CABG alone or associated with procedures of the ascending aorta and with valve replacement. Inflammation has been implicated as a possible reason for troponin release even in the absence of myocardial injury. Lower troponin levels are reported following off-pump CABG and non-CABG procedures. This makes diagnosis of postoperative MI more difficult (Januzzi, 2009). It is recommended that a CABG-related MI be diagnosed based on biomarkers that are elevated more than five times the upper limit of normal for the first 72 hours after surgery and when the elevated biomarkers accompany either new pathological Q waves, new left bundle branch block, confirmed occlusion of a graft or native artery, or imaging that suggests loss of viable myocardial tissue (Thygesen, Alpert, & White, 2007).

Patients with suspected MI or persistent ischemia follow the same course as uncomplicated postoperative patients, with beta blockade and intravenous nitroglycerin being administered to them if the blood pressure permits (Zafari, 2014). Serial troponin levels should be obtained and monitored as well as 12-lead ECG for the presence of new Q waves. Intra-aortic balloon pump therapy is suggested to diminish inotrope use, infarct size, and myocardial oxygen demand (Parissis, Soo, & Al-Alao, 2012).

Cardiac Arrest

Cardiac arrest is the most serious complication of any cardiac surgery procedure, with the incidence of occurrence estimated to be 0.7% to 2.9% (Gologorsky et al., 2010). It can occur unexpectedly at any time from the OR until discharge. It must be managed immediately and in accordance with American Heart Association and advanced cardiac life support (ACLS) standards (Bojar, 2011). Potential causes for unexpected cardiac arrest in an otherwise hemodynamically stable patient include mechanical issues such as bleeding/cardiac tamponade and acute graft closure; ventricular arrhythmias are another common scenario. Overall mortality rates for cardiac arrest following cardiac surgery are 30% to 75%, and survival is much more likely when bleeding or tamponade is the inciting factor (Bojar, 2011).

As resuscitation efforts are started, evaluation for potential causes—including those unique to cardiac surgery patients—should begin. Checking the position of the endotracheal tube, signs of hypovolemia, patient temperature, chest tube drainage, proper ventilator functioning, results from chest radiograph (for widened mediastinum, tension pneumothorax, or tamponade), arterial blood gas, and electrolytes may help identify the underlying cause of cardiac arrest. Noting the infusion rates of vasoactive agents may provide additional clues. Treating and reversing the cause is the priority here, occurring simultaneously with an established protocol for high-quality cardiopulmonary resuscitation, epinephrine, early defibrillation, and emergency chest reentry. Because of the need for this emergent and highly organized approach to resuscitation following cardiac arrest in the cardiac surgery population, hospitals in Europe have adopted cardiac surgery-specific protocols designed to assist staff with

Box 13-2   Internal Defibrillation Procedure

1. Follow the procedure for chest reentry.
2. Follow the procedures for advanced cardiac life support (ACLS).
3. Prepare the defibrillator for internal defibrillation by gathering sterile internal defibrillation paddles.
4. Assist with positioning the internal paddles on the heart.
   a. One paddle is placed over the right atrium or right ventricle.
   b. The other paddle is placed over the apex of the heart.
5. Charge the defibrillator paddles (5–20 joules).
6. Verify providers are clear of the patient and all equipment before defibrillation.
7. Assess the patient's cardiac rhythm for conversion and presence of pulse.
8. If needed, repeat the defibrillation, following ACLS guidelines.
9. Assist with transport to the operating room or closure at the bedside.
10. Monitor the patient's neurologic, cardiac, and pulmonary status until stable.

resuscitation efforts. The Cardiac Surgery Advanced Life Support (CALS) course has been linked to improved patient outcomes. The CALS guidelines have yet to be endorsed by the American Heart Association. **Box 13-2** lists the steps for internal defibrillation.

PULMONARY COMPLICATIONS

Virtually all patients undergoing cardiac surgical procedures will have some degree of postoperative respiratory dysfunction; however, the majority will overcome it without major disruption in oxygenation or ventilation (Bojar, 2011). Cardiac surgery patients are at risk for developing postoperative pulmonary complications due to a number of factors. Preoperative factors include age over 65 years, female gender, recent smoking, chronic obstructive pulmonary disease (COPD), congestive heart failure, diabetes, hypercarbia, and use of vasoactive drug support. Intraoperative risk factors include phrenic nerve injury, aortic cross-clamping, use of IABP, and duration of CPB. Postoperative risk factors that have been identified include presence of bacteremia, endocarditis, gastrointestinal (GI) hemorrhage, acute

kidney injury, sternal infection, stroke, new-onset atrial fibrillation (AF), anemia, and reoperation for postoperative bleeding (Jensen & Yang, 2007; Ji et al., 2013). Protocols have been developed and are widely utilized that allow for rapid weaning and successful extubation for the majority of cardiac surgery patients (Kiessling et al., 2013).

Preoperative identification of patients with pulmonary risk factors should facilitate provision of proper perioperative intervention. Early identification and intervention to maximize lung function prior to surgery can prevent the incidence of most postoperative pulmonary dysfunction.

Developing an understanding of the postoperative changes in pulmonary function, routine pulmonary management, and contributory factors of pulmonary dysfunction allows for the early identification and management of such problems.

Postoperative Effects on Pulmonary Function

Respiratory complications are noted to be among the top contributors of postoperative morbidity for the cardiac surgery patient. The development of pulmonary dysfunction after cardiac surgery is associated with inconsistencies in gas exchange, ventilation/perfusion mismatch, decreased functional residual capacity, and pulmonary shunting. Patients will often manifest signs of respiratory dysfunction including shortness of breath, tachypnea, and decreased oxygen saturation. Dysfunction may be related to use of general anesthesia and neuromuscular blocking agents, a decreased vital capacity from a median sternotomy, and thoracic manipulation. Atelectasis, increased capillary leak, and inflammation for CPB may also contribute to pulmonary dysfunction, as will administration of blood products and crystalloids during surgery (Roekaert & Heijmar, 2012). **Table 13-4** lists other factors contributing to higher risk of pulmonary dysfunction.

Atelectasis

Atelectasis occurs in most patients who undergo general anesthesia. Collapse of the individual alveoli, particularly in the dependent parts of the lungs leading to atelectasis, is prevalent in cardiac surgery patients. The absence of traditional ventilation while on CPB as well as deliberate intraoperative lung collapse all contribute to this problem, with the incidence of atelectasis reported to be as high as 98% (Nakazato, Takeda, Tanaka, & Sakamoto, 2012). The development of atelectasis is thought to be due to intraoperative displacement of the diaphragm from a sternotomy, lack of lung activity while the patient is on CPB, and from high oxygen concentration during surgery. In patients undergoing CPB, atelectasis is related to increased extravascular lung water, which changes surfactant activity, causes activation of the inflammatory process, and results in coagulation. This results in decreased gas exchange, changes in ventilation-to-perfusion ratio, decreased functional residual capacity, increased shunt, and hypoxemia (Padovani & Cavenaghi, 2011). Decreased oxygenation and lung compliance result, continue into the postoperative

period, and can have a substantial impact on patient recovery. Areas of atelectasis can lead to an increased risk of postoperative respiratory infection. Pneumonia is a common hospital-acquired infection in postoperative cardiac surgery patients and is a leading cause of morbidity and mortality in these patients (Padovani & Cavenaghi, 2011).

Techniques or devices that encourage patients to inspire deeply are beneficial. The aim of therapy is to produce a large and sustained increase in the transpulmonary pressure, thereby distending the lung and re-expanding the collapsed alveoli. Several alveolar recruitment methods while intubated include increased levels of positive end expiratory pressure (PEEP) for short periods of time (sustained inflation) (Padovani & Cavenaghi, 2011). Once extubated, methods such as noninvasive ventilation, nebulization, deep-breathing exercises, incentive spirometry, and chest physiotherapy have been shown to be helpful in reexpansion of the collapsed lung units (Madappa, 2014; Nakazato et al., 2012). Vigorous pulmonary toileting along with early ambulation are generally effective therapies for the postoperative cardiac surgery patient who is recovering from atelectasis.

Pleural Effusion

Postoperative pleural effusions, or fluid collections in the pleural space, occur in about 60% of cardiac surgery patients, occurring more frequently in those who undergo takedown of the internal thoracic artery (ITA) (Bojar, 2011). Causes of pleural effusions in postoperative cardiac surgery patients include heart failure, postpericardiotomy syndrome, pneumonia, pulmonary embolism, chylothorax, hemothorax, and erosion of a central venous catheter through central venous structures, or they can be related to the surgical procedure (Heffner, 2013). Chest tubes left in place at the end of the cardiac surgery procedure are often strategically placed to avoid postoperative pleural effusions. Pleural

| Table 13-4 Factors Contributing to Development of Pulmonary Dysfunction After Cardiac Surgery ||
Contributing Factors	Effects on Pulmonary System
General anesthesia Paralytics Narcotics Supine positioning	Decreased central respiratory drive leading to decreased use of respiratory muscles Upward shift of diaphragm Chest wall relaxation Changes in compliance of chest wall
Cardiopulmonary bypass	Pulmonary edema from fluid overload and hemodilution Interstitial pulmonary edema from a systemic inflammatory response, which produces capillary leak Complement activation, release of cytokines, and neutrophil activation, which cause increased endothelial permeability Insufficient alveolar distention to activate production of surfactant, which may lead to alveolar collapse, retention of secretions, and atelectasis
Cooling for myocardial protection	Phrenic nerve injury
Median sternotomy incision and chest tubes	Chest wall splinting, which reduces the patient's ability to take deep breaths
Use of ITA for coronary artery bypass conduit	Use of ITA requires pleural dissection, which causes a potential decrease in chest wall compliance
Sternal or thoracotomy incisional pain Obesity Age Diaphragmatic injury Smoking history History of COPD, heart failure	Decreased respiratory muscle use

COPD, chronic obstructive pulmonary disease; ITA, internal thoracic artery.

Sources: Data from Jensen, L., & Yang, L. (2007). Risk factors for postoperative pulmonary complications in coronary artery bypass graft surgery patients. *European Journal of Cardiovascular Nursing, 6*(3), 241–246; Ji, Q., Mei, Y., Wang, X., Feng, J., Cai, J., & Ding, W. (2013). Risk factors for pulmonary complications following cardiac surgery with cardiopulmonary bypass. *International Journal of Medical Sciences, 10*(11), 1578–1583; Roekaert, S., & Heijmar, J. (2012). Postoperative considerations in cardiac surgery. In C. Narin (Ed.), *Perioperative considerations in cardiac surgery*. Retrieved from http://www.intechopen.com/books/howtoreference/perioperative-considerations-in-cardiac-surgery/-early-postoperative-care-after-cardiac-surgery

effusions are easily diagnosed on a chest radiograph.

Patients with small pleural effusions (less than two intercostal spaces [ICSs] on a chest radiograph) are usually asymptomatic. A small percentage of patients with an ITA (7%) and saphenous vein (2%) CABG procedures have pleural effusions that can be seen in more than two ICSs. Pleural effusions are typically left-sided (Heffner, 2013). Small pleural effusions will likely resolve on their own, with the body reabsorbing the fluid collection (Mullen-Fortino & O'Brien, 2008). Diuretics can also be used when pleural effusions are bilateral and appear to be related to congestive heart failure. Moderate to large effusions may occupy more than 25% of the lung and may cause activity-limiting dyspnea and require intervention. In this situation, a thoracentesis or chest tube insertion is indicated (Bojar, 2011).

Phrenic Nerve Injury

There has been a decline in phrenic nerve injury with diaphragmatic dysfunction as a result of improved techniques used in cardiac surgical procedures. The incidence is reported at 11%. Historically, the primary etiology of this morbid complication was cold injury to the phrenic nerve caused from the use of ice in the pericardial region as a method of myocardial protection. Phrenic nerve injury is also thought to be related to the pleurotomy required for ITA harvesting; this results in more chest wall trauma, pain, and decreased ability to cough and deep breathe (Kamanger, 2013). Ice is not used routinely in the pericardium anymore; however, phrenic nerve injury may also occur with the takedown of the ITA. Dissection of the ITA may also decrease blood supply to the intercostal muscles, which may result in injury to the phrenic nerve (Kamanger, 2013).

Signs and symptoms depend on whether the paralysis is unilateral or bilateral. Unilateral phrenic nerve injuries rarely produce significant respiratory symptoms, and patients can usually be extubated without difficulty. Some patients may be asymptomatic at rest but develop dyspnea on exertion and activity intolerance. If the patient has a history of lung disease, dyspnea at rest may be present; orthopnea may occur. In contrast, bilateral phrenic nerve injury, although rare, results in paradoxical breathing, tachypnea, shallow respirations, dyspnea, and carbon dioxide retention when attempts are made at extubation. Symptoms may increase when the patient is in a supine position. Other symptoms may include anxiety, insomnia, morning headache, extreme sleepiness during the day,

and poor sleep. Gastrointestinal symptoms such as dyspepsia, regurgitation, nausea, and epigastric pain may occur. Arterial blood gas analysis will reveal hypoxia and progressive hypercarbia. The hypoxia is related to atelectasis and ventilation/perfusion mismatching. Chest radiograph may reveal an elevated hemidiaphragm at end-expiration with spontaneous ventilation, small lung volumes, and atelectasis; these will not be apparent while the patient is mechanically ventilated owing to the effects of the positive-pressure ventilation. Treatment may involve plication of the diaphragm, which attempts to stabilize the diaphragmatic muscle and prevents paradoxical motion with breathing. Phrenic pacing, diaphragmatic pacing, or noninvasive ventilation at night may be required. A tracheostomy with positive-pressure ventilation may be required if less invasive methods are not successful. Inspiratory muscle strength and endurance training may be successful. Nerve reconstruction techniques may be attempted on some patients (Kamangar, 2013). Many patients improve with chest physiotherapy and prevention and treatment of pneumonia (Kamanger, 2013). Phrenic nerve injury is discussed in more detail in Chapter 11.

Pneumothorax

A pneumothorax is air in the pleural space. If a pleural space is opened at the time of surgery (e.g., during the takedown of an ITA), a chest tube must be placed to drain both air and fluid to avoid complications (Bojar, 2011). A small PTX can also occur because of direct injury to the lung during surgery, central venous cannulation, or barotrauma during positive-pressure ventilation. This is usually noted in the immediate postoperative period and detected on the initial postoperative chest radiograph (Stark, 2013). The incidence of PTX may increase in patients with pre-existing bullous lung disease or in those requiring high levels of PEEP. A PTX that is small will usually reabsorb on its own and can be monitored with serial chest radiographs. A chest tube must be inserted for any large PTX because it could potentially enlarge with the use of positive-pressure ventilation (Bojar, 2011).

It is not uncommon for a tension PTX to develop following cardiac surgery. The most common causes are regional block, airway instrumentation, and central line placement. Patients with COPD are at greater risk. It is rare, but it can also occur intraoperatively. Signs may be masked during general anesthesia. When the patient is admitted to the ICU, peak airway pressures are elevated; more pressure is required to deliver the same tidal volume. Expiratory volumes are decreased and are due to air leaking into the pleural space. An increase in end-expiratory pressure will be noted even in patients not receiving PEEP (Jain, Arora, Juneja, Mehta, & Trehan, 2014). In this situation, the patient acutely decompensates. Although breath sounds may be diminished, it may be difficult to assess given ventilator sounds and various alarms in the unit. Other signs and symptoms of tension PTX can include distended neck veins, hypotension, and tracheal deviation away from the collapsed lung. If the patient is hemodynamically unstable and a tension PTX is suspected, decompression with a 16-gauge needle at the second intercostal space, midclavicular line, is indicated. A rush of air and an improvement in hemodynamics confirm the diagnosis (Jain et al., 2014). A chest radiograph should be obtained to assess the involved structures and the severity of the tension PTX. Treatment also includes immediate placement of a chest tube, usually at the fifth intercostal space, anterior axillary line, for the residual PTX (Daley, 2014).

Prolonged Mechanical Ventilation

A small number of patients will require prolonged mechanical ventilation after cardiac surgery. Prolonged mechanical ventilation beyond 48 hours occurs in about 5% to 10% of patients and is usually the result of cardiac or hemodynamic dysfunction, surgical reexploration, neurologic complications, or acute renal failure (Bojar, 2011). These patients typically do not have gas exchange or oxygenation issues but require an airway support because of critical illness. Prolonged mechanical ventilation is discussed in detail in Chapter 11.

Acute Respiratory Distress Syndrome

Acute respiratory distress syndrome (ARDS) is characterized by inflammation of the lung parenchyma and increased microvascular permeability, which causes leakage of fluid into the alveolar space, hypoxemia, increased work of breathing, and pulmonary infiltrates on chest radiograph. This syndrome usually becomes evident within the first 24–48 hours following cardiac surgery and can be a direct result of the acute inflammatory reaction and systemic response seen with CPB. The reported incidence of patients developing ARDS after cardiac surgery is up to 20%; mortality rates are as high as 80% (Mazzeffi & Rock, 2012). Previous cardiac surgery, shock, and excessive administration of blood products are important predictive factors for this complication (Milot et al., 2001). Transfusion-related acute lung injury (TRALI) presents a similar clinical picture to that of ARDS, resulting in diffuse pulmonary edema due to increased alveolar permeability. Transfusion-related acute lung injury is thought to be an immune-mediated response between donor plasma antibodies and the recipient leukocyte antigens; criteria defining TRALI include hypoxemia with increased oxygen requirements, along with the development of pulmonary infiltrates within 6 hours of transfusion (Bojar, 2011).

Treatment of ARDS and TRALI is mainly supportive, with maintenance of adequate oxygenation being the primary goal. The use of smaller tidal volumes (6 mL/kg) and PEEP has been associated with improved outcomes. Use of judicious fluid administration, minimizing administration of blood products, nutrition, and early mobility may improve outcomes as well (Stephens, Shah, & Whitman, 2013).

Pneumonia

Postoperative pneumonia is the most common infection following cardiac surgery. It usually occurs within 5 days of surgery but may develop within the first 24–48 hours (Conde, 2012). The reported incidence of postoperative pneumonia is 3% to 5% (Silvestry, 2014). As discussed in Chapter 11, patients with persistent LV failure are also at risk for development of pneumonia. Additionally, patients with perioperative renal failure and those who receive excessive blood product administration are also at a higher risk because of the additional fluid volume burden on the pulmonary system. Other identified independent predictors of postoperative pneumonia include COPD, postoperative AF, diabetes, smoking, older age, longer ICU length of stay (LOS), hypertension, preoperative corticosteroid use, and length of CPB time (Acker et al., 2011; Silvestry, 2014; Topal, 2012). Patients with incisional pain from either a sternotomy or thoracotomy are also at risk for developing pneumonia if the pain interferes with effective coughing and deep breathing (Silvestry, 2014).

Signs and symptoms may include fever, elevated white blood cell count, increased pulmonary secretions, and pulmonary infiltrates on chest radiograph. Hypoxemia may develop with associated increased oxygen requirements (Conde, 2012).

Aggressive use of incentive spirometry, chest physiotherapy, and early mobilization are all strategies to avoid postoperative pneumonia in the cardiac surgery population. Finally, one key to the avoidance of postoperative pneumonia is to follow evidence-based guidelines for the prevention and management of ventilator-associated conditions (VACs). Basic strategies for avoidance of VACs are oral hygiene using chlorhexidine solution, keeping patients semirecumbent, avoiding gastric over-distention, early nutrition, and daily sedation interruption for early weaning and extubation from the ventilator. These guidelines can be accessed in their entirety from the American Association of Critical-Care Nurses website (http://www.aacn.org/), in the "Practice Alerts" section.

HEMATOLOGIC COMPLICATIONS

Bleeding

Bleeding and clotting are common postoperative scenarios in the cardiac surgery patient population. Severe bleeding (i.e., bleeding requiring transfusion of more than 10 units of packed red blood cells) is reported to occur in up to 5% of patients. It is typically related to incomplete hemostasis, heparin used during CPB, decreased circulating clotting factors, hypothermia, dilutional decrease in platelets, coagulopathies, or platelet dysfunction (Silvestry, 2014). Postoperative bleeding typically subsides within the first few hours; however, 1% to 3% of patients will require mediastinal reexploration (Bojar, 2011). Typically, bleeding following cardiac surgery can be classified into two categories: surgical versus nonsurgical (coagulopathy). The etiology of postoperative bleeding may be surgical incision sites, platelet inhibition from exposure to preoperative antiplatelet drugs, platelet dysfunction from exposure to the CPB circuit, the effects of heparin, or a combination of these. Excessive bleeding is defined as loss of more than 500 mL of blood in the first postoperative hour. Bleeding is a significant contributor to postoperative morbidity and mortality; therefore prompt assessment and treatment in the ICU are critical. Administration of blood products may be enough to correct bleeding caused from coagulopathies. However, bleeding that persists despite correction of coagulation factors will require return to the OR for early mediastinal reexploration (Bojar, 2011; Ferraris et al., 2011). Usual sources of surgical bleeding include, but are not limited to, coronary anastomoses sites, saphenous vein branches, ITA takedown sites or the ITAs themselves, cannulation sites, or sternal wire sites.

Bleeding following cardiac surgery typically leads to administration of blood products (Silvestry, 2014). Packed red blood cells are often used to maintain adequate hemodynamic parameters, and to correct hemoglobin to ensure adequate and tissue oxygen delivery. Additionally, fresh frozen plasma, platelets, and cryoprecipitate are often required to correct other postoperative coagulopathies. It has been projected that cardiac surgery operations account for 15% of the nation's blood supply annually, with approximately 30% of all patients who undergo CABG requiring a blood transfusion (Ferraris et al., 2011). More importantly, evidence suggests that this number is increasing because of the changing age and acuity of our patients, as well as the complexity of the surgical procedures being offered (Ferraris et al., 2011).

There are various risk factors that predispose patients to postoperative bleeding following cardiac surgery. These are summarized in **Table 13-5**.

Quantitative assessment of postoperative bleeding is critical to document the extent of hemorrhage and the associated patient response while rectifying the situation. General guidelines for excessive mediastinal bleeding are characterized by continuous chest tube output of greater than 200 mL/hr for 2 hours. Making sure the chest tubes remain patent and documentation of the color and consistency of chest tube output are important. Additionally, accurate and frequent documentation (every

15–30 minutes) of blood loss will be key to keeping up with volume replacement when excessive bleeding is occurring. Assessment of hemodynamics using a pulmonary artery catheter is important to provide information about filling pressures and CO. Maintenance of adequate hemodynamics is crucial. This is generally accomplished through administration of crystalloid and colloid solutions along with administration of packed red blood cells to keep hemoglobin 8 g/dL or above (Bojar, 2011; Ferraris et al., 2011). Typical indications for surgical reexploration are blood loss greater than 200 mL/hr for 4 hours, 300 mL/hr for 2–3 hours, 400 mL/hr for 1 hour, or 500 mL/hr for 1 hour (Bojar, 2011; Ferraris et al., 2011). Additionally, surgical reexploration should be reconsidered when there is acute onset of bleeding (> 300 mL/hr) after a period of minimal bleeding had been noted (Bojar, 2011).

In addition to hemodynamics, coagulation studies should be monitored. Prothrombin time (PT)/activated partial thromboplastin time (aPTT), international normalized ratio (INR), fibrinogen level, platelet function testing, or thromboelastogram (TEG) should be obtained and trended so that platelets, cryoprecipitate, and fresh frozen plasma can be administered to correct abnormalities in platelets, fibrinogen, and coagulation factors, respectively (Enriquez & Shore-Lesserson, 2009). Additionally, medications that improve platelet function (e.g., desmopressin [DDAVP®]) or prevent fibrinolysis (e.g., epsilon-aminocaproic acid [Amicar®]) may also help in improving postoperative coagulopathy (Silvestry, 2014). Protamine sulfate is also administered to reverse the heparin given during CPB. Therefore, activated clotting times and TEG may be utilized to assess for heparin rebound or incomplete reversal as a factor in postoperative bleeding. There are several potential side effects related to protamine sulfate infusion—bradycardia and hypotension being most common.

Table 13-5   Risk Factors for Postoperative Bleeding Following Cardiac Surgery

Patient-Related Risk Factors

Advanced age

Females or those with small BSA

Advanced cardiac disease, LV dysfunction, shock, or any combination of these

Preoperative anemia

Known coagulopathies (e.g., Von Willebrand's disease, hemophilia)

Other extracardiac comorbidities—renal or hepatic disease, thrombocytopenia

Preoperative Medications

High-dose aspirin

Antiplatelet drugs such as clopidogrel (Plavix®), prasugrel (Effient®), and ticagrelor (Brilinta®)

Low-molecular-weight heparin or fondaparinux within 24 hours of procedure

Incomplete reversal of INR off warfarin

Emergency surgery while on glycoprotein IIb/IIIa inhibitors eptifibatide (Integrilin®) or abciximab (ReoPro®)

Surgical Procedure–Related Risk Factors

Complex procedures—combined CABG/valve and others with long CPB time, circulatory arrest

Emergent procedures

Reoperations

Use of bilateral ITAs

Heparin rebound or incomplete reversal of heparin with protamine

BSA, body surface area; CABG, coronary artery bypass grafting; CPB, cardiopulmonary bypass; INR, international normalized ratio; ITAs, internal thoracic arteries; LV, left ventricular

Sources: Bojar, R. (2011). *Manual of perioperative care in adult cardiac surgery* (5th ed.). Hoboken, NJ: Blackwell; Ferraris, V., Brown, J., Despotis, G., Hammon, J., Reece, T., Saha, S., . . . Clough, E. (2011). 2011 update to the Society of Thoracic Surgeons and the Society of Cardiovascular Anesthesiologists Blood Conservation Clinical Practice Guidelines. *Annals of Thoracic Surgery, 91*, 944–982.

A frequently used medication that may help in patients with severe and uncontrollable bleeding is factor VIIa. Recombinant activated factor VIIa provides a sudden surge of thrombin-expediting platelet activation and fibrin clot formation and produces a rapid improvement in the INR (Bojar, 2011), although evidence suggests that recombinant factor VIIa may be helpful in achieving hemostasis at the site of vessel injury, thereby reducing transfusion requirements. Activated platelets are present throughout the body following CPB. Therefore, systemic thrombosis may occur in 5% to 10% of patients (Bojar, 2011). Current recommendations exist for dosing factor VIIa for use in cardiac surgery patients (60 µg/kg) because it is expensive. There are specific dosing guidelines that are critical to avoid complications (e.g., acute graft closure) (Ferraris et al., 2011). Factor VIIa is discussed in more detail in Chapter 12.

Thrombosis

Patients who have undergone CABG procedures are also at risk for developing clots.

This is believed to be related to increased platelet activity. Aspirin may not be effective in mitigating clot formation (Silvestry, 2014).

Heparin-Induced Thrombocytopenia (HIT)

Thrombocytopenia is common following CPB. It affects 35% of high-risk postoperative patients (Rezende et al., 2011). In one study, 31.5% of patients developed a platelet count at least 33% lower than baseline (Chandra et al., 2013). In another study, HIT was present in 0.3% of cardiac surgery patients; secondary thrombocytopenia was present in 8.7% of patients. Patients with HIT had a mortality rate of 11.1% (vs. 4.5% of patients with thrombocytopenia and 4% of patients with secondary thrombocytopenia) (Seigerman, Cavallaro, Hagaki, Chung, & Chikwe, 2014).

This condition has numerous etiologies in cardiac surgery patients. Predictors of HIT include female gender, congestive heart failure, cardiac insufficiency, atrial fibrillation, hepatic disease, and chronic kidney injury. Heparin-induced thrombocytopenia is associated with increased risk of death, stroke, amputation, acute kidney injury, respiratory failure, and need for a tracheostomy (Seigerman et al., 2014). Factors such as effects of the CPB circuitry (e.g., mechanical destruction of platelets), hemodilution, platelet dysfunction, depletion of platelets, intravascular devices, use of IABP therapy, and effects of medications (e.g., antibiotics, antiarrhythmics) are common causes of thrombocytopenia in this population. A multitude of medications used in the cardiac surgery setting can also cause thrombocytopenia. One medication of significance is heparin, which is used to counteract exposure of the blood to the surfaces of the CPB machines (Bojar, 2011).

Heparin-induced thrombocytopenia is a prothrombotic disorder of coagulation caused by platelet-activating, heparin-dependent antibodies. The platelet activation effect leads to excessive thrombin generatic, evolving into a hypercoagulable state eliciting both venous and arterial thrombosis. Patients undergoing cardiac surgery are at a higher risk for HIT secondary to the large systemic dose and long exposure to unfractionated heparin required for both preoperative and intraoperative systemic anticoagulation (Selleng, Markentin, & Greinacher, 2007). Heparin-induced thrombocytopenia develops in approximately 1% of all inpatients receiving heparin. However, major thrombotic complications can be avoided when HIT is suspected by using alternative direct thrombin inhibitors for anticoagulation (e.g., bivalirudin [Angiomax®] and argatroban). The diagnosis of HIT should be considered when the platelet count falls to less than 150,000 mm^3 or by greater than 50% of the baseline count between 3 and 14 days of exposure. Laboratory testing with platelet factor-4/heparin enzyme-linked immunosorbent assay (ELISA) antibody and serotonin release assay are necessary to identify whether the patient has acquired the antibodies (Eke, 2014). When HIT is suspected, all heparin products must be discontinued, including use of heparin-coated vascular access catheters and heparin flushes for intravenous lines. Non-heparin anticoagulants (direct thrombin inhibitors), such as argatroban, should be administered even when confirmatory lab results are not yet available to prevent new thrombosis. Argatroban has been approved by the U.S. Food and Drug Administration for prevention and treatment of HIT (Eke, 2014).

Correlation of laboratory data with clinical symptoms is important for an accurate diagnosis. Careful and thorough assessment for areas of new thrombosis should occur by monitoring skin temperature, color, sensation, and peripheral pulses. In addition, ongoing recognition of signs and symptoms of stroke, MI, pulmonary embolism, and renal impairment are important, because they signal a much more serious complication of HIT. Postoperative care should include use of measures to prevent venous thrombotic events, including early mobility (ambulation if possible), isometric exercises, sequential compression devices, graduated compression stockings, or combinations of these interventions (Mullen-Fortino & O'Brien, 2008).

RENAL COMPLICATIONS

Cardiac surgery–associated acute kidney injury (CSA-AKI) is a common and serious complication of the use of CPB and is among the top two causes of AKI in the ICU (Mao et al., 2013). The incidence of postoperative renal complications is reported as high as 30%, and mortality rates for those developing CSA-AKI requiring dialysis can be upwards of 55% (Mao et al., 2013; Silvestry, 2014). In addition, AKI following cardiac surgery has been correlated with poor quality of life, longer lengths of hospital stay, and decreased long-term survival (Lagercrantz, Lindblom, & Sartipy, 2010). The associated mortality rate following cardiac surgery is 1% to 5%, depending on the type of cardiac surgery and preoperative comorbidities (Silvestry, 2014). Data from 1998 suggest that the costs associated with AKI following cardiac surgery were hundreds of millions of dollars (Mangano, Diamondstone, & Ramsey, 1998).

Preoperative risk factors for development of AKI include increased age, female gender, reduced LV function or moderate to advanced heart failure, diabetes mellitus, COPD, peripheral vascular disease, emergent or reoperative surgery, advanced atherosclerotic disease, preoperative use of contrast media, decreased creatinine clearance (glomerular filtration rate < 60 mL/min), and elevated creatinine levels (> 1.5 mg/dL) (Bojar, 2011; Mao et al., 2013; Silvestry, 2014).

Long duration of CPB is thought to put the patient at risk for AKI. It is believed to be related to renal artery vasoconstriction, hypothermia, loss of pulsatile blood flow while on CPB, and atheroembolic disease (Silvestry, 2014). There are also several intraoperative measures that should be employed to avoid renal complications and preserve renal blood flow during cardiac surgical procedures. Development of CSA-AKI is associated with a variety of factors. The most critical factor is maintenance of adequate mean perfusion pressures to ensure renal perfusion while on CPB. For that reason, keeping the CPB run as short as possible, off-pump coronary artery surgery, or minimally invasive procedures are good options for preservation of renal function. Additional intraoperative measures include optimizing hemodynamics both before and after the initiation of CPB through the use of vasopressors and administration of antifibrinolytics to minimize perioperative bleeding (Bojar, 2011). Avoidance of nephrotoxic agents (e.g., aminoglycosides, angiotensin-converting enzyme inhibitors, and contrast media) in the immediate postoperative period is also suggested (Silvestry, 2014).

Postoperatively, aggressive intervention and early recognition of CSA-AKI may prevent serious and permanent renal damage. The ICU nurse plays a key role in the optimization of hemodynamics. This can often be challenging in the early postoperative phase when rewarming occurs and fluid shifts may cause extreme blood pressure lability. Additionally, prompt identification of reduced urine output, worsening tissue edema, and discontinuation of any potential nephrotoxic drugs are key to renal function preservation. In nonoliguric renal failure, treatment should be directed toward restriction of fluids, administration of diuretics, and close electrolyte monitoring and replacement. Although loop diuretics such as furosemide have not been shown to improve renal function or recovery, they have been shown to increase urine output and prevent the progression to oliguric renal failure (Bojar, 2011).

Likewise, administration of renal dose dopamine remains controversial, because data do not support improved survival or prevention of renal failure with this therapy. Further, there are no supportive data for the use of aggressive dialysis, although some unease exists that renal function may be augmented with these techniques. Dialysis should be considered with signs and symptoms of uremia, fluid overload, and electrolyte abnormalities (vs. blood urea nitrogen and creatinine levels) (Silvestry, 2014).

Fortunately, only a small percentage (1% to 5%) of patients with CSA-AKI require initiation of renal replacement therapy (RRT) (Mao et al., 2013). Although optimal timing to initiate RRT following cardiac surgery remains uncertain, recent data suggest that once oliguric renal failure that is resistant to diuretics occurs, RRT should be instituted as soon as possible (Bojar, 2011; Mao et al., 2013). The most common forms of RRT used following cardiac surgery include intermittent hemodialysis and continuous venovenous hemofiltration. Regardless of the type of RRT utilized, placement of special vascular access catheters is required. Additionally, patient care is centered on managing the fluid and electrolyte shifts caused by this treatment. The ICU nurse plays a key role in the monitoring and treatment of metabolic acidosis, hyper-/hypokalemia, hypomagnesemia, hypocalcemia, and hyperglycemia. The care of these patients can be quite challenging; therefore, prompt treatment of the underlying cause is critical.

Maintenance of glycemic control (blood sugar < 180 mg/dL) has been linked to improved outcomes and prevention of serious infection. Likewise, early nutritional intervention and support during critical illness have been shown to improve patient recovery by reducing the risk of development of other additional serious postoperative complications (Abunnaja, Cuviello, & Sanchez, 2012).

GASTROINTESTINAL COMPLICATIONS

Gastrointestinal (GI) complications occur in 1% to 3% of all patients undergoing cardiac surgical procedures, and the mortality rate averages around 25% (Bojar, 2011). The pathophysiology of the most serious GI complications is related to perioperative low CO, which produces vasoconstriction, hypoxia, and hypoperfusion resulting in intestinal ischemia. Other GI complications include paralytic ileus, GI hemorrhage secondary to gastritis or perforated peptic ulcer disease, acute pancreatitis, acute cholecystitis, and acute hepatic failure (Dong et al., 2012).

Predictive factors for the development of GI complications include advanced age, chronic kidney disease, history of peptic ulcer disease, poor LV function, reoperations or prolonged CPB, the use of an IABP, prolonged mechanical ventilation, and AF (Bojar, 2011; Dong et al., 2012).

Most GI complications are difficult to diagnose because of their atypical symptoms, and the presence of incisional pain often makes it difficult to accurately describe their symptoms. All of these factors may delay diagnosis or treatment leading to serious and often fatal sequelae of respiratory failure, renal failure, sepsis, and shock.

Overall, the mortality rate is 50% among patients who develop serious GI complications related to visceral or splanchnic hypoperfusion and ischemia (Dong et al., 2012). This hypoperfusion stems from low CO. Therefore, as with most complications of cardiac surgery, prevention, early recognition, and intervention are key, and maintenance of adequate perfusion pressure while on CPB is critical. Additionally, the presence of atheromatous disease of the aorta and perioperative paroxysmal atrial fibrillation also places the patient at high risk for development of serious embolic/ischemic GI complications.

Postoperatively, all patients return to the ICU with a nasogastric tube in place, which typically remains in place until after extubation. Administration of anti-acid medications (e.g., famotidine [Pepcid®] or ranitidine [Zantac®]) is standard for all patients admitted to the ICU; proton pump inhibitors (e.g., pantoprazole [Protonix®] or esomeprazole [Nexium®]) are often added for those patients with a history of peptic ulcer disease to prevent serious complications. Postoperatively, diet is advanced as tolerated, but the ICU nurse should monitor the patient for presence and changes in bowel sounds, abdominal pain or distention, nausea, and vomiting. Initial treatment of suspected GI complications is conservative—nothing administered orally (NPO) and supportive care with intravenous fluids and medications. If GI complications are suspected, diagnostic lab tests—complete blood count, comprehensive metabolic panel, liver function tests, amylase and lipase, and lactic acid levels—should be performed. An abdominal radiograph, computed tomography scan, or both may be obtained. Once a diagnosis has been made, early surgical intervention via a laparotomy is warranted and may be life-saving in those patients who are attempting to compensate for ischemic bowel or a major GI-induced sepsis or bleed (Dong et al., 2012).

NEUROLOGIC COMPLICATIONS

Cardiac surgery patients may develop any of a wide range of neurologic complications. The reported incidence is 2% to 6% in this patient population (Silvestry, 2014). Neurologic complications resulting in central nervous system injury may be divided into two types. Type I is a focal injury such as stroke or encephalopathy. Type II is a neurocognitive insult—memory deficit, a notable decline in intellectual function, and seizure. The risk of developing a type I complication is more likely in procedures where CPB is utilized or in those patients with advanced age or undergoing valvular surgery (Bojar, 2011).

Preoperative risk factors for neurologic complications include prior stroke or transient ischemic attack, carotid artery disease, increased age, female gender, smoking, atrial fibrillations, and atherosclerosis of the ascending aorta (Bojar, 2011). Neurologic complications following cardiac surgery are discussed in detail in Chapter 16.

SYSTEMIC INFLAMMATORY RESPONSE TO CARDIAC SURGERY

The body's complement system is composed of more than 30 proteins; activation of this system and the resulting inflammatory response can have serious effects on the cardiac surgery patient (Stahl, Shernan, Smith, & Levy, 2012). Inflammation is the body's response to the disruption within the tissues and involves a series of controlled humoral and cellular reactions. Complement activation during cardiac surgery can be triggered by a number of mechanisms: tissue trauma during the procedure and the resulting release of plasmin; intravenous administration of protamine following CPB; and, most recently, cardiac dysrhythmias have been directly correlated with high levels of C-reactive protein markers following CABG (Stahl et al., 2012). Additionally, a very specific activator of the response can be seen as a result of CPB when a patient's blood comes into contact with the foreign surface of the CPB circuit.

The systemic inflammatory response is characterized by the release of pro-inflammatory factors such as interleukins 6 and 8 (IL-6 and IL-8) and tumor necrosis factor, and it has been directly linked to several postoperative complications. This inflammatory response has been directly correlated to myocardial ischemia and reperfusion injury, pulmonary dysfunction, ARDS, and severe systemic peripheral vasodilation, often requiring vasopressor support (Stahl et al., 2012).

Current recommendations for treatment call for supportive care until the inflammatory response resolves. Much research is being conducted on specific complement pathway inhibitors. Investigational studies are being conducted to both identify a genetic component to complement response and specific pathway inhibitors to improve outcomes. Likewise, the use of statins (e.g., atorvastatin [Lipitor®] or simvastatin [Zocor®]) has been shown to play a role in the reduction of oxidative stress and C-reactive protein and may diminish the associated inflammatory response (Martinez-Comendador, Alvarez, Sierra, Teijeira, & Adrio, 2013). Additionally, advances in CPB technology have resulted in the routine use of heparin-coated circuits, thereby making them more biocompatible, reducing the complement and platelet activation and local immune response (Bojar, 2011).

INFECTIOUS COMPLICATIONS

Infectious complications occur in 5% to 20% of all cardiac surgery cases, increasing postoperative mortality and prolonging hospital LOS (Cove, Spelman, & MacLaren, 2012). The most common infections following cardiac surgery are respiratory, surgical site, and those related to devices such as urinary catheters. Several prophylactic measures are taken to minimize a patient's risk for a perioperative infection. Antibiotics administered just prior to skin incision reduce the incidence of mediastinitis. Similarly, the use of preoperative intranasal mupirocin and chlorhexidine oral rinses have been shown to reduce staphylococcal and other nosocomial respiratory infections (Bojar, 2011).

Surgical site infections (SSIs) following cardiac surgery can present in varying forms of severity, affecting both the graft harvest sites as well as the sternal incision. These infections can be classified as either superficial—limited to the skin or subcutaneous tissue—or deep—involving the sternal bone, substernal space, or mediastinum (mediastinitis) (Cove et al., 2012). Fortunately, deep sternal wound infections (DSWIs) occur in less than 2% of patients, as they are potentially lethal—carrying a 50% mortality rate when they are present (Cove et al., 2012). Identified risk factors for this complication include increased body mass index (BMI), diabetes, COPD, duration of surgery, use of an IABP, older age, previous cardiac surgery, LVEF 30% or less, peripheral vascular disease, administration of blood products, and impaired nutritional status. Additional surgical factors that may lead to DSWI include the use of bilateral ITA grafts, prolonged surgery or CPB time (more than 90 minutes), excessive mediastinal bleeding or reexploration, and hyperglycemia in the ICU (Al-Zaur, Ammouri, Al-Hassan, & Amr, 2010; Ariyaratnam, Bland, & Loubani, 2010; Floros et al., 2011; Kubota et al., 2013).

Diligence related to glycemic control—maintenance of glucose levels less than 180 mg/dL for the first two postoperative days—has been shown to improve surgical mortality and is therefore one of the core measures of quality following cardiac surgical procedures. The ICU nurse should monitor the patient for purulent discharge from the wound, fever, increased pain or tenderness of the chest wall, or an unstable sternum. In addition to adhering to facility-specific wound care policies, administration of prophylactic antibiotic therapy for 48 hours and tight glycemic control help to minimize the likelihood of serious infections. Wound care is discussed in detail in Chapter 18.

SUMMARY

The initial 24-hour period following cardiac surgery is a challenging and tenuous time. Patients have high levels of vulnerability and instability in the initial postoperative period. While there is some degree of predictability in terms of the postoperative trajectory, the trends toward increasing age and number of preoperative comorbidities in these patients have increased the level of complexity associated with this population. Most patients, despite their initial instability, are successfully extubated within 6–12 hours and discharged from the ICU within 24 hours, and have an overall hospital LOS of 4–7 days (Bojar, 2011).

The role of ICU nurses cannot be overemphasized in terms of their influence in reducing the likelihood of critical events associated with postoperative complications. High levels of clinical judgment, adherence to evidence-based practice guidelines, and caring practices are essential competencies. Prevention and prompt recognition of postoperative complications are pivotal to help ensure optimal patient outcomes.

CASE STUDY

A 77-year-old female patient with a history of ST-segment elevation MI involving the inferior wall, mitral regurgitation, diabetes, hypertension, body mass index of 35 kg/m^2, 1-pack per day of tobacco, COPD, and doxorubicin-induced cardiomyopathy is admitted. She underwent on-pump CABG for 3-vessel disease with mitral valve replacement. Her intraoperative course was uneventful except for slightly prolonged CPB time. She was admitted to the cardiovascular ICU postoperatively. Admitting hemodynamic parameters are as follows: BP 150/92, HR 116, PAP 40/22 mmHg, CVP 16 mmHg, SVR 1,600 dynes/sec/cm^{-5}, CI 1.8 L/min/m^2.

Critical Thinking Questions

1. What risk factors does this patient have for low cardiac output syndrome?
2. What factors should the nurse consider when determining whether this patient is at risk for postoperative pulmonary complications?
3. Why is this patient at risk for hematologic complications?

Answers to Critical Thinking Questions

1. Age, combined CABG/valve procedure, prolonged CPB time.
2. Female gender, smoking history, diabetes, prolonged CPB time, heart failure, general anesthesia, neuromuscular blocking agents, obesity, supine positioning, median sternotomy, low LVEF. She may be at risk for prolonged mechanical ventilation, atelectasis, and pneumonia.
3. This patient is at risk for bleeding from exposure to CPB circuitry, heparin effects, advanced age, female, LV dysfunction, combined CABG/valve procedure, and prolonged CPB time.

SELF-ASSESSMENT QUESTIONS

1. Which of the following patients is at greatest risk for development of complications following cardiac surgery? A:
   a. 72-year-old having first cardiac surgery with LVEF 45%
   b. 66-year-old with diabetes having CABG/valve surgery with LVEF 35%
   c. 57-year-old with renal dysfunction and LVEF 50%
   d. 68-year-old with delirium and LVEF 40%

2. Patients with a history of which of the following rhythms is at greatest risk for developing complications following cardiac surgery?
   a.
   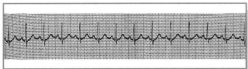
   b.
   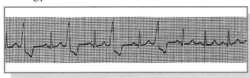
   c.
   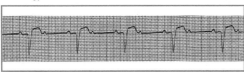
   d.
   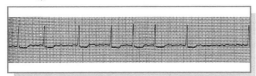

3. Which of the following statements indicates that the patient has an understanding of upcoming cardiac surgery?
   a. "I am looking forward to the surgery being over. My heart will contract much better right after it is over."
   b. "I opted not to have bypass with my surgery. I don't want my vital signs to be unstable after surgery."
   c. "My blood vessels may be dilated for a while after surgery. I may need medicine to help with that."
   d. "If my blood pressure is good right after surgery, I will know I am out of the woods."

4. Which of the following is a sign of exhausted compensatory mechanisms when decreased ventricular function is present?
   a. Cardiac output 6 L/minute
   b. Heart rate 50
   c. Capillary refill time 4 sec
   d. Urine output 0.5 mL/kg/hr

5. Which of the following arterial blood gas results may be found in a patient with decreased ventricular function following cardiac surgery?

	pH	pCO_2	HCO_3
a.	7.28	35	18
b.	7.48	30	22
c.	7.50	40	28
d.	7.30	50	25

6. Which of the following hemodynamic parameters is optimal in a postoperative cardiac surgery patient?
   a. HR 105
   b. CI 2.5 $L/min/m^2$
   c. CVP 17 mmHg
   d. SVR 1,200 $dynes/sec/cm^{-5}$

7. For which of the following should the nurse observe in a patient who underwent aortic valve replacement?
   a. MAP 75 mmHg
   b. CO 1.8 L/minute
   c. HR 50
   d. SvO_2 70%

8. Which of the following interventions should the nurse anticipate for a patient whose cardiac index is 2.2 $L/min/m^2$ following cardiac surgery?

a. Prevention of hypothermia
b. Mechanical ventilation
c. Treatment of bradycardia
d. Withholding sedation and analgesia

9. Which of the following may be a cause of postoperative hemodynamics including a CVP 1 mmHg and PAOP 6 mmHg?
   a. Increased LV compliance
   b. Vasoconstriction during rewarming
   c. Hypothermia
   d. Increased vasomotor tone

10. Which of the following sets of hemodynamic parameters should the nurse anticipate in a patient with diastolic dysfunction following cardiac surgery?

	PAOP (mmHg)	CO (L/min)
a.	20	6
b.	7	9
c.	5	4
d.	18	3.5

Answers to Self-Assessment Questions

1. b	6. b
2. d	7. b
3. c	8. b
4. c	9. c
5. a	10. d

Clinical Inquiry Box

Questions: What is the incidence of pulmonary complications following open heart surgery and what are the predisposing factors?

Reference: Al-Qubati, F. A. A. Damag, A., & Noman, T. (2013). Incidence and outcome of pulmonary complications after open cardiac surgery, Thowra Hospital, Cardiac Center, Sana'a, Yemen. *Egyptian Journal of Chest Diseases and Tuberculosis, 62*(4), 775–780.

Objectives: To determine the incidence of pulmonary complications after open heart surgery and identify their predisposing factors.

Method: Prospective study

Results: The incidence of pulmonary complications was 15.08% with an associated mortality rate of 18.5%. Pulmonary complications occurred in 2.23% of patients who underwent valve replacement and 5.05% of patients with congenital heart disease. The incidence of ARDS was 3.35% with an associated mortality rate of 66.6%, pneumonia occurred in 2.79%, atelectasis occurred in 3.35%, pleural effusion occurred in 2.27%, and pneumothorax occurred in 0.55%. Most predisposing factors included massive blood transfusion, reexploration for control of postoperative bleeding, CPB, and increased length of stay in the ICU.

Conclusion: Cardiopulmonary bypass time kept as short as possible and PEEP 7–8 cmH$_2$O during mechanical ventilation help prevent ARDS. Prophylactic use of broad spectrum antibiotics will help prevent infection. Early ambulation and physiotherapy are recommended.

REFERENCES

Abunnaja, A., Cuviello, A., & Sanchez, J. A. (2012). Enteral and parenteral nutrition in the perioperative period: State of the art. *Nutrients, 5*, 608–623.

Acker, M. A., Argenziano, M., Puskas, J. D., Ferguson, B. F., Gilijns, A. C., & Blackstone, E. H. (2011). Abstract 12247: Infections after cardiac surgery: Initial experience from the Cardiothoracic Surgical Trials Network. *Circulation, 124*, A12247.

Al-Attar, N. (2011). *Postoperative myocardial infarction*. Retrieved from http://www.escardio.org/communities/councils/ccp/e-journal/volume10/Pages/Postoperative- myocardial-infarction-Nawwar-Al-Attar.aspx#.VKlfKSeodKo

Al-Zaur, I. M., Ammouri, A. A., Al-Hassan, M. A., & Amr, A. A. (2010). Risk factors for deep sternal wound injuries after cardiac surgery in Jordan. *Journal of Clinical Nursing, 19*(13–14), 1873–1881.

Alsaddique, A. A., Royse, C. F., Fouda, M. A., & Royse, A. G. (2012). *Diastolic heart failure after cardiac surgery*. Retrieved from http://cdn.intechopen.com/pdfs-wm/32299.pdf

Ariyaratnam, P., Bland, M., & Loubani, M. (2010). Risk factors and mortality associated with deep sternal wound injuries following coronary bypass surgery with or without concomitant procedures in a UK population: A basis for a new risk model. *Interactive Cardiovascular and Thoracic Surgery, 11*, 543–546.

Beebe, R., & Myers, J. (2011). Heart failure. In R. Beebe & J. Myers (Eds.), *Professional paramedic: Medical emergencies, maternal health, and pediatrics* (pp. 66–97). Clifton Park, NY: Delmar.

Bojar, R. (2011). *Manual of perioperative care in adult cardiac surgery* (5th ed). Hoboken, NJ: Blackwell.

Čanádyová, J., Zmeko, D., & Mikráček, A. (2012). Re-exploration for bleeding or tamponade after cardiac operation. *Interactive Cardiovascular and Thoracic Surgery, 14*(6), 704–707.

Chandra, A. B., Mittal, N., Sanbidi, S., Belur, A., Pathak, S., Pathak, H., . . . Xu, Y. (2013). Low incidence of clinically significant heparin-induced thrombocytopenia after cardiopulmonary bypass surgery. *Journal of Blood Disorders & Transfusion, 5*, 180. doi: 10.4172/2155-9864.1000180

Conde, M. V. (2012). *Overview of management of postoperative pulmonary complications*. Retrieved from http://www.uptodate.com/contents/overview-of-the-management-of-postoperative-pulmonary-complications?source=search_result&search=overview+of+management+of+postoperative+pulmonary+complications&selectedTitle=1~150

Cool, S.-C., Thomas, M., Nolan, J., & Parr, M. (2014). Cardiac surgery—postoperative care. In S.-C. Cool, M. Thomas, J. Nolan, & M. Parr (Eds.), *Key clinical topics in critical care* (pp. 90–95). London: J. P. Medical Ltd.

Cove, M., Spellman, D., & MacLaren, G. (2012). Infectious complications of cardiac surgery: A clinical review. *Journal of Cardiothoracic and Vascular Anesthesia, 26*(6), 1094–1100.

Daley, B. J. (2014). *Pneumothorax treatment and management*. Retrieved from http://emedicine.medscape.com/article/424547-treatment

Dong, G., Liu, C, Xu, B., Jing, H., Li, D., & Wu, H. (2012). Postoperative abdominal complications after cardiopulmonary bypass. *Journal of Cardiothoracic Surgery, 7*(108), 1–5.

Eke, S. (2014). *Heparin-induced thrombocytopenia*. Retrieved from http://emedicine.medscape.com/article/1357846-overview

Enriquez, L. J., & Shore-Lesserson, L. (2009). Point-of-care coagulation testing and transfusion algorithms. *British Journal of Anaesthesia, 103*(Suppl. 1), i14–122.

Ferraris, V., Brown, J., Despotis, G., Hammon, J., Reece, T., Saha, S., . . . Clough, E. (2011). 2011 update to the Society of Thoracic Surgeons and the Society of Cardiovascular Anesthesiologists Blood Conservation Clinical Practice Guidelines. *Annals of Thoracic Surgery, 91*, 944–982.

Floerchinger, B., Camboni, D., Schopka, S., Kolat, P., Hilker, M., & Schmid, C. (2013). Delayed cardiac tamponade after open heart surgery—Is supplemental CT imaging reasonable? *Journal of Cardiothoracic Surgery, 8*, 158.

Floros, P., Sawhney, R., Vrtik, M., Hinton-Bayre, A., Weimers, P., Senewirathe, S., . . . Shah, P. (2011). Risk factors and management approach for deep sternal wound infections after cardiac surgery at a tertiary medical centre. *Heart, Lung and Circulation, 20*(11), 712–717.

Gologorsky, E., Macedo, F. I. B., Carvalho, E. M., Gologorsky, A., Ricci, M., & Salerno, T. A. (2010). Postoperative cardiac arrest after heart surgery: Does extracorporeal perfusion support a paradigm change in management? *Anesthesiology Research and Practice, 2010*. Article # 937215. Retrieved from http://www.hindawi.com/journals/arp/2010/937215/

Guarracino, F., Baldassarri, R., & Pinsky, M. R. (2013). Ventriculo-arterial decoupling in acutely altered hemodynamic status. In J.-L. Vincent (Ed.), *2013 annual update in intensive care and emergency medicine* (pp. 225–236). New York, NY: Springer.

Haddad, F., Couture, P., Tousignant, C., & Denault, A. Y. (2009). The right ventricle in cardiac surgery, a perioperative perspective: II. Pathophysiology, clinical importance, and management. *Anesthesia & Analgesia, 18*(2), 422–433.

Heffner, J. E. (2013). *Pleural effusions following cardiac surgery*. Retrieved from http://www.uptodate.com/contents/pleural-effusions-following-cardiac-surgery

Helgadottir, S., Sigurdsson, M. I., Ingvarsdottir, I. L., Arnar, D. O., & Gudbjartsson, T. (2012). Atrial fibrillation following cardiac surgery: Risk analysis and long-term survival. *Journal of Cardiovascular Surgery, 7*(87), 1749–1753.

Jain, A., Arora, D., Juneja, R., Mehta, Y., & Trehan, N. (2014). Life-threatening tension pneumothorax during cardiac surgery: A case report. *Heart, Lung and Vessels, 6*(3), 204–207.

Januzzi, J. L. (2009). Troponin testing after cardiac surgery. *HSR Proceedings in Intensive Care & Cardiovascular Anesthesia, 1*(3), 22–32.

Jensen, L., & Yang, L. (2007). Risk factors for postoperative pulmonary complications in coronary artery bypass graft surgery patients. *European Journal of Cardiovascular Nursing, 6*(3), 241–246.

Ji, Q., Mei, Y., Wang, X., Feng, J., Cai, J., & Ding, W. (2013). Risk factors for pulmonary complications following cardiac surgery with cardiopulmonary bypass. *International Journal of Medical Sciences, 10*(11), 1578–1583.

Ji, Z., Mei, Y., Wang, X., Feng, J., Cai, J., Xie, S., . . . Hu, D. (2008). Study on the risk factors of postoperative hypoxemia in patients undergoing coronary artery bypass grafting. *Circulation, 72*(18), 1975–1980.

Kamanger, N. (2013). *Diaphragmatic paralysis*. Retrieved from http://www.emedicine.medscape.com/article/298200-followup

Khalpey, Z. I., Ganim, R. B., & Rawn, J. D. (2008). Postoperative care of cardiac surgery patients. In L. H. Cohn (Ed.), *Cardiac surgery in the adult* (pp. 465–486). New York, NY: McGraw-Hill.

Kiessling, A. H., Huneke, P., Reyher, C., Bingold, T., Zierer, A., & Moritz, A. (2013). Risk factor analysis for fast track protocol failure. *Journal of Cardiothoracic Surgery, 8*, 47. Retrieved from http://www.cardiothoracicsurgery.org/content/8/1/47

Klabunde, R. E. (2013). *Ventricular and atrial hypertrophy and dilation*. Retrieved from http://www.cvphysiology.com/Heart%20Failure/HF009.htm

Kouchoukos, N. T., Blackstone, E. H., Hanley, F. L., & Kirklin, J. K. (2013). Postoperative care. In N. T. Kouchoukos, E. H. Blackstone, F. L. Hanley, & J. K. Kirklin (Eds.), *Kirklin/Barratt-Boyes cardiac surgery* (4th ed., pp. 189–250). Philadelphia, PA: Elsevier.

Kraut, J. A., & Madias, N. E. (2010). Metabolic acidosis: Pathophysiology, diagnosis and management. *Nature Reviews: Nephrology, 6*(5), 274–285.

Kubota, H., Miyata, H., Motomura, N., Ono, M., Takamoto, S., Harii, K., . . . Kyo, S. (2013). Deep sternal wound infections after cardiac surgery. *Journal of Cardiothoracic Surgery, 8*, 132. Retrieved from http://www.cardiothoracicsurgery.org/content/8/1/132

Lagercrantz, E., Lindblom, D., & Sartipy, U. (2010). Survival and quality of life in cardiac surgery patients with prolonged intensive care. *Annals of Thoracic Surgery, 89*, 490–496.

Levitov, A., & Marik, P. E. (2011). Echocardiographic assessment of preload responsiveness in critically ill patients. *Cardiology Research and Practice, 2012*. Article ID 819696. Retrieved from http://www.hindawi.com/journals/crp/2012/819696/

Lim, C. C. S., Cuculi, F., van Gaal, W. J., Testa, L., Arnold, J. R., Karamitsosi, T., . . . Banning, A. P. (2011). Early diagnosis of perioperative myocardial infarction after coronary artery bypass grafting: A study using biomarkers and cardiac magnetic resonance imaging. *Annals of Thoracic Surgery, 92*, 2046–2053.

Madappa, T. (2014). *Atelectasis treatment and management*. Retrieved from http://emedicine.medscape.com/article/296468-treatment

Maesen, B., Nijs, J., Maessen, J., Allessie, M., & Schotten, U. (2012). Post-operative atrial fibrillation: A maze of mechanisms. *Eurospace, 14*(2), 159–174.

Mangano, C. M., Diamondstone, L. S., & Ramsey, J. G. (1998). Renal dysfunction after myocardial revascularization: Risk factors, adverse outcomes, and hospital resource utilization. *Annals of Internal Medicine, 128*, 194–203.

Mao, H., Katz, N., Ariyanon, W., Blanca-Mantos, L., Adýbelli, Z., Giuliani, A., . . . Ronco, C. (2013). Cardiac surgery-associated acute kidney injury. *Cardiorenal Medicine, 3*, 178–199.

Martinez-Comendador, J., Alvarez, J. R., Sierra, J., Teijeira, E., & Adrio, B. (2013). Preoperative statin therapy in cardiac surgery is more effective in patients who display preoperative activation of the inflammatory system. *Texas Heart Institute Journal, 40*(1), 42–49.

Mazzeffi, M., & Rock, P. (2012). Should we prone cardiac surgery patients with acute respiratory distress syndrome? *Annals of Thoracic Surgery, 97*(3), 1122.

Milot, J., Perron, J., Lacasse, Y., Letourneau, L., Cartier, P., & Maltais, F. (2001). Incidence and predictors of ARDS after cardiac surgery. *Chest, 119*(3), 884–888.

Mullen-Fortino, M., & O'Brien, N. (2008). Caring for a patient after coronary artery bypass graft surgery. *Nursing, 38*(3), 46–52.

Nair, S. G. (2010). Atrial fibrillation after cardiac surgery. *Annals of Cardiac Anaesthesia, 13*(3), 196–205.

Nakazato, K., Takeda, S., Tanaka, K., & Sakamoto, A. (2012). Aggressive treatment with noninvasive ventilation for mild hypoxemic respiratory failure after cardiovascular surgery: Retrospective observational study. *Journal of Cardiothoracic Surgery, 7.* Retrieved from http://cardiothoracicsurgery.org/content/pdf/1749-8090-7-41.pdf

Neto, J. D. C., Neto, J. A. L., Simões, M. A. C., & Stolf, N. A. G. (2010). Coronary-artery spasm after coronary artery bypass graft without extracorporeal circulation. Diagnostic and management. *Revista Brasileira de Cirurgia Cardiovascular, 25*(3), 410–414.

Padovani, C., & Cavenaghi, O. M. (2011). Alveolar recruitment in patients in the immediate postoperative period of cardiac surgery. *Revista Brasileira de Cirurgia Cardiovascular, 26*(1), 116–121.

Parissis, H., Soo, A., & Al-Alao, B. (2012). Intra-aortic balloon pump (IABP): From the old trends and studies to the current "extended" indications of its use. *Journal of Cardiothoracic Surgery, 7,* 128. doi: 10.1186/1749-8090-6-147

Peretto, G., Durante, A., Limite, L., & Cianflone, D. (2014). Postoperative arrhythmias after cardiac surgery: Incidence, risk factors and therapeutic management. *Cardiology Research and Practice, 2014,* 615987. Retrieved from http://dx.doi.org/10.1155/2014/615987

Rezende, E., Moralis, G., Silva, J. M., Jr., de Oliveria, A. M. R. R., Souza, J. M., Toledo, D. O., . . . Brandão, E. M. (2011). Thrombocytopenia in cardiac surgery: Diagnostic and prognostic importance. *Revista Brasileira de Cirurgia Cardiovascular, 26*(1), 47–55.

Rodrigues, A. J., Evora, P. M., & Evora, P. R. B. (2014). *Use of inhaled nitric oxide in cardiac surgery: What is going on?* Retrieved from http://www.intechopen.com/books/cardiac-surgery-a-commitment-to-science-technology-and-creativity/use-of-inhaled-nitric-oxide-in-cardiac-surgery-what-is-going-on-

Roekaert, S., & Heijmar, J. (2012). Postoperative considerations in cardiac surgery. In C. Narin (Ed.), *Perioperative considerations in cardiac surgery.* Retrieved from http://www.intechopen.com/books/howtoreference/perioperative-considerations-in-cardiac-surgery/-early-postoperative-care-after-cardiac-surgery

Rosas, M. M., Giocoechea-Turcott, E. W., Ortiz, P. L., Salazar, A., & Palma, B. A. (2012). Glycemic control in cardiac surgery. In C. Narin (Ed.), *Perioperative considerations in cardiac surgery* (pp. 247–264). Retrieved from http://www.intechopen.com/books/perioperative-considerations-in-cardiac-surgery/glycemic-control-in-cardiac-surgery

Schiavone, W. A. (2013). Cardiac tamponade: 12 pearls. *Cleveland Clinic Journal of Medicine, 80*(2), 109–116.

Seigerman, M., Cavallaro, P., Hagaki, S., Chung, I., & Chikwe, J. (2014). Incidence and outcomes of heparin-induced thrombocytopenia in patients undergoing cardiac surgery in North America: An analysis of the nationwide inpatient sample. *Journal of Cardiothoracic and Vascular Anesthesia, 28*(1), 98–102.

Selleng, K., Markentin, T., & Greinacher, A. (2007). Heparin induced thrombocytopenia in intensive care unit patients. *Critical Care Medicine, 35*(4), 1165–1176.

Shavelle, D. M. (2014). *Clinical syndromes of stunned or hibernating myocardium.* Retrieved from http://www.uptodate.com/contents/clinical-syndromes-of-stunned-or-hibernating-myocardium

Shen, J., Lall, S., Zheng, V., Buckley, P., Damiano, R. J., Jr., & Schuessler, R. B. (2011). The persistent problem of new-onset postoperative atrial fibrillation: A single-institution experience over two decades. *Journal of Thoracic and Cardiovascular Surgery, 141,* 559–570.

Sherwood, L. (2012). Cardiac physiology. In L. Sherwood (Ed.), *Fundamentals of human physiology* (pp. 225–259). Belmont, CA: Brooks/ Cole.

Silvestry, F. E. (2014). *Postoperative complications among patients undergoing cardiac surgery.* Retrieved from http://www.uptodate.com/ contents/postoperative-complications- among-patients-undergoing-cardiac-surgery

Singla, N., Warltier, D. C., Gandhi, S. D., Sladen, R. N., Aronson, S., . . . Corwin, H. L. (2008). Treatment of acute postoperative hypertension in cardiac surgery patients: An efficacy study of clevidipine. Assessing its postoperative antihypertensive effect in cardiac surgery–2 (ESCAPE-2), a randomized, double-blind, placebo-controlled trial. *Anesthesia & Analgesia, 107*(1), 59–67.

Stahl, G., Shernan, S., Smith, P., & Levy, J. (2012). Complement activation and cardiac surgery: A novel target for improving outcomes. *Anesthesia & Analgesia, 115*(4), 759–771.

Stark, P. (2013). *Imaging of pneumothorax.* Retrieved from http://www.uptodate.com/contents/ imaging-of-pneumothorax

Stephens, R. S., Shah, A. S., & Whitman, G. J. (2013). Lung injury and acute respiratory distress syndrome after cardiac surgery. *Annals of Thoracic Surgery, 95*(3), 1122–1129.

Thygesen, K., Alpert, J. S., & White, H. D. (2007). Universal definition of myocardial infarction. *Circulation, 116,* 2634–2653.

Topal, A. E. (2012). Risk factors for the development of pneumonia post cardiac surgery. *Cardiovascular Journal of Africa, 23*(4), 212–215.

Vlahakes, G. J. (2012). Right ventricular failure following cardiac surgery. *Cardiology Clinics, 30*(2), 283–289.

Wilson, S. F. (2012). Perfusion. In J. F. Giddens (Ed.), *Concepts for nursing practice—Pageburst E-Book on VitalSource.* Retrieved from http:// www.elsevieradvantage.com/samplechapters/9780323083775/Sample_Chapter.pdf

Yarlagadda, C. (2014). *Cardiac tamponade: Clinical presentation.* Retrieved from http://emedicine. medscape.com/article/152083-overview

Zafari, A. M. (2014). *Myocardial infarction treatment and management.* Retrieved from http://emedicine.medscape.com/article/155919-treatment

WEB RESOURCES

Median sternotomy: http://www.youtube.com/ watch?v=r7RsB0BA4EI:

Heparin-induced thrombocytopenia: https://www .youtube.com/watch?v=SWT5nZjnk_w

Sepsis development and progression: http://www .youtube.com/watch?v=HoxoeP-l5Uw

Chapter 14

Pain Management

Noreen O'Connor Peyatt

INTRODUCTION

One of the most common inquiries patients have prior to surgery is how much pain they will experience postoperatively (Vadivelu, Mitra, & Naravan, 2010). According to patients, pain following intrathoracic, abdominal, and gastric surgeries ranks among the most severe and lasts anywhere between 2 and 8 days (D'Arcy, 2011). Patients undergoing cardiac surgery also reveal that postoperative pain relief is a significant concern, and it is one of the most clinically challenging problems for nurses caring for these patients. Pain following cardiac surgery may be associated with the sternotomy, trauma caused by thoracic cage retractors, graft sites, chest tubes, mechanical ventilation, endotracheal tube suctioning, dressing changes, and even the use of air mattresses (Aslan, Badir, Arli, & Cakmakci, 2010). Unrelieved postoperative pain is associated with increased length of stay (LOS) and decreased patient satisfaction (Viscusi, 2012). Healthcare providers acknowledge that unrelieved postoperative pain can have deleterious effects on cardiac surgery outcomes. In the changing world of health care, decreasing length of stay, improving patient outcomes, and increasing patient satisfaction are imperative.

Inadequate pain relief may contribute to numerous complications in the postoperative period. The stress of unrelieved pain on the cardiovascular system results in activation of the sympathetic nervous system (SNS). This SNS activation produces a variety of unwanted effects. Postoperatively, these unwanted effects include hypercoagulation, tachycardia, hypertension, and increased myocardial workload and oxygen demand (Wells, Pasero, & McCaffery, 2008). Additionally, patients may suffer from atelectasis, pneumonia, inability to move bronchial secretions, muscle weakness, hyperglycemia, confusion, and an overwhelming stress response (Joshi & Jagadeesh, 2013). Aggressive pain control is essential in preventing these complications and improving outcomes. Cardiac morbidity is the primary cause of death following anesthesia and surgery (Wells et al., 2008).

Despite these potentially devastating complications, recent reviews report only modest success in effectively managing postoperative pain. An historic look at the undertreatment of pain reveals a landmark study in 1973 by Marks and Sachar in which the authors described that greater than 70% of hospitalized patients experienced moderate to severe pain (Wells et al., 2008). More than 40 years later, patients continue to describe inadequate pain control, and recent studies report pain is underestimated, undermedicated, and underrelieved (Bunchungmongkol & Pipanmekaporn, 2013). In a frequently cited study, a random sample of patients described the postoperative pain experience. Incredibly, approximately 80% of the patients surveyed indicated they experienced unrelieved postoperative pain (Apfelbaum, Chen, Mehta, & Gan, 2003). Despite significant advances in care, an estimated 50% to 70% of patients still experience moderate to severe postoperative pain (Pogatzki-Zhan, Zahn, & Brennan, 2007). Adding insult to injury, the incidence of chronic pain following cardiac surgery ranges from 21% to 55% (Cogan, 2010).

A prospective study of 200 patients who underwent open heart surgery revealed that the majority experienced moderate postoperative pain. In addition, those same patients reported significant pain in two or more sites that did not decrease during the first 2 days postoperatively (Mueller et al., 2000). Another study of patients following cardiac surgery reported that more than 77% of patients recalled having postoperative pain (Gélinas, 2007). Surveys of cardiac surgery patients at a Midwest academic medical center reflected lower than anticipated patient satisfaction ratings. Pain management became the focus of a multidisciplinary cardiovascular surgery team after recognizing that poor patient satisfaction was related to inadequate pain relief. The team sought to decrease stress, pain, and anxiety through a systematic approach to managing pain. As a result of their efforts, the center experienced excellent clinical outcomes, improved patient satisfaction, and high levels of technical expertise (Cutshall et al., 2007). This demonstrates that adequate pain relief is possible.

Although significant numbers of research studies support the presence of unmanaged postsurgical pain despite advances in pain management, little to no progress has been made in reducing the incidence of postoperative cardiac surgery pain (Gélinas, 2007). One possible contributor to inadequate pain management is the lack of regular reassessments following administration of analgesics. In one study, only 4.4% of pain-related interventions had associated reassessments targeting efficacy of an analgesic intervention (Bucknall, Manias, & Botti, 2007).

Other data support that while there is a high incidence of patients reporting moderate to severe levels of pain following cardiac surgery, those individuals receive only a small percentage of their prescribed or allotted analgesic dosage. Despite ordering and availability of analgesics by providers, some patients receive less than half of the amount of analgesic ordered (Vadivelu et al., 2010).

Presence of pain following cardiac surgery has implications for optimal recovery. In addition to surgical pain, patients report incidental pain associated with repositioning, coughing and deep breathing, using the incentive spirometer, moving or turning in bed, and getting up (Cogan, 2010; Gélinas, 2007).

Pain management requires effective and efficient assessment, treatment, and evaluation by all members of the healthcare team, with nurses playing a fundamental role. Nurses are essential advocates for patients who are experiencing pain. Nurses help ensure that patients receive the best possible pain and symptom management. To be an effective patient advocate, nurses must be able to recognize pain, be available, be ready to act, be empathetic instead of judgmental, and be willing to educate not only the patient but also the healthcare team (Pasero & McCaffery, 2011; St. Marie, 2010).

WHAT IS PAIN?

According to the International Association for the Study of Pain (IASP; 2008), "pain is an unpleasant sensory and emotional experience associated with actual or potential tissue damage, or described in terms of such damage" (p. 34). The subcommittee on Taxonomy of IASP first defined pain in 1979.

This definition continues to be used in the literature and practice (Gélinas, 2007; IASP, 2008). Pain is subjective and uniquely experienced by the individual patient (Ranger & Campbell-Yeo, 2008). Multiple factors, including previous pain experience, culture, mood, and coping skills, influence an individual's pain experience (Pasero & McCaffery, 2011; St. Marie, 2010). "The patient's experience of pain is seen as involving far more than a localized sensation; it encompasses what this sensation means to him" (McCaffery, 1972, p. 7).

Pain is subjective (Pasero & McCaffery, 2011; St. Marie, 2010; IASP, 2008). The patient's self-report of pain is the most reliable indicator of its presence. Pain is described as "whatever the person says it is and exists whenever he says it does" (McCaffery, 1972, p. 8). However, the inability to communicate does not preclude the fact the patient may still be experiencing pain. The use of the word "says" does not mean the patient must verbalize existence of pain. All patient behaviors—whether voluntary or involuntary, verbal or nonverbal—may indicate presence of pain (McCaffery, 1972). Measures must be taken to appropriately assess and treat patients who may be unable to verbally report pain (Gélinas, 2007; Herr et al., 2006; IASP, 2008; Pasero & McCaffery, 2011).

PAIN PATHWAYS AND PROCESSES

A specialized system, called the nociceptive system, mediates the sensory experience of acute pain. The term *nociception* describes the process by which information about an unpleasant or painful stimulus transmits from the periphery to the brain. Nociception is the total neural activity that occurs prior to the cognitive processes that enable individuals to identify or experience a sensation as pain. Nociception is necessary in order for

an individual to experience pain. Four unique processes comprise the process of nociception: transduction, transmission, perception, and modulation (St. Marie, 2010). The nociceptive process begins with the initial tissue injury, whether real or perceived.

Transduction, the first step in the nociceptive process, is the conversion of noxious stimuli into electrical energy or nerve impulses. Transduction occurs at nociceptors, or nerve endings that are activated by powerful stimuli. Noxious stimuli such as pressure, temperature extremes, mechanical insults such as a surgical incision, or irritant chemicals trigger the release of numerous chemicals. Chemical release includes bradykinin, histamine, and prostaglandins, which activate or sensitize the nociceptors. Some analgesic therapies work by preventing or modifying transduction. Local anesthetics and antiepileptic drugs block peripheral sodium channels and thus inhibit the production of the action potentials. Nonsteroidal antiinflammatory drugs (NSAIDs) inhibit the production of prostaglandins that would otherwise sensitize nociceptors (Dubin & Patapoutian, 2010).

Transmission is the actual conduction of painful impulses from the nociceptors in the periphery to the spinal cord and brain via two types of primary afferent neurons: myelinated A-delta fibers and unmyelinated C fibers. The A-delta fibers rapidly produce acute, sharp pain, while the C fibers conduct the impulse more slowly, thereby producing diffuse, dull, aching pain. From the nociceptor, the action potential travels to the dorsal root ganglia and then to the dorsal horn of the spinal cord. The location where nerve fibers enter the spinal cord helps to explain the pattern of pain sensed in cutaneous tissues. The primary afferent neurons release excitatory neurotransmitters such as glutamate in the spinal cord. These transmitters activate spinal neurons that send axons across the spinal cord and up ascending pain pathways via the spinothalamic tracts to the thalamus. Fibers synapse in the thalamus and make connections with other parts of the brain including the limbic system. Some medications exert their analgesic effects by regulating the release of neurotransmitters. Opioids work at the level of the spinal cord and bind to presynaptic receptors, decreasing calcium conduction and thus the release of neurotransmitters in the dorsal horn (Dubin & Patapoutian, 2010; Pasero & McCaffery, 2011; St. Marie, 2010).

Perception is the process by which a conscious individual recognizes the sensation of pain. Perception occurs as the brain processes the information. The spinal cord sends the information carried by the free nerve ending to the thalamus, and the information is then sent to the cortical areas of the brain where pain perception occurs. Sensory information about the pain combines with emotional, cognitive, and sociocultural determinants to create the pain experience. Many interventions can affect the perception of pain. For example, cognitive strategies such as distraction, relaxation, hypnosis, and imagery are effective pain-reducing therapies that operate at this level of the pain pathway and are useful pain management techniques (Dubin & Patapoutian, 2010; Pasero & McCaffery, 2011).

Modulation, the final step, occurs when stimuli are either enhanced or inhibited by the hypothalamus, pons, and somatosensory cortex so as to process and transmit a pain sensation (Dubin & Patapoutian, 2010; Pasero & McCaffery, 2011; St. Marie, 2010). Modulation involves both the peripheral and central nervous systems and many different neurochemicals. Endogenous opioids in the peripheral and central nervous systems and the central inhibitory neurotransmitters norepinephrine and serotonin are significant components in modulating pain impulses (Pasero & McCaffery, 2011; St. Marie, 2010). An example of modulation is the use of

antidepressants for the management of pain. Some antidepressants block the reuptake of the neurotransmitters, norepinephrine and serotonin, making them available in the fight against pain (Pasero & McCaffery, 2011; St. Marie, 2010). **Figure 14-1** depicts the pain physiology process.

Smoking serves as a nicotine-delivery vehicle and produces changes in physiology. Exposure to systemic nicotine has consistent antinociceptive effects. Chronic exposure of nicotine causes the endogenous opioid system to change in ways that may affect processing of nociceptive stimuli. Smoking can produce changes in central nervous system function that persist long after subjects stop smoking. Smokers have been found to complain of greater pain intensity and an increased number of painful sites overall as well as chronic pain. Nicotine withdrawal is thought to enhance perception of pain. Smoking also causes changes in the neuroendocrine system that could modulate pain perception. Smoking is thought to impair oxygen delivery to tissues by increasing sympathetic outflow and carboxyhemoglobin levels. Hence, smoking may accelerate degenerative processes that interfere with wound healing. Evidence supports that an increase in postoperative analgesic requirements should be anticipated in cigarette smokers (Shi, Weingarten, Mantilla, Hooten, & Warner, 2010).

TYPES OF PAIN

There are two major classifications of pain: nociceptive and neuropathic. Understanding the type of pain experienced by the patient is key to providing the most effective treatment. Nociceptive pain occurs with direct stimulation of pain receptors. Examples of this type of pain include tissue injury or inflammation. Nociceptive pain can be further classified as either somatic or visceral. Somatic pain refers to the stimulation of pain in the cutaneous

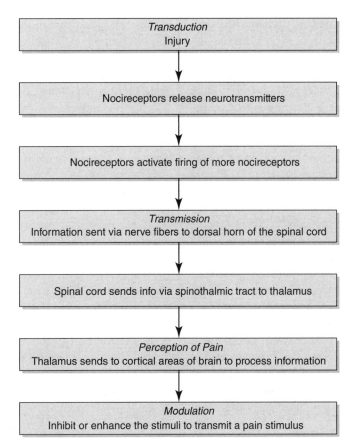

Figure 14-1 Pathophysiology of pain.

and deep layers of skin. Patients are able to localize this pain, which often comprises acute pain due to surgery. Somatic pain often responds best to NSAIDs or acetaminophen. Visceral pain refers to pain resulting from infiltration or compression of the abdominal or thoracic viscera. Patients often have difficulty localizing visceral pain because the pain is referred to another part of the body. Opioids often work well in the treatment of visceral pain (Pasero & McCaffery, 2011).

Postoperative cardiac surgery patients are likely to experience pain from a variety of sources. Incisions from sternotomy, thoracotomy and graft sites, required invasive procedures, tissue retraction and dissection, turning, and presence and removal of chest tubes are some of the identified etiologies (Aslan et al., 2010; Gélinas, 2007). Data have shown that patients who underwent painful procedures (e.g., chest tube removal) and were not premedicated for pain subsequently reported moderate to high levels of pain (Aslan et al., 2010).

Neuropathic pain is primarily caused by a dysfunction in the nervous system that can occur either centrally or peripherally. Neuropathic pain is often the consequence of an injury to the nervous system that results in sustained abnormal sensory processing. Patients often describe this pain as burning, fire, stinging, and electric. Examples of neuropathic pain include diabetic neuropathy and phantom pain (Pasero & McCaffery, 2011).

Pain is further categorized as acute or chronic. Acute pain typically has a sudden onset and serves as a warning signal to the body. Acute pain usually results from an insult or injury, and as the insult or injury resolves, so should the pain. Acute pain may last for a moment or it can be more severe and last weeks to months. Experts agree that, by definition, acute pain duration is less than 6 months (Pasero & McCaffery, 2011). On the other hand, chronic pain, also referred to as persistent pain, persists beyond the time of tissue healing. On average, chronic pain lasts greater than 6 months and is sometimes difficult to manage. Chronic pain often affects function and, therefore, quality of life (Pasero & McCaffery, 2011). Acute and chronic pain can be visualized as a continuum instead of two distinct categories (St. Marie, 2010). For patients who undergo cardiac surgery, healthcare providers' focus remains on acute, nociceptive pain.

Unfortunately, patients who undergo cardiac surgery have a significant risk for developing chronic pain. The incidence of chronic pain following cardiac surgery ranges from 21% to 55% (Cogan, 2010). Over time, the patient's pain characteristics may progress from acute, nociceptive pain to chronic, neuropathic pain in origin. This pain is often the result of nerve damage associated with sternal incisions and retractions. Approximately 30% to 44% of patients who undergo thoracotomy exhibit chronic pain 6 months to a year after surgery has been reported (Cerfolio, Bryant, Bass, & Bartolucci, 2003; Jensen & Andersen, 2004). The risk of developing chronic pain seems to be reduced if postoperative pain is adequately managed (Cogan, 2010), placing greater emphasis on the need to control pain in the acute postoperative period.

In another study of cardiac surgery patients, 29% of patients experienced persistent pain from any site (lasting at least 2 months postoperatively), and 25% reported persistent sternotomy pain. Other sites of pain included the shoulder, back, and neck. Pain intensity in these patients was mild, with 7% of the study participants reporting that the pain interfered with activities of daily living (ADLs). There was no significant difference in the incidence in those patients who received postoperative high thoracic epidural anesthesia and opioids (Ho, Royse, Royse, Penberthy, & McRae, 2002; Mueller et al., 2000).

These findings were corroborated in another study of cardiac surgery patients. Patients who reported moderate to severe postoperative pain were the same patients who reported chronic post-sternotomy pain more frequently (Lahtinen, Kokki, & Hynynen, 2006).

Research indicates that individuals who experience uncontrolled acute pain for long periods of time have a greater probability of developing chronic pain (St. Marie, 2010). One hypothesis for this phenomenon suggests that a neurophysiologic link results in glial activation following nerve or tissue injury. The signaling molecules involved in glial activation are ATP; CX3CL (fractalkine); CCL1 (monocyte chemotactic protein-1); the pro-inflammatory cytokines interleukin 1-beta (IL-1β), interleukin 6 (IL-6), tumor necrosis factor alpha (TNF-α), and substance P (SP); and glutamate (St. Marie, 2010). This supports the belief that individuals require early cessation of pain in order to prevent progression to a state of chronic pain. Clearly, early recognition and treatment of acute pain is of prime importance.

PAIN ASSESSMENT

Pain assessment is the cornerstone of good pain management. Precise and methodical assessment of pain is necessary to determine the most efficacious treatment regimen for patients presenting with pain. The national pain management standards, as delineated by The Joint Commission, require the prompt management of pain once identified (Wells et al., 2008). According to The Joint Commission (2012), "a comprehensive pain assessment is conducted as appropriate to the individual's condition and the scope of care, treatment and services provided." The expectation is for healthcare providers to perform an initial pain assessment and, based on the need of the patient, perform regular reassessments. For Joint Commission–accredited organizations, this is mandatory. Having national standards also implies the risk of legal liability if pain is poorly managed. Consumers have the right to have their pain adequately assessed and managed, and there are instances of legal action for poor pain management (Furrow, 2001).

Typically, during screening, the provider inquires about the patient's present pain state and history of pain. Pain history should always include the use of analgesics, dosing, and efficacy. The progression to a more detailed assessment is determined following the initial screening. Assessment of pain focuses on several key components including the location, intensity, quality, and duration of the pain; effective pain relief techniques; and the patient's perception of an acceptable pain level or comfort goal (Pasero & McCaffery, 2011). Pain assessment is a continuous cycle of assessment, intervention, and reassessment. In order to successfully manage pain, the nurse must first ask about the pain, accept the subjective report of pain, intervene to relieve the pain in accordance with the patient's comfort goal, reassess pain following any intervention, and advocate for changes in the pain management regime as needed (Pasero & McCaffery, 2011).

A variety of pain assessment tools exist to aid in the assessment of pain. Self-report of pain is the gold standard for verbal patients. Nurses regularly use pain intensity scales, in clinical practice, to elicit patient's self-report. Use of pain rating scales facilitates the identification of pain intensity over time and helps to evaluate the effectiveness of pain-relieving interventions (Pasero & McCaffery, 2011). Pasero and McCaffery (2011) evaluated numerous pain intensity rating scales for use in cognitively intact adolescent and adult patients. The numeric rating scale (NRS) and FACES pain rating scale are two of the most frequently used tools in daily clinical practice.

Use of the NRS typically involves a horizontal line with a 0–5 scale or 0–10 scale. The healthcare provider anchors the scale by explaining that zero is no pain and the opposite end of the scale is the worst imaginable pain. This scale is well established with good validity and reliability. Although healthcare providers often present the scale verbally without providing a visual copy for the patient, research shows that the use of the written copy results in better patient understanding (Herr, 2011). A survey of healthcare professionals indicated that 70% prefer use of the 0–10 scale for clinical practice (Pasero & McCaffery, 2011). In a recent literature review comparing studies of the NRS, verbal rating scales, and visual analog scales (VASs), the authors report that the NRS showed better overall compliance and was easy to use (Hjermstad et al., 2011). The 0–10 NRS is available in many languages.

Developed originally for use in children, the FACES pain scale is appropriate for use with some adults. The FACES scale is gender, age, and culture neutral. This scale is also translated into several languages. According to Herr (2011), the FACES pain scale is preferred among African American and Asian adults. The FACES scale contains brief words below the faces to better describe pain. The anchor for zero is still no pain with the opposite end of the scale indicating "hurts worst" (Pasero & McCaffery, 2011).

Pain Assessment in Patients Who Are Unable to Communicate

Assessment of pain for patients who are unable to communicate can be challenging for nurses. The identification of pain in non-verbal patients can be tedious. It requires obtaining data from various sources in order to make a clinical judgment that validates a diagnosis of pain (Herr, 2011). Healthcare providers must not assume that noncommunicative patients are not in pain (Pasero & McCaffery, 2011). A good rule of thumb is to assume pain is present in nonverbal hospitalized patients and then perform a thorough pain assessment to determine if intervention is required (Pasero, 2009).

Utilization of a behavioral observation pain assessment tool may be necessary based on the patient's condition. Behavioral assessment tools measure behaviors labeled as indicative of pain. The Checklist of Nonverbal Pain Indicators, the Behavioral Pain Scale, and the Critical-Care Pain Observation Tool (CPOT) are valid and reliable tools that measure the presence or absence of pain (Herr, 2011; Pasero & McCaffery, 2011). Observable behaviors include facial expressions, body movements, ease of breathing, vocalization, and/or muscle tension. Each observed behavior is scored and the patient receives a total score that correlates with the presence or absence of pain (Herr, 2011). This score helps guide the healthcare provider in the management of pain.

The American Society for Pain Management Nursing (Jarzyna et al., 2011) recommends use of a hierarchical approach for pain assessment. First, all attempts must be made to obtain a patient self-report of pain, the gold standard of pain assessment. Explanation as to the inability of obtaining a self-report should be documented, and further assessment should ensue. A search for the potential cause of pain is conducted, with the provider assuming that pain is present.

Behavioral observation is the best approach to assessment when the patient is unable to self-report. Pain behaviors, however, are not always indicative of pain intensity. Healthcare providers may consider pain reports provided by family members or significant others because they can often identify subtle changes in the patient's status (Pasero & McCaffery, 2011). However, research indicates that discrepancies often exist between patient self-report and reports given by other observers. Others often underestimate pain or mistake non-pain behaviors as indicative of pain. Therefore, one must consider all aspects of an assessment and perhaps perform an analgesic trial, monitoring the patient's response to the medication (Herr, 2011).

Preoperative Baseline Assessment

Optimal postoperative pain management begins with the preoperative pain assessment. To optimally manage postoperative pain, nurses should obtain a thorough preoperative health history that encompasses topics related to the patient's current and past experiences with pain. Many factors can affect a patient's response and perception of pain—for example, smoking history, fatigue, sleep deprivation, fear, anxiety, depression, anger, misinformation, altered mental status, educational level, cultural background, ethnic background, and pain experience (Pasero & McCaffery, 2011; St. Marie, 2010). Past experiences should alert the nurse to factors that may directly affect the patient's response to the current treatment, including medications that have been effective in the past, acceptable pain levels, concerns about pain, and educational needs. Healthcare providers must understand that for patients with a history of chronic pain or opioid dependence, postoperative pain management may be more difficult (D'Arcy, 2011). Discussions focusing on the patient's expectations help the nurse and patient to mutually develop a plan of care related to pain that includes desirable, predictable outcomes (Pasero & McCaffery, 2011).

The pain assessment process includes multiple components: initial assessment, treatment, reassessment, and evaluation. Optimal goals include adequate pain management, manageable side effects, and assurance of safety (Dunwoody, Krenzischek, Pasero, Rathmell, & Polomano, 2008). Dimensions of the assessment should include the pain's location, description, intensity, duration, alleviating and aggravating factors, associative factors, and impact on ADLs. To identify the location and obtain a description of the pain, the nurse should ask patients to describe the pain in their own words and to point to the location of pain (Pasero & McCaffery, 2011; St. Marie, 2010). Identifying the best pain assessment tool for the patient preoperatively can help the patient provide the most reliable information regarding pain intensity in the postoperative period (Gélinas, 2007). This may contribute to more effective pain management and, subsequently, increased patient satisfaction.

Determining the duration of pain includes asking questions concerning the timing of when the pain starts, how long it lasts, and which factors alleviate it. Healthcare providers should also inquire about factors that aggravate the pain. Additionally, determining if any associated factors exist can assist the nurse in developing a more comprehensive treatment plan. For example, do nausea and vomiting accompany the pain? Treatment may need to include measures that control these associated factors. Determining how the pain affects the individual's activities of daily living provides supplemental information about how the pain interferes with normal functioning. The nurse can develop treatment strategies to target specific challenges the patient faces

related to ADLs (Pasero & McCaffery, 2011; St. Marie, 2010).

Although a considerable amount of research on pain over the past several decades exists, only a small percentage of the studies focus on patients undergoing cardiac surgery. In such investigations, the focus was on pain intensity, but other important pain factors were not addressed. Mueller and colleagues (2000) evaluated the pain in postoperative patients following cardiac surgery and found that pain intensity was highest during the first 2 postoperative days and lowest on days 3 and 7. Age was the only demographic variable that affected pain in this study; patients over the age of 60 had lower pain intensity scores on the second postoperative day than did patients younger than age 60. Pain location varied, with patients reporting more shoulder pain on day 7. Pain distribution did not vary in this study.

The baseline assessment also provides the opportunity to discuss postoperative pain management techniques such as patient-controlled analgesia (PCA), epidural analgesia, and nerve blocks. The nurse has the chance to provide education and help frame expectations for the postoperative period. Patients may have numerous questions and anxiety about postoperative pain. The nurse is in a unique position to assist in decreasing anxiety and fear that surround pain, and thus increase the success of postoperative pain management (D'Arcy, 2011).

Reassessment of Pain

Following the initial pain assessment and the subsequent pain treatment, regular reassessment of the patient helps determine if the interventions provided are effective or need modification. Reassessment of pain entails comparing pain behaviors and vocalizations exhibited after the intervention to the pain observed during the initial assessment (Pasero & McCaffery, 2011). In order to determine efficacy of interventions, nurses must make reassessment after any treatment a priority. Reassessments must be comprehensive, timely, and include the presence of adverse side effects. In addition, the reassessment should include whether or not the patient's comfort goal is met (Gordon et al., 2008).

Organizations can assist with ensuring assessment and reassessment compliance by implementing documentation systems that support the nurse to complete the task. Electronic documentation systems that promote ease of obtaining pain assessments before and after interventions will help guide the nurse in completing this crucial component of the care plan and help improve patient outcomes. Electronic documentation systems help promote uniformity, allow data collection and analysis, and promote real-time documentation. Additionally, the ability to easily visualize trends is helpful to all healthcare providers and can assist in making necessary changes to an analgesic regimen (Wang, Hailey, & Yu, 2011).

Little research exists in the areas of reevaluation of pain and the measurement tools used to determine the patient's comfort. One study, however, found a significant lack of pain reassessment by nurses. The authors proposed that knowledge, time, and workload may be factors that limit effective reassessment of pain. Interestingly, these researchers found that nurses tended to be more focused on surgical pain; therefore, the nurses did not consider other complaints of pain a priority, resulting in delayed treatment (Bucknall et al., 2007). Nurses must be educated regarding the potential gap in pain control measures due to periods of increased and uncontrolled pain that result directly from lack of timely reevaluation (Polomano, Dunwoody, Krenzischek, & Rathmell, 2008).

PHASES OF PAIN

The patient experiences pain through three phases: anticipation, presence, and aftermath. The nurse's responsibility is to intervene and assist the patient with each pain phase (Pasero & McCaffery, 2011). During the anticipation phase, interventions should focus on patient education and the reduction of anxiety. Research supports that anxiety increases intensity of pain scores (Pasero & McCaffery, 2011; St. Marie, 2010). Anxiety can often be relieved with knowledge that pain may occur and the development of a realistic plan to manage it when it does. Preoperative discussion of comfort goals and realistic techniques to achieve the goals are essential to successful postoperative reduction of pain and anxiety (Pasero & McCaffery, 2011).

The presence of pain is the phase where interventions can directly affect the patient's level of comfort and pain intensity. Physiologically, the management of pain revolves around altering the source and perception of pain and blocking the transmission of pain impulses within the nervous system. Different pharmacologic and nonpharmacologic agents perform differently in relation to the pathology of pain. One strategy is to block or limit the effect of local mediators at the site of injury and decrease inflammation. Nonsteroidal anti-inflammatory drugs are able to block specific mediator production such as prostaglandin, thereby decreasing the inflammatory response. Other medications such as clonidine (Catapres®) block the release of epinephrine from the nerve fibers. A second strategy involves limiting transmission to the secondary neurons in the dorsal horn. The action potential can be blocked or inhibited by local anesthetics and some anticonvulsants such as phenytoin (Dilantin®). Opioids also are used to inhibit both synapses at the dorsal horn. Additionally, nonpharmacologic interventions such as massage and application of heat or cold may inhibit transmission of pain-related messages. The final strategy in pain management is to enhance the inhibition of the pain sensation. Opioids are the agents of choice in such a case because they will affect both the primary and secondary neurons. Tricyclic antidepressants can have the same effect by interfering with serotonin uptake and primary neuron transmission (Lome, 2005).

PREEMPTIVE ANALGESIA

Preemptive analgesia is the administration of analgesics prior to insult or injury. The goal is to prevent the sensitization to pain, especially prior to surgical intervention (Pasero & McCaffery, 2011). Recent evidence suggests that the administration of preoperative analgesics may indeed help to decrease the sensitization to postoperative pain. This decreased sensitization of nociceptors indicates that preemptive analgesic use has the possibility of greater efficacy than the same treatment administered postoperatively (Dhal & Moiniche, 2004). Researchers theorized that the administration of preemptive analgesia would decrease postoperative pain and also prevent the development of chronic pain. Dhal and Moiniche (2004) performed a literature review to examine studies in which patients received preemptive NSAIDs prior to surgery. They reported that in six of eight studies, patients experienced lower postoperative pain scores and required less opiates.

Data indicate the benefit of preemptive analgesia might be realized for as long as 1 year after surgery. Effective administration of preemptive analgesia involves the use of various medications and routes of administration. Use of preemptive analgesia includes opiates, local anesthetics, NSAIDs, acetaminophen, antidepressants, and gamma-aminobutyric acid; analgesic therapies target the expected postoperative pain. Depending on the surgical procedure, administration of preemptive analgesia may be oral, intravenous, or epidural or in the form of a nerve block (Dhal & Moiniche, 2004).

One study demonstrated that patients who received a single dose of oral gabapentin prior to cardiac surgery required significantly less morphine postoperatively. In addition to decreased morphine consumption, patients reported considerably lower postoperative pain scores and nausea (Menda et al., 2010). Another study on preemptive use of gabapentin (Neurontin®) prior to coronary artery bypass graft (CABG) surgery describes similar results. Patients who received a single dose of gabapentin preoperatively had substantially lower pain scores and required less tramadol in the postoperative period; however, no significant difference existed in pain scores at 1 and 3 months (Ucak et al., 2011). Despite positive outcomes reported in the literature, the general consensus among researchers is that the use of preemptive analgesia is not beneficial; however, this is not an indication to abandon ongoing research (Pasero & McCaffery, 2011). Some studies clearly demonstrate the benefit of preemptive analgesia. The results regarding the use of aggressive analgesics perioperatively and postoperatively are clear.

MANAGEMENT OF PAIN

In 1784, a surgeon by the name of James Monroe first described the advantage of postoperative opium use:

> Opium . . . is highly expedient to abate the smarting of the wound after the operation is over, and to induce sleep; but the stronger dose we dare venture to give has little or no effect in mitigating the suffering of the patient during the operation. (Sattari, Baghdadchi, Kheyri, Khakzadi, & Mashayekhi, 2013, p. 373)

For centuries healthcare providers have strived to provide acceptable postoperative pain management. Adequate pain management is essential for the well-being of all patients and is a fundamental human right (Brennan, Carr, & Cousins, 2007; D'Arcy, 2011). The consequences of inadequate pain management include physiologic, psychological, social, and economic ramifications. Physiologically, unrelieved pain results in many adverse effects, including increased heart rate, systemic vascular resistance, and increased circulating catecholamines. These effects place patients at greater risk for myocardial ischemia, stroke, and bleeding. Additionally, chronic pain decreases mobility, alters sleep patterns, causes immune dysfunction, and creates dependence on medication and codependence on family members. In terms of psychological effects, studies show that patients with chronic pain are four times more likely to suffer from depression and anxiety. Social and economic factors include the inability or decreased ability to work. This change in work status directly affects the individual's socioeconomic status, impacts unemployment and disability, and increases dependence on government benefits (Brennan et al., 2007; Sattari et al., 2013).

Opioids, non-opioids, and other analgesics used as adjuvant therapies are the mainstays in pain management (D'Arcy, 2011; Pasero & McCaffery, 2011). Treatment modalities may differ, depending on whether the goal is treating acute versus chronic pain, or nociceptive versus neuropathic pain. Healthcare providers must be cognizant that patients respond uniquely to medications; patients may metabolize medications rapidly, moderately, or slowly. How a patient metabolizes the medication should influence dosing regimens because genetics play an important role in how patients respond to medications (D'Arcy, 2011).

Traditionally, pain management strategies have applied the World Health Organization's (WHO) cancer pain treatment ladder in attempts to manage postoperative pain. This ladder suggests that the first step in treating mild pain should include using non-opioids with or without adjuvant medications. Step two entails the addition of opioids to the adjuvants for mild to moderate pain. Step three involves continuing opioid use for moderate to severe pain. Postoperative pain reaches its highest level initially after the surgery, but then rapidly improves (Li, 2008).

In one study, Reimer-Kent (2003) developed a pain management guideline using the WHO ladder to prevent pain following cardiac surgery. Under this guideline, most patients received acetaminophen around the clock; 89% of patients received an NSAID, and all patients received intermittent morphine. The morphine was converted from the intravenous route of administration to an oral preparation on the second postoperative day. The amount of morphine administered declined significantly by the second postoperative day. Effective pain relief was reported in 95% of the patients in this study.

Evidence-based guidelines must direct efforts to manage postoperative pain related to site-specific surgeries. Rosenquist and Rosenburg (2003) gathered a multidisciplinary group to review and grade the evidence and then provide recommendations along these lines. The authors developed an algorithmic approach to pain assessment with a flow diagram outlining the key considerations prior to, during, and after the treatment of pain. Site-specific pain management recommendations were provided regarding the use of pharmacologic and nonpharmacologic therapy. **Table 14-1** summarizes these recommendations for pain management in conjunction with cardiothoracic surgery.

The use of intravenous opioids is the preferred method of managing pain in the immediate postoperative period for patients who undergo CABG surgery. These

Table 14-1	Recommended Surgery-Specific Pain Management Modalities
Surgical Procedure	**Preferred Modality and Route of Administration**

Thoracotomy	**Pharmacologic**
	• **Opioids administered:** PO, IV, PCA, epidural, intrathecal
	   * **CAUTION:** *IM administration is not recommended for pain management due to painful administration, unreliable absorption, and rapid decrease in action.*
	• **NSAIDs administered:** PO, IV
	   * **CAUTION:** *Do not administer NSAIDs if patient has actual or potential risk for bleeding.*
	• **Local anesthetics administered:** Epidural, intrathecal, regional
	
	Nonpharmacologic
	• Application of cold
	• TENS
	• Cognitive/behavioral (patient dependent)

CABG	**Pharmacologic**
	• **Opioids administered:** PO, IV, PCA, intrathecal
	   * **CAUTION:** *IM administration is not recommended for pain management due to painful administration, unreliable absorption, and rapid decrease in action.*
	• **NSAIDs administered:** PO, IV
	   * **CAUTION:** *Do not administer NSAIDs if patient has actual or potential risk for bleeding or renal hypoperfusion.*
	
	Nonpharmacologic
	• Massage

CABG, coronary artery bypass grafting; IM, intramuscular; IV, intravenous; NSAIDs, nonsteroidal anti-inflammatory drugs; PCA, patient-controlled analgesia; PO, by mouth; TENS, transcutaneous electrical nerve stimulation.

Sources: Cogan, J. (2010). Pain management after cardiac surgery. *Seminars in Cardiothoracic and Vascular Anesthesia, 14*(3), 201–204; Cutshall, S. M., Fenske, L. L., Kelly, R. F., Phillips, B. R., Sundt, T. M., & Bauer, B. A. (2007). Creation of a healing enhancement program at an academic medical center. *Complementary Therapies in Clinical Practice, 13*(4), 217–223; Pasero, C., & McCaffery, M. (2011). *Pain assessment and pharmacologic management.* St. Louis, MO: Mosby; Rosenquist, R. W., & Rosenburg, J. (2003). Postoperative pain guidelines. *Regional Anesthesia and Pain Medicine, 28*(4), 279–288.

medications can be delivered via nurse or patient-controlled methods. The use of PCA devices allows for the administration of small, frequent doses of opioids by the patient. One advantage is the ability to obtain and maintain a steady state. Another advantage is the psychological benefit related to the self-administration of analgesia (D'Arcy, 2011). In a study by Sattari and colleagues (2013), postoperative cardiac surgery patients received intravenous morphine and an NSAID either orally or rectally. Although these patients reported moderate pain, they also reported satisfaction with pain management. Additionally, other studies demonstrate the effective use of morphine for various postoperative cardiac surgery patients (Coventry, Siffleet, & Williams, 2006).

Multimodal Analgesia

The use of multimodal analgesic therapy is fundamental to exceptional pain management and is strongly endorsed by experts in the field of pain management (D'Arcy, 2011; Pasero & McCaffery, 2011). The theory of multimodal analgesia is to maximize the efficacy of individual agents to create a synergistic analgesic effect. In turn, the synergy should decrease the dose of medications, thereby decreasing associated side effects and increasing analgesia (Young & Buvanendran, 2012). Proponents of multimodal analgesia stress the importance of procedure-specific approaches. An example is the use of continuous epidural analgesia that combines opiate and local anesthetic. Dosing requirements in the epidural space are significantly lower than intravenous or oral routes of administration. In turn, patients often experience decreased side effects with improved analgesia. Despite evidence showing the benefits of multimodal analgesia, the technique continues to be underused (White & Kehlet, 2010).

Epidural and local anesthetics are the preferred methods for managing pain in patients who are undergoing a thoracotomy (Chaney, 2009). Agreement exists that epidural use in these patients provides an excellent method for pain control during the acute pain phase (Chaney, 2009; Ng & Swanevelder, 2007). Other reported benefits of epidural analgesia include earlier extubation and enhanced pulmonary function (Chaney, 2009). Some conflicting data exist regarding enhanced pulmonary function with epidural pain management following thoracotomy. Some data suggest that while pain management may be effective and this may lead to earlier extubation, pulmonary function may not be enhanced with epidural pain management (Asenjo & Carli, 2009).

Data are inconsistent regarding the benefits of thoracic epidural anesthesia. In one study involving cardiac surgery patients, participants received either 1) thoracic epidural analgesia in combination with general anesthesia, followed by postoperative patient-controlled thoracic epidural analgesia, or 2) general anesthesia, followed by PCA with intravenous morphine. No differences between these two groups were observed in terms of pain relief, pulmonary function, ambulation, level of sedation, LOS, or quality of recovery. The study authors did conclude, however, that thoracic epidural anesthesia decreases stress response and pain scores (Hansdottir et al., 2006). The major concern when using epidural analgesia is the potential for development of an epidural hematoma. When this strategy is used, the intensive care unit (ICU) nurse must monitor for and report lower extremity motor weakness (Mehta & Kumar, 2004). The use of thoracic epidurals is not without risk. Risks include failure of the catheter to provide the desired analgesia, hematoma, and motor block; nursing tasks for care and monitoring increase with epidural analgesia. According to Chaney (2009), the only clear benefit of thoracic epidurals in patients undergoing cardiac surgery is improved pain management.

The use of intrathecal morphine has been reported to be effective in the management of postoperative cardiac surgery pain. In one study, patients undergoing on-pump bypass who received intrathecal morphine prior to induction of general anesthesia were extubated earlier and had a shorter ICU length of stay than did a comparison group of patients who did not receive the intrathecal injection prior to induction (Yapici et al., 2008).

An additional method of pain management for CABG patients is the use of intravenous

NSAIDs (Acharya & Dunning, 2010). The use of NSAIDs in conjunction with opioids in other surgical procedures is well established. Nonsteroidal anti-inflammatory drugs are opioid sparing and provide excellent pain relief (White & Kehlet, 2010). Data suggest that administering NSAIDs results in reduced pain scores, less opioid requirements, and no differences in mortality or incidence of serious side effects (Acharya & Dunning, 2010; White & Kehlet, 2010).

Despite the potential advantages of postoperative NSAID use, its use is limited in cardiac surgery patients due to the potential for troublesome side effects. The actual occurrence of side effects tends to depend on whether the medication inhibits cyclooxygenase 1 or 2 (COX-1 or COX-2), or both. Serious side effects, including sternal wound infections, myocardial ischemia, infarction, stroke, and pulmonary embolus, have been reported with the use of COX-2 inhibitors; as a consequence, these medications are not recommended for patients deemed to have an increased cardiac risk (White & Kehlet, 2010).

Another promising addition to the multimodal therapy tool kit is the use of acetaminophen. The effective use of oral acetaminophen as an analgesic and antipyretic is well documented; however, the recent approval of intravenous (IV) acetaminophen by the U.S. Food and Drug Administration adds a new dimension to managing pain. Acetaminophen has an advantage over other analgesic agents because, in appropriate weight-based doses, it is safe. As a non-opiate, acetaminophen use does not result in respiratory depression, sedation, constipation, ileus, or pruritus, nor does it have the potential renal or hematologic complications associated with NSAID administration. Moreover, the risk of addiction or diversion is nonexistent (Young & Buvanendran, 2012).

A European study of more than 600 patients undergoing outpatient surgery revealed that the patients received a single dose of IV acetaminophen (1 g) prior to the end of surgery; of those patients, almost 50% received a single dose of acetaminophen for postoperative pain management with good results (Silihoglu et al., 2009). A retrospective study involving more than 400 cardiac surgery patients who received IV acetaminophen 1 g every 6 hours postoperatively, compared to matched control patients who did not receive IV acetaminophen, demonstrated the effectiveness of IV acetaminophen. The group of patients receiving IV acetaminophen experienced less time on the ventilator, decreased stay in the ICU, and overall decreased LOS in the hospital.

Research supports the use of IV acetaminophen as an adjunct in the postoperative period; however, some organizations have limited the prescribing due to cost concerns. Although cost is always a concern, the current research demonstrates improved outcomes and shorter lengths of stay. Cautious use of acetaminophen is warranted in patients with liver dysfunction, those with a history of alcohol abuse, severely malnourished patients, and the elderly. In addition, nurses must be cognizant of other acetaminophen-containing medications (Young & Buvanendran, 2012).

PAIN SEQUELAE

Inadequate postoperative pain management may lead to numerous complications and poor patient outcomes. Unrelieved acute pain can have hemodynamic, metabolic, and hemostatic consequences. Patients in pain are less likely to ambulate, delaying early mobilization and increasing the risk for thromboembolic complications. Patients who experience pain, especially following cardiac surgery, may not perform respiratory exercises, such as coughing, deep breathing, or incentive spirometry, leading to an increased risk of pneumonia. Increases in autonomic activity may lead to slowing of the gastrointestinal system and resultant postoperative ileus; urinary retention may also be a problem. Furthermore, poor pain management contributes to increased length of stay in the hospital and decreased patient satisfaction. When pain is unrelieved, patients may become anxious, irritable, and agitated, and experience altered sleep cycles (Dunwoody et al., 2008; Pasero & McCaffery, 2011; St. Marie, 2010).

NONPHARMACOLOGIC PAIN MANAGEMENT

Use of nonpharmacologic interventions to augment pain control range from relaxation techniques to application of heat or cold to use of transcutaneous electrical nerve stimulation (TENS). The success of relaxation techniques typically is patient dependent, although results appear to be better if patients learn the techniques preoperatively (Rosenquist & Rosenburg, 2003). Unfortunately, little research exists related to the use of nonpharmacologic techniques following cardiac surgery; however, the research does support the benefit of various nonpharmacologic methods in improving pain management overall.

The use of music to augment pain management appears in the literature and does show some promise. In a review of studies from 1995 through 2007, it was found that 42 studies were conducted to assess the efficacy of music as a means of pain control. Roughly half the studies showed that pain reduction might be achieved through the use of music. Of the 42 studies, 7 were conducted with cardiothoracic surgery patients (Nilsson, 2008). A study of postoperative cardiac surgery patients combined analgesics with the use of sedative music for 30 minutes. Results showed a reduction in anxiety and pain as compared to patients receiving the usual course of treatment (Voss et al., 2004). A more recent study explored the effects of music chosen by the patients on their self-reported pain intensity and physiologic pain indicators following open heart surgery. The patients in the music group had significantly lower pain scores and increased oxygen saturation. The researchers concluded that the addition of music is a harmless, effective, and easy technique to help diminish the potentially detrimental effects of pain following open heart surgery (Özer, Özlü, Arslan, & Günes, 2013). A study in patients who underwent CABG surgery revealed a correlation between use of slow, deep breathing and medication administration during painful procedures such as chest tube removal and a decrease in pain scores immediately following the procedure and 15 minutes later (Friesner, Curry, & Moddeman, 2006).

In a study of postoperative cardiac surgery patients, those who used TENS experienced less pain related to coughing and experienced improved chest wall mechanics, tidal volume, and vital capacity (Cipriano, Carvalho, Bernardelli, & Peres, 2008). However, the use of TENS in patients with an implanted cardioverter defibrillator may result in an inappropriate shock and must be used with extreme caution and under the guidance of a healthcare provider (Holmgren, Carlsson, Mannheimer, & Edvardsson, 2008).

The addition and implementation of massage therapy in postoperative cardiac surgery patients helps promote comfort and reduce pain. Research suggests providing massage helps decrease pain and anxiety in postsurgical patients and may be used as an alternative intervention when other nursing and medical treatments are not effective in reducing pain (Anderson & Cutshall, 2007). A randomized trial of more than 150 patients who underwent elective cardiac surgery compared the use of massage to rest. The researchers reported significant reductions in pain, anxiety, and muscle tension in the patients who received therapeutic massage. Additionally, the massage patients reported increased relaxation and satisfaction with pain management (Braun et al., 2012). Massage also improves mood following cardiac surgery and is a complementary nursing intervention that is simple and inexpensive (Babaee, Shafiei, Sadeghi, Nik, & Valiani, 2012).

SPECIAL CONSIDERATIONS

Pain is a unique, subjective, individualized experience. Nevertheless, some elements that affect the response to pain management techniques may apply across certain groups of people. Recognition of these special considerations may assist the nurse with managing an individual's pain. The special considerations for pain management discussed here are gender differences, cultural influences, and older age.

Gender

Researchers in the study of pain management understand that clear differences exist between the way men and women experience pain, and they recognize the importance of acknowledging these differences. Women tend to have a lower threshold for pain than men (Aubrun, Salvi, Coriat, & Riou, 2005). Evidence clearly suggests that the perception of pain is different for men and women and that women have a higher incidence of undertreatment for pain (Fillingim, King, Ribeiro-Dasilva, Rahim-Williams, & Riley, 2009; Pasero & McCaffery, 2011). In a study of more than 4,000 postoperative patients, the authors measured pain scores and total amount of morphine administered to obtain pain relief. Slightly less than 50% of the patients were female; however, the female patients required significantly more morphine overall and reported higher pain scores. The difference in morphine requirements was slightly more than 10% between men and women (Aubrun et al., 2005). Several studies

utilizing video vignettes discovered that nurses were more likely to undertreat pain in women than in men and healthcare providers were more likely to provide optimal pain treatment regimens for men than women (Pasero & McCaffery, 2011). Gender bias in the treatment of pain is concerning. Research demonstrates that, very often, women experiencing chest pain are much less likely than men to receive invasive and noninvasive diagnostic procedures. Additionally, women are far less likely to receive interventional cardiac procedures when presenting with complaints of chest pain (Fillingim et al., 2009). A frequently cited study indicated that, following cardiac surgery, women were more likely to receive sedating medications while prescriptions for men more likely included analgesics (Evrard & Balthazart, 2004).

Psychological factors also play a part in the role of gender differences. Psychosocial factors shape an individual's expectations, emotions, and social learning (Fillingim et al., 2009). Societal norms in how children of both genders are raised, for example, play a part in their pain experience (Bernardes, Keogh, & Lima, 2008; Fillingim et al., 2009). Stereotypical norms accept that women may show more emotion around pain while men are less verbal and more stoic.

When studying pain differences reflective of gender, researchers measure gender personality traits in relation to pain. For example, persons identified as possessing more feminine characteristics (women) report experiencing more pain than men. Additionally, reports point to the fact that men—that is, those persons with more masculine traits—report a higher tolerance of pain (Bernardes et al., 2008). Gender-related differences exist among pain beliefs, expectations, and behaviors. Gender role expectations can account for the fact that males predominately underreport pain and women are more apt to verbalize pain. Additionally, males demonstrate greater pain endurance, whereas women report a lower threshold and tolerance, resulting in their greater willingness to report pain (Fillingim et al., 2009). Similarly, studies suggest that women were more likely to experience severe pain and on a more frequent basis. In a study of cardiac surgery patients, female patients rated their pain on a VAS higher than did their male counterparts (Miller & Newton, 2006). Some differences in the reports of pain between males and females may be related to the issue of willingness to make a self-report. Males and females have different behaviors regarding the expression of and response to pain (Miller & Newton, 2006).

These data on gender differences are corroborated through studies in other patients who have undergone cardiac surgery. Compared to males, females more frequently report less improvement in pain scores or higher pain intensity (Decker & Perry, 2003; Watt-Watson et al., 2004; Yorke, McLean, & Wallis, 2004), report lower health-related quality of life after cardiac surgery (Gjeilo, Wahba, Klepstad, Lydersen, & Stenseth, 2008), and experience a more difficult recovery (Vaccarino et al., 2003).

Conclusions regarding gender differences and recovery from cardiac surgery are inconsistent. King (2000), for example, reported fewer differences between males and females in terms of short-term recovery following cardiac surgery but stressed the importance of ongoing research.

Differences between males and females in the response to analgesia are well documented in the literature. Some studies show greater morphine potency but slower onset of pain relief in females. Additionally, researchers reported that NSAIDs have refractory effects in women when doses exceed 800 mg. Pharmacokinetics may play a role in these differences, although studies to date have not shown any significance in clinical practice. One explanation may be that the differences are related to the specific drugs, rather than to whole categories of drugs (Giles & Walker, 2000).

Greenspan and colleagues (2007) suggest the need to explore numerous variables and their influence on gender-related pain responses. These variables include comorbidities, culture, disability, medications, coping, and physical variables. In order to appropriately respond to an individual's pain experience, nurses need to be sensitive to various societal norms and communication patterns related to gender and recognize the potential differences in reports of pain and their own potential biases (Miller & Newton, 2006). Healthcare providers must be mindful of the potential gender differences that exist between males and females and appreciate the influence psychology and society have on the tolerance, perception, and expression of pain (Fillingim et al., 2009).

Race, Ethnicity, and Culture

Distinguishing differences among the definitions of race, ethnicity, and culture has proved difficult in the literature, with many of the terms being used interchangeably. The literature debates whether the term *race* is a biological or social concept. Typically, race is predominantly used to collect data regarding health disparities. There is no globally accepted definition of race; however, the National Institutes of Health has adopted the use of five racial categories to collect its data (Ezenwa, Ameringer, Ward, & Serlin, 2006).

By comparison, "ethnicity" refers to a group of people who share ancestry, social background, culture, and traditions that are sustained over a period of time and provide a sense of identity for group members. Typically, self-identification is the best approach to assigning individuals to a particular ethnic group (Lasch, 2002).

Finally, "culture" seems to be derived from behavioral and attitudinal norms in relation to belief systems. Culture is viewed as a factor influencing healthcare practices and illness beliefs. In terms of the pain experience, then, culture affects all areas related to pain, including expression, reporting, and management (Lasch, 2002).

Given that there are differences in the way these terms are used and studied, findings in this arena must be reviewed carefully. For example, a study of patients experiencing low back pain found that immigrated Latinos in New York showed pain responses more similar to the responses of a New England Latino group than to the responses of a group in Puerto Rico. The authors concluded that the pain response is shaped by culture (Morris, 2001).

Questions often arise as to whether race, ethnicity, and culture affect how different groups biologically experience pain or how the factors influence the perception of pain. Additionally, culture can influence how the caregiver assesses and treats the pain of persons from different ethnic backgrounds.

Authors of several studies have reported that racial and ethnic minorities are at higher risk for undertreatment of pain (Pasero & McCaffery, 2011; St. Marie, 2010). In general, research shows significant differences in terms of the amount of opiate analgesics administered to patients who were white as compared to those who were Hispanic or black (Heins, Heins, Costello, Huang, & Mishra, 2006; Tamayo-Sarrer, Hinze, Cydulka, & Baker, 2003; Terrell, Hui, Castelluccio, McGrath, & Miller, 2010). In these cases, patients who were white received higher amounts of opiates than did patients of other races. A systematic review of studies investigating the influence of race on analgesic administration further demonstrates disparities in pain management related to ethnicity and race in the United States

(Cintron & Morrison, 2006; Pasero & McCaffery, 2011). The lesson for nurses is that care must be taken to acknowledge potential differences related to race, ethnicity, and culture in how pain is experienced, including the awareness that people are individuals with individual needs.

The Elderly Population

The optimal treatment of pain is a complex endeavor but may be even more complicated in the elderly population. This difference may be explained by elderly patients' tendency to underreport pain, difficulty communicating, and caregiver biases regarding the use of pain medication in the older patient (Pasero & McCaffery, 2011).

Although older patients may not experience changes in the perception of pain, some physiologic changes do occur with aging that must be considered when utilizing pain medications. In particular, physiologic changes related to renal and liver function may affect the way the older patient metabolizes and eliminates pain medication, resulting in a longer duration of action and the risk for oversedation (Burgess & Burgess, 2008; Pasero & McCaffery, 2011; St. Marie, 2010). For this reason, care must be taken when prescribing, administering, and monitoring the effects of pain medications in the elderly population (Pasero & McCaffery, 2011).

Assessment is crucial for managing pain in the older patient. The pain scale chosen is important to the individual functioning of the older patient, and the same scale should be used consistently when assessing a particular patient to ensure reliability of the results (Pasero & McCaffery, 2011; St. Marie, 2010). Trying different scales to determine the best fit for individual patients is a good strategy. Often, older patients have more success using simple word scales, such as "none," "mild," "moderate," and "severe," than with a numeric scale or a VAS. Often, if the older patient has any cognitive impairment, rating pain may be difficult. The FACES scale, which seems to be easily used, often produces unreliable results with the elderly. The faces are often seen by these individuals as representing moods like sadness instead of pain, which results in understated pain intensity (Burgess & Burgess, 2008).

Additional challenges in using pain scales in the elderly population relate to vision and hearing loss, which are more prevalent in older individuals. It is critical that the nurse assess for these deficits and utilize assistive devices as appropriate (Pasero & McCaffery, 2011).

For the patient with vision impairment, the use of a verbal reporting scale might be best; in contrast, hearing-impaired patients may prefer to use a printed scale that they can point or gesture toward. Depending on the severity of cognitive impairment, the use of "yes" or "no" questions with a behavioral observation scale may be the best option. Studies have found that the use of proxy reports, relying on the assessment of a family member or on nursing judgment of the pain, often leads to underestimation of the actual pain experienced (Pasero & McCaffery, 2011).

The older patient's view of pain and pain management may also be a barrier to the effective assessment and treatment of pain. Many older patients may fear addiction to painkillers and, therefore, underreport their pain. Preparing patients for pain management following surgery provides nurses with a unique opportunity to educate patients and their families about pain, tolerance, dependence, addiction, the patient's disease process, and various pain control techniques (Goldstein & Morrison, 2005). Clearly exploring fears related to addiction and educating about the differences between psychological addiction and physiologic dependence may assist in decreasing fear and anxiety.

Treatment strategies for the older patient can include medication regimens in which the patient does not have to request treatment. Options to consider may include nerve blocks, epidural analgesia, and around-the-clock dosing of pain medications; ongoing, vigilant nursing assessment will be crucial to the success of these regimens. Opioids are the most widely utilized therapy with surgical patients, though their dosing needs to be considered carefully. Typically, if communication deficits are present, nurses may be fearful of postoperative delirium and withhold opioids. Nevertheless, even though these medications may potentially contribute to postoperative delirium, recent studies suggest that patients with higher pain scores and uncontrolled pain are more likely to develop delirium (Burgess & Burgess, 2008). Further complicating matters is the fact that research shows unrelieved acute pain may result in altered mental status. Pasero and McCaffery (2011) advocate to "assume pain is present" in older patients exhibiting increased agitation.

The level of postoperative pain following cardiac surgery in relation to age has been investigated; results have been inconsistent, however. In one study, patients older than age 60 received less analgesic therapy than younger patients. Yorke and colleagues (2004) found that older postoperative cardiac surgery patients received less analgesic therapy and were refused pain medication more often than were younger patients. In contrast, Decker and Perry (2003) reported higher levels of self-reported pain in older patients. Ultimately, comprehensive patient education regarding the importance of managing pain, attentive nursing assessment, and systematic evaluation of analgesic effectiveness can promote the best possible pain management.

SUMMARY

Frequent patient assessment is the key to outstanding management of pain (Pasero & McCaffery, 2011). Without systematic assessment and reassessment, it becomes impossible to adequately and expertly treat pain. Exceptional pain assessment and management following cardiac surgery are essential to ensuring improved patient outcomes. Knowledge that assessment techniques may need adjustment when providing care to nonverbal and elderly patients may allow for more optimal pain control. Acknowledging the differences in pain perception related to gender and culture allows the nurse to recognize trends and avoid biases when dealing with different groups of people. Recognizing the unique and subjective nature of the pain experience will assist in maximizing positive outcomes for pain management. This multifaceted process involves the timely assessment of pain, appropriate interventions, reassessment, and ongoing evaluation of the pain management regimen.

The use of multimodal analgesia techniques provides superior dynamic pain relief and helps diminish analgesic side effects during the postoperative period (Pasero & McCaffery, 2011). The addition of nonpharmacologic techniques aimed at augmenting pain management provides nurses with a relatively simple addition to the arsenal of available modalities. Healthcare providers must focus on pain management that is acceptable to the patient and remember that inadequate postoperative pain management may contribute to the development of chronic pain syndromes (Cogan, 2010). In today's ever-changing healthcare environment, diminishing complications, decreasing length of stay, and increasing patient satisfaction are imperative to the success of organizations. Good pain management can assist in meeting these goals.

CASE STUDY

A 64-year-old patient with a history of coronary artery disease, myocardial infarction with multi-vessel stents, hyperlipidemia, hypertension, and diabetes underwent an off-pump CABG procedure with median sternotomy and saphenous vein harvesting. Upon completion of surgery, the patient was transferred to the cardiovascular intensive care unit. Upon admission, data are as follows: Vital signs were BP 140/80, HR 115, RR 18, temperature 36°C, CVP 3 mmHg, SpO_2 97%. Chest tube has 150 mL bloody drainage. Ventilator settings: SIMV 10 Vt 550 mL, PEEP 5 cmH$_2$0, Rate 12, Pressure Support 5 cmH$_2$0. The patient is intubated but reversed from anesthesia. An infusion of propofol (Diprivan®) is initiated at 3 mg/kg/hour. The patient grimaces when suctioned, turned, and upon the initiation of early mobility.

Critical Thinking Questions

1. What tool should the nurse use to assess this patient's pain at this time?
2. What is/are the etiologic factor(s) of this patient's pain?
3. What treatment modalities should the nurse anticipate using and why?

Answers to Critical Thinking Questions

1. A behavioral rating scale or FACES rating scale should be used at this time because the patient is sedated on a propofol infusion. At this time, the patient is unable to self-report pain levels. The CPOT may be used. Physiologic parameters are not ideal to use in this patient because vital signs are influenced by the cardiac surgery procedure performed and by the associated postoperative inflammatory process.

2. Sources of this patient's pain may include the midsternotomy incision, saphenous vein harvesting, turning and positioning, early mobility, presence of the chest tube, lying on the operating room table during surgery, or any combination of these factors. The patient may also have dysarthria, a heightened skin sensation. This can occur in the early postoperative period and is often associated with a sternotomy.

3. An opioid is indicated for this postoperative pain. Nonsteroidal anti-inflammatory drugs are not ideal at this time if they can interfere with platelet function and cause additional postoperative bleeding. Weight-based intravenous acetaminophen may be administered if the patient's liver function tests are within range. This latter intervention may decrease the amount of postoperative opioids that may be required.

SELF-ASSESSMENT QUESTIONS

1. Which of the following statements is true regarding pain following cardiac surgery?
   a. The pain decreases over the first few postoperative days.
   b. Mild to moderate levels of pain can be expected.
   c. With advances in intraoperative anesthesia care, less than half of cardiac surgery patients experience postoperative pain.
   d. Patients receive less than half of the analgesics prescribed.

2. Which of the following types of pain is of primary concern immediately following cardiac surgery?
   a. Acute, visceral
   b. Chronic, somatic
   c. Chronic, neuropathic
   d. Acute, nociceptive

3. Your cardiac surgery patient is experiencing persistent sternotomy pain but is reluctant to take pain medication.

Which of the following is the nurse's best response?
   a. "If you don't let us help you with your pain, you will develop chronic pain."
   b. "Pro-inflammatory cytokines are mostly causing you to have pain."
   c. "What about taking pain medications is of concern to you?"
   d. "We can wait until your pain level is higher, if you prefer."

4. Which of the following should the nurse use as the initial step to perform a pain assessment of a cardiac surgery patient?
   a. Search for and identify sources of pain.
   b. Ask the patient to quantify the pain level.
   c. Observe the patient for physiologic signs of pain.
   d. Ask family members about the patient's level of pain.

5. Which of the following is a consequence of unrelieved pain?
   a. Decreased circulating catecholamines
   b. Increased systemic vascular resistance
   c. Decreased amounts of interleukins

d. Increased production of anti-inflammatory mediators

6. Which of the following is a physiologic strategy to decrease pain levels?
   a. Increase prostaglandin levels
   b. Increase release of epinephrine from nerve fibers
   c. Decrease serotonin uptake
   d. Decrease inhibition of primary and secondary neurons

7. Which of the following is the first step in the World Health Organization pain management ladder that can be used for cardiac surgery patients?
   a. Non-opioid
   b. Adjuvant agent
   c. Opioid
   d. Nonpharmacologic intervention

8. Which of the following is the preferred method to manage pain of patients who undergo coronary artery bypass grafting surgery in the immediate postoperative period?
   a. Morphine
   b. Phenytoin (Dilantin®)

c. Ibuprofen (Motrin®)
d. Amitriptyline (Elavil®)

9. Your patient is receiving celecoxib (Celebrex®) following cardiac surgery. For which of the following complications is the patient at increased risk?
   a. Sternal wound infection
   b. Hyperglycemia
   c. Pulmonary edema
   d. Hypokalemia

10. Your patient has undergone a thoracotomy. Which of the following should the nurse anticipate using as the preferred method of pain management?
    a. PCA with an opioid
    b. Epidural with local anesthetic
    c. Oral or IV NSAID
    d. Application of heat

Answers to Self-Assessment Questions

1. d	6. c
2. d	7. a
3. c	8. a
4. b	9. a
5. b	10. b

Clinical Inquiry Box

Question: What are nurses' learning needs to prepare patients for managing pain before and after discharge home following cardiac surgery?

Reference: Leegaard, M., Watt-Watson, J., McGillion, M., Costello, J., Elgie-Watson, J., & Partridge, K. (2011). Nurses' education needs for pain management of post-cardiac surgery patients: A qualitative study. *Journal of Cardiovascular Nursing, 26*(4), 312–320.

Objective: To determine nurses' learning needs to prepare patients for managing pain before and after discharge home following cardiac surgery

Method: Focus groups study. Twenty-seven participants were asked about their perceptions of patient education, needs for pain management following cardiac surgery, and approaches to help nurses meet these needs. The Pain Beliefs Scale was used to capture participants' misbeliefs about pain.

Results: Pain management challenges in the hospital were identified, especially related to patient age, patient concerns regarding use of opioids, need for multiple management strategies, and preparing patients to manage pain at home. Brief in services, hands-on learning, lunch-and-learn sessions, and designated education days were the most useful education strategies.

Conclusion: Most common pain knowledge gaps were identified.

REFERENCES

Acharya, M., & Dunning, J. (2010). Does the use of non-steroidal anti-inflammatory drugs after cardiac surgery increase the risk of renal failure? *Interactive Cardiovascular and Thoracic Surgery*, *11*, 461–467.

Anderson, P. G., & Cutshall, S. M. (2007). Massage therapy: A comfort intervention for cardiac surgery patients. *Clinical Nurse Specialist*, *21*(3), 161–167.

Apfelbaum, J. L., Chen, C., Mehta, S. S., & Gan, T. J. (2003). Postoperative pain experience: Results from a national survey suggest postoperative pain continues to be undermanaged. *Anesthesia & Analgesia*, *97*(2), 534–540.

Asenjo, F., & Carli, F. (2009). Neural blockade for abdominal and thoracic (non-vascular) surgery. In M. J. Cousins, D. B. Carr, T. T. Horlocker, & P. O. Bridenbaugh (Eds.), *Cousin's & Bridenbaugh's neural blockade on clinical anesthesia and pain medicine* (4th ed., pp. 520–532). Philadelphia, PA: Lippincott Williams & Wilkins.

Aslan, F. E., Badir, A., Arli, S. K., & Cakmakci, H. (2010). Patients' experience of pain after cardiac surgery. *Contemporary Nurse*, *34*(1), 48–54.

Aubrun, F., Salvi, N. S., Coriat, P., & Riou, B. (2005). Sex and age related differences in morphine requirements for postoperative pain relief. *Anesthesiology*, *103*(1), 156–160.

Babaee, S., Shafiei, Z., Sadeghi, M. M., Nik, A. Y., & Valiani, M. (2012). Effectiveness of massage therapy on the mood of patients after open-heart surgery. *Iranian Journal of Nursing and Midwifery Research*, *17*(2, Suppl. 1), S120–S124.

Bernardes, S. F., Keogh, E., & Lima, M. L. (2008). Bridging the gap between pain and gender research: A selective literature review. *European Journal of Pain*, *12*(4), 427–440.

Braun, L. A., Stanguts, C., Casanelia, L., Sptizer, O., Paul, E., Vardaxis, N. J., . . . Rosenfeldt, F. (2012). Massage therapy for cardiac surgery patients—a randomized trial. *Journal of Thoracic and Cardiovascular Surgery*, *144*(6), 1453–1459.

Brennan, F., Carr, D., & Cousins, M. (2007). Pain management: A fundamental right. *Anesthesia & Analgesia*, *105*(1), 205–221.

Bucknall, T., Manias, E., & Botti, M. (2007). Nurses' reassessment of postoperative pain after analgesic administration. *Clinical Journal of Pain*, *23*(1), 1–6.

Bunchungmongkol, N., & Pipanmekaporn, T. (2013). Quality assessment of postoperative pain management following adult cardiac surgery. *European Journal of Anaesthesiology*, *30*, 226.

Burgess, F. W., & Burgess, T. A. (2008). Pain management in the elderly surgical patient. *Medicine & Health*, *91*(1), 11–14.

Cerfolio, R. J., Bryant, A. S., Bass, C. S., & Bartolucci, A. A. (2003). A prospective, double-blinded, randomized trial evaluating the use of preemptive analgesia of the skin before thoracotomy. *Annals of Thoracic Surgery*, *76*(4), 1055–1058.

Chaney, M. A. (2009). Thoracic epidural analgesia in cardiac surgery—the current standing. *Annals of Cardiac Anaesthesia*, *12*(1), 1–3.

Cintron, A., & Morrison, R. S. (2006). Pain and ethnicity in the United States: A systematic review. *Journal of Palliative Medicine*, *9*(6), 1454–1473.

Cipriano, G., Carvalho, C. A., Bernardelli, G. F., & Peres, P. A. (2008). Short-term transcutaneous electrical nerve stimulation after cardiac surgery: Effect on pain, pulmonary function and electrical muscle activity. *Interactive Cardiovascular and Thoracic Surgery*, *7*(4), 539–543.

Cogan, J. (2010). Pain management after cardiac surgery. *Seminars in Cardiothoracic and Vascular Anesthesia*, *14*(3), 201–204.

Coventry, L. L., Siffleet, J. M., & Williams, A. M. (2006). Review of analgesia use in the intensive care unit after heart surgery. *Critical Care and Resuscitation*, *8*(2), 135–140.

Cutshall, S. M., Fenske, L. L., Kelly, R. F., Phillips, B. R., Sundt, T. M., & Bauer, B. A. (2007). Creation of a healing enhancement program at an academic medical center. *Complementary Therapies in Clinical Practice*, *13*(4), 217–223.

D'Arcy, Y. (2011). New thinking about postoperative pain management. *OR Nurse*, *5*(6), 28–36.

Decker, S., & Perry, A. G. (2003). The development and testing of the PATCOA to assess pain in confused older adults. *Pain Management Nursing*, *4*(2), 77–86.

Dhal, J. B., & Moiniche, S. (2004). Pre-emptive analgesia. *British Medical Bulletin, 71*(1), 13-27.

Dubin, A. E., & Patapoutian, A. (2010). Nociceptors: The sensors of the pain pathway. *The Journal of Clinical Investigation, 120*(11), 3760-3772.

Dunwoody, C. J., Krenzischek, D. A., Pasero, C., Rathmell, J. P., & Polomano, R. C. (2008). Assessment, physiological monitoring, and consequences of inadequately treated acute pain. *Pain Management Nursing, 9*(1), 11-21.

Evrard, H. C., & Balthazart, J. (2004). Rapid regulation of pain by estrogens synthesized in spinal dorsal horn neurons. *Journal of Neuroscience, 24*, 7225-7229.

Ezenwa, M. O., Ameringer, S., Ward, S. E., & Serlin, R. C. (2006). Racial and ethnic disparities in pain management. *Journal of Nursing Scholarship, 38*(3), 225-233.

Fillingim, R. B., King, C. D., Ribeiro-Dasilva, M. C., Rahim-Williams, B., & Riley, J. L. (2009). Sex, gender, and pain: A review of recent clinical and experimental findings. *The Journal of Pain, 10*(5), 447-485.

Friesner, S. A., Curry, D. M., & Moddeman, G. R. (2006). Comparison of two pain management strategies during chest tube removal: Relaxation exercise with opioids and opioids alone. *Heart & Lung, 35*(4), 269-276.

Furrow, B. R. (2001). Pain management and provider liability: No more excuses. *The Journal of Law, Medicine & Ethics, 29*(1), 28-51.

Gélinas, C. (2007). Management of pain in cardiac surgery ICU patients: Have we improved over time? *Intensive and Critical Care Nursing, 23*(5), 298-303.

Giles, B. E., & Walker, J. S. (2000). Sex differences in pain and analgesia. *Pain Reviews, 7*(3-4), 181-193.

Gjeilo, K. H., Wahba, A., Klepstad, P., Lydersen, S., & Stenseth, R. (2008). The role of sex in health-related quality of life after cardiac surgery: A prospective study. *European Journal of Cardiovascular Prevention & Rehabilitation, 15*(4), 448-452.

Goldstein, N. E., & Morrison, R. S. (2005). Treatment of pain in older adults. *Critical Reviews in Oncology/Hematology, 54*(2), 157-164.

Gordon, D. B., Rees, S. M., McCausland, M. P., Pellino, T. A., Sanford-Ring, S., Smith-Helmenstine, J., . . . Danis, D. M. (2008). Improving reassessment and documentation of pain management. *The Joint Commission Journal on Quality and Patient Safety, 34*(9), 509-517.

Greenspan, J. D., Craft, R. M., LeResche, L., Arendt-Nielsen, L., Berkley, K. J., Fillingim, R. B., . . . Traub, R. J. (2007). Studying sex and gender differences in pain and analgesia: A consensus report. *Pain, 132*(Suppl. 1), S26-S45.

Hansdottir, V., Philip, J., Olsen, M. F., Eduard, C., Houltz, E., & Ricksten, S. E. (2006). Thoracic epidural versus intravenous patient-controlled analgesia after cardiac surgery: A randomized controlled trial on length of hospital stay and patient-perceived quality of recovery. *Anesthesiology, 104*(1), 142-151.

Heins, J. K., Heins, A., Costello, M., Huang, K., & Mishra, S. (2006). Disparities in analgesia and opioid prescribing practices for patients with musculoskeletal pain in the emergency department. *Journal of Emergency Nursing, 32*(3), 219-224.

Herr, K. (2011). Pain assessment strategies in older patients. *The Journal of Pain, 12*(3, Suppl. 1), S3-S13.

Herr, K., Coyne, P. J., Key, T., Manworren, R., McCaffery, M., Merkel, S., . . . Wild, L. (2006). Pain assessment in the nonverbal patient: Position statement with clinical practice recommendations. *Pain Management Nursing, 7*(2), 44-52.

Hjermstad, M. J., Fayers, P. M., Haugen, D. F., Caraceni, A., Hanks, G. W., Loge, J. H., . . . Kaasa, S. (2011). Studies comparing numerical rating scales, verbal rating scales, and visual analogue scales for assessment of pain intensity in adults: A systematic literature review. *Journal of Pain and Symptom Management, 41*(6), 1073-1093.

Ho, S. C., Royse, C. F., Royse, A. G., Penberthy, A., & McRae, R. (2002). Persistent pain after cardiac surgery: An audit of high thoracic epidural and primary opioid analgesia therapies. *Anesthesia & Analgesia, 95*(4), 820-823.

Holmgren, C., Carlsson, T., Mannheimer, C., & Edvardsson, N. (2008). Risk of interference from transcutaneous electrical nerve stimulation on the sensing function of implantable defibrillators. *Pacing and Clinical Electrophysiology, 31*(2), 151–158.

International Association for the Study of Pain. (2008). *IASP pain taxonomy.* Retrieved from http://www.iasp-pain.org/Taxonomy

Jarzyna, D., Jungquist, C. R., Pasero, C., Willens, J. S., Nisbet, A., Oakes, L., . . . Polomano, R. C. (2011). American Society for Pain Management nursing guidelines on monitoring for opioid-induced sedation and respiratory depression. *Pain Management Nursing, 12*(3), 118–145.

Jensen, M. K., & Andersen, C. (2004). Can chronic poststernotomy pain after cardiac valve replacement be reduced using thoracic epidural analgesia? *Acta Anaesthesiologica Scandinavica, 48*(7), 871–874.

Joint Commission. (2012). *Provision of care, treatment, and services (CAMH/hospitals).* Retrieved from http://www.jointcommission.org/mobile/standards_information/jcfaqdetails.aspx?Standar dsFAQId=471&StandardsFAQChapterId=78

Joshi, S. S., & Jagadeesh, A. M. (2013). Efficacy of perioperative pregabalin in acute and chronic post-operative pain after off-pump coronary artery bypass surgery: A randomized, double-blinded placebo controlled trial. *Annals of Cardiac Anaesthesia, 16*(3), 180–185.

King, K. M. (2000). Gender and short-term recovery from cardiac surgery. *Nursing Research, 49*(1), 29–36.

Lahtinen, P., Kokki, H., & Hynynen, M. (2006). Pain after cardiac surgery: A prospective cohort study of 1-year incidence and intensity. *Anesthesiology, 105*(4), 794–800.

Lasch, K. E. (2002). Culture and pain. *Pain: Clinical updates, International Association of the Study of Pain,* 10(5). Retrieved from http://www.iasp-pain.org/

Li, J. M. (2008). Pain management in the hospitalized patient. *Medical Clinics of North America, 92*(2), 371–385.

Lome, B. (2005). Acute pain and the critically ill trauma patient. *Critical Care Nursing Quarterly, 28*(2), 200–207.

McCaffery, M. (1972). *Nursing management of the patient with pain.* Philadelphia, PA: Lippincott.

Mehta, Y., & Kumar, S. (2004). New horizons for critical care in cardiac surgery. *Indian Journal of Critical Care Medicine, 8*(1), 11–13.

Menda, F., Koner, O., Sayin, M., Ergenoglu, M., Kucukaksu, S., & Aykac, B. (2010). Effects of single-dose gabapentin on postoperative pain and morphine consumption after cardiac surgery. *Journal of Cardiothoracic and Vascular Anesthesia, 24*(5), 808–813.

Miller, C., & Newton, S. (2006). Pain perception and expression: The influence of gender, personal self-efficacy, and lifespan socialization. *Pain Management Nursing, 7*(4), 148–152.

Morris, D. B. (2001). Ethnicity and pain. *Pain: Clinical Updates: International Association of the Study of Pain,* 9(4). Retrieved from http://www.iasp-pain.org/

Mueller, X. M., Tinguely, F., Tavaearai, H. T., Revelly, J.-P., Chioléro, R., & von Segesser, L. K. (2000). Pain location, distribution, and intensity after cardiac surgery. *Chest, 118*(2), 391–396.

Ng, A., & Swanevelder, J. (2007). Pain relief after thoracotomy: Is epidural analgesia the optimal technique? *British Journal of Anaesthesia, 98*(2), 159–162.

Nilsson, U. (2008). The anxiety and pain-reducing effects of music interventions: A systemic review. *AORN, 87*(4), 780–807.

Özer, N., Özlü, Z. K., Arslan, S., & Günes, N. (2013). Effect of music on postoperative pain and physiologic parameters of patients after open heart surgery. *Pain Management Nursing, 14*(1), 20–28.

Pasero, C. (2009). Challenges in pain assessment. *Journal of PeriAnesthesia Nursing, 24,* 50–54.

Pasero, C., & McCaffery, M. (2011). *Pain assessment and pharmacologic management.* St. Louis, MO: Mosby.

Pogatzki-Zahn, E. M., Zahn, P. K., & Brennan, T. J. (2007). Postoperative pain—Clinical implications of basic research. *Best Practice & Research Clinical Anaesthesiology, 21*(1), 3–13.

Polomano, R. C., Dunwoody, C. J., Krenzischek, D. A., & Rathmell, J. P. (2008). Perspective on pain management in the 21st century. *Pain Management Nursing, 9*(1), S3–S10.

Ranger, M., & Campbell-Yeo, M. (2008). Temperament and pain response: A review of the literature. *Pain Management Nursing, 9*(1), 2–9.

Reimer-Kent, J. (2003). From theory to practice: Preventing pain after cardiac surgery. *American Journal of Critical Care, 12*(2), 136–143.

Rosenquist, R. W., & Rosenburg, J. (2003). Postoperative pain guidelines. *Regional Anesthesia & Pain Medicine, 28*(4), 279–288.

Sattari, M., Baghdadchi, M. E., Kheyri, M., Khakzadi, H., & Mashayekhi, S. O. (2013) Study of patient pain management after heart surgery. *Advanced Pharmaceutical Bulletin, 3*(2), 373–377.

Shi, Y., Weingarten, T. N., Mantilla, C. B., Hooten, W. M., & Warner, D. O. (2010). Smoking and pain: Pathophysiology and clinical implications. *Anesthesiology, 113*(4), 977–992.

Silihoglu, Z., Yildirim, M., Demiroluk, S., Kaya, G., Karatas, A., Ertem, M., . . . Aytac, E. (2009). Evaluation of intravenous paracetamol administration on postoperative pain and recovery characteristics in patients undergoing laparoscopic cholecystectomy. *Surgical, Laparoscopy, Endoscopy Percutaneous Techniques, 19*(4), 321–321.

St. Marie, B. (2010). *Core curriculum for pain management nursing* (2nd ed.). St. Louis, MO: Kendall Hunt.

Tamayo-Sarrer, J. H., Hinze, S. W., Cydulka, R. K., & Baker, D. W. (2003). Racial and ethnic disparities in the emergency department analgesic prescription. *American Journal of Public Health, 93*(12), 2067–2073.

Terrell, K. M., Hui, S. L., Castelluccio, P., McGrath, R. B., & Miller, D. K. (2010). Analgesic prescribing for patients who are discharged from an emergency department. *Pain Medicine, 11*(7), 1072–1077.

Ucak, A., Onan, B., Sen, H., Selcuk, I., Turan, A., & Yilmaz, A. (2011). The effects of gabapentin on acute and chronic postoperative pain after coronary artery bypass graft surgery. *Journal of Cardiothoracic and Vascular Anesthesia, 25*(5), 824–829.

Vaccarino, V., Lin, Z. Q., Kasl, S. V., Mattera, J. A., Roumanis, S. A., Abramson, J. L., & Krumholz, H. M. (2003). Gender differences in recovery after coronary artery bypass surgery.

Journal of the American College of Cardiology, 41(2), 307–314.

Vadivelu, N., Mitra, S., & Naravan, D. (2010). Recent advances in post-operative pain management. *Yale Journal of Biology and Medicine, 83*(1), 11–25.

Viscusi, E. R. (2012). *IV acetaminophen improves pain management and reduces opioid requirements in surgical patients: A review of the clinical data and case-based presentations.* Retrieved from http://www.anesthesiologynews.com/download/SR122_WM.pdf

Voss, J. A., Good, M., Yates, B., Baun, M. M., Thompson, A., & Hertzog, M. (2004). Sedative music reduces anxiety and pain during chair rest after open heart surgery. *Pain, 112*(1–2), 197–203.

Wang, N., Hailey, D., & Yu, P. (2011). Quality of nursing documentation and approaches to its evaluation: A mixed method systematic review. *Journal of Advanced Nursing, 67*(9), 1858–1875.

Watt-Watson, J., Stevens, B., Katz, J., Costello, J., Reid, G., J., & David, T. (2004). Impact of preoperative education on pain outcomes after coronary artery bypass graft surgery. *Pain, 109*(1–2), 73–85.

Wells, N., Pasero, C., & McCaffery, M. (2008). Improving the quality of care through pain assessment and management In R. G. Hughes (Ed.), *Patient safety and quality: An evidence-based handbook for nurses* (pp. 470–497). Rockville, MD: Agency for Healthcare Research and Quality.

White, P. F., & Kehlet, H. (2010). Improving postoperative pain management. *Anesthesiology, 112*(1), 220–225.

Yapici, D., Altunkan, Z. O., Atici, S., Bilgin, E., Doruk, N., Cinel, I., . . . Oral, U. (2008). Postoperative effects of low-dose intrathecal morphine in coronary artery bypass surgery. *Journal of Cardiac Surgery, 23*(2), 140–145.

Yorke, J., McLean, B., & Wallis, M. (2004). Patient's perceptions of pain management after cardiac surgery in an Australian critical care unit. *Heart & Lung, 33*(1), 33–41.

Young, A., & Buvanendran, A. (2012). Recent advances in multimodal analgesia. *Anesthesiology Clinics, 30*(1), 91–100.

WEB RESOURCES

American Academy of Pain Management: http://www.aapainmanage.org/

Pain Management Nursing: http://www.painmanagementnursing.org/

American Pain Society: http://www.ampainsoc.org/

National Pain Foundation: http://www.nationalpainfoundation.org/default.asp

International Association for the Study of Pain (IASP): https://members.iasp-pain.org/

American Society for Pain Management Nursing (ASPMN): http://www.aspmn.org/

Daily Pain Diary: https://www.caremark.com/Imagebank/Health_Diaries/DailyPainDiary.pdf Inside look at Chronic Pain: http://www.or-live.com/distributors/nlm-flash/chp_1867/rnh.cfm?id=704

Transcutaneous Electrical Nerve Stimulation (TENS): https://www.intelihealth.com/article/learn-about-transcutaneous-electrical-nerve-stimulation-tens

Chapter 15

Postoperative Dysrhythmias

Roberta Kaplow

INTRODUCTION

Dysrhythmias following cardiac surgery are known complications and account for high mortality rates, increased hospital length of stay (LOS), and costs. The length of time the dysrhythmias last, ventricular response rate, patient's baseline cardiac function, and presence of comorbidities will impact the clinical significance of the dysrhythmias. Management includes identifying and treating the underlying cause(s) as well as pharmacologic and nonpharmacologic interventions. If the dysrhythmia is self-limiting, treatment may not be necessary, depending on the patient's hemodynamic response. However, treatment may be necessary if systemic infections or persistent pericardial effusion encompass the clinical situation (Peretto, Durante, Limite, & Cianflone, 2014).

Patients may have dysrhythmias prior to surgery or develop them intraoperatively or postoperatively. The origins of dysrhythmias include the atrium, atrioventricular (AV) node, or ventricle. This chapter discusses the most commonly encountered postoperative dysrhythmias (PODs), including their incidence, etiology, and suggested management.

INCIDENCE

The incidence of dysrhythmias can be as high as 60% in cardiac surgery patients depending upon the type (Helgadottir, Sigurdsson, Ingvarsdottir, Arnar, & Gudbjartsson, 2012; Maesen, Nijs, Maessen, Allessie, & Schotten, 2012; Shen et al., 2011). Dysrhythmias may compromise cardiac output (CO) by as much as 15% to 25% (Silvestry, 2014) when they interfere with diastolic filling. It is essential that the nurse working in the intensive care unit (ICU) with postoperative cardiac surgery patients be proficient in identifying and possibly eradicating potential causes and promptly recognizing potentially life-threatening dysrhythmias. Assessment of the patient requires evaluation of cardiac rhythm, its effects on systemic perfusion, and etiologic factors.

ETIOLOGY

Several potential etiologic factors related to postoperative cardiac surgery dysrhythmias have been identified. The trauma associated with cardiac surgery itself places the patient at risk for the development of PODs. In addition, advanced age has been implicated in their development. This is felt to be related to changes in structure and electrophysiology associated with aging (Peretto et al., 2014). Examples include enlargement of the atria or increased atrial pressures. Others at risk include those with a history of severe stenosis of the right coronary artery, disease of the sinoatrial (SA) or AV node, or mitral valve disease. These changes have predisposed elderly patients to postoperative atrial tachyarrhythmias, especially postoperative atrial fibrillation (POAF) (Peretto et al., 2014). Patients with a history of chronic obstructive pulmonary disease (COPD) or stroke are also at increased risk for PODs (Maesen et al., 2012; Peretto et al., 2014).

Dysrhythmias in postoperative cardiac surgery patients may result from fluid overload–induced acute atrial enlargement, respiratory complications, electrolyte disturbances (e.g., hypokalemia, hyperkalemia, hypomagnesemia), surgical trauma (inadequate cardioprotection during bypass procedures), hypothermia, hyperadrenergic state, acid–base imbalance, anxiety, or pain. Presence of hypoxia, hypercarbia, excess catecholamines, and use of instrumentation in the operating room may also precipitate the development of PODs. Further, cardiopulmonary bypass (CPB), the amount of cross-clamp time, type of cardioplegia used, and coronary artery bypass grafting (CABG) procedures put the patient at risk for the development of PODs (Peretto et al., 2014).

Postoperative dysrhythmias are anticipated following cardiac transplant procedures as well. They are thought to be due to ischemia of the donor heart, extensive suture lines, rejection, augmented atherosclerosis, and procedure-associated denervation (Dasari et al., 2010; Peretto et al., 2014). The incidence is reported at 4% to 24% of heart transplant patients (Maesen et al., 2012; Peretto et al., 2014).

ATRIAL DYSRHYTHMIAS

Atrial dysrhythmias are the most commonly encountered rhythm abnormalities in the postoperative CABG patient. The overall incidence of atrial dysrhythmias is reported to be as high as 60%. A higher incidence is reported in patients who undergo valve surgery than CABG (Helgadottir et al., 2012; Maesen

et al., 2012; Shen et al., 2011). The incidence of development of atrial dysrhythmias is reported to be 29% to 44% in patients undergoing CABG alone (Helgadottir et al., 2012; Maesen et al., 2012; Nair, 2010; Shen et al., 2011), as high as 40% in patients undergoing valve replacements (Nair, 2010), and 50% to 64% following CABG and valve surgery combined (Helgadottir et al., 2012; Nair, 2010). Atrial dysrhythmias that may develop in the postoperative cardiac surgery patient may include sinus tachycardia, premature atrial contractions (PACs), atrial fibrillation (AF), and atrial flutter.

Sinus tachycardia is a common dysrhythmia following surgery in general, with cardiac surgery being no exception. It can be attributed to the normal stress response. As a general guideline, treatment of sinus tachycardia should focus on ameliorating its underlying cause. Etiology of sinus tachycardia may include pain, fever, anxiety, anemia, medications (e.g., catecholamines), hypermetabolic state (e.g., sepsis), or an increase in adrenergic tone (e.g., in a patient taking a beta blocker preoperatively). The presence of sinus tachycardia is not likely to cause adverse effects if the patient has normal left ventricular (LV) function, and treatment is usually not indicated (Peretto et al., 2014).

Premature atrial contractions may also develop in the postoperative cardiac surgery patient. These abnormal beats are usually not clinically significant and rarely require treatment. However, PACs can predispose patients to POAF (Hashemzadeh, Dehdilani, & Dehdilani, 2013). Eighty-seven percent of postoperative cardiac surgery patients were found to have had PACs prior to the onset of POAF. These patients showed either a pattern of sustained uniform PAC activity or spontaneous bursts of high PAC activity interspaced with relatively quiet periods of PAC activity prior to AF (Bashour et al., 2004). If characteristic PAC patterns predict POAF, pharmacologic interventions with agents used to treat

POAF could be initiated when the characteristic PAC pattern is first detected. During the highest POAF risk period (postoperative days 1–5), nurses should maintain a high level of vigilance for potential intervention.

Atrial fibrillation is the most common dysrhythmia that may occur in the postoperative cardiac surgery patient (Gu, Wei, Huang, & Yin, 2012). In one study, the overall rate of patients who developed POAF was 44%. In this study, of the patients who underwent aortic valve replacement, CABG, or off-pump coronary artery bypass grafting (OPCAB), 74%, 44%, and 35%, respectively, developed POAF. The patients who developed POAF were older, more often female, had a lower ejection fraction (EF), and were less likely to be smokers. In that same study, the overall 5-year survival was significantly higher in patients who did not develop POAF (Helgadottir et al., 2012). Previous data suggest a POAF incidence rate of 30% to 50% (Echahidi, Pibarot, O'Hara, & Mathieu, 2008).

Postoperative atrial fibrillation is often self-limiting, with the majority of patients with new-onset POAF converting back to normal sinus rhythm (NSR) within 6 to 8 weeks postoperatively (Peretto et al., 2014). The peak onset of occurrence of POAF is 2–4 days following surgery (Helgadottir et al., 2012; Koniari, Apostolakis, Rogkakou, Baikoussis, & Dougenis, 2010; Maesen et al., 2012; Nair, 2010; Peretto et al., 2014; Rho, 2009), with some reporting a small percentage of patients (6%) developing POAF after 6 days (Maesen et al., 2012).

Data suggest that up to 30% of patients who develop POAF did not have a history of this dysrhythmia. The majority transition back to NSR within 12 hours, and 80% convert back within 24 hours (Peretto et al., 2014). Incidence data are variable and depend on the type of procedure performed. Patients who undergo OPCAB have less risk of developing POAF. This is felt to be related to the development of less inflammation as

compared with on-pump procedures (Peretto et al., 2014; Tomic et al., 2005).

The pathophysiology of AF involves the rapid release of multiple impulses from the atrium to the AV node; however, the AV node can respond to only a few of these impulses. In AF, the patient's heart does not contract with maximum efficiency. The rapid quivering of the atria may result in hemodynamic compromise from decreased atrial filling and the atrial kick that can normally contribute as much as 25% of CO (Silvestry, 2014). Loss of atrial kick can result in increased pulmonary pressure. This is seen more often in patients with decreased diastolic function (Peretto et al., 2014). In patients with normal LV function, however, AF is generally well tolerated (Koniari et al., 2010; Peretto et al., 2014). Because the blood lingers in the atria with AF, small clots may develop, which places the patient at risk for stroke.

Risk Factors for POAF

Many studies have attempted to determine the etiology of AF in the postoperative cardiac surgery patient. The cause of POAF is multifactorial (Maesen et al., 2012). A patient's demographic data and medical history provide insight into the probability of PODs.

Risk factors may be categorized into preoperative, intraoperative, and postoperative risks. The primary predictor of POAF is age (Maesen et al., 2012). As the body ages, structural and size changes of the atria predispose the individual to develop atrial dysrhythmias. Preoperative risks may also include atrial fibrosis; history of rheumatic heart disease; valve disease; right coronary artery stenosis; increased LV diastolic pressure; hypertension; acute coronary syndrome; heart disease (e.g., LV hypertrophy); enlargement of the left atrium; dilation of the right atrium and right ventricle; history of heart failure, which results in atrial stretch from volume overload; COPD; diabetes mellitus;

pulmonary hypertension; tachycardia; hypokalemia; hypomagnesemia; hypothyroidism;
preoperative beta blocker withdrawal; preoperative use of digoxin or milrinone; and
obesity (Fleming et al., 2008; Koniari et al.,
2010; Maesen et al., 2012; Nair, 2010; Peretto
et al., 2014; Zacharias et al., 2005). The presence of pericardial effusion, pericarditis, acute
enlargement of the atria, and ischemia has
been frequently implicated in the development of POAF (Maesen et al., 2012; Peretto
et al., 2014). Surprisingly, some data suggest that current smokers were less likely to
develop dysrhythmias following CABG. This
phenomenon is thought to be related to the
"hyperadrenergic stimulation" from nicotine
in current smokers. This was found not to be
true of patients who smoked in the past (Al-
Sarraf et al., 2010; Yun, Bazar, Lee, Gerber, &
Daniel, 2005). These data are not consistent.

Intraoperative risks that have been identified include sympathetic stimulation from
catecholamines, fluid losses, anemia, pain,
or administration of adrenergic agents. Sympathetic stimulation leads to an increase in
heart rate and contractility from beta-1 receptor stimulation. Sympathetic stimulation also
leads to an increase in excitability and automaticity (the heart's inherent ability to initiate a beat). Patients with POAF have higher
levels of norepinephrine as compared to
patients who do not develop POAF. There is
also an associated shortened atrial refractori-
ness associated with sympathetic stimulation.
This can put the patient at risk to develop a
POD (Maesen et al., 2012).

Inflammation associated with cardiac
surgery has been suggested as a mechanism
contributing to development of POAF. Inflammation leads to the release of pro-inflammatory mediators. This is manifested with
elevated white blood cell, monocyte, and neutrophil counts (Maesen et al., 2012). A systemic
inflammatory response may develop from CPB.

Oxidative stress is another suggested etiologic factor for POAF related to cardiac
surgery. A consequence of CPB is ischemia.
During reperfusion, there is an increased production of reactive oxygen species (from pro-
oxidants [vs. antioxidants]). This can result in
myocardial stunning, tissue damage, and cell
death. The degree of oxidative stress depends
on the extent of ischemia and left ventricular
ejection fraction (LVEF) (Maesen et al., 2012).

Cross-clamping without adequate atrial
protection, bicaval venous cannulation, metabolic imbalances, fluid and electrolyte shifts,
cardioplegia, the surgical incision, and the
surgical procedure itself have also been implicated (Hall, Smith, & Rocker, 2007; Koniari
et al., 2010; Maesen et al., 2012; Nair, 2010;
Peretto et al., 2014; Rho, 2009). Patients who
underwent OPCAB were reported to have a
lower incidence of POAF. This is thought to
be related to CPB-associated systemic inflammatory effect (Helgadottir et al., 2012). These
effects are not consistently reported in the
literature (Maesen et al., 2012).

Postoperative factors that have been implicated in the development of POAF include
hemodynamic compromise (e.g., secondary
to heart failure, myocardial infarction [MI],
venous thrombotic events [VTEs], bleeding
from anticoagulation), administration of
beta-1 agonists (e.g., dopamine [Intropin®],
dobutamine [Dobutrex®]), hypomagnesemia,
extubation, increased sympathetic and parasympathetic tone, and an exaggerated inflammatory response (Hall et al., 2007; Koniari et
al., 2010; Nair, 2010; Rho, 2009). Fluid shifts
from the interstitium to the vascular space
can cause atrial stretch, which can put the
patient at risk for POAF (Nair, 2010). Data
from one study suggest that patients who
receive dexmedetomidine (Precedex®) following cardiac surgery were less likely to develop
postoperative atrial dysrhythmias when compared to those who received propofol (Dipri-
van®) (Vlessides, 2012). This is thought to be
related to dexmedetomidine's anti-inflammatory properties, which are typical in alpha-2
agonists.

Complications of POAF

A number of consequences of POAF following cardiac surgery have been reported. Development of POAF has been reported to result in increased LOS (Helgadottir et al., 2012; Maesen et al., 2012; Nair, 2010; Rho, 2009); increased LOS in the ICU (Helgadottir et al., 2012; Rho, 2009); postoperative mortality (Helgadottir et al., 2012; Maesen et al., 2012); increased 5-year mortality (Helgadottir et al., 2012); hemodynamic instability (Koniari et al., 2010; Maesen et al., 2012); increased risk of stroke (Arsenault et al., 2013; Koniari et al., 2010; Maesen et al., 2012; Nair, 2010); increased costs (Rho, 2009); renal failure (Nair, 2010); heart failure (Nair, 2010); decreased cognitive function lasting up to 6 weeks (Nair, 2010); MI (Nair, 2010); need for a permanent pacemaker, tracheostomy, or intra-aortic balloon pump (Nair, 2010); and increased postoperative bleeding (Nair, 2010). Patients who developed POAF also received more transfusions while bleeding was somewhat increased (Helgadottir et al., 2012).

Prevention of POAF

Prevention of POAF is essential to help decrease LOS and overall mortality (Koniari et al., 2010). The individual patient scenario, potential adverse events, and cost should be considered when deciding on the appropriate intervention to prevent POAF (Arsenault et al., 2013). No single agent or combination of agents has entirely eradicated POAF. Use of prophylaxis for POAF is supported in the literature. However, lack of published clinical guidelines and the negative inotropic effects of a number of the agents have thus far resulted in prophylactic measures not being implemented consistently (Helgadottir et al., 2012).

Pharmacotherapy

Patients who are at high risk for the development of POAF may receive preventive antiarrhythmic therapy. Consideration should be given to renal function and the side effects of the agents when deciding if preventive strategies are warranted.

Beta Blockers

The use of beta blockers to prevent POAF is supported by international guidelines, but these are not consistently followed (Gajulapalli & Rader, 2012; Lutz, Panchagnula, & Barker, 2011; Nair, 2010). Data demonstrate that beta blockers are efficacious in helping to prevent POAF. Beta blockers are considered the first choice to prevent POAF and should be used unless contraindicated (Arsenault et al., 2013; Fleming et al., 2008; Koniari et al., 2010; Wu et al., 2013). Their use has also been shown to decrease mortality rates (Ferguson, Coombs, & Peterson, 2002; Koniari et al., 2010). Beta blockers should be administered on the morning of surgery, unless contraindicated (Nair, 2010). Contraindications to beta blocker use include hemodynamic compromise, use of inotropes, and presence of heart block (i.e., first-degree AV block with a PR interval greater than 0.24 second, second- or third-degree AV block).

Sotalol

Sotalol (Betapace®) is a class III agent (potassium channel blocker), which causes an increase in repolarization time. It also has beta blocker properties. Sotalol may be more effective in reducing the incidence of POAF with fewer associated side effects than beta blockers. Some data suggest better efficacy than a beta blocker (Sanjuán et al., 2004). Administration should begin 1–2 days preoperatively or within 4 hours postoperatively (Peretto et al., 2014). However, because there is a potential for proarrhythmic effects with sotalol, beta blockers have been reported as safer to administer for the prevention of POAF (Koniari et al., 2010). Administration of sotalol may prolong the QT interval (Nair,

2010). Sotalol is contraindicated in patients with heart failure (Callahan, 2011).

Amiodarone

Amiodarone (Cordarone®) prolongs both the duration and the refractory period of the myocardial cell action potential. It possesses mild alpha, beta, and calcium channel blocking effects. Because of the wide range of effects, amiodarone has been shown to be effective in decreasing incidence of AF (Clark, Hodge, Ressler, & Lee, 2011). Amiodarone may be useful when use of beta blockers is not feasible (Koniari et al., 2010). Amiodarone has been shown to be effective to decrease the incidence of POAF by up to 50% (Peretto et al., 2014; Wu et al., 2013) but not affect mortality rates (Nair, 2010). A variety of administration schedules and routes of administration are reported. It is unclear if amiodarone is more effective than a beta blocker to prevent POAF (Peretto et al., 2014). An infusion may be started if the patient is at high risk for POAF (e.g., age older than 65 years, history of COPD or heart failure, or prolonged CPB time) (Nair, 2010). Beta blockers and amiodarone may also be used in combination for this purpose. Because amiodarone has properties from all four classes of cardiac medications, hypotension and bradycardia are possible (Nair, 2010).

Magnesium

Hypomagnesemia is a risk factor for the development of POAF. Low magnesium levels may last up to 4 days after cardiac surgery. As such, administration of magnesium for prophylaxis has been evaluated. In some studies, statistically significant differences in the incidence of POAF have been reported in patients who received prophylactic magnesium administration (Gu et al., 2012; Hazelrigg et al., 2004; Koniari et al., 2010; Zangrillo et al., 2005). Statistically

significant differences in the incidence of POAF are not consistently reported (Arsenault et al., 2013; Kohno, Koyanagi, Kasegawa, & Miyazaki, 2005). Administration of magnesium is not consistently recommended in guidelines. In one study, the combination of magnesium with beta blockers did not decrease the incidence of POAF following CABG versus beta blocker therapy alone. There was no decrease in LOS or mortality rate with combination therapy. In fact, the postoperative adverse events reported were higher in patients who received combination therapy (Wu et al., 2013).

Nonsteroidal Anti-Inflammatory Drugs

Nonsteroidal anti-inflammatory drugs (NSAIDs) have been studied to determine if they decrease the incidence of POAF. The thinking behind such an intervention is that an inflammatory process is strongly associated with cardiac arrhythmias (Granier, Massin, & Pasquie, 2013). Some preliminary evidence suggests that NSAIDs may be helpful in preventing POAF (Davis, Packard, & Hilleman, 2010; Koniari et al., 2010). In an observational cohort of 4,657 patients undergoing CABG, Mathew and colleagues (2004) identified the use of NSAIDs as a protective factor against POAF. Chereku and colleagues (2004) published the results of an open-label randomized trial of 100 patients undergoing CABG. Systematic use of ketorolac and ibuprofen significantly decreased the incidence of POAF from 28.6% to 9.8%, without any major mortality or morbidity compared with control group. Larger trials to support this suggestion are needed (Davis et al., 2010).

Corticosteroids

Administration of corticosteroids has been evaluated to determine if there is an associated decrease in the incidence of POAF following a patient's first CABG procedure or aortic valve replacement. In one study, patients received hydrocortisone 100 mg or placebo. In another, patients received methylprednisolone 1 g preoperatively and dexamethasone (Decadron®) 4 mg postoperatively every 6 hours for 24 hours. While the incidence of POAF was decreased in both studies, the LOS and complication rates were higher in the latter study of patients receiving methylprednisolone and Decadron (Halonen et al., 2007; Prasongsukarn et al., 2005). In a meta-analysis, Ho and Tan (2009) studied the effect of corticosteroids on the prevention of postoperative complications. Among the 50 randomized controlled studies, 16 studies with 1,479 patients addressed the question of POAF. Findings indicate that prophylactic use of corticosteroids before cardiac surgery reduced the risk of POAF from 35.1% to 25.1% ($p < 0.01$). Nurses should consider the impact of corticosteroids on an increase in hyperglycemia and a potential for postoperative infection.

N-acetylcysteine

Administration of N-acetylcysteine (NAC) has been demonstrated to be effective in reducing the incidence of POAF in patients undergoing CABG, valve surgery, or a combination of these procedures (Ozaydin et al., 2008). As described earlier, a consequence of CPB is ischemia that results in oxidative stress. An increasing body of evidence demonstrates that oxidative stress and inflammatory reaction play an important role in the pathophysiology of POAF. N-acetylcysteine has proven to decrease serum levels of molecular markers of cellular oxidative stress in patients undergoing heart surgery. Administration of NAC, which has antioxidant properties, may decrease the incidence of POAF (Maesen et al., 2012). The duration of NAC administration should be until postoperative days 2–3 when the inflammatory cytokines levels are the highest, corresponding to the day of the highest incidence of POAF (Liu, Xu, & Fan, 2014).

Other Antioxidants

Nitric oxide (NO) and vitamin C have also been shown to hinder oxidative stress in patients who are undergoing CABG. Results from one study suggested that inspired NO gas has an antioxidant property that reduces the levels of cell death and is not associated with significantly worse physiologic outcomes (Elahi, Worner, Khan, & Matata, 2009; Maesen et al., 2012).

Statins

It has been suggested that preoperative administration of a statin may decrease the incidence of POAF. A recent meta-analysis of postoperative mortality and morbidity in patients on preoperative statin therapy gives a 1.2% and 4.4% absolute reduction in 30-day mortality for cardiac and vascular surgery, respectively (Hindler et al., 2006). This is felt to be related to the antioxidant and decreased inflammatory effect of these agents and that they may diminish myocardial perfusion injury following cardiac surgery (Helgadottir et al., 2012; Liakopoulos et al., 2009; Patti et al., 2006). These data are not consistent as some suggest that preoperative administration of statins does not decrease the incidence of POAF (Virani et al., 2008).

Electrical Therapy: Atrial Pacing

Data suggest that right atrial pacing decreases the incidence of POAF (Burgess, Kilborn, & Keech, 2006; Singhal & Kejriwal, 2010). This translated to decreased LOS and hospital costs (Arsenault et al., 2013). When treatment continued for 96 hours following cardiac surgery, biatrial pacing was effective in preventing POAF following CABG (Fan et al., 2000). Biatrial pacing is a complex therapy to use. As such, it is less well established (Nair, 2010).

Atrial Dysrhythmias Following Cardiac Transplant

In the cardiac transplant patient, there is a reported lower incidence of PODs than with other cardiac surgeries. Factors that have been implicated in the development of POAF include ischemia, denervation, pericardial inflammation, potential drug interactions with immunosuppression, autonomic hypersensitivity, primary graft failure, early rejection, administration of inotropes, ventricular dysfunction, valve regurgitation, systemic inflammation, allograft vasculopathy, and a focal trigger from superior or inferior vena cava or coronary sinus. Atrial flutter is reported to be the most common dysrhythmia noted on patient follow up. It may be due to rejection, atrial remodeling (same causes as AF), atrial suture lines, conduction barriers, or issues related to recipient-to-donor atrial conduction (Thajudeen et al., 2012).

Treatment of POAF

Treatment of AF focuses on control of rate and rhythm. Several treatment strategies for the management of AF have been reported. Ultimately, intervention to bring about a conversion from AF to NSR is most desirable. Management strategies of POAF include heart rate control with either medications or electricity (e.g., synchronized cardioversion [SCV]). The latter may not be necessary given the percentage of patients who convert to NSR on their own (Peretto et al., 2014). Knowing the factors that predispose the patient to developing AF, the nurse should attempt to anticipate the occurrence of this complication and be prepared to quickly respond to the dysrhythmias and convert the patient to NSR. A detailed preoperative history is important in preventing postoperative dysrhythmias. Analysis of the electrocardiogram will reveal the presence of preexisting conditions such as LV hypertrophy.

A rapid assessment of the patient's hemodynamic status is essential to help determine the appropriate treatment strategy (Rho, 2009). If the patient is stable, pharmacotherapy may be attempted. If unstable (e.g., presence of hypotension, mental status changes, chest pain, shortness of breath, heart failure symptoms, or cold and clammy skin), SCV is indicated. There is a reported conversion rate to NSR in 95% of cases (Rho, 2009).

Development of POAF becomes clinically significant due to the resultant decreases in diastolic filling and CO. Hypotension and ischemia result from the associated increase in myocardial oxygen consumption. Patients typically become symptomatic when they develop POAF with a rapid ventricular response (Peretto et al., 2014). When a cardiac surgery patient develops POAF, hemodynamic stability status, possible underlying causes, and goals of treatment are all key considerations that need to be identified promptly. Antiarrhythmic therapy and consideration of antithrombotic therapy to prevent a VTE are the mainstays of therapy (Peretto et al., 2014).

Establishment of hemodynamic stability should be the principal goal of therapy. Hemodynamic stability may need to be attained by controlling rate, rhythm, or both; the former is usually all that is required. The pharmacologic agents used to prevent or treat postoperative dysrhythmias are discussed in detail in Chapter 12.

Agents recommended by the American College of Cardiology, European Society of Cardiology, and the American Heart Association that are used to control heart rate associated with POAF include beta blockers and amiodarone. Digoxin is not currently recommended and has limited use following cardiac surgery (Nair, 2010). The use of beta blockers has been reported to decrease the incidence of POAF from 30–40% to 12–16% in patients who underwent CABG. Similarly, a decrease from 37–50% to 15–20% is reported in patients who have undergone valve procedures. Beta blockers also decrease the ventricular response rate when POAF develops. Patients seem to derive the most benefit when beta blocker therapy is initiated preoperatively or in the immediate postoperative period (Peretto et al., 2014).

Some data suggest that carvedilol (Coreg®) is more effective than metoprolol (Lopressor®) (Haghjoo et al., 2007). Beta-1 selective agents may be preferred in patients where bronchoconstriction is not desirable. Carvedilol blocks alpha₁ receptors and has a vasodilator effect, so its use results in little change in the hemodynamic profiles of patients. Carvedilol may be used to control the ventricular rate of AF.

Patients who are beta blocker naïve will typically remain on therapy at least until their first postoperative ambulatory visit. Those who were on beta blockers in the past (e.g., for MI, heart failure, hypertension) should remain on long-term therapy (Peretto et al., 2014).

Amiodarone may also be used to decrease the ventricular response rate of POAF. If the patient has undergone SCV, has converted after delivery of one shock, and is on an amiodarone infusion, it may be discontinued after 7 days (Nair, 2010).

Anticoagulation

Patients who develop POAF that lasts more than 48 hours are at risk for a VTE. The risk increases further in patients with mitral valve disease secondary to rheumatic fever, previous VTE, hypertension, or heart failure. Data are not consistent regarding the usefulness of anticoagulation in preventing stroke in these patients. Conversion to NSR may be challenging in patients with valve disease (Peretto et al., 2014).

Administration of anticoagulants in the postoperative cardiac surgery period carries the risk of increased bleeding and cardiac tamponade. Given that POAF is typically self-limiting, the provider should weigh the risks and benefits of anticoagulation (Peretto et al., 2014). Up to 80% of patients who develop POAF after cardiac surgery convert to NSR within 24 hours; that percentage increases to 90% in 6–8 weeks (Peretto et al., 2014). If the patient has normal LV function, long-term therapy is usually not required. However, if the patient has POAF that has lasted more than 48 hours and anticoagulation is deemed necessary, a heparin infusion followed by oral anticoagulants is recommended (Nair, 2010). Patients with POAF following cardiac surgery may be discharged on oral anticoagulants and antiarrhythmic therapy (Peretto et al., 2014).

Rhythm Control

If patients are symptomatic following rate control for POAF, rate control cannot be accomplished, or based on patient preference, attempts to eradicate POAF should be considered (Nair, 2010). This may be accomplished with either use of pharmacotherapy or electricity. Rhythm control is not essential if the patient has hemodynamic stability. This is especially true for elderly patients (Nair, 2010).

Procainamide (Pronestyl®) is a class Ia agent (sodium channel blocker). It may be used to help convert the patient to NSR. Side effects may include hypotension, QT interval prolongation, and gastrointestinal and lupus-like side effects. Procainamide administration may result in an increased ventricular rate if no other agents to slow the rate of AV conduction have been administered (Nair, 2010). Procainamide is reportedly effective up to 60% of the time (Peretto et al., 2014).

Ibutilide (Corvert®) is a class III antiarrhythmic (potassium channel blocker). It may be used to convert patients with POAF following cardiac surgery. Ibutilide is administered as an intravenous bolus and may be repeated once. The ICU nurse must monitor the patient for development of torsades de pointes if ibutilide is used because QT prolongation is possible (Nair, 2010; Nair, George, & Koshy, 2011). In one study, ibutilide was noted to be as effective as amiodarone in converting a patient out of POAF, but the amount of time it took to convert was lower in patients who received ibutilide. Further, the authors reported fewer hemodynamic effects with ibutilide; more patients who received amiodarone developed hypotension (Bernard et al., 2003).

Dofetilide (Tikosyn®), another class III antiarrhythmic, may be used to convert patients with POAF following cardiac surgery (Peretto et al., 2014). A number of drug–drug interactions are reported with dofetilide (Callahan, 2011).

Despite hypomagnesemia being identified as a potential risk factor for the development of POAF, supplementation with magnesium has revealed conflicting results with regard to its management. Data suggest that adequate serum magnesium levels should be maintained with care not to cause hypermagnesemia (Peretto et al., 2014).

In addition to pharmacotherapy, a number of other approaches have been employed, including SCV and surgical interventions (e.g., Cox Maze III, Ex-Maze procedure, or cryoablation). The Cox Maze III procedure continues to have a success rate up to 90% (Weimer et al., 2012).

Ablative techniques that electrically separate the pulmonary veins from the atria have been used to ensure that impulses are not conducted. Single radiofrequency ablation (RFA) may be tried in patients who did not successfully convert to NSR with one or two drugs. Efficacy of single RFA is reported as high as 80% in patients with paroxysmal AF and up to 60% in patients with persistent POAF (Lindsay, 2012; Peretto et al., 2014). This procedure may also be performed concomitantly with cardiac surgery in patients with preoperative AF. While ablative methods

do not have as high a success rate as some other surgical approaches, they are simpler, cost-effective, and have a reported correction rate of 53.1% for patients undergoing a single ablation procedure and 79.8% for patients undergoing multiple procedures (Ganesan et al., 2013). Surgical treatment of AF is discussed in more detail in Chapters 3 and 7.

VENTRICULAR DYSRHYTHMIAS

Three dysrhythmias of ventricular origin have been reported in the postoperative cardiac surgery patient: premature ventricular contractions (PVCs), ventricular tachycardia (VT), and ventricular fibrillation (VF). A number of risk factors for the development of postoperative ventricular arrhythmias (POVAs) have been cited in the literature.

Patients found to be at lower risk had a higher EF, mild (as opposed to more than mild) COPD, and were undergoing off-pump surgery. Patients at higher risk were older, were undergoing emergent surgery, had a lower EF, had a history of peripheral vascular disease (PVD), had problematic ischemia, had LV dysfunction, had preoperative hypotension, experienced hemodynamic changes, experienced shifts in electrolytes during cardiac surgery, or had long on-pump time (El-Chami et al., 2012).

Ventricular dysrhythmias are less common than dysrhythmias of atrial origin in patients having undergone cardiac surgery and may be indicative of myocardial dysfunction. Current data suggest the incidence of PVCs and paroxysmal VT to be up to 3.2% (El-Chami et al., 2012). This rate is considered low given the use of inotropes, fluid and electrolyte shifts, and ischemia and reperfusion associated with cardiac surgery. In fact, cardiac surgery has been called a "stress test" given the presence of the reversible causes of VT and VF (Frankel, 2012).

Ventricular dysrhythmias are of clinical concern because of the potential for associated hemodynamic instability. Loss of the atrial kick may decrease CO. Further, their presence can impact patient outcomes. Postoperative ventricular arrhythmias are associated with a higher mortality rate prior to hospital discharge and within 1 year following cardiac surgery. Specifically, data suggest an 18.5% 1-year mortality rate following hospital discharge (El-Chami et al., 2012; Frankel, 2012).

Premature Ventricular Contractions

Premature ventricular contractions can be considered clinically insignificant unless they become frequent (more than 30/min), are multifocal, or the patient is close to developing R on T. In this case, ventricular function may be impacted (Peretto et al., 2014). Premature ventricular contractions usually do not require intervention if the patient has normal LV function and normal metabolic and electrolyte levels. Any of these etiologies require correction if present. For example, alterations in potassium level may be the underlying cause of PVCs and would require optimization (Peretto et al., 2014). Administration of dobutamine (Dobutrex®) has been implicated in the development of ventricular escape beats in up to 15% of patients who underwent cardiac surgery. In addition, infusion of milrinone (Primacor®), a phosphodiesterase inhibitor, has been implicated in the development of PVCs and paroxysmal VT in up to 17% of patients (Peretto et al., 2014).

In addition to treating the underlying cause, treatment of clinically significant PVCs may include pharmacotherapy. While lidocaine (Xylocaine®) has been effective in decreasing the number of PVCs that cause hemodynamic instability, no improvement in mortality has been reported and it is considered potentially harmful. Use of overdrive pacing, dual chamber pacing, and implantable cardioverter defibrillators (ICDs) has not impacted patient prognosis. Development of postoperative PVCs does not seem to impact patient outcome (Peretto et al., 2014).

Ventricular Tachycardia and Ventricular Fibrillation

The incidence of VT or VF following cardiac surgery is 0.4% to 3% (Gajulapalli & Rader, 2012; Peretto et al., 2014). In one report, predictors of postoperative VT or VF included older age, lower EF, emergent surgery, and history of PVD. Patients who received off-pump procedures were less likely to develop POVAs (El-Chami et al., 2012). Other patients at risk are reported to include those with LV dysfunction, structural heart disease, heart failure, hemodynamic instability, electrolyte imbalance, decreased oxygen levels, hypovolemia, ischemia, MI, reperfusion after CPB, use of inotropes or antiarrhythmics, and acute graft closure. In the immediate postoperative period, hemodynamic instability, electrolyte or acid–base imbalance, hypoxia, anemia, or new ischemia put the patient at risk for VT or VF (Gajulapalli & Rader, 2012; Peretto et al., 2014). Sequelae of CPB include inflammation, oxidative stress, shifts in electrolytes, release of vasoactive substances, and peripheral and cerebral emboli (El-Chami et al., 2012).

The development of paroxysmal VT has not been shown to impact patient outcome. However, postoperative cardiac surgery patients who develop sustained VT have a mortality rate as high as 50% (Gajulapalli & Rader, 2012). There is also a reported recurrence rate of up to 40% in patients discharged from the hospital and a 2-year mortality rate due to cardiac issues as high as 20% (Peretto et al., 2014).

Management of Postoperative Ventricular Dysrhythmias

Patients who develop paroxysmal VT who remain hemodynamically stable and who are otherwise asymptomatic do not necessarily need to be treated aside from treating the underlying cause. Patients who develop sustained VT should be treated with either medication (if asymptomatic) or SCV if symptomatic (Peretto et al., 2014). Medications include amiodarone and procainamide.

In patients with VT and a pulse, amiodarone is indicated as the first-line therapy. A bolus of 150 mg over 10–15 minutes is recommended (American Heart Association, 2011). Additional doses of 150 mg may be administered. The nurse should observe for hypotension and bradycardia. Amiodarone is reported to be better tolerated than other antiarrhythmic therapies in patients with systolic dysfunction (Peretto et al., 2014). If patients convert to NSR, it has been suggested that they be started on long-term beta blocker or angiotensin-converting enzyme inhibitor therapy as better long-term survival has been reported (Gajulapalli & Rader, 2012).

Procainamide may be used as a second-line therapy. A loading dose of 20–50 mg/min up to 17 mg/kg can be followed by a continuous infusion of 1–4 mg/min. Patients with renal dysfunction may be excluded from this therapy due to an associated buildup of a toxic metabolite, N-acetyl-procainamide (Gajulapalli & Rader, 2012; Peretto et al., 2014). The nurse should observe the patient for development of hypotension and for QRS widening while the patient is receiving procainamide. Therapy should be stopped if the QRS widens by 50%, hypotension develops, or the maximum dose has been received.

Sotalol may also be used to treat VT with a pulse if the patient is stable. Because sotalol has proarrhythmic effects, the nurse should observe the patient for development of torsades de pointes.

Sustained VT may also be treated with electricity. Patients with epicardial pacing wires still in place may be treated with pacing if they develop VT with a slower rate. It is possible for a patient's condition to worsen to a VT with a more rapid ventricular response or VF. Because of this, equipment should be readily available in case SCV (for unstable VT) or defibrillation (for VF or pulseless VT) is required (Gajulapalli & Rader, 2012; Peretto et al., 2014).

Emergency CPB may be initiated in the cardiovascular ICU if patients do not respond to conventional therapies (Gajulapalli & Rader, 2012). A survival rate of 56% has been reported with this intervention. No mediastinitis has been reported as a complication.

Implantation of an ICD should be considered in patients requiring long-term therapy. These may include patients who do not have a reversible cause such as those with paroxysmal VT, history of MI, LVEF less than 40%, or those who have induced ventricular arrhythmias with electrophysiology studies (Peretto et al., 2014). Guidelines for ICD placement do not include patients with an LVEF higher than 35% and those who underwent a revascularization procedure within 90 days (El-Chami et al., 2012). If a patient converted to NSR and had no prior risk factors, electrophysiology studies should be performed. If VT or VF is induced, an ICD should be considered (Gajulapalli & Rader, 2012).

Ventricular fibrillation should be treated with immediate defibrillation per advanced cardiac life support (ACLS) protocol, cardiopulmonary resuscitation, administration of epinephrine and antiarrhythmic agents, and eradication of the underlying cause. The amount of energy used for defibrillation depends on how the energy is delivered—monophasic or biphasic, although the latter is presently more common (American Heart Association, 2011).

Amiodarone is indicated as first-line therapy for refractory pulseless VT and VF. A bolus of 300 mg may be followed by a continuous infusion of 1 mg/min for the first 6 hours post-resuscitation and 0.5 mg/min for the next 18 hours. Additional boluses of 150 mg may be administered as indicated (American Heart Association, 2011; Peretto et al., 2014).

BRADYARRHYTHMIAS

Following cardiac surgery, development of bradyarrhythmias is common. These rhythms may include sick sinus syndrome (SSS), second-degree AV block Type II, sinus pauses, sinus bradycardia, or complete heart block (Gajulapalli & Rader, 2012; Peretto et al., 2014). Bradyarrhythmias are most common in patients who have undergone valve surgery. It may also occur following CABG. Development of this complication is believed to be related to surgical injury and edema (Peretto et al., 2014).

The overall incidence of bradyarrhythmias following CABG is 0.8–3.4% and 2–4% following valve surgery. The development of symptomatic bradycardia is higher in patients who undergo tricuspid or aortic valve procedures. Up to 21% of patients who undergo a heart transplant may develop dysfunction of the SA node and 4% to 5% may develop AV block. Both groups may require pacemaker therapy (Gajulapalli & Rader, 2012). In one study, the incidence of symptomatic bradycardia, second-degree AV block, and complete heart block was 8%, 6.4% and 7%, respectively. Most of these patients underwent either CABG, mitral valve replacement, aortic valve replacement, or mitral and aortic valve replacement (Emkanjoo et al., 2008). Presence of a heart block may also be associated with an inferior wall MI. Other identified risk factors for high degrees of AV block include older age, history of left bundle branch block, calcification of a valve, removal of LV aneurysm, stenosis of the left main coronary artery, larger number of vessels bypassed, CPB time, increased vagal tone during the surgical procedure, type of anesthesia, and presence of postoperative pain (Gajulapalli & Rader, 2012; Peretto et al., 2014). Other factors identified include medications (e.g., digoxin, amiodarone, calcium channel blockers, and beta blockers) and certain surgical approaches. Patients undergoing procedures involving some specific approaches experienced second-degree AV block Type II and complete heart block. Some additional patients developed SSS or persistent sinus bradycardia or junctional rhythm (Peretto et al., 2014).

Following heart transplant, development of SSS is common. Up to 21% of these patients require insertion of a permanent pacemaker. Patients at risk for development of bradyarrhythmias following heart transplant include the donor being of older age, higher donor ischemic time, patients who have undergone biatrial (versus bicaval) transplant, and increased cross-clamp time (Gajulapalli & Rader, 2012; Peretto et al., 2014).

Management of Bradyarrhythmias

Treatment of the underlying cause of the bradyarrhythmia is essential. This may include discontinuing the medications that may cause AV block. Referral to a current ACLS manual is suggested (Gajulapalli & Rader, 2012). Management of bradyarrhythmias usually entails use of a temporary pacemaker. The epicardial wires that are oftentimes left in place following the initial cardiac surgery are used for this purpose. Of the patients who develop complete heart block, up to 100% will require insertion of a permanent pacemaker. It is typical for patients with persistent SSS or complete heart block lasting more than 5 to 7 days to receive a permanent pacemaker (Brignole et al., 2013). This time allows edema of the conduction system to resolve (Gajulapalli & Rader, 2012). A permanent pacemaker has been required in up to 24% of patients following cardiac surgery (Peretto et al., 2014). Until a permanent pacemaker can be inserted, transcutaneous or transvenous pacing or a pulmonary artery catheter with a pacing port may also be used.

Management of Bradydysrhythmias Following Cardiac Transplant

A significant difference exists in the pharmacologic management of bradydysrhythmias following cardiac transplant and the approaches used in patients who undergo other cardiac surgical procedures and develop postoperative dysrhythmias. Patients may develop bradycardia following a heart transplant due to sympathetic denervation, SA node ischemia, ischemia of the graft, and medications used during surgery (Thajudeen et al., 2012). Bradycardia may develop as a consequence of the incision made in the SA node during surgery. Atropine will not be effective in this instance because of the severing of the vagus nerve.

Management with a pacemaker should be the primary treatment. Pacemakers also give the patient the needed atrial kick and augment CO. Intravenous inotropic support may be used in asymptomatic patients. Agents such as isoproterenol (Isuprel®), theophylline (Theo-Dur®), or terbutaline (Brethine®) may be used to increase heart rate of the newly implanted heart. If the bradyarrhythmia persists, consideration should be given to implanting a pacemaker. The patient should also be evaluated for rejection with endomyocardial biopsy (Thajudeen et al., 2012).

EPICARDIAL PACEMAKERS

Placement of epicardial pacing wires facilitates temporary pacing following cardiac surgery. Pacing electrodes are attached directly to the atria, the ventricles, or both during surgery. The wires are inserted in the event that the patient develops bradycardia, second-degree AV block Type II, complete heart block, prolonged AV delay, bifascicular block with first-degree AV block, prolonged QT syndrome, junctional tachycardia, supraventricular tachycardia, atrial flutter with a rate less than 320–340/min, or junctional rhythm, all of which require better conduction control to resolve. The wires are then secured to the epicardium and brought out through the skin. Depending on the surgeon's preference, the patient may have one or two sets of pacing wires emplaced. Generally, the ventricular and atrial wires exit the skin to the left and right of the sternum, respectively. It is essential for the ICU nurse to secure the leads to the patient's chest or abdomen, have a pacemaker generator with new batteries readily available, and ensure that all wiring and connections are tight and free of fraying. The ends of the pacer wires should be covered, insulated, and protected with a clean, dry dressing. Gloves should be worn when handling the wires, and other electrical appliances should be kept away from the ends to prevent electrical interference (Reade, 2007).

Epicardial pacing wires should be removed following the discontinuation of heparin and before warfarin (Coumadin®) therapy is initiated. The patient should be observed for a few hours for the development of tamponade because there is a small risk of this complication. Other complications associated with epicardial pacing wire removal are ventricular dysrhythmias and damage to the anastomoses (Reade, 2007).

SUMMARY

Nurses caring for patients who have undergone cardiac surgery must understand which patients are at risk for the development of dysrhythmias, know how to identify these dysrhythmias, be able to prevent their occurrence, and implement early treatment to correct any irregular rhythm that does arise. While it may be difficult to isolate the underlying cause of a postoperative dysrhythmia, correction of possible etiologies is an essential component of successful management. As part of the clinical patient assessment, the ICU nurse should note the duration of the dysrhythmia as well as any associated hemodynamic effects.

CASE STUDY

A 71-year-old male patient is admitted to the ICU immediately following aortic valve repair. His history includes myocardial infarction, heart failure with an LVEF of 30%, and peripheral vascular disease. He is discharged from the ICU on the second postoperative day and transferred to a cardiac surgery step-down unit. On postoperative day 3, the patient developed a 45-sec run of monomorphic ventricular tachycardia. He remained asymptomatic throughout the event, reporting palpitations only.

Critical Thinking Questions

1. Which factors might predispose this patient to paroxysmal ventricular tachycardia?
2. Which prophylactic treatment could have been utilized to reduce the incidence of rhythm problems?
3. What is the best method to manage paroxysmal ventricular tachycardia postoperatively in this patient?

Answers to Critical Thinking Questions

1. Aortic valve replacement, patient age, history of MI, heart failure with low LVEF, and peripheral vascular disease.
2. Ensure the patient's serum electrolytes are within acceptable range, maintain optimal oxygenation, and optimize fluid volume status.
3. Determine if the patient is symptomatic or asymptomatic. Treat the underlying cause, if possible. Follow ACLS guidelines published by the American Heart Association.

SELF-ASSESSMENT QUESTIONS

1. Presence of which of the following places the patient at risk for dysrhythmias following cardiac surgery?
   a. Fever
   b. Dehydration
   c. Hypomagnesemia
   d. Hypoadrenergic state

2. Which of the following rhythms is most commonly encountered following coronary artery bypass graft surgery?

   a.

   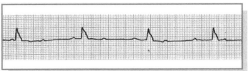

b.

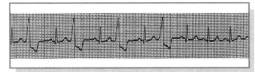

c.

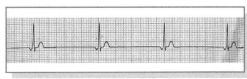

d.

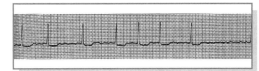

3. Your postoperative valve surgery patient develops atrial fibrillation. For which of the following other complications should the nurse observe?
   a. Seizures
   b. Atelectasis
   c. Acute kidney injury
   d. Heart failure

4. Which of the following patients is at greatest risk for developing atrial fibrillation following cardiac surgery? A:
   a. 50-year-old with decreased adrenergic tone
   b. 60-year-old with hypermagnesemia
   c. 65-year-old with pericarditis
   d. 40-year-old with atrial enlargement

5. Following orthotopic heart transplant, you note presence of two P waves. Which of the following is indicated?
   a. Continue to monitor
   b. Anticipate ventricular pacing
   c. Administer atropine 0.5 mg IV
   d. Evaluate potassium level

6. Which of the following is the initial treatment of postoperative atrial fibrillation?
   a. Digoxin
   b. Ibutilide
   c. Metoprolol
   d. Amiodarone

7. Prophylaxis for postoperative atrial fibrillation with beta blockers may be indicated for which of the following patients?
   a. Patients receiving inotropes
   b. Patients with PR interval > 0.24 sec
   c. Patients with second-degree AV block Type II
   d. Patients who underwent valve surgery

8. Your postoperative cardiac surgery patient develops supraventricular tachycardia. For which of the following patients is adenosine indicated initially?
   a. Patients with atrial flutter
   b. Patients who underwent heart transplantation
   c. Patients with a history of bronchial asthma
   d. Patients who had repair of the aortic valve

9. Which of the following patients who underwent cardiac surgery is at greatest risk for the development of ventricular tachycardia or ventricular fibrillation? A(n):
   a. 80-year-old with history of COPD and LVEF 40%
   b. 60-year-old with history of bradycardia and LVEF 50%
   c. 75-year-old with history of hypotension and LVEF 45%
   d. 50-year-old with history of left coronary artery stenosis and LVEF 55%

10. The patient with which of the following sets of hemodynamic parameters is at greatest risk for the development of monomorphic ventricular tachycardia?

	BP	PAP
a.	90/65	14/9
b.	150/85	50/35
c.	146/82	20/8
d.	84/50	64/42

Answers to Self-Assessment Questions

1. c	6. c
2. d	7. d
3. d	8. d
4. c	9. a
5. a	10. b

Clinical Inquiry Box

Question: Does administration of a statin decrease the incidence of postoperative atrial fibrillation following cardiac surgery in patients who are also treated with a beta blocker?

Reference: Mithani, S., Akbar, M. S., Johnson, D. J., Kuskowski, M., Apple, K. K., Bonawitz-Conlin, J., . . . Bloomfield, H. E. (2009). Dose dependent effect of statins on postoperative atrial fibrillation after cardiac surgery among patients treated with beta blockers. *Journal of Cardiothoracic Surgery, 4,* 61. doi: 10.1186/1749-8090-4-61

Objective: To determine if administration of a statin decreases the incidence of postoperative atrial fibrillation following cardiac surgery in patients who are also treated with a beta blocker.

Method: A retrospective review of 1,936 patients who underwent CABG or valve surgery in a veteran's medical center. All patients had received a beta blocker postoperatively; 92% received the beta blocker within 24 hours of cardiac surgery.

Results: There was no statistically significant difference in the incidence of POAF between patients taking statins and those who were not. In subgroup analysis, it was determined that there was a statistically significant difference in the incidence in POAF in patients taking more than 20 mg of simvastatin daily when compared to patients taking lower doses.

Conclusion: Patients who underwent cardiac surgery who were being treated with postoperative beta blockers had a decreased chance of developing POAF if taking a statin at higher dose levels.

REFERENCES

Al-Sarraf, N., Thalib, L., Hughes, A., Houlihan, M., Tolan, M., Young, V., . . . McGovern, E. (2010). The risk of arrhythmias following coronary artery bypass surgery: Do smokers have a paradox effect? *Interactive Cardiovascular and Thoracic Surgery, 11*(5), 550–555.

American Heart Association. (2011). *Advanced cardiovascular life support provider manual.* Dallas, TX: Author.

Arsenault, K. A., Yusuf, A. M., Crystal, E., Healey, J. S., Morillo, C. A., Nair, G. M., . . . Whitlock, R. P. (2013). Interventions for preventing post-operative atrial fibrillation in patients undergoing heart surgery. *Cochrane Database of Systematic Reviews, 1,* CD003611.

Bashour, C. A., Visinescu, M., Gopakumaran, B., Wazni, O., Carangio, F., Yared, J-P., . . . Starr, N. (2004). Characterization of premature atrial contraction activity prior to the onset of postoperative atrial fibrillation in cardiac surgery patients. *Chest, 126*(4, MeetingAbstracts), 831S–832S.

Bernard, E. O., Schmid, E. R., Schmidlin, D., Scharf, C., Candinas, R., & Germann, R. (2003). Ibutilide versus amiodarone in atrial fibrillation: A double-blinded, randomized study. *Critical Care Medicine, 31,* 1031–1034.

Brignole, M., Auricchio, A., Baron-Esquivas, G., Bordachar, P., Boriani, G., Breithardt, O.-A., . . . Vardas, P. E. (2013). 2013 ESC guidelines on cardiac pacing and cardiac resynchronization therapy. *European Heart Journal, 34,* 2281–2329.

Burgess, B. C., Kilborn, M. J., & Keech, A. C. (2006). Interventions for prevention of postoperative atrial fibrillation and its complications after cardiac surgery: A meta-analysis. *European Heart Journal, 27,* 2846–2857.

Callahan, T. (2011). Managing newly diagnosed atrial fibrillation: Rate, rhythm, and risk. *Cleveland Clinical Journal of Medicine, 78*(4), 258–264.

Cheruku, K. K., Ghani, A., Ahmad, F., Pappas, P., Silverman, P. R., Zelinger, A., . . . Silver, M. A. (2004). Efficacy of nonsteroidal anti-inflammatory medications for prevention of atrial fibrillation following coronary artery bypass graft surgery. *Preventive Cardiology, 7,* 13–18.

Clark, T. R., Hodge, D., Ressler, E., & Lee, M. (2011). *Antiarrhythmic agents: Dronedarone (Multaq®) and Amiodarone.* Retrieved from http://www.ihs.gov/nptc/documents/NPTC%20Amiodarone-Dronedarone%20Monograph.pdf

Dasari, T. W., Pavlovic-Surjancev, B., Patel, N., Williams, A. A., Ezidinma, P., Rupani, A., . . .

Heroux, A. L. (2010). Incidence, risk factors, and clinical outcomes of atrial fibrillation and atrial flutter after heart transplantation. *American Journal of Cardiology, 106*(5), 737–741.

Davis, E. M., Packard, K. A., & Hilleman, D. E. (2010). Pharmacologic prophylaxis of postoperative atrial fibrillation in patients undergoing cardiac surgery: Beyond beta blockers. *Pharmacotherapy, 30*(7), 274e–318e.

Echahidi, N., Pibarot, P., O'Hara, G., & Mathieu, P. (2008). Mechanisms, prevention, and treatment of atrial fibrillation after cardiac surgery. *Journal of the American College of Cardiology, 51*(8), 793–801.

El-Chami, M. F., Sawaya, F. J., Kilgo, P., Stein, W., Halkos, M., Thourani, V., . . . Leon, A. R. (2012). Ventricular arrhythmia after cardiac surgery: Incidence, predictors, and outcomes. *Journal of the American College of Cardiology, 80*, 2664–2671.

Elahi, M. M., Worner, M., Khan, J. S., & Matata, B. M. (2009). Inspired nitric oxide and modulation of oxidative stress during cardiac surgery. *Current Drug Safety, 4*(3), 188–198.

Emkanjoo, Z., Mirza-Ali, M., Alizadeh, A., Hosseini, S., Jorat, M. V., Nikoo, M. H., . . . Sadr-Ameli, M. A. (2008). Predictors and frequency of conduction disturbances after open-heart surgery. *Indian Pacing Electrophysiology Journal, 8*(1), 14–21.

Fan, K., Lee, K. L., Chiu, C. S., Lee, J. W. T., He, G.-W., Cheung, D., . . . Lau, C.-P. (2000). Effects of biatrial pacing in prevention of postoperative atrial fibrillation after coronary artery bypass surgery. *Circulation, 102*, 755–760.

Ferguson, T. B., Jr., Coombs, L. P., & Peterson, E. D. (2002). Preoperative beta-blocker use and mortality and morbidity following CABG surgery in North America. *Journal of the American Medical Association, 287*(17), 2221–2227.

Fleming, G. A., Marray, K. T., Yu, C., Burbe, J. G., Petracek, M. R., Moff, S. J., . . . Pretorius, M. (2008). Milrinone use is associated with postoperative atrial fibrillation after cardiac surgery. *Circulation, 118*(16), 1619–1625.

Frankel, D. S. (2012). Ventricular arrhythmias after cardiac surgery: Failing the stress test. *American College of Cardiology, 60*(25), 2672–2673.

Gajulapalli, R. D., & Rader, F. (2012). *Post operative arrhythmias, Special topics in cardiac surgery.*

Retrieved from http://www.intechopen.com/books/special-topics-in-cardiac-surgery/post-operative-arrhythmias

Ganesan, A. N., Shipp, N. J., Brooks, A. G., Kuklik, P., Lau, D. H., Lim, H. S., . . . Sanders, P. (2013). Long-term outcomes of catheter ablation of atrial fibrillation: A systematic review and meta-analysis. *Journal of the American Heart Association, 2*, e004549. Retrieved from http://jaha.ahajournals.org/content/2/2/e004549.full

Granier, M., Massin, F., & Pasquie, J.-P. (2013). Pro- and anti-arrhythmic effects of anti-inflammatory drugs. *Anti-Inflammatory & Anti-Allergy Agents in Medicinal Chemistry, 12*, 83–93.

Gu, W. J., Wei, C. Y., Huang, D. Q., & Yin, R. X. (2012). Meta-analysis of randomized controlled trials on the efficacy of thoracic epidural anesthesia in preventing atrial fibrillation after coronary artery bypass grafting. *BMC Cardiovascular Disorders, 12*, 67.

Haghjoo, M., Saravi, M., Hashemi, M. J., Hosseini, S., Givtaj, N., Ghafarinejad, M. H., . . . Sadr-Ameli, M. A. (2007). Optimal beta-blocker for prevention of atrial fibrillation after on-pump coronary artery bypass graft surgery: Carvedilol versus metoprolol. *Heart Rhythm, 4*(9), 1170–1174.

Hall, R. I., Smith, M. S., & Rocker, G. (2007). The systemic inflammatory response to cardiopulmonary bypass: Pathophysiological, therapeutic, and pharmacological considerations. *Anesthesia & Analgesia, 85*, 766–782.

Halonen, J., Halonen, P., Järvinen, O., Taskinen, P., Auvinen, T., Tarkka, M., . . . Hakala, T. (2007). Corticosteroids for the prevention of atrial fibrillation after cardiac surgery: A randomized controlled trial. *Journal of the American Medical Association, 297*(14), 1562–1567.

Hashemzadeh, K., Dehdilani, M., & Dehdilani, M. (2013). Postoperative atrial fibrillation following open cardiac surgery: Predisposing factors and complications. *Journal of Cardiovascular and Thoracic Research, 5*(3), 101–107.

Hazelrigg, S. R., Boley, T. M., Cetindag, I. B., Mouton, K. P., Trammell, G. L., . . . Verhulst, S. (2004). The efficacy of supplemental magnesium in reducing atrial fibrillation after coronary artery bypass grafting. *Annals of Thoracic Surgery, 77*, 824–830.

Helgadottir, S., Sigurdsson, M. I., Ingvarsdottir, I. L., Arnar, D. O., & Gudbjartsson, T. (2012). Atrial fibrillation following cardiac surgery: Risk analysis and long-term survival. *Journal of Cardiovascular Surgery, 7*(87), 1749-1753.

Hindler, K., Shaw, A. D., Samuels, J., Fulton, S., Collard, C. D., & Riedel, B. (2006). Improved postoperative outcomes associated with preoperative statin therapy. *Anesthesiology, 105*(6), 1260-1272.

Ho, K. M., & Tan, J. A. (2009). Benefits and risks of corticosteroid prophylaxis in adult cardiac surgery: A dose-response meta-analysis. *Circulation, 119*(4), 1853-1866.

Kohno, H., Koyanagi, T., Kasegawa, H., & Miyazaki, M. (2005). Three-day magnesium administration prevents atrial fibrillation after coronary artery bypass grafting. *Annals of Thoracic Surgery, 79*, 117-126.

Koniari, I., Apostolakis, E., Rogkakou, C., Baikoussis, N. G., & Dougenis, D. (2010). Pharmacologic prophylaxis for atrial fibrillation following cardiac surgery: A systematic review. *Journal of Cardiothoracic Surgery, 5*, 121. Retrieved from http://www.ncbi.nlm.nih.gov/pmc/articles/PMC3006380/

Liakopoulos, O. J., Coi, Y.- H., Kuhn, E. W., Wittwer, T., Borys, M., Madershahian, N., . . . Wahlers, T. (2009). Statins for prevention of atrial fibrillation after cardiac surgery: A systematic literature review. *The Journal of Thoracic and Cardiovascular Surgery, 138*(3), 678-686.

Lindsay, B. D. (2012). Atrial fibrillation: New drugs, devices, and procedures. *Cleveland Clinic Journal of Medicine, 79*(8), 553-559.

Liu, X.-H., Xu, C.-Y., & Fan, G.-H. (2014). Efficacy of N-acetylcysteine in preventing atrial fibrillation after cardiac surgery: A meta-analysis of published randomized controlled trials. *BMC Cardiovascular Disorders, 14*, 52. doi:10.1186/1471-2261-14-52. Retrieved from http://www.biomedcentral.com/1471-2261/14/52

Lutz, J. M., Panchagnula, U., & Barker, J. M. (2011). Prophylaxis against atrial fibrillation after cardiac surgery. Effective, but not routinely used. A survey of cardiothoracic units in the United Kingdom. *Journal of Cardiothoracic and Vascular Anesthesia, 25*(1), 90-94.

Maesen, B., Nijs, J., Maessen, J., Allessie, M., & Schotten, U. (2012). Post-operative atrial fibrillation: A maze of mechanisms. *Eurospace, 14*(2), 159-174.

Mathew, J. P., Fontes, M. L., Tudor, I. C., Ramsay, J., Duke, P., Mazer, C. D., . . . Mangano, D. T. (2004). A multicenter risk index for atrial fibrillation after cardiac surgery. *Journal of the American Medical Association, 291*, 1720-1729.

Nair, M., George, L. K., & Koshy, S. K. G. (2011). Safety and efficacy of ibutilide in cardioversion of atrial flutter and fibrillation. *Journal of the American Board of Family Medicine, 24*(1), 86-92.

Nair, S. G. (2010). Atrial fibrillation after cardiac surgery. *Annals of Cardiac Surgery, 13*(3), 196-205.

Ozaydin, M., Peker, O., Erdogan, D., Kapan, S., Turker, Y., Varol, E., . . . Ibrisim, E. (2008). N-acetylcysteine for the prevention of postoperative atrial fibrillation: A prospective, randomized, placebo-controlled pilot study. *European Heart Journal, 29*(5), 625-631.

Patti, G., Chello, M., Candura, D., Pasceri, V., D'Ambrosio, A., Covino, E., . . . DiSciascio, G. (2006). Randomized trial of atorvastatin for reduction of postoperative atrial fibrillation in patients undergoing cardiac surgery: Results of the ARMYDA-3 (Atorvastatin for Reduction of MYocardial Dysrhythmia After cardiac surgery) study. *Circulation, 114*(4), 1455-1461.

Peretto, G., Durante, A., Limite, L. R., & Cianflone, D. (2014). Postoperative arrhythmias after cardiac surgery: Incidence, risk factors, and therapeutic management. *Cardiology Research and Practice, 2014*, 1-15.

Prasongsukarn, K., Abel, J. G., Jamieson, W. R., Cheung, A., Russell, J. A., Walley, K. R., . . . Lichtenstein, S. V. (2005). The effects of steroids on the occurrence of postoperative atrial fibrillation after coronary artery bypass grafting surgery: A prospective randomized trial. *Journal of Thoracic and Cardiovascular Surgery, 130*(1), 93-98.

Reade, M. C. (2007). Temporary epicardial pacing after cardiac surgery: A practical review. *Anaesthesia, 62*(3), 264-271.

Rho, R. W. (2009). The management of atrial fibrillation after cardiac surgery. *Heart, 95*, 422-429.

Sanjuán, R., Blasco, M., Carbonell, N., Jordá, A., Nuñez, J., Martínez-León, J., . . . Otero, E. (2004). Preoperative use of sotalol versus atenolol for atrial fibrillation after cardiac surgery. *Annals of Thoracic Surgery, 77*(3), 838–843.

Shen, J., Lall, S., Zheng, V., Buckley, P., Damiano, R. J., Jr., & Schuessler, R. B. (2011). The persistent problem of new-onset postoperative atrial fibrillation: A single-institution experience over two decades. *Journal of Thoracic and Cardiovascular Surgery, 141*, 559–570.

Silvestry, F. E. (2014). *Postoperative complications among patients undergoing cardiac surgery.* Retrieved from http://www.uptodate.com/contents/postoperative-complications-among-patients-undergoing-cardiac-surgery

Singhal, P., & Kejriwal, N. (2010). Right atrial pacing for prevention of postoperative atrial fibrillation following coronary artery bypass grafting: A prospective observational trial. *Heart, Lung and Circulation, 19*(7), 395–399.

Thajudeen, A., Stecker, E. C., Shehata, M., Patel, J., Wang, X., McAnulty, J. H., Jr., . . . Chugh, S. S. (2012). Arrhythmias after heart transplantation: Mechanisms and management. *Journal of the American Heart Association, 1*, e001461. Retrieved from http://jaha.ahajournals.org/content/1/2/e001461.full

Tomic, V., Russwurm, S., Möller, E., Claus, R. A., Blaess, M., Brunkhorst, F., . . . Bauer, M. (2005). Transcriptomic and protemic patterns of systemic inflammation in on-pump and off-pump coronary artery bypass grafting. *Circulation, 112*(19), 2912–2920.

Virani, S. S., Nambi, V., Razavi, M., Lee, V. V., Elayda, M., Wilson, J. M., . . . Ballantyne, C. M. (2008). Preoperative statin therapy is not associated with a decrease in the incidence of postoperative atrial fibrillation in patients undergoing cardiac surgery. *American Heart Journal, 155*, 541–546.

Vlessides, M. (2012). Dex after heart surgery may reduce risk of arrhythmias. *Clinical Anesthesiology, 38*, 9.

Weimer, T., Schena, S., Bailey, M. S., Maniar, H. S., Schuessler, R. B., Cox, J. L., . . . Damiano, R. J. (2012). The Cox-Maze procedure for lone atrial fibrillation: A single-center experience over 2 decades. *Circulation, 5*, 8–14.

Wu, X., Wang, C., Zhu, J., Zhang, C., Zhang, Y., & Gao, Y. (2013). Meta-analysis of randomized controlled trials on magnesium in addition to beta-blocker for prevention of postoperative atrial arrhythmias after coronary artery bypass grafting. *BMC Cardiovascular Disorders, 13*, 5.

Yun, A. J., Bazar, K. A., Lee, P. Y., Gerber, A., & Daniel, S. M. (2005). The smoking gun: Many conditions associated with tobacco exposure may be attributable to paradoxical compensatory autonomic responses to nicotine. *Medical Hypotheses, 64*(6), 1073–1079.

Zacharias, A., Schwann, T. A., Riordan, C. J., Durham, S. J., Shah, A. S., & Habib, R. H. (2005). Obesity and risk of new-onset atrial fibrillation after cardiac surgery. *Circulation, 101*, 1403–1408.

Zangrillo, A., Landoni, G., Sparacio, D., Pappalardo, F., Bove, T., Cerchierini, E., . . . Crescenzi, G. (2005). Perioperative magnesium supplementation to prevent atrial fibrillation after off-pump coronary artery surgery: A randomized controlled study. *Journal of Cardiothoracic and Vascular Anesthesia, 19*(6), 723–728.

WEB RESOURCES

A guide to reading and understanding EKG interpretation: http://students.med.nyu.edu/erclub/ekghome.html

ECG Interpretation and Clinical Significance: http://www.google.com/url?sa=t&rct=j&q=&esrc=s&frm=1&source=web&cd=7&ved=0CE4QFjAG&url=http%3A%2F%2Fhighered.mheducation.com%2Fsites%2Fdl%2Ffree%2F007351098x%2F451682%2Fsample_ch05.pdf&ei=dR7UU8KSBOfksATZlILgCw&usg=AFQjCNH2pEAxSwRh3gyW58JB3hMRIdb4yg

Catheter ablation—Treatment of atrial fibrillation: http://www.youtube.com/watch?v=lP1hPiE_2y8

Watch a Live Case of AFib Ablation: How to Fix Long-Standing Persistent AFib: http://www.youtube.com/watch?v=pnO2oNXa9-s

Chapter 16

Neurologic Complications

Myra F. Ellis and Roberta Kaplow

INTRODUCTION

A significant number of patients who undergo coronary artery bypass grafting (CABG) and other types of cardiac surgery develop adverse temporary or permanent neurologic complications. Neurologic complications following cardiac surgery are considered severe because they affect mortality and, for survivors, quality of life. In addition, neurologic complications dramatically increase the length of hospitalization and costs associated with cardiac surgery.

Neurologic complications cover a wide range of disorders, from debilitating stroke or coma to encephalopathy, delirium, and neurocognitive dysfunction. Adverse cerebral outcomes can be divided into two types: Type I and Type II. Type I deficits include stroke and major focal neurologic deficits, transient ischemic attacks (TIA), stupor, and coma. Type II deficits include decline in intellectual function, deficits in memory, neurocognitive dysfunction, delirium, and seizure without evidence of focal deficit. Also, coma is sometimes seen (Silvestry, 2014).

Other neurologic complications have also been reported following cardiac surgery, including injuries to the brachial plexus, phrenic nerve, cranial nerves, other peripheral nerves, and visual pathways. These injuries occur less frequently and are usually less serious, but nevertheless contribute to overall patient discomfort and morbidity.

The reported incidence of adverse cerebral outcomes varies widely, from 0.4% to 80%, depending on how the deficit is defined. The incidence of neurologic dysfunction following CABG is 2% to 6%. This incidence is about equally divided between stroke and encephalopathy. The incidence of both types of deficits increases with age (Silvestry, 2014). Valve surgeries and combined CABG and valve surgeries have higher risk of stroke than CABG alone (O'Brien et al., 2009). Surprisingly, the incidence of neurologic complications remains unchanged despite a decrease in mortality rate for cardiac surgery patients (Roekaerts & Heijmans, 2012).

Neurologic complications are the second leading cause of morbidity and mortality in postoperative cardiac surgery patients; heart failure is the leading cause (McGarvey, Cheung, & Stecker, 2013). Postoperative neurologic complications have been attributed to patient-specific factors, emboli, hypoperfusion, and metabolic derangements.

Studies suggest that elderly patients with comorbidities and cardiovascular disease may benefit more from surgical treatment than from medical management. Technological advances of cardiopulmonary bypass (CPB) and other improvements, as well as increased life expectancy for the population as a whole, have allowed the benefits of cardiac surgery to be offered more frequently to older patients with more comorbidities. Unfortunately, elderly patients are at increased risk for pathophysiologic stress, including neurologic dysfunction, following cardiac surgery (Roekaerts & Heijmans, 2012). However, data suggest that patients in their 80s have exceptional survival and do better when they are discharged home rather than to a lower level care facility (Society of Thoracic Surgeons, 2012). This chapter discusses the incidence and extent of neurologic complications following cardiac surgery, offers evidence-based strategies for prevention of these undesirable sequelae, and describes nursing management of patients with adverse neurologic outcomes.

DESCRIPTION OF NEUROLOGIC COMPLICATIONS

Type I Neurologic Deficits

Type I complications occur in approximately 3% of patients and usually involve a stroke (Silvestry, 2014). The incidence is variable depending on procedure. For example, earlier data reveal the risk of early stroke reported at 4.8% in patients undergoing isolated aortic valve replacement, 8.8% for patients undergoing mitral valve replacement, and 9.7% of patients undergoing multi-valve surgery. Further, patients who undergo CABG had a reported risk of 3.8%, while patients having a combined CABG and valve procedure have a 7.4% risk (Bucerius et al., 2003). These stroke symptoms may include hemiparesis, hemiplegia, aphasia, dysarthria, hand incoordination, and changes in the visual field (Roekaerts & Heijmans, 2012).

Risk Factors for Neurologic Complications

A number of risk factors have been implicated in adverse neurologic outcomes. These factors incorporate a combination of patient risk factors, intraoperative variables, and postoperative events. Importantly, the additive effect of variables significantly increases a patient's risk. Identification of risk factors has led to predictive models that allow stroke probability to be calculated for individual patients (McKhann, Grega, Borowicz, Baumgartner, & Selnes, 2006). Risk factors are summarized in **Table 16-1**.

In addition to those listed in Table 16-1, cerebral dysfunction is another noted risk factor. This latter factor makes the brain more prone to injury. Decreased perfusion to the brain may be secondary to systemic hypoperfusion or decreased cerebral blood flow (Roekaerts & Heijmans, 2012; Silvestry, 2014). The Society of Thoracic Surgeons (2014) has developed a risk calculator that is available online. It predicts the risk of stroke for patients undergoing CABG, valve surgery, and a combination of these.

Risk factors for stroke within the first 30 days of cardiac surgery have also been reported. These include long duration of mechanical ventilation (greater than 30.5 hours), history of stroke with paresis, atrial fibrillation (AF), low hematocrit (less than 28%), mean perfusion pressure during CPB (less than 70 mmHg), time to regain consciousness postoperatively (longer than 14.5 hours), and long aortic cross-clamping time (Baranowska et al., 2012).

Type II Neurologic Deficits

Type II neurologic deficits occur in approximately 3% of patients (Silvestry, 2014). Type II injuries also carry important implications for both long- and short-term disability and are associated with increased length of hospital stay, higher hospital costs, and an increased likelihood of discharge to places other than home (McGarvey et al., 2013).

Type II deficits usually dissipate slowly but progressively. Patients typically return to their baseline 3 to 12 months after surgery. Postoperative encephalopathy, however, is associated with poor short-term outcomes (e.g., increased length of stay [LOS], three times

Table 16-1	Significant Risk Factors for Type I and Type II Neurologic Complications
Risk Factors	
Types I and II	Advanced age, especially older than 70 years
	History of pulmonary disease
	History of or existing hypertension
	Peripheral vascular disease
	Prior cardiac surgery
Type I	Moderate to severe proximal aortic atherosclerosis of proximal or ascending aorta
	Significant atherosclerosis of intracerebral arteries
	Stenosis of the circumflex artery greater than 70%
	Carotid vascular disease
	History of neurologic deficit
	LCOS
	Pre-existing cardiovascular disease
	Peripheral artery disease
	Diabetes mellitus
	Preoperative or postoperative AF
	Recent MI
	Female gender
	History of unstable angina
	Use of left ventricular venting procedure
	Use of intra-aortic balloon pump
	Moderate to severe LV dysfunction
	Previous stroke or TIA
	Development of left mural thrombus
	Complex surgical procedures
	Prolonged CPB time
	Hemodynamic instability
	Lower BSA
	Previously elevated serum creatinine level
	On-pump arrest
Type II	History of excessive alcohol consumption
	Postoperative dysrhythmias
	Metabolic conditions
	Heart failure
	Intraoperative hypotension
	Prolonged oxygen desaturation

AF, atrial fibrillation; BSA, body surface area; CPB, cardiopulmonary bypass; LCOS, low cardiac output syndrome; LV, left ventricular; MI, myocardial infarction; TIA, transient ischemic attack.

Sources: Data from Hillis, L. D., Smith, P. K., Anderson, J. L., Bittl, J. A., Bridges, C. R., Byrne, J. G., . . . Winniford, M. D. (2011). 2011 ACCF/AHA guideline for coronary artery bypass graft surgery. A report of the American College of Cardiology Foundation/American Heart Association Task Force on Practice Guidelines. Developed in collaboration with the American Association for Thoracic Surgery, Society of Cardiovascular Anesthesiologists, and Society of Thoracic Surgeons. *Journal of the American College of Cardiology, 58*(24), e123–210. doi: 10.1016/j.jacc.2011.08.009; McDonagh, D. L., Berger, M., Mathew, J. P., Graffagnino, C., Milano, C. A., & Newman, M. F. (2014). Neurological complications of cardiac surgery. *Lancet Neurology, 13*(5), 490-502; McGarvey, M. L., Cheung, A. T., & Stecker, M. M. (2013). *Neurologic complications of cardiac surgery*. Retrieved from http://www.uptodate.com/contents/neurologic-complications-of-cardiac-surgery?source=search_result&search=neurologic+complications+of+cardiac+surgery; Roekaerts, P. M. H. J., & Heijmans, J. H. (2012). Early postoperative care after cardiac surgery. In C. Narin (Ed.), *Perioperative considerations in cardiac surgery*. Retrieved from http://www.intechopen.com/books/perioperative-considerations-in-cardiac-surgery/-early-postoperative-care-after-cardiac-surgery-; Silvestry, F. E. (2014). *Postoperative complications among patients undergoing cardiac surgery*. Retrieved from http://www.uptodate.com/contents/postoperative-complications-among-patients-undergoing-cardiac-surgery; Whitlock, R., Healey, J. S., Connolly, S. J., Wang, J., Danter, M. R., Tu, J. V., . . . Yusuf, S. (2014). Predictors of early and late stroke following cardiac surgery. *Canadian Medical Journal*. Retrieved from http://www.cmaj.ca/content/early/2014/07/21/cmaj.131214

higher mortality rate, and less likelihood to be discharged to home) (McGarvey et al., 2013).

Termed *post-perfusion syndrome*, *post-pump syndrome*, and *pump head*, type II deficits are thought to be due to cerebral microemboli that develop with manipulation of the heart and aorta, especially during cannulation and clamping of the aorta. Intraoperative hypotension may also lead to cerebral injury and cognitive decline. Systemic inflammation and general anesthesia have also been implicated (McGarvey et al., 2013). Data from one study suggested that a drop in mean arterial pressure of 27 mmHg or more during surgery resulted in a decrease of 1.4 points on the Mini Mental Status Exam (Gottesman et al., 2010).

Data suggest that cognitive decline that occurs following cardiac surgery may be related to a variation in the gene apolipoprotein E4 (ApoE4). The variation may be identified with genetic testing. Being aware of the presence of the ApoE4 genotype may help patients make more informed decisions about cardiac surgery and increase the predictability of cognitive decline 5 years postoperatively. Genetic implications of cardiac surgery are discussed in detail in Chapter 21.

Predictors for Types I and II Deficits

Older age, especially older than 70 years, is a strong predictor for both Type I and Type II deficits. A history of significant hypertension has also been linked to both types of adverse neurologic outcomes following cardiac surgery. In addition, patients undergoing combined open chamber procedures and coronary artery surgery are at greatest risk for adverse neurologic outcomes; these complications are equally divided between Type I and Type II deficits (Martin, de Melo, & de Sousa, 2008).

Predictors for Type I Deficits

Moderate to severe proximal aortic atherosclerosis, as identified by intraoperative palpation, is the single greatest marker for a Type I neurologic deficit. The risk for Type I deficits increases in the presence of aortic lesions, with these kinds of complications being more prevalent in older patients (Martin et al., 2008). Atherosclerotic emboli are likely mobilized by manipulation of the aorta.

In a large prospective review, it has been shown that 30% to 40% of strokes occur intraoperatively, with the remainder occurring 1–2 days after surgery (Tarakji, Sabik, Bhudia, Batizy, & Blackstone, 2011). Strokes are uncommon after the first week. Different mechanisms are believed to be responsible for early versus late stroke. Cerebral hypoperfusion and atheroembolization are thought to be responsible for intraoperative or early-onset stroke. Cardiogenic embolism, especially associated with AF, low cardiac output (CO), and postoperative hypercoagulopathy are the most common etiologies of delayed ischemic stroke (Hillis et al., 2011).

Predictors for Type II Deficits

Factors that are associated with Type II deficits are listed in Table 16-1. Although a recent study linked aortic atherosclerosis to delirium (Nina et al., 2012), earlier studies did not show a strong correlation between the two, suggesting an etiology related to pathology of the microcirculation in the brain, rather than embolization (Hogue, Palin, & Arrowsmith, 2006). Other factors linked to Type II deficits include certain genetic factors (American Society of Anesthesiologists, 2013; Mathew et al., 2007). Type II deficits are seen more commonly in patients who have experienced periods of hypoperfusion or hypotension (Grocott, Homi, & Puskas, 2005).

UNDERLYING PATHOPHYSIOLOGY

The precise mechanisms of cerebral injury following cardiac surgery are not fully understood. Numerous factors inherent to cardiac surgery play a role in adverse neurologic outcomes. These complications have been attributed primarily to the presence of ascending aortic atherosclerosis and the effects of CPB. Reported mechanisms are the embolization of gas and particulate matter, inadequate cerebral perfusion, and large fluctuations in hemodynamic parameters (Hillis et al., 2011).

Patients who undergo cardiac surgery experience a profound systemic inflammatory response, especially when CPB is used. One of the effects of the systemic inflammatory response related to CPB is the development of clots. Cardiopulmonary bypass activates the intrinsic and extrinsic pathways of the coagulation system secondary to factors including hypothermia, pumps propelling blood through the circuit, and exposure of blood to the artificial surfaces of the bypass circuit (Durandy, 2014). Cognitive decline has been linked to surgeries other than cardiac procedures in elderly patients (Hillis et al., 2011). Notably, exposure to general anesthetic agents may contribute to cognitive decline. In addition, postoperative hyperthermia and cerebral edema have been linked to poor neurologic outcomes, although these complications may be an effect of processes that resulted in cerebral injury itself, rather than being directly responsible for the neurologic deficit (Grocott & Yoshitani, 2007).

STRATEGIES FOR NEUROPROTECTION DURING CARDIAC SURGERY

Careful preoperative screening can help identify patients who are at higher risk for developing neurologic complications. For example, a biomarker known as N-methyl-D-aspartate (NMDA) receptor antibody (NR2Ab) is predictive of severe neurologic adverse events after CPB. The NMDA receptor is the primary excitatory amino acid receptor of the central nervous system (CNS). When nerve cells are damaged from ischemia, a process begins that causes nerve cells to undergo programmed cell death. During this time, NR2 receptors are ruined and NR2 peptides are released into the bloodstream. The peptides cause the development of autoantibodies (NR2Ab), which are possible biomarkers of neurologic complications such as stroke and cerebral ischemia (Weissman, Khunteev, & Dambinova, n.d.). A number of strategies have been suggested to minimize patients' risk of experiencing neurologic deficits following cardiac surgery.

Avoiding Injury

Many strategies to reduce complications during cardiac surgery focus on avoiding injury. As previously stated, atherosclerosis is an important predictor of stroke. The surgeon can identify high-risk patients intraoperatively with the use of epiaortic ultrasound or transesophageal echocardiogram (TEE) to modify cannulation sites and avoid atheroma (fatty deposits in arteries). Epiaortic ultrasound imaging is superior to direct palpation or TEE and is defined as Class IIa in the 2011 American College of Cardiology Foundation (ACCF)/American Heart Association (AHA) guideline for CABG (Hillis et al., 2011; Likosky et al., 2012). Single cross-clamp technique and the use of an internal thoracic artery–Y (ITA-Y) graft for proximal anastomosis to avoid aortic manipulation are also intraoperative strategies to minimize atheroembolism (Yang, Zhang, Gu, & Wei, 2012). In patients with severe atherosclerosis, other options for surgery may be employed, such as off-pump coronary artery bypass grafting (OPCAB) or replacement of the ascending aorta under deep hypothermic circulatory arrest. Data are not consistent in showing benefit with avoidance of CPB. The ACCF/AHA CABG guideline does not find enough evidence to conclude that OPCAB is better for limiting neurologic deficits (Hillis et al., 2011). Off-pump coronary artery bypass grafting is discussed in detail in Chapter 7. Concentration has changed to evaluating patient-related factors for neurologic complications (McGarvey et al., 2013).

Other strategies shown to reduce neurologic injury include emboli reduction with the use of cell saver to process shed mediastinal blood, post-pump arterial filters, and acid–base balance management with the alpha-stat method, de-airing procedures, and minimizing aortic trauma in patients with a severely calcified aorta. Hyperglycemia, hypotension, and hyperthermia during rewarming have all been linked to adverse neurologic outcomes and should be avoided (McGarvey et al., 2013). During preoperative screening, if patients have significant carotid stenosis, consideration may be given to preoperative stenting or a combined CABG with carotid endarterectomy procedure (McGarvey et al., 2013).

Initial data suggest that intraoperative multimodal brain monitoring may decrease the incidence of neurologic complications (Zanatta et al., 2011). Several modes of cerebral monitoring exist. These methods may help reveal cerebral hypoperfusion and hypoxia, which contribute to intraoperative brain injury. Examples of methods available include near-infrared cerebral oximetry, jugular bulb oximetry, electroencephalogram (EEG), somatosensory-evoked potentials, and transcranial Doppler ultrasound (Arnaoutakis & Baumgartner, 2013).

Minimizing Injury

Other strategies to reduce neurologic complications focus on minimizing the extent of injury. These measures include rapid treatment of AF and early identification of and intervention for ischemic brain lesions. Some evidence suggests that increasing blood pressure to increase cerebral blood flow may help to minimize infarction size (McGarvey et al., 2013).

DIAGNOSIS AND TREATMENT OF CNS INJURY

Nurses who care for postoperative cardiac surgery patients should be able to recognize those patients who are at increased risk for CNS injury and differentiate between the various types of neurologic deficits. Care includes interval assessments of neurologic function and changes to the plan of care to enhance neurologic recovery.

Stroke

Stroke is a devastating complication following cardiac surgery (McGarvey et al., 2013). Postoperative stroke is a leading cause of death following CPB. The incidence of stroke has been reported to range from 1% to 5%. Valve surgery poses even higher risk for stroke. This is thought to be potentially related to air embolism (McDonagh et al., 2014). There is variability in incidence of stroke attributed to differences in patient populations, surgical procedure, and data collection methods. Increased rates of stroke and encephalopathy are attributed to increased numbers of high-risk patients undergoing cardiac surgery (e.g., those with a previous stroke, hypertension, diabetes, AF, or valvular disease) (Whitlock et al., 2014).

Postoperative cardiac surgery stroke is categorized into two types—early and late. Early stroke occurs in 24 hours or earlier following cardiac surgery; late stroke occurs more than 24 hours after CPB. Early stroke is associated with increased mortality rate and discharge to a skilled rehabilitation facility. In-hospital mortality for early (41%) and late stroke (13%) is higher than for patients with no postoperative stroke (Lisle et al., 2008).

Most of the strokes following cardiac surgery are ischemic in nature (Henke & Eigsti, 2003). A small percentage (5%) of patients with ischemic strokes, however, experience hemorrhagic alteration or conversion. Intracranial hemorrhage with associated clinical significance is rare following cardiac surgery (McGarvey et al., 2013). Strokes that occur later in the postoperative period are more often associated with dysrhythmias, especially AF; valve surgery; use of a ventricular assist device; low CO; or postoperative hypercoagulopathy (Hillis et al., 2011).

Presence of carotid artery disease may be a risk factor for postoperative cardiac surgery stroke. Specifically, those with symptomatic carotid stenosis, bilateral asymptomatic stenosis, and unilateral asymptomatic stenosis with contralateral carotid occlusion may be at increased risk. The quality of supportive data regarding this is considered to be poor, however (Lazar, Wilson, & Messé, 2013).

Cardiac surgery causes an inflammatory response that can result in disruption of the blood–brain barrier (BBB) and neurologic dysfunction. Data from model studies have revealed that CPB leads to opening of the BBB. This disruption can be detected on magnetic resonance imaging (MRI). The BBB may be open during surgery or in the immediate postoperative period. It closes shortly thereafter. Cerebral ischemia is associated with opening of the BBB. Further studies are needed in this area (Merino et al., 2013).

Postoperative cardiac surgery patients who develop a stroke have higher mortality rates and longer hospital stays (McGarvey et al., 2013). The mortality rate in postoperative CABG patients who develop stroke is 10-fold higher than those without it (Hillis et al., 2011). Mortality rates are higher in patients who develop an intraoperative versus postoperative stroke (41% versus 13%). Patients who have a stroke following cardiac surgery are also likely to have focal deficits and are more likely to be discharged to a place other than home (McGarvey et al., 2013).

Suspicion for stroke occurs when the patient fails to awaken, move extremities, follow commands after discontinuation of sedation, or any combination of these in the first 6 postoperative hours (McKhann et al., 2006). The onset of focal findings such as facial droop, hemiparesis, aphasia, visual disturbances, or pupil change may also indicate stroke. Assessment is often difficult in the immediate postoperative period, however, and is confounded by the patient's emergence from anesthesia and the effects of postoperative medications.

A postoperative stroke may go unnoticed in the first 24 to 48 hours after surgery until anesthesia has worn off and the patient has been weaned off of mechanical ventilation (Dafer, 2006; McGarvey et al., 2013). Diagnosis of stroke is made based on the presence of findings on the physical exam and diffusion-weighted MRI results (Lazar et al., 2013). Patients suspected of having a stroke should be evaluated by a neurologist and undergo brain imaging.

Brain MRI—specifically, diffusion-weighted imaging—is the most accurate neuroimaging technique available; it is able to detect microemboli-related events. It will confirm presence of a cerebral infarction and identify other unsuspected infarcted areas. It may help determine etiology of the stroke (e.g., embolism) (McGarvey et al., 2013). Unfortunately, MRI is often impractical in postoperative cardiac surgery patients due to the presence of metallic implants such as valves, defibrillators, pacemakers, or surgical metal (e.g., epicardial pacing wires). An alternative imaging modality, head computed tomography (CT), can be used in such cases (Oliveira-Filho & Koroshetz, 2013).

Another complication, though rare, is perioperative vision loss, which can occur at a rate of 0.2% (Newman, 2008). It is thought to occur from an interruption of the blood supply to the optic nerve heads, which are supplied by branches of the ophthalmic artery. The loss of vision is called ischemic optic neuropathy (ION). It is further delineated as posterior ION (PION) or anterior

ION (AION). Anterior ION is more prevalent among cardiac surgery and heart valve replacement patients, while PION is seen with spine and neck procedures. Multiple factors have been associated with ION: long duration in the prone position, high volume of blood loss, hypotension (especially intraoperatively), anemia, hypoxia, excessive fluid replacement, use of vasoconstrictor agents, elevated venous pressure, and patient risk factors. Those patients most at risk have a history of smoking, vascular disease, diabetes, hypertension, and carotid artery disease (American Society of Anesthesiologists Task Force on Perioperative Visual Loss, 2012).

Neurologic assessments of cardiac surgery patients should be conducted at regular intervals in the postoperative period. This review includes assessment of the patient's level of consciousness (LOC) and motor movement. As mentioned earlier, medications given during the intraoperative period can make accurate assessment more difficult. If deficits are suspected, a full neurologic assessment should be performed. The National Institutes of Health Stroke Scale (NIHSS) outlines a complete evaluation for stroke. The NIHSS assessment includes LOC, best gaze, visual fields, facial palsy, motor function of arms and legs, limb ataxia, sensory, best language, dysarthria, extinction, and inattention (National Institute of Neurological Disorders and Stroke, n.d.).

Treatment of Stroke

Treatment of stroke is primarily supportive in nature. Prompt recognition and intervention are essential. The initial goals are to stabilize the patient, treat the underlying cause, determine if the stroke is ischemic in nature with either a noncontrast CT or MRI of the brain. Assessment of vital signs, obtaining appropriate laboratory and other diagnostic data (e.g., electrocardiogram [ECG], complete blood count, cardiac enzymes with troponin,

comprehensive metabolic profile, and coagulation profile), and treating volume depletion and any electrolyte imbalances are also indicated (Silvestry, 2014).

Management of ischemic perioperative stroke following cardiac surgery is similar to management of stroke in other patient populations; however, the use of tissue plasminogen activator (t-PA) is contraindicated following cardiac surgery due to the significant risk of bleeding (McGarvey et al., 2013). Monitoring the patient's neurologic, hematologic, and respiratory status is essential. Nursing care is guided by the specific neurologic deficits observed in the patient. Evidence-based guidelines have been published for the management of stroke (Jauch et al., 2013).

BLOOD PRESSURE SUPPORT

Blood pressure lowering is not recommended unless the systolic blood pressure is greater than 220 mmHg or diastolic blood pressure is greater than 120 mmHg, or the patient is at risk for aortic dissection, acute myocardial infarction (MI), or heart failure. Care should be taken to gradually decrease blood pressure to a specified target because the other extreme—hypotension—worsens neurologic outcome. Periods of hypotension should be similarly avoided so as to maintain adequate cerebral perfusion. If hypotension does develop, placement of the patient in supine position and administration of intravenous fluids is recommended. If needed, pressors (e.g., phenylephrine [Neosynephrine®]) may be added. Judicious volume expansion is recommended for patients who are normotensive (McGarvey et al., 2013).

OXYGENATION SUPPORT

Supporting adequate tissue oxygenation is important in patients who are experiencing cerebral ischemia. Patients with acute stroke may have abnormal breathing patterns and may need increased support to prevent hypoxia, which can worsen brain injury. Endotracheal intubation may be necessary if concerns arise about airway protection, pulmonary edema, or the patient's ability to maintain adequate oxygenation. Pneumonia is among the leading complications of stroke. It occurs in 5% to 9% of patients. The incidence is higher in patients with ischemic stroke (Chalela, 2012), so optimal nursing management includes measures to prevent ventilator-associated conditions. Oxygen saturation levels of at least 92% should be maintained. Hyperbaric oxygen may be considered if the patient is stable and has a suspected air embolism (McGarvey et al., 2013).

TEMPERATURE MANAGEMENT

Increased body temperature is associated with increased morbidity and mortality in acute stroke patients. It is important to assess these patients for sources of hyperthermia, which may be related to brain injury or secondary infections. In such cases, patients may benefit from measures that lower their body temperature. Interventions to accomplish this goal may include the administration of antipyretics and application of cooling devices (McGarvey et al., 2013).

Hypothermia protects against cerebral ischemia. Although the neuroprotective benefits of hypothermia are well known, it is only suggested that there is a malfunction in those protective benefits (Joshi et al., 2010).

GLYCEMIC CONTROL

Hypoglycemia may mimic symptoms of stroke and may exacerbate brain injury. Initial assessment of the patient upon presentation of stroke symptoms should include measurement of serum glucose and correction of hypoglycemia.

Conversely, hyperglycemia is associated with poorer outcomes following stroke and should be avoided (McGarvey et al., 2013). Researchers hypothesize that hyperglycemia increases the infarct size associated with a stroke and elevates cerebral lactate levels,

which results in acidosis of brain tissue and decreases the function of the mitochondria of the penumbra (an ischemic area that is still viable, located adjacent to the area affected by the stroke). Hyperglycemia is also reported to disrupt the blood–brain barrier, which puts the patient at risk of developing cerebral edema; this complication, in turn, promotes brain cell death in the stroke-affected area. All of these factors influence morbidity and mortality following a stroke (Kim, Moon, Gee, Choi, & Ho, 2011). Blood glucose levels less than 60 mg/dL should be treated with an appropriate hypoglycemia protocol. Similarly, blood glucose levels greater than 180 mg/dL should be treated with an insulin infusion (McGarvey et al., 2013).

The AHA/American Stroke Association guidelines for management of acute stroke recommend treating hyperglycemia with a goal of serum glucose in the range of 140 to 180 mg/dL. A systematic review of 11 trials of more than 1,500 patients with acute ischemic stroke who were randomized to tight glycemic control or usual care showed no difference between groups in mortality or neurologic outcome. There was a higher rate of treatment for symptomatic hypoglycemia in the intervention group (Bellolio, Gilmore, & Ganti, 2014). Careful titration and control of serum glucose levels are key nursing measures and are usually best accomplished with an insulin infusion.

ANTI-PLATELET THERAPY

Although studies have failed to confirm the efficacy of anticoagulation following CABG and fibrinolysis is contraindicated in patients who have undergone this surgical procedure, administration of aspirin and clopidogrel (Plavix®) has been shown to decrease neurologic complications following CABG and improve outcomes following stroke. If not contraindicated, anti-platelet therapy is recommended in postoperative cardiac surgery patients (McGarvey et al., 2013).

Prevention of Secondary Complications

Stroke following cardiac surgery increases both intensive care unit (ICU) and overall hospital LOS. Patients who experience this neurologic complication are at increased risk for secondary complications and have a three-fold to six-fold increased risk of death. Mortality rates in the range of 14% to 30% have been reported in hospitalized patients who follow this course (McGarvey et al., 2013). Anticipation of complications allows the ICU nurse to develop a plan of care to reduce the risk of stroke and its sequelae. Common secondary complications include aspiration, pneumonia, venous thrombotic events, urinary tract infections, and skin breakdown.

Encephalopathy and Delirium

Postoperative cardiac surgery patients are at greater risk for not only a stroke, but also encephalopathy. *Encephalopathy* is a generic term that refers to several types of brain dysfunction. Encephalopathy is common after cardiac surgery. Patients typically manifest disorientation, confusion, lethargy, agitation, paranoia, or hallucinations.

The etiology is multifactorial and may be due to inflammation of the brain, cerebral hypoperfusion, hypoxia, metabolic derangements, use of psychotropic drugs for anesthesia, pain control with opioids, or any combination of these. Temporary resedation may be useful until the patient is oriented and calm. This condition is usually temporary and is associated with longer LOS and higher mortality rates (Makhann, Gottesman, Grega, Baumgartner, & Selnes, 2011; Roekaerts & Heijmans, 2012). Risk factors identified in the literature include aortic cross-clamping, CPB, ventilation time, serum creatinine, age, MI, diabetes, emergent surgery, lung disease, and an abnormal ECG (Nina et al., 2012).

By definition, delirium is a disturbance of consciousness with reduced ability to focus, sustain, or shift attention; it is a change in cognition or development of a perceptual disturbance that is not accounted for by a pre-existing dementia. It develops over a short period of time (hours to days) and varies during the day. Delirium is more common in older patients (Silvestry, 2014). The incidence of this complication has been reported to range from 3% to 52% (Koster, Hensens, Schuurmans, & van der Palen, 2011). The incidence of delirium following vascular and cardiac surgery is twice the rate of other surgical patients (Gottesman et al., 2010). Patients who develop postoperative delirium are more likely to develop respiratory insufficiency, sternal instability necessitating surgical revision, and sternal wound infection (Koster et al., 2011).

A review of 5,034 consecutive patients who had cardiac surgery at a single center showed delirium to be an independent predictor of death up to 10 years postoperatively, especially in younger patients and those who did not have a stroke (Gottesman et al., 2010). Intensive care unit and hospital LOS, mortality, and development of post-ICU cognitive impairment are increased in patients who experience delirium (Barr et al., 2013).

Recommendations regarding assessing and treating delirium are based on clinical observation (Silvestry, 2014). Suggested preventive measures include minimizing sensory deprivation and administration of benzodiazepines or narcotics postoperatively, avoiding disruption of the sleep–wake cycle, checking for withdrawal symptoms, monitoring serum electrolytes and renal and liver function, and observing for metabolic encephalopathies (McGarvey et al., 2013).

Delirium is a "disturbance of consciousness with inattention that is accompanied by changes in cognition or perceptual disturbance and has an acute onset with a fluctuating course" (Chang, Tsai, Lin, Chen, & Liu, 2008, p. 568). It is the most common neurologic complication following cardiac surgery

(Alejaldre, Delgado-Mederos, Santos, & Marti-Fabrogas, 2010). This condition develops over the course of hours to days and may be life-threatening. An estimated 3% to 52% of postoperative cardiac surgery patients develop delirium (Koster et al., 2011). The incidence is higher in those patients with preexisting psychological disorders; diabetes; substantial prior alcohol use; left ventricular ejection fraction (LVEF) less than 30%; cardiogenic shock; MI; memory complaints; advanced age (older than 65-70 years); elevated EUROscore (Andrade, Moraes, & Andrade, 2014); history of stroke; peripheral vascular disease; low serum albumin level; low CO; use of intra-aortic balloon pump therapy or inotropic medications; preoperative cognitive decline; urgent surgery; AF; receipt of antihypertensive, anticholinergic, or antidepressant agents; receipt of benzodiazepines, opioids, or statins; and preoperative delirium. Use of fentanyl or ketamine has also been implicated in delirium (Koster et al., 2011; Tse et al., 2012).

Reported intraoperative risk factors for delirium include hemofiltration, longer duration of CPB, use of diazepam, duration of anesthesia, lactate levels, need for inotropes following CPB, and reinstitution of CPB (Norkienė, Ringaitienė, Kuzminstáitė, Šipylaitė, 2013).

Postoperative use of opioids, dexmedetomidine (Precedex®), or rivastigmine (Exelon®) as well as transfusion of more than 2 liters of packed red blood cells, acute postoperative infection, hematocrit less than 30%, prolonged use of inotropic agents, or electrolyte abnormalities have been implicated in the development of postoperative delirium (Koster et al., 2011; Tse et al., 2012). Postoperative encephalopathy may be related to the development of microemboli, cerebral edema secondary to the inflammatory response, inadequate temperature regulation, or cerebral hypoperfusion (Henke & Eigsti, 2003).

Symptoms of delirium include an inability to maintain attention, changing LOC, cognitive deficits, memory impairment, illusions, hallucinations, inappropriate speech, and motor abnormalities (Hakim, Othman, & Naoum, 2012). Focal neurologic findings are not present in delirium. Early detection and treatment of delirium are important aspects of the nursing care of postoperative cardiac surgery patients and may limit this complication's severity or prevent it altogether.

Agitation often accompanies postoperative delirium. It is defined as extreme motor or vocal behavior that is disruptive, is unsafe for the patient and staff, or interferes with the delivery of patient care and medical therapies. Examples of agitation in hospitalized patients may include screaming, shouting, moaning, combativeness (e.g., biting, kicking, hitting, scratching), pulling out tubes and disconnecting monitoring devices, and getting out of bed. Delirium and agitation often present together and may be difficult to distinguish.

Treatment of Delirium

Delirium after cardiac surgery is common and multifactorial. As such, it is important for ICU nurses to recognize patients who are at risk of developing this neurologic complication and adjust their care to reduce or prevent postoperative delirium. The main aspects of managing delirium include identifying and treating the underlying causes, providing environmental changes (quiet and well lit), reorienting (e.g., with use of calendars, clocks, family photos) and communicating with the patient often, and minimizing pharmacologic interventions. Modifying sleep–wake cycles with medications, correcting sensory deficits (e.g., with glasses or hearing aids, as applicable), and administering fluids and proper nutrition have been suggested. If severe, constant observation is recommended (Koster et al., 2011). Early mobilization of adult ICU patients has been shown to reduce the incidence and duration of delirium (Alagiakrishnan, 2014;

Barr et al., 2013; Francis, 2014). The multidisciplinary Clinical Practice Guidelines for the Management of Pain, Agitation, and Delirium in Adult Patients in the ICU summarize best practices for managing delirium and improving clinical outcomes (Barr et al., 2013). Best practices for prevention and treatment are summarized in **Table 16-2**.

IDENTIFICATION AND TREATMENT OF THE CAUSE

Routine monitoring for delirium is recommended in adult ICU patients. The Confusion Assessment Method for the ICU and the Intensive Care Delirium Screening Checklist are the most valid and reliable tools for monitoring delirium in the ICU (Barr et al., 2013). Administration of risperidone (Risperdal®), a newer neuroleptic with fewer reported adverse events than haloperidol (Haldol®), has been shown to decrease the incidence of delirium in older patients who underwent on-pump cardiac surgery (Hakim et al., 2012).

In patients experiencing postoperative delirium, a thorough examination must be made to identify and allow for correction of possible causes. The underlying causes of delirium may be metabolic derangements including electrolyte disorders, drug or alcohol withdrawal, nutritional deficiencies, or medications. Careful review of medications with emphasis on new medications is warranted whenever delirium presents. Attempts should be made to avoid use of drugs that impair reality, such as benzodiazepines or barbiturates, in postoperative patients.

Analgesics are often associated with mental status changes. Undertreatment of pain, however, may contribute to increased stress and sleep deprivation, thereby exacerbating postoperative delirium. The ICU nurse should closely monitor patients to avoid adverse effects from analgesics. Special care should be given to administering narcotics in the elderly population because glomerular filtration rate decreases with age (Wooten, 2012).

ENVIRONMENTAL AND SUPPORTIVE MEASURES

Environmental interventions include minimizing or eliminating factors that exacerbate delirium. In the ICU, patients are frequently exposed to interruptions in sleep patterns, noise, and excessive environmental stimulation (Koster et al., 2011). Transfer to a progressive care unit should be made as soon as medically feasible and often results in abatement of delirium-related symptoms. In addition, care should be taken to reduce sensory

---

Table 16-2   Best Practices for Prevention of Delirium

- Target risk factors that might trigger an episode.
- Perform early mobilization.
- Provide adequate fluids.
- Provide stimulating activities and familiar objects.
- Encourage the use of eyeglasses and hearing aids, if applicable.
- Use simple and regular communication about people, current place, and time.
- Provide mobility and range-of-motion exercises.
- Reduce noise and avoid sleep interruptions.
- Provide appropriate pain management and offer nondrug treatment for sleep problems or anxiety.
- Do not use either haloperidol or atypical antipsychotics to prevent delirium.

Sources: Data from Barr, J., Fraser, G. L., Puntillo, K., Ely, E. W., Gelinas, C., Dasta, J. F., . . . Jaeschke, R. (2013). Clinical practice guidelines for the management of pain, agitation, and delirium in adult patients in the intensive care unit. *Critical Care Medicine, 41*(1), 263–306; Francis, J. (2014). Delirium and acute confusional states: Prevention, treatment and prognosis. Retrieved from http://www.uptodate.com/contents/delirium-and-acute-confusionalstates-prevention-treatment-and-prognosis

impairment and to return patients' glasses or hearing aids as soon as practical. In all cases, nurses should focus on providing patients with reorientation and reassurance.

In extreme cases of agitation, restraints may be needed to ensure the patient's safety. Attendance at the bedside by family members or sitters is preferable to the use of physical restraints. Sitters may participate in orienting activities by talking to the patient, engaging in frequent touch, and making eye contact.

DRUG THERAPY

Pharmacologic interventions may be necessary in patients with postoperative delirium, especially when agitation is present. Despite the prevalence of postoperative delirium, only a limited number of agents to treat this complication have been studied in postoperative patients.

Haloperidol (Haldol®) is a first-generation, high-potency neuroleptic that has been frequently used in the treatment of delirium in the ICU. Because of the side effects of haloperidol, use of newer neuroleptic agents (e.g., risperidone, olanzapine [Zyprexa®], quetiapine [Seroquel®]) have been suggested for treatment of psychotic symptoms. This group of agents is associated with the development of extrapyramidal symptoms, tardive dyskinesia, and neuroleptic malignant syndrome (Alagiakrishnan, 2014). The latter syndrome includes symptoms of high fever, diaphoresis, labile blood pressure, stupor, muscle rigidity, and autonomic dysfunction (National Institute of Neurological

Disorders and Stroke, 2014). There is no evidence that haloperidol decreases the duration of delirium in adult ICU patients, and the current 2013 guidelines do not recommend the use of haloperidol due to lack of clinical data to support its use (Barr et al., 2013). Haloperidol has been linked to cardiac dysrhythmias, including torsades de pointes, and should be avoided in patients with known risk (Barr et al., 2013). Continuous infusion of dexmedetomidine is recommended for mechanically ventilated patients with delirium who require continuous sedation and have delirium that is unrelated to alcohol or benzodiazepine withdrawal. Dexmedetomidine is indicated to decrease the duration of delirium in these patients (Barr et al., 2013).

Patients who do receive antipsychotic therapy with haloperidol should have ECG monitoring, including measurement of the QT interval (see **Box 16-1**). A QT interval of greater than 450 milliseconds or more than 25% over baseline warrants close monitoring and possibly a reduction or discontinuation of haloperidol, although QT prolongation may not always precede dysrhythmias (McAuley, 2014).

Treatment of delirium with benzodiazepines is reserved for patients who are experiencing withdrawal from alcohol or sedative hypnotics. Patients who are unable to tolerate high doses of antipsychotic medications may benefit from combined benzodiazepine therapy (Alagiakrishnan, 2014). Benzodiazepine use may be a risk factor in the development of delirium (Barr et al., 2013).

Box 16-1   Measuring QT Intervals

$\dfrac{QT}{\sqrt{RR}}$ (the number of seconds between R waves)

Each small box in ECG paper equals 0.04 sec. Each large box equals 0.20 sec.

Seizures

Seizures are a rare neurologic complication following cardiac surgery, occurring in 0.5% to 3.5% of patients following CABG (McGarvey et al., 2013). They most often accompany cerebral insult from hypoxia or emboli (air or particulate). Seizures may also be caused by hypoxemia, hyponatremia, hypoglycemia, stroke, or medication overdoses, especially overdoses of lidocaine (Xylocaine®) or procainamide (Pronestyl®) (McGarvey et al., 2013). Lysine analogs such as tranexamic acid and epsilon-aminocaproic acid are used in antifibrinolytic therapy for cardiac surgery patients and have been associated with postoperative seizures (Manji et al., 2012; Martin et al., 2011).

In one study of patients who developed seizures following cardiac surgery, a five-times higher mortality rate was reported when compared to patients who did not develop postoperative seizures (29% vs. 6%) (Goldstone et al., 2011).

A thorough examination for contributing factors, evaluation by a neurologist, CT scan, and EEG should be performed, and administration of anticonvulsant therapy should be considered (Kouchoukos, Blackstone, Hanley, & Kirklin, 2012). An EEG is recommended for patients who are unresponsive 18 to 24 hours after surgery to determine if seizure activity is occurring without motor manifestations. Preventive measures include preventing electrolyte abnormalities (e.g., hyponatremia, hypomagnesemia, and hypocalcemia), withdrawal of medications (e.g., benzodiazepines, barbiturates), and toxic levels of lidocaine (McGarvey et al., 2013).

Cognitive Decline

Cognitive decline is commonplace following cardiac surgery, with a reported incidence of 48% of patients. This impairment persists for at least 30% of patients for up to 6 weeks and up to 6 months for 25% of patients (Sun, Lindsay, Monsein, Hill, & Corso, 2012). Typical cognitive disturbances include mild difficulty with memory, problem solving, attention, and ability to learn.

Data are inconclusive as to whether preoperative education is effective in augmenting physical and psychological recovery following cardiac surgery. Some researchers have found no decrease in anxiety, pain, or LOS, while others show interventions are effective (Guo, 2015). To ensure that education is provided, the ICU nurse should prepare patients and families for the possibility that the patient may experience some cognitive decline and reassure them that most patients experience improvement in these symptoms if they do occur. In addition, both patients and families should be taught about subtle changes and symptoms for which to observe. Neurocognitive deficits usually resolve gradually and most patients return to their baseline neurocognitive function in 3–12 months after surgery (Fontes et al., 2013; McGarvey et al., 2013).

Anxiety and Depression

Data on postoperative cardiac surgery patients suggest that the presence of anxiety and depression are present in 30% to 40% of patients undergoing cardiac surgery (Tully & Baker, 2012). These symptoms each account for a twofold increase in hospital readmissions (Suls & Bunde, 2005). Aside from their physiologic impact in the immediate postoperative period, these conditions are reported to have negative effects on long-term quality of life (Tully, Baker, Turnbull, Winefield, & Knight, 2009). Both the immediate and long-term effects may increase the risk of death following cardiac surgery (Cserép et al., 2012).

Minor depressive episodes have been found in 13% to 18% of CABG patients; these conditions were not present preoperatively (Tully & Baker, 2012). Data suggest a correlation between the presence of symptoms of depression and the chance of hospital readmission for cardiac issues within 6 months of discharge following CABG (Oxlad, Stubberfield, Stuklis, Edwards, & Wade, 2006; Suls & Bunde, 2005). In one study, major depressive symptoms were associated with a twofold risk of cardiac events. These data were reported after adjusting for LVEF, gender differences, increased LOS, New York Heart Association class, number of vessels involved, and living alone (Connerey, Shapiro, McLaughlin, Bagiella, & Sloan, 2001). Of 62,665 patients who underwent CABG in another study, 9% of patients with major depression had an increase in hospital mortality (Dao et al., 2010). Depression is also reported to be a predisposing factor that increases the risk of delirium in cardiac surgery patients (Sockalingam et al., 2005). Depression is a major predictor of whether patients will participate in and complete cardiac rehabilitation (Hillis et al., 2011).

Depression occurs commonly after cardiac surgery and may last for months postoperatively. Although it may be severe in rare cases, depression is usually mild, disappears spontaneously, and is treated short term. Pharmacologic intervention is typically implemented. The ICU nurse should be aware of the proarrhythmic and cardiotoxic effects of tricyclic antidepressants (Ha & Wong, 2011). Selective serotonin reuptake inhibitors (SSRIs) are thought to be safer. However, some data suggest an increase in bleeding (Kim et al., 2009), renal complications, and ventilation time (Xiong et al., 2006) with SSRIs. Nonpsychological education interventions have reported little impact on depression or anxiety; however, interventions that provided information and emotional support were found to be effective (Sorlie, Busund, Sexton, & Sorlie, 2007). These latter data are not consistent (Lie, Arnesen, Sandrik, Hamilton, & Bunch, 2007) and could not be generalized to patients who underwent CABG procedures (Sebregts, Falger, Appels, Kester, & Bär, 2005).

Anxiety has variable effects on postoperative cardiac surgery outcomes (Leentjens, Maclullich, & Meagher, 2008; Sockalingam et al., 2005). Anxiety is high for patients preoperatively due to fear of dying. Upcoming surgery is the primary etiology; however, anxiety levels do not return to baseline levels postoperatively. There is increased risk of short-term and long-term mortality when this occurs (Tully & Baker, 2012).

Generalized anxiety disorder and panic disorder are the two most common conditions found. They occur in up to 11% of CABG patients. Post-traumatic stress disorder (PTSD) has recently been reported in CABG patients. The PTSD is felt to be related to surgery and hospital stressors (Dao et al., 2010).

In one study of patients admitted for CABG surgery, 92% had mild preoperative anxiety and 8% had major anxiety. Each of these patients was readmitted to the hospital within 6 months of discharge. In that same study, 72% of CABG surgery patients had depression preoperatively and were readmitted to the hospital. Depressive symptoms worsened in some of these patients, but most patients with preoperative depression experienced a resolution or reduction of their symptoms after CABG (Murphy et al., 2008).

The ICU nurse should collaborate with members of the multidisciplinary team to help ensure early recognition and prompt management of anxiety and depression in postoperative cardiac surgery patients.

OTHER NEUROLOGIC INJURIES

Although central neurologic complications receive more attention and have a greater impact on patient recovery, several other neurologic complications associated with cardiac surgery bear mentioning. These include, but are not limited to, injuries to the brachial plexus, phrenic nerve, and recurrent laryngeal nerve.

Brachial Plexus Injury

The brachial plexus includes divisions of the fifth and eighth cranial nerves and the first thoracic nerve; it forms the peripheral nerves that innervate structures of the upper extremities. The brachial plexus passes over the first rib and under the clavicle, with cords that pass downward into the axilla (Gray, 2000). The location and structure of the brachial plexus make it susceptible to injury by direct puncture, stretch, fractures, or displacement of the first rib.

Several prospective studies on cardiac surgery patients reported a 2% to 15% incidence of injuries to the brachial plexus and identified risk factors for this type of complication. Pertinent etiologic factors include sternal retraction, first rib fractures, use of internal thoracic artery (ITA) retractors, ITA dissection, positioning during surgery, central venous catheter placement, and advanced patient age (McGarvey et al., 2013).

Sensory and motor symptoms associated with this type of injury will vary, depending on the site of the nerve damage. Brachial plexus injury often presents as paresthesia of the fourth and fifth digits on the affected side and discoordination of an upper extremity, but may also cause pain and weakness. The presence of pain is consistent with a peripheral injury; in contrast, the presence of confusion, cranial nerve involvement, or hemiparesis is typically consistent with a central injury (McGarvey et al., 2013). Patients often report symptoms several days postoperatively. These subtle injuries may be overlooked owing to the emphasis placed on more serious issues in the immediate postoperative period. Any patient complaints suggestive of brachial plexus damage should be reported to the surgeon, and a full assessment of motor and sensory function should be performed for the muscles affected by the brachial plexus.

The symptoms of brachial plexus injuries may persist for several months, but generally resolve without treatment (Grocott, Clark, Homi, & Sharma, 2004). In rare cases, prolonged recovery with residual symptoms has been reported. It is important to reassure patients that brachial plexus injury is generally transient—most patients are symptom-free at discharge. In any patient who experiences this type of injury, collaboration with a physical therapist is indicated to augment the patient's strength and flexibility. Nerve conduction studies and electromyography are indicated in patients who fail to recover from symptoms within 3 weeks (McGarvey et al., 2013).

Phrenic Nerve Injury

Damage to one or both phrenic nerves may occur during cardiac surgery. This complication, which is usually related to the application of topical hypothermia, sternal retraction, or surgical trauma during left ITA dissection (Aposoudou & Johnson, 2009), occurs in 1% to 30% of patients (McGarvey et al., 2013). The phrenic nerve traverses the thoracic cavity to provide denervation to the diaphragm. The left phrenic nerve runs between the lung and mediastinal aspect of the pleura along the pericardium. The right phrenic nerve is deeper in the thoracic cavity, running lateral to the right subclavian vein (Gray, 2000).

Diagnosis of phrenic nerve damage may be made by chest radiograph, fluoroscopy, spirometry, ultrasound, or nerve conduction studies. The reported incidence of phrenic nerve dysfunction is decreasing because of the decreased use of iced slush and the use of foam insulation (McGarvey et al., 2013).

Paralysis of the diaphragm results in immobility or paradoxical movement of the affected side. Most patients have unilateral phrenic nerve injury, commonly on the same side as the ITA harvest (McGarvey et al., 2013). Unilateral phrenic nerve palsy is usually associated with minimal symptoms because of the recruitment of accessory muscles. The most common complaints include nocturnal orthopnea or dyspnea on exertion.

Phrenic nerve neuropathies generally resolve in 3 months to 1 year following cardiac surgery, but may take 2 years or longer to subside completely (McGarvey et al., 2013). In patients with underlying lung disease (e.g., chronic obstructive pulmonary disease), the consequences may be more serious. Deterioration in lung function and extended hospital stays have been reported in these individuals (Aguirre et al., 2013; Bojar, 2011). Bilateral phrenic nerve paralysis is a rare and serious complication of cardiac surgery that carries a significant associated mortality. The first indication may be difficulty in weaning the patient with normal lung function from mechanical ventilation. Bilateral phrenic neuropathy has a much longer recovery time. These patients may compensate with accessory muscle use during the day but experience respiratory insufficiency at night. Prolonged ventilatory support may be necessary (McGarvey et al., 2013).

Recurrent Laryngeal Nerve Neuropathy

The left recurrent laryngeal nerve lies in close proximity to the parietal pleura as it encircles the aortic arch (Gray, 2000). Vocal cord paralysis as a result of injury to this nerve is less common than injury to the brachial plexus or phrenic nerve, with a reported incidence of approximately 10% (Yuan, 2012).

The left recurrent laryngeal nerve may be injured during cardiac surgery if the pleura is opened and large amounts of ice slush are placed in the pleural cavity. Other sources of injury to the left recurrent laryngeal nerve include tracheal intubation, central line placement, and cardioversion (Yuan, 2012). Hoarseness developed 0 to 7 days after surgery. In most cases, the left side is involved; few are bilateral. For those patients who developed this complication, cardiac surgery included replacement of the aorta, CABG, valve replacement, or heart transplantation. Of these patients, more than 70% had resolved hoarseness (Yuan, 2012).

For the nurse caring for postoperative cardiac surgery patients, it is important to observe patients with a weak or ineffective cough, respiratory insufficiency, or hoarseness following extubation, as these may be indications of recurrent laryngeal nerve neuropathy and not laryngeal edema. Dysphagia, change in voice quality, inefficient cough, and throat clearing are often associated with vocal cord paralysis. Other symptoms included stridor, aspiration, respiratory distress/failure, poor feeding, failure to be extubated, difficulty weaning from nasal continuous positive airway pressure, delayed swallowing, and decreased laryngeal closure. Patients in whom this complication is suspected should remain NPO until further evaluation is performed because these patients are at risk for aspiration and pneumonia (Yuan, 2012). Patients with unilateral vocal cord paralysis may demonstrate respiratory insufficiency, stridor, and signs of airway obstruction. In postoperative cardiac surgery patients, these symptoms are often attributed—erroneously—to cardiac or respiratory dysfunction. It is essential that the ICU nurse identify these symptoms both correctly and promptly to avoid patient decompensation and reintubation (Hamdan, Moukarbel, Farhat, & Obeid, 2002).

A definitive diagnosis is made by performing laryngoscopy in a spontaneously breathing patient. Recovery following unilateral vocal cord paralysis usually takes 8 to 12 months; for some patients, however, the damage is permanent. Most patients recover with conservative treatment, but occasionally patients may require reintubation, tracheostomy, vocal cord medialization (an implant to provide bulk to the vocal cord), or any combination of these measures (Yuan, 2012).

Treatment includes the use of Gelfoam® /Teflon® injections, intravenous steroid therapy, speech therapy, or a type I thyroplasty (Yuan, 2012).

Intercostal Nerve Injury

Intercostal thoracic artery harvesting may cause injury to the anterior intercostal nerves. Symptoms may include numbness, tenderness, pain with light touch, or persistent burning pain over the sternum or left anterolateral aspect of the chest wall. Although symptoms typically resolve within 4 months, in some patients symptoms may last as long as 28 months (McGarvey et al., 2013).

Other Peripheral Neuropathies

Other, less common peripheral neuropathies have also been reported. The outcomes of postoperative neuropathies depend on the type and location of the injury as well as its severity. The symptoms rarely last more than 4 months, and improvement is gradual (Aposoudou & Johnson, 2009).

Horner's syndrome is rare following cardiac surgery. It is characterized by miosis, ptosis, and anhidrosis (inability to sweat); is reported after median sternotomy (Imamaki et al., 2006); and is thought to result from damage to the cervical sympathetic chain. Such damage occurs from a first rib fracture (Ahmadi, Saxena, Wilson, & Bunton, 2013).

Upper extremity neuropathies occur in 2% to 15% of patients. They are thought to be due to either brachial plexus traction, brachial plexus compression between the clavicle and first rib during sternal retraction, injury to the nerve during harvesting of the ITA, hypothermia, or hemodynamic changes that occur during CPB (McGarvey et al., 2013). Risk factors that have been identified for peripheral nerve injuries include general and epidural anesthesia, hypertension, tobacco use, and diabetes (Welch et al., 2009).

Patients report numbness, weakness, pain, and discoordination of an upper extremity; decreased reflexes are found. The symptoms usually resolve in 3 weeks. Conservative treatment (e.g., physical therapy to increase strength and flexibility) is indicated (McGarvey et al., 2013).

Axonal injury is less common. It is associated with neurologic symptoms that last a longer time. If improvement in neuropathy is not seen after 3 weeks, electromyography and nerve conduction studies should be performed to confirm diagnosis, identify the injury site, determine the degree of nerve disruption, and provide a precise prognosis for recovery (McGarvey et al., 2013).

SUMMARY

Neurologic complications following cardiac surgery present an important medical complication. Many are associated with longer lengths of ICU and hospital stay, as well as poorer long-term outcomes. Despite advances in cardiac surgery, neurologic complication rates are increasing. Intensive care unit nurses caring for postoperative cardiac surgery patients should be able to recognize which patients are at increased risk for these complications and plan their care so as to prevent these complications from occurring, minimize the associated detrimental effects, and help ensure effective symptom management. Preventive strategies may include maintaining adequate blood pressure, avoiding development of shock, preventing infection, and administering albumin (Chang et al., 2008). Although management of neurologic complications is primarily supportive in nature, early recognition and prompt intervention may minimize complications (Silvestry, 2014).

CASE STUDY

A 77-year-old patient with a body surface area (BSA) of 1.3 kg/m^2, history of hypertension, diabetes, atrial fibrillation, peripheral vascular disease, hyperlipidemia, carotid stenosis with subsequent carotid endarterectomy, and an LVEF of 35% underwent an on-pump CABG for triple-vessel disease. Her intraoperative course was complicated by hemodynamic instability that was managed with fluids and low-dose pressors. After the patient awakened from anesthesia and was extubated in the ICU, a mild facial droop, hemiparesis, and aphasia were noted.

Critical Thinking Questions

1. What risk factors were present for the patient's postoperative condition?
2. Why is cardiopulmonary bypass a risk factor for this patient's condition?
3. What treatment is appropriate for the patient at this time?

Answers to Critical Thinking Questions

1. Older age, atrial fibrillation, low LVEF, low BSA, hypertension, and intraoperative hemodynamic instability are all risk factors for a stroke.
2. Patients who undergo cardiac surgery experience a profound systemic inflammatory response, especially when CPB is used. One of the effects of the systemic inflammatory response related to CPB is the development of clots. Cardiopulmonary bypass activates the intrinsic and extrinsic pathways of the coagulation system secondary to factors including hypothermia, pumps propelling blood through the circuit, and exposure of blood to the artificial surfaces of the bypass circuit.
3. Stabilize vital signs, administer oxygen to attain and maintain SpO$_2$ of at least 92%, restore normovolemia with fluids, correct any electrolyte imbalances, maintain blood glucose greater than 60 and less than 180 mg/dL, institute aspiration precautions, keep head of bed at least 30 degrees unless contraindicated, maintain normothermia, administer aspirin or clopidogrel, and prevent additional complications (e.g., pneumonia, venous thrombotic events, urinary tract infection, pressure ulcers).

SELF-ASSESSMENT QUESTIONS

1. Your postoperative coronary artery bypass graft with cardiopulmonary bypass patient has a history of alcohol consumption and postoperative dysrhythmias. For which of the following is the patient at risk?
   a. Transient ischemic attack
   b. Coma
   c. Focal neurologic deficits
   d. Agitation

2. Your elderly patient with a history of diabetes and unstable angina has aortic atherosclerosis. For which of the following is the patient at risk?
   a. Stroke
   b. Disorientation
   c. Seizure
   d. Memory deficits

3. Your patient has a history of heart failure, peripheral vascular disease, hypertension, and prior coronary artery bypass grafting. For which of the following is the patient at risk?
   a. Stroke
   b. Memory deficits
   c. Coma
   d. Stupor

4. Which of the following conditions places the patient at increased risk for adverse neurologic outcomes?
   a. Blood glucose 70 mg/dL
   b. Blood pressure 130/50
   c. Temperature 101°F
   d. Serum sodium level 130 mEq/L

5. Which of the following about strokes occurring following cardiac surgery is true?
   a. Those that occur within the first postoperative day are often associated with valve surgery.
   b. The risk of stroke is less if patients awaken neurologically intact.
   c. The majority of strokes are manifested within 1 to 2 days of surgery.
   d. Most strokes involve intracranial hemorrhage.

6. Which of the following patients is at greatest risk of a stroke following cardiac surgery?
   a. A patient with hypothermia
   b. A patient with atrial fibrillation
   c. A patient with increased cardiac output
   d. A patient with decreased pulmonary artery pressures

7. Which of the following are signs of catastrophic stroke?
   a. Hypotension with tachycardia
   b. Constricted pupils

   c. Failure to follow commands after sedation has been discontinued
   d. Posturing

8. Which of the following should the nurse include in the care of patients following a stroke after cardiac surgery?
   a. Maintaining systolic blood pressure between 160 and 180 mmHg
   b. Gradual temperature warming
   c. Keeping blood glucose levels between 110 and 180 mg/dL
   d. Administering daily aspirin

9. Your 68-year-old patient with an LVEF of 25% underwent cardiac surgery. On postoperative day 2, new cognitive deficits, disorientation, agitation, and combativeness are noted. Which of the following should management of this patient include?
   a. Hourly neuro checks
   b. Minimizing use of narcotic analgesics
   c. Administering barbiturates
   d. Replacing the patient's hearing aid

10. Which of the following places the postoperative cardiac surgery patient at risk for seizures?
    a. Serum sodium level 129 mEq/L
    b. Serum glucose 140 mg/dL
    c. Oxygen saturation 92%
    d. Hemoglobin 8.3 g/dL

Answers to Self-Assessment Questions

1. d	6. b
2. a	7. d
3. b	8. d
4. c	9. d
5. c	10. a

Clinical Inquiry Box

Question: Does teaching caregivers delirium prevention strategies decrease the incidence and duration of postoperative delirium in cardiac surgery patients?

Reference: Mailhot, T., Cossette, S., Bourbonnais, A., Cote, J., Denault, A., Cote, M. C., . . . Guertin, M. C. (2014). Evaluation of a nurse mentoring intervention to family caregivers in the management of delirium after cardiac surgery (MENTOR_D): A study protocol for a randomized controlled pilot trial. *Trials, 15*(1), 306. doi: 10.1186/1745-6215-15-306

Objective: This proposed randomized pilot trial examines the use of an experimental nursing intervention to help family caregivers manage post-cardiac surgery delirium in their relatives.

Method: In this randomized pilot study, cardiac surgery patients were divided into two groups to receive usual care (control group) or an experimental intervention aimed at reducing delirium severity (intervention group). The nurse taught family caregivers delirium prevention strategies, how to recognize delirium, and supportive interventions to offer during delirium episodes. Data were collected from standard delirium assessments, medical records, questionnaires, and a novel measure of delirium.

Discussion: Delirium affects a larger percentage of cardiac surgery patients, and few proven strategies to treat or reduce the incidence exist. New strategies for early detection, monitoring, and management of delirium are needed. This proposed study offers a novel patient-/family-centered nursing intervention that may improve recognition and management of delirium after cardiac surgery.

REFERENCES

Aguirre, V. J., Sinha, P., Zimmet, A., Lee, G. A., Kwa, L., & Rosenfeldt, F. (2013). Phrenic nerve injury during cardiac surgery: Mechanisms, management and prevention. *Heart, Lung and Circulation, 22*(11), 895–902.

Ahmadi, O., Saxena, P., Wilson, P. K. J., & Bunton, R. W. (2013). First rib fracture and Horner's syndrome: A rare clinical entity. *Annals of Thoracic Surgery, 95*(1), 355.

Alagiakrishnan, K. (2014). *Delirium treatment & management.* Retrieved from http://emedicine.medscape.com/article/288890-treatment

Alejaldre, A., Delgado-Mederos, R., Santos, M. A., & Marti-Fabrogas, J. (2010). Cerebrovascular complications after heart transplantation. *Current Cardiology Reviews, 6*(3), 214–217.

American Society of Anesthesiologists. (2013). *People born with a certain gene more likely to suffer long-term cognitive decline after heart surgery.* Retrieved from https://www.asahq.org/For-the-Public-and-Media/Press-Room/Anesthesiology-and-Other-Scientific-Press-Releases/Cognitive-Decline-After-Heart-Surgery.aspx

American Society of Anesthesiologists Task Force on Perioperative Visual Loss. (2012). Practice advisory for perioperative visual loss associated with spine surgery: An updated report by the American Society of Anaesthesiologists Task Force on Perioperative Visual Loss. *Anesthesiology, 116*(2), 274–285.

Andrade, I. N., Moraes Neto, F. R., & Andrade, T. G. (2014). Use of EuroSCORE as a predictor of morbidity after cardiac surgery. *Revista Brasileira de Cirurgia Cardiovascular, 29*(1), 9–15.

Aposoudou, J., & Johnson, J. S. (2009). Postoperative neuropathy after cardiac surgery. In G. Shorten, S. F. Dierforf, G. Iohon, C. J. O'Connor, & C. W. Hogue (Eds.), *Case-based anesthesia: Clinical learning guides.* Philadelphia, PA: Lippincott Williams & Wilkins.

Arnaoutakis, G. J., & Baumgartner, W. A. (2013). Coronary artery bypass. In L. Kanser, J. L. Kron, & T. L. Spray (Eds.), *Cardiothoracic surgery* (3rd ed., pp. 390–395). Philadelphia, PA: Lippincott Williams & Wilkins.

Baranowska, K., Juszczyk, G., Dmitruk, I., Knapp, M., Tycińska, A., Jakubów, P., . . . Himle, T. (2012). Risk factors of neurological complications in cardiac surgery. *Kardiologia Polska, 70*(8), 811–818.

Barr, J., Fraser, G. L., Puntillo, K., Ely, E. W., Gélinas, C., Dasta, J. F., . . . Jaeschke, R. (2013). Clinical practice guidelines for the management of pain, agitation, and delirium in adult patients in the intensive care unit. *Critical Care Medicine, 41*(1), 263–306.

Bellolio, M. F., Gilmore, R. M., & Ganti, L. (2014). Insulin for glycaemic control in acute ischaemic stroke. *Cochrane Database of Systematic Reviews, 1*, CD005346. doi: 10.1002/14651858. CD005346.pub4

Bojar, R. M. (2011). Post-ICU care and other complications. In R. M. Bojar (Ed.), *Manual of perioperative care in adult cardiac surgery* (pp. 641–726). Hoboken, NJ: Blackwell.

Bucerius, J., Gummert, J. F., Borger, M. A., Walther, T., Doll, N., Onnasch, J. F., . . . Mohr, F. W. (2003). Stroke after cardiac surgery: A risk factor analysis of 16,184 consecutive adult patients. *Annals of Thoracic Surgery, 75*(2), 472–478.

Chalela, J. A. (2012). *Stroke-related pulmonary complications and abnormal respiratory patterns.* Retrieved from http://uptodate.com/contents/stroke-related-pulmonary-complications-and-abnormal-respiratory-patterns

Chang, Y.-L., Tsai, Y.-F., Lin, P.-J., Chen, M.-C., & Liu, C.-Y. (2008). Prevalence and risk factors for postoperative delirium in a cardiovascular intensive care unit. *American Journal of Critical Care, 17*(6), 567–575.

Connerney, I., Shapiro, P. A., McLaughlin, J. S., Bagiella, E., & Sloan, R. P. (2001). Relation between depression after coronary artery bypass surgery and 12-month outcome: A prospective study. *Lancet, 358*(9295), 1766–1771.

Cserép, Z., Losoncz, E., Balog, P., Sziki-Török, T., Juhász, B., Kertai, M. D., . . . Székely, A. (2012). The impact of preoperative anxiety and education level on long-term mortality after cardiac surgery. *Journal of Cardiothoracic Surgery, 7.* Retrieved from http://www.cardiothoracicsurgery.org/content/7/1/86

Dafer, R. M. (2006). Risk estimates of stroke after coronary artery bypass graft and carotid endarderctomy. *Neurology Clinics, 24*, 795–806.

Dao, T. K., Chu, D., Springer, J., Gopaldos, R. R., Menefee, D. S., Anderson, T., . . . Nguyen, Q. (2010). Clinical depression, posttraumatic stress disorder, and comorbid depression and posttraumatic stress disorder as risk factors in in-hospital mortality after coronary artery bypass grafting surgery. *The Journal of Thoracic and Cardiovascular Surgery, 140*(3), 606–610.

Durandy, Y. (2014). Minimizing systemic inflammation during cardiopulmonary bypass in the pediatric population. *Artificial Organs, 38*, 11–18.

Fontes, M. T., Swift, R. C., Phillips-Bute, B., Podgoreanu, M. V., Stafford-Smith, M., Newman, M. F., . . . Mathew, J. P. (2013). Predictors of cognitive recovery after cardiac surgery. *Anesthesia & Analgesia, 116*(2), 435–442.

Francis, J. (2014). *Delirium and acute confusional states: Prevention, treatment and prognosis.* Retrieved from http://www.uptodate.com/contents/delirium-and-acute-confusional-states-prevention-treatment-and-prognosis

Goldstone, A. B., Bronster, D. J., Anyanwu, A. C., Goldstein, M. A., Filsoufi, F., Adams, D. H., . . . Chikwe, J. (2011). Predictors and outcomes of seizures after cardiac surgery: A multivariable analysis of 2578 patients. *Annals of Thoracic Surgery, 91*(2), 514–518.

Gottesman, R. F., Grega, M. A., Bailey, M. M., Pham, L. D., Zeger, S. L., Baumgartner, W. A., . . . McKhann, G. M. (2010). Delirium after coronary artery bypass graft surgery and late mortality. *Annals of Neurology, 67*(3), 338–344.

Gray, H. (2000). Neurology. In *Anatomy of the human body.* Retrieved from http://www.bartleby.com/107/

Grocott, H. P., Clark, J. A., Homi, H. M., & Sharma, A. (2004). "Other" neurologic complications after cardiac surgery. *Seminars in Cardiothoracic and Vascular Anesthesia, 8*(3), 213–226.

Grocott, H. P., Homi, H. M., & Puskas, F. (2005). Cognitive dysfunction after cardiac surgery: Revisiting etiology. *Seminars in Cardiothoracic and Vascular Anesthesia, 9*(2), 123–129.

Grocott, H. P., & Yoshitani, K. (2007). Neuroprotection during cardiac surgery. *Journal of Anesthesia, 21*(3), 367–377.

Guo, P. (2015). Preoperative education interventions to reduce anxiety and improve recovery among cardiac surgery patients: A review of randomized controlled trials. *Journal of Clinical Nursing, 24*(1–2), 34–46.

Ha, J. H., & Wong, C. K. (2011). Pharmacologic treatment of depression in patients with myocardial infarction. *Journal of Geriatric Cardiology, 8*, 121–126.

Hakim, S. M., Othman, A. I., & Naoum, D. O. (2012). Early treatment with risperidone for subsyndromal delirium after on-pump cardiac surgery in the elderly: A randomized trial. *Anesthesiology, 16*(5), 987–997.

Hamdan, A. L., Moukarbel, R. V., Farhat, F., & Obeid, M. (2002). Vocal cord paralysis after open-heart surgery. *European Journal of Cardio-Thoracic Surgery, 21*(4), 671–674.

Henke, K., & Eigsti, J. (2003). After cardiopulmonary bypass: Watching for complications. *Nursing, 33*(3), 32cc1–32cc4.

Hillis, L. D., Smith, P. K., Anderson, J. L., Bittl, J. A., Bridges, C. R., Byrne, J. G., . . . Winniford, M. D. (2011). 2011 ACCF/AHA guideline for coronary artery bypass graft surgery: A report of the American College of Cardiology Foundation/American Heart Association Task Force on Practice Guidelines. Developed in collaboration with the American Association for Thoracic Surgery, Society of Cardiovascular Anesthesiologists, and Society of Thoracic Surgeons. *Journal of the American College of Cardiology, 58*(24), e123–210.

Hogue, C. W., Palin, C. A., & Arrowsmith, J. E. (2006). Cardiopulmonary bypass management and neurologic outcomes: An evidence-based appraisal of current practices. *Anesthesia & Analgesia, 103*(1), 21–37.

Imamaki, M., Ishida, A., Shimura, H., Kohno, A., Ishida, K., Sakurai, M., . . . Miyazaki, M. (2006). A case complicated with Horner's syndrome after off-pump coronary artery bypass. *Annals of Thoracic and Cardiovascular Surgery, 12*, 113–115.

Jauch, E. C., Saver, J. L., Adams, H. P., Bruno, A., Connors, J. J., Demaerschalk, B. M., . . . Yonas, H. (2013). Guidelines for the early management of patients with acute ischemic stroke. *Stroke, 44*(3), 870–947.

Joshi, B., Brady, K., Lee, J., Easley, B., Paingrahi, R., Smielewski, P., . . . Hogue, C. W. (2010). Impaired autoregulation of cerebral blood flow during rewarming from hypothermic cardiopulmonary bypass and its potential association with stroke. *Anesthesia & Analgesia, 110*(2), 321–328.

Kim, D. H., Daskalakis, C., Whellan, D. J., Whitman, I. R., Hohmann, S., Medvedev, S., . . . Kraft, W. K. (2009). Safety of selective serotonin reuptake inhibitor in adults undergoing coronary artery bypass grafting. *American Journal of Cardiology, 103*(10), 1391–1395.

Kim, D. W., Moon, Y., Gee, N. H., Choi, J. W., & Oh, J. (2011). Blood-brain barrier disruption is involved in seizure and hemianopia in nonketotic hyperglycemia. *Neurologist, 17*(3), 164–166.

Koster, S., Hensens, A. G., Schuurmans, M. J., & van der Palen, J. (2011). Risk factors for delirium after cardiac surgery: A systematic review. *European Journal of Cardiovascular Nursing, 10*(4), 197–204.

Kouchoukos, N. T., Blackstone, E. H., Hanley, F. L., & Kirklin, J. K. (2012). Postoperative care. In N. T. Kouchoukos, E. H. Blackstone, F. L. Hanley, & J. K. Kirklin (Eds.), *Kirklin/Barratt-Boyes cardiac surgery* (4th ed., pp. 189–250). Philadelphia, PA: Elsevier Saunders.

Lazar, H. L., Wilson, C. A., & Messé, S. R. (2013). *Coronary artery bypass grafting in patients with cerebrovascular disease.* Retrieved from http://www.uptodate.com/contents/coronary-artery-bypass-grafting-in-patients-with-cerebrovascular-disease

Leentjens, A. F., Maclullich, A. M., & Meagher, D. J. (2008). Delirium, Cinderella no more . . .? *Journal of Psychosomatic Research, 65*, 20S.

Lie, I., Arnesen, H., Sandrik, L., Hamilton, G., & Bunch, E. H. (2007). Effects of a home-based intervention program on anxiety and depression 6 months after coronary artery bypass grafting: A randomized controlled trial. *Journal of Psychosomatic Research, 62*(4), 411–418.

Likosky, D. S., Dacey, L. J., Leavitt, B. J., Sardella, G. L., Russo, L., . . . Ross, C. S. (2012). Abstract 328: The importance of using single aortic clamp technique to reduce brain injury after coronary artery bypass grafting. *Circulation: Cardiovascular Quality and Outcomes, 5,* A328. Retrieved from http://circoutcomes.ahajournals.org/cgi/content/meeting_abstract/5/3_MeetingAbstracts2012/A328

Lisle, T. C., Barrett, K. M., Gazoni, L. M., Surenson, B. R., Scott, C. D., Kazemi, A., . . . Johnston, K. C. (2008). Timing of stroke after cardiopulmonary bypass determines mortality. *Annals of Thoracic Surgery, 85*(5), 1556–1563.

Makhann, G. M., Gottesman, R. F., Grega, M. A., Baumgartner, W. A., & Selnes, O. A. (2011). Neurological and cognitive sequelae of cardiac surgery. In R. S. Bonser, D. Pagano, & A. Hauerich (Eds.), *Brain protection in cardiac surgery. Volume 1.* (pp. 19–28). London: Springer-Verlag.

Manji, R. A., Grocott, H. P., Leake, J., Ariano, R. E., Manji, J. S., Menkis, A. H., . . . Jacobsohn, E. (2012). Seizures following cardiac surgery: The impact of tranexamic acid and other risk factors. *Canadian Journal of Anaesthesia, 59*(1), 6–13.

Martin, J. F., de Melo, C. V., & de Sousa, L. P. (2008). Cognitive decline after cardiac surgery. *Revista Brasileira de Cirurgia Cardiovascular, 23*(2), 245–255.

Martin, K., Knorr, J., Breuer, T., Gertler, R., Macguill, M., Lange, R., . . . Wiesner, G. (2011). Seizures after open heart surgery: Comparison of epsilon-aminocaproic acid and tranexamic acid. *Journal of Cardiothoracic and Vascular Anesthesia, 25*(1), 20–25.

Mathew, J. P., Podgoreanu, M. V., Grocott, H. A, White, W. D., Morris, R. W., Stafford-Smith, M., . . . Newman, M. F. (2007). Genetic variants in P-selectin and C-reactive protein influence susceptibility to cognitive decline after cardiac surgery. *Journal of the American College of Cardiology, 49*(19), 1934–1942.

McAuley, D. (2014). *Haloperidol LACTATE (Haldol®)*. Retrieved from http://www.globalrph.com/haloperidol_dilution.htm

McDonagh, D. L., Berger, M., Mathew, J. P., Graffagnino, C., Milano, C. A., & Newman, M. F. (2014). Neurological complications of cardiac surgery. *Lancet Neurology, 13*(5), 490–502.

McGarvey, M. L., Cheung, A. T., & Stecker, M. M. (2013). *Neurologic complications of cardiac surgery.* Retrieved from http://www.uptodate.com/contents/neurologic-complications-of-cardiac-surgery?source=search_result&search=neurologic+complications+of+cardiac+surgery

McKhann, G. M., Grega, M. A., Borowicz, L. M., Baumgartner, W. A., & Selnes, O. A. (2006). Stroke and encephalopathy after cardiac surgery: An update. *Stroke, 37*(2), 562–571.

Merino, J. G., Latour, L. L., Tso, A., Lee, K. Y., Dang, D. W., Davis, R. A., . . . Warach, S. (2013). Blood-brain barrier disruption after cardiac surgery. *American Journal of Neuroradiology, 34,* 518–523.

Murphy, B. M., Elliott, P. C., Higgins, R. O., Le Grande, M. R., Worcheter, M. U., & Goble, A. J. (2008). Anxiety and depression after coronary artery bypass graft surgery: Most get better, some get worse. *European Journal of Cardiovascular Prevention & Rehabilitation, 15*(4), 434–440.

National Institute of Neurological Disorders and Stroke. (2014). *NINDS Neuroleptic malignant syndrome information page.* Retrieved from http://www.ninds.nih.gov/disorders/neuroleptic_syndrome/neuroleptic_syndrome.htm

National Institute of Neurological Disorders and Stroke. (n.d). *Stroke.* Retrieved from http://stroke.nih.gov/documents/NIH_stroke_scale_Booklet.pdf

Newman, N. J. (2008). Perioperative visual loss after nonocular surgeries. *American Journal of Ophthalmology, 145,* 604–610.

Nina, V. J., Rocha, M. I., Rodrugues, R. F., Oliveira, V. C., Teixeira, J. L., Figueredo, S. D., . . . Sousa, C. A. C. (2012). Assessment of CABDEAL scores as predictor of neurologic dysfunction after on-pump coronary artery bypass grafting surgery. *Revista Brasileira de Cirurgia Cardiovascular, 27*(3), 429–435.

Norkienė, I., Ringaitienė, D., Kuzminstáitė, V., & Šipylaitė, J. (2013). Incidence and risk factors of early delirium after cardiac surgery. *BioMed Research International, 2013.* Article ID 323491.

O'Brien, S. M., Shahian, D. M., Filardo, G., Ferraris, V. A., Haan, C. K., Rich, J. B., . . . Anderson, R. P. (2009). The Society of Thoracic Surgeons 2008 cardiac surgery risk models: Part 2—isolated valve surgery. *Annals of Thoracic Surgery, 88*(Suppl. 1), S23–42.

Oliveira-Filho, J., & Koroshetz, W. J. (2013). *Neuroimaging of acute ischemic stroke.* Retrieved from http://www.uptodate.com/contents/neuroimaging-of-acute-ischemic-stroke

Oxlad, M., Stubberfield, J., Stuklis, R., Edwards, J., & Wade, T. D. (2006). Psychological risk factors for cardiac-related hospital readmission within 6 months of coronary artery bypass graft surgery. *Journal of Psychosomatic Research, 61*(6), 775–781.

Roekaerts, P. M. H. J., & Heijmans, J. H. (2012). Early postoperative care after cardiac surgery. In C. Narin (Ed.), *Perioperative considerations in cardiac surgery*. Retrieved from http://www.intechopen.com/books/perioperative-considerations-in-cardiac-surgery/-early-postoperative-care-after-cardiac-surgery-

Sebregts, E. H., Falger, P. R., Appels, A., Kester, A. D., & Bär, F. W. (2005). Psychological effects of a short behavior modification program in patients with acute myocardial infarction or coronary artery bypass grafting: A randomized controlled trial. *Journal of Psychosomatic Research, 58*(5), 417–424.

Silvestry, F. E. (2014). *Postoperative complications among patients undergoing cardiac surgery*. Retrieved from http://www.uptodate.com/contents/postoperative-complications-among-patients-undergoing-cardiac-surgery

Society of Thoracic Surgeons. (2012). *People older than 80 fare well after valve replacement surgery*. Retrieved from http://www.sts.org/news/people-older-80-fare-well-after-valve-replacement-surgery

Society of Thoracic Surgeons. (2014). *Risk calculator*. Retrieved from http://www.sts.org/quality-research-patient-safety/quality/risk-calculator-and-models/risk-calculator

Sockalingam, S., Parekh, N., Bogoch, I. I., Sun, J., Mahtani, R., Beach, C., . . . Bhalerao, S. (2005). Delirium in the postoperative cardiac patient: A review. *Journal of Cardiac Surgery, 20*(6), 560–567.

Sorlie, T., Busund, R., Sexton, H., & Sorlie, D. (2007). Video information combined with individualized information sessions: Effects on emotional well-being following coronary artery bypass surgery. A randomized trial. *Patient Education and Counseling, 65*(2), 180–188.

Suls, J., & Bunde, J. (2005). Anger, anxiety and depression as risk factors for cardiovascular disease: The problems and implications of overlapping affective dispositions. *Psychological Bulletin, 131*(2), 260–300.

Sun, X., Lindsay, J., Monsein, L. H., Hill, P. C., & Corso, P. J. (2012). Silent brain injury after cardiac surgery: A review. *Journal of the American College of Cardiology, 60*(9), 791–797.

Tarakji, K. G., Sabik, J. F., III, Bhudia, S. K., Batizy, L. H., & Blackstone, E. H. (2011). Temporal onset, risk factors, and outcomes associated with stroke after coronary artery bypass grafting. *Journal of the American Medical Association, 305*(4), 381–390.

Tse, L., Schwarz, S. K. W., Bowering, J. B., Moore, R. L., Burns, K. D., Richford, C. M., . . . Ban, A. M. (2012). Pharmacologic risk factors for delirium after cardiac surgery: A review. *Current Neuropharmacology, 10*(3), 181–196.

Tully, P. J., & Baker, R. A. (2012). Depression, anxiety, and cardiac morbidity outcomes after coronary artery bypass surgery: A contemporary and practical review. *Journal of Geriatric Cardiology, 9*(2), 197–208.

Tully, P. J., Baker, R. A., Turnbull, D. A., Winefield, A. R., & Knight, J. L. (2009). Negative emotions and quality of life six months after cardiac surgery: The dominant role of depression not anxiety symptoms. *Journal of Behavioral Medicine, 32*(6), 510–522.

Weissman, J. D., Khunteev, G. A., & Dambinova, S. A. (n.d.). Biomarkers in acute stroke. *MAG Journal,* 20–22. Retrieved from http://www.plosone.org/article/fetchSingleRepresentation.action?uri=info:doi/10.1371/journal.pone.0042362.s001

Welch, M. B., Brummett, C. M., Welch, T. D., Tremper, K. K., Guglani, P., & Mashour, G. A. (2009). Perioperative peripheral nerve injuries: A retrospective study of 380,680 cases during a 10-year period at a single institution. *Anesthesiology, 111*(3), 490.

Whitlock, R., Healey, J. S., Connolly, S. J., Wang, J., Danter, M. R., Tu, J. V., . . . Yusuf, S. (2014). Predictors of early and late stroke following cardiac surgery. *Canadian Medical Journal*. Retrieved from http://www.cmaj.ca/content/early/2014/07/21/cmaj.131214

Wooten, J. M. (2012). Pharmacotherapy considerations in elderly patients. *Southern Medical Journal, 105*(8), 437–445.

Xiong, G. J., Jiang, W., Clare, R., Shaw, L. K., Smith, P. K., Mahaffey, K. W., . . . Newby, L. K. (2006). Prognosis of patients taking selective serotonin reuptake inhibitors before coronary artery bypass grafting. *American Journal of Cardiology, 98*(1), 42–47.

Yang, J.-F., Zhang, H.-C., Ga, C.-X., & Wei, H. (2012). Total arterial off-pump coronary revascularization with a bilateral internal mammary artery y graft (208 cases). *Journal of Surgical Technique and Case Report, 4*(1), 10–14.

Yuan, S.-M. (2012). Hoarseness subsequent to cardiovascular surgery, intervention maneuver, and endotracheal intubation: The so-called iatrogenic Ortner's (cardiovocal) syndrome. *Cardiology Journal, 19*(6), 560–566.

Zanatta, P., Messerotti Benvenuti, S., Bosco, E., Baldanzi, F., Palomba, D., & Valfrè, C. (2011). Multimodal brain monitoring reduces major neurologic complications in cardiac surgery. *Journal of Cardiothoracic and Vascular Anesthesia, 25*(6), 1076–1085.

Chapter 17

Fluid and Electrolyte Imbalances Following Cardiac Surgery

Vicki Morelock

INTRODUCTION

Numerous factors increase the cardiac surgery patient's predisposition for postoperative fluid and electrolyte imbalances. These include anesthesia, induced hypothermia, physiologic effects of cardiopulmonary bypass (CPB) techniques, cardioplegia, hemodilution, and rapid fluid and electrolyte shifts across fluid compartments following CPB. A systemic inflammatory response post bypass (vasoplegia), postoperative myocardial stunning, ischemia or infarct, shock-like syndrome resulting in potential renal insult, use of positive and negative inotropic agents, degree of oxygenation and oxygen delivery to the tissues, and third spacing are additional factors affecting the hemodynamic, fluid, and electrolyte indices. Peripheral vascular tone, intraoperative and postoperative volume repletion, the rewarming process that follows hypothermia, stress associated with surgery including sympathetic stimulation from pain and anxiety, and rhythm conduction changes such as bradycardia, tachycardia, or dysrhythmias also affect fluid balance and electrolyte shifting. Comorbidities such as diabetes, hypertension, smoking, chronic obstructive pulmonary disease (COPD), chronic kidney disease changes, and normal aging (elderly) must be taken into account when treating cardiac surgery patients (Khalpey et al., 2012).

This chapter provides an overview of some of the common acid–base and fluid and electrolyte imbalances, treatments for these alterations, and the intensive care unit (ICU) nurse's role in caring for these patients in the immediate postoperative period. The chapter concludes with a brief look at acute kidney injury (AKI) and its treatment implications as they relate to the patient who has undergone cardiac surgery.

FLUID AND ELECTROLYTE DISTRIBUTION

Slightly more than half of the average adult's body weight is made up of fluid—55% to 60% of body weight in men, 50% to 55% of body weight in women, and slightly less in older adults (Haljamae, 2011; Huether, 2010). The term "fluid" refers to both water and substances such as electrolytes that are dissolved in it. Electrolytes are substances that develop a positive (cation) or negative (anion) electrical charge when dissolved in body fluid (Felver, 2010; Huether, 2010).

Fluids are found in both the intracellular and extracellular compartments of the body. Intracellular fluid (ICF) accounts for approximately two-thirds of all body fluids. It is located primarily in skeletal muscle mass and provides nutrients for daily cellular metabolism. Intracellular fluid contains high levels of potassium and phosphorus, and has a moderate amount of magnesium and proteins

(Huether, 2010). Extracellular fluid (ECF) is further divided into intravascular fluid (plasma) and interstitial fluid (between the cells). Extracellular fluid is more easily lost than ICF because of its location. Electrolyte values that are reported reflect plasma levels and represent ECF. They have a circadian rhythm to them (e.g., potassium elevates during the hours a person is active and reaches its trough when the person sleeps [Felver, 2010]).

FACTORS AFFECTING FLUID VOLUME DISTRIBUTION

Fluid balance and homeostasis are maintained by several body systems, including the heart, lungs, endocrine system, and renal system. Additionally, the pituitary, adrenal, and parathyroid glands all play important roles in maintaining fluid balance and composition. Without a properly functioning cardiovascular system, blood could not be pumped to the kidneys. The renal system requires approximately 25% of cardiac output (CO) for adequate function to occur. The goals for patients are to maintain adequate oxygen delivery to all the tissues and minimize stress on the body. This is accomplished with maintaining a mixed venous oxygen (O_2) greater than 60%, a mean arterial pressure (MAP) greater than 65 mmHg, and a cardiac index (CI) greater than 2 L/min/m² for most patients (Khalpey et al., 2012).

Without proper lung function, blood is inadequately oxygenated, carbon dioxide (CO_2) is not removed through exhalation, and insensible water loss does not occur. The lungs act as the first line of defense against acid–base imbalances. Without all three body systems functioning in harmony, acid–base, fluid, and electrolyte disturbances will occur.

Fluid exchange takes place between the intracellular and extracellular compartments according to differences in hydrostatic pressure and colloid osmotic pressure (COP). Surgery causes a decrease in COP by causing

increased capillary permeability, which results in fluid shifts from the vasculature to the interstitium (Huether, 2010).

The endocrine system causes sodium and water retention and potassium excretion by stimulating production of antidiuretic hormone (ADH) in response to surgical trauma. Antidiuretic hormone secretion causes the kidneys to reabsorb water with a subsequent decrease in diuresis and serum sodium concentration in the postoperative period. Increased production of renin and aldosterone leads to sodium retention and potassium excretion (Huether, 2010). Cortisol, which is secreted in response to stress, inhibits production of stress-related mediators (tumor necrosis factor 1, cytokines, and growth factors), contributing to postoperative fluid homeostasis by maintaining capillary integrity and decreasing fluid shifts seen with an inflammatory process (Forshee, Clayton, & McCance, 2010).

During and following CPB, the body experiences an increase in interstitial volume, sodium retention, and potassium excretion. Plasma COP decreases over this same period. Depending on the length of the case, the interstitial compartment may swell 8% to 33% (Hammon & Hines, 2012).

ACID–BASE IMBALANCES

Acid–base balance is determined by the arterial blood pH (hydrogen ion concentration; normal range 7.35–7.45), arterial carbon dioxide (pCO_2; normal range 35–45 mmHg), partial pressure of oxygen (pO_2) in arterial blood (normal range 80–100 mmHg), and bicarbonate (HCO_3) value (normal range 22–26 mEq/L). **Table 17-1** provides a brief overview of arterial blood gas (ABG) values and their interpretive implications.

The human body desires to maintain a state of homeostasis at all times. When changes in pH occur, buffer systems are activated to assist the body to normalize pH. As

Table 17-1	Arterial Blood Gas Values and Interpretation	
Lab Parameter	**Normal Value**	**Results and Implications**
pH	7.35–7.45	< 7.35 = acidosis
		> 7.45 = alkalosis
		If compensation is suspected and the pH is within normal limits, look at the "end" where the pH falls: Is it closer to the acidosis side or the alkalosis side?
HCO_3	22–26 mEq/L	< 22 = metabolic acidosis
		> 26 = metabolic alkalosis
pCO_2	35–45 mmHg	< 35 = respiratory alkalosis
		> 45 = respiratory acidosis
pO_2	80–100 mmHg	< 80 = possible hypoxemia

changes in pH occur, cellular responses are stimulated immediately. When the cellular responses are inadequate to handle the resultant change in pH, the respiratory system will provide compensation; if needed, the renal system will activate its compensatory mechanisms as well. Arterial blood gas changes that are primarily driven by the kidneys may take days to appear, whereas changes caused by the respiratory system will occur in a matter of minutes (MacKusick, 2007).

Acidosis

Respiratory Acidosis

Respiratory acidosis may occur in the immediate postoperative period following cardiac surgery and is a direct result of inadequate ventilation or sedation causing hypoventilation and hypercarbia (Huether, 2010). **Table 17-2** lists common causes of respiratory acidosis in the postoperative cardiac surgery patient. Evaluation of ABG results and observation for signs and symptoms are essential roles of the ICU nurse. Early signs and symptoms of respiratory acidosis

may include headache, restlessness, blurred vision, and anxiety. If the condition continues, the patient may develop dizziness, confusion, weakness, palpitations, tetany, convulsions, coma, or ventricular fibrillation (VF) (Huether, 2010).

Treatment of respiratory acidosis will vary according to the cause, but generally focuses on improving the patient's ventilation/perfusion (V/Q) status. Conventional interventions performed by the ICU nurse include frequent pulmonary hygiene; use of incentive spirometry; and encouraging turning, coughing, and deep breathing. Titration of sedation may be indicated if it will not cause excessive patient discomfort. If the patient is on mechanical ventilation, respiratory acidosis can be corrected by increasing the patient's minute ventilation; this goal can be accomplished by increasing the preset rate or tidal volume. If the patient is not on mechanical ventilation and conventional interventions are not successful in correcting the respiratory acidosis, depending on the patient's clinical status and ABG results, intubation and mechanical support may be required (Lemmer & Vlahakes, 2010).

Table 17-2   Common Causes of Respiratory Acidosis in the Postoperative Cardiac Surgery Patient

Central respiratory depression:

- Cardiac arrest with resultant cerebral hypoxia
- Obesity
- Use of opiates, sedatives, or anesthesia

Pulmonary issues:

- Acute respiratory distress syndrome
- Aspiration, pneumonia, airway obstruction, or any combination of these
- Asthma
- Atelectasis
- Bronchospasm or laryngospasm
- Pneumothorax
- Pulmonary edema
- Pulmonary embolism
- Restrictive lung diseases

Increased CO_2 production:

- Shivering
- Sepsis

Hypoventilation secondary to the following conditions:

- Pain
- Sternal incision
- Residual anesthesia
- Awakening with inadequate analgesia and impaired respiratory mechanics
- Side effects of opiates

Other:

- Inadequate mechanical ventilation (user error)
- Inadequate ventilation/perfusion ratio (decreased ventilation)
- Neuromuscular blocking agents

Sources: Data from Gerhardt, M. A. (2007). Postoperative care of the cardiac surgical patient. In F. A. Hensley, D. E. Martin, & G. P. Gravlee (Eds.), *A practical approach to cardiac anesthesia* (pp. 261–288). Philadelphia, PA: Lippincott Williams & Wilkins; and Huether, S. E. (2010). The cellular environment: Fluids and electrolytes, acids and bases. In K. L. McCance, S. E. Huether, V. L. Brashers, & N. S. Rote, (Eds.), *Pathophysiology: The biologic basis for disease in adults and children* (6th ed., pp. 96–125). Maryland Heights, MO: Mosby Elsevier.

Metabolic Acidosis

Because a state of electrical neutrality must be maintained within the body at all times, patients with a metabolic acidosis must retain a positive ion (cation) to adjust for the increasing bicarbonate. This goal is accomplished by the renal system, which accumulates positively charged potassium ions. Hyperkalemia frequently accompanies a metabolic acidosis (unless the metabolic acidosis is caused by lactic acidosis or diarrhea). It has been suggested that when acid (hydrogen ion) levels are high in the blood, the body attempts to compensate by causing muscles to take up the excess hydrogen. In order to maintain neutrality, in exchange for the hydrogen ions, potassium is transferred into the blood. Signs and symptoms of metabolic acidosis may include headache and lethargy, followed by confusion and drowsiness leading to coma. Other symptoms include nausea, vomiting, or both; abdominal discomfort; and warm, flushed skin from peripheral vasodilation. Cardiac output may decrease as myocardial contractility is depressed. Hypotension and dysrhythmias may occur (Huether, 2010). Because of the contractility issues commonly associated with metabolic acidosis and the potential for hyperkalemia, the ICU nurse should monitor for dysrhythmias in patients who develop this imbalance. **Table 17-3** lists common causes of metabolic acidosis seen in the postoperative cardiac surgery patient.

Metabolic acidosis is generally classified as having either a high or normal anion gap. Bicarbonate and chloride are considered the major anions in the body. To calculate the plasma anion gap, subtract chloride and bicarbonate from sodium (Pollock & Funk, 2013). In cases where a metabolic acidosis is accompanied by a loss of bicarbonate with retention of chloride to maintain balance, a normal anion gap metabolic acidosis state is present. The most common causes of normal anion gap acidosis include renal tubular acidosis,

Table 17-3   Common Causes of Metabolic Acidosis in the Postoperative Cardiac Surgery Patient

Hemodynamics

- Decreased cardiac output
- Inadequate systemic perfusion
- Decreased cardiac function
- Decreased peripheral perfusion
- Hypotension
- Hypovolemia
- Vasoconstriction from hypothermia

Physiologic conditions (increasing acids)

- Sepsis
- Renal failure
- Renal tubular acidosis
- Regional ischemia
- Diabetic ketoacidosis
- Splanchnic ischemia
- Anaerobic metabolism

Sources: Data from Gerhardt, M. A. (2007). Postoperative care of the cardiac surgical patient. In F. A. Hensley, D. E. Martin, & G. P. Gravlee (Eds.), *A practical approach to cardiac anesthesia* (pp. 261–288). Philadelphia, PA: Lippincott Williams & Wilkins; and Huether, S. E. (2010). The cellular environment: Fluids and electrolytes, acids and bases. In K. L. McCance, S. E. Huether, V. L. Brashers, & N. S. Rote, (Eds.), *Pathophysiology: The biologic basis for disease in adults and children* (6th ed., pp. 96–125). Maryland Heights, MO: Mosby Elsevier.

excessive administration of isotonic solutions, and diarrhea (Huether, 2010). In cases where the concentration of anions (other than chloride) increases (thereby destroying the electrical neutrality of the body), a high anion gap acidosis is said to exist (Huether, 2010). Lactic acidosis, renal failure, and diabetic ketoacidosis (DKA) are the most common causes of high anion gap acidosis.

Alkalosis

Respiratory Alkalosis

Respiratory alkalosis occurs when there is alveolar hyperventilation causing hypocapnia (Huether, 2010). **Table 17-4** lists common

causes of respiratory alkalosis seen in the postoperative cardiac surgery patient. When respiratory alkalosis is seen early in the postoperative period, it is related to ventilator-induced hyperventilation. When it is seen later in the postoperative course, respiratory alkalosis is arising as a compensatory mechanism (e.g., in response to diuretic therapy) (Lemmer & Vlahakes, 2010).

Signs and symptoms of respiratory alkalosis may include lightheadedness, inability to concentrate, dizziness, confusion, headache,

Table 17-4   Common Causes of Respiratory Alkalosis in the Postoperative Cardiac Surgery Patient

Hyperventilation secondary to the following conditions:

- Anxiety or fear
- Pain or generalized discomfort

Increased oxygen demand as a result of the following conditions:

- Fever
- Bacteremia (especially with Gram-negative organisms)
- Sepsis

Pulmonary disorders

- Pneumonia
- Pulmonary edema
- Pulmonary embolism
- V/Q mismatch (increased ventilation, decreased perfusion)

Medications: Respiratory stimulants

- User error
- Inappropriate ventilator settings
- Hyperventilation during transfer from operating room

Sources: Data from Gerhardt, M. A. (2007). Postoperative care of the cardiac surgical patient. In F. A. Hensley, D. E. Martin, & G. P. Gravlee (Eds.), *A practical approach to cardiac anesthesia* (pp. 261–288). Philadelphia, PA: Lippincott Williams & Wilkins; and Huether, S. E. (2010). The cellular environment: Fluids and electrolytes, acids and bases. In K. L. McCance, S. E. Huether, V. L. Brashers, & N. S. Rote, (Eds.), *Pathophysiology: The biologic basis for disease in adults and children* (6th ed., pp. 96–125). Maryland Heights, MO: Mosby Elsevier.

Table 17-5   Common Causes of Metabolic Alkalosis in the Postoperative Cardiac Surgery Patient
Adrenal disorders: hyperaldosteronism
Hypokalemia
Hypochloremia
Excessive diuretic administration
Nasogastric suctioning
Overuse of potassium-wasting drugs (e.g., increased use of thiazide diuretics)
Vomiting
Massive transfusions (from citrate)
Source: Data from Huether, S. E. (2010). The cellular environment: Fluids and electrolytes, acids and bases. In K. L. McCance, S. E. Huether, V. L. Brashers, & N. S. Rote, (Eds.), *Pathophysiology: The biologic basis for disease in adults and children* (6th ed., pp. 96-125). Maryland Heights, MO: Mosby Elsevier.

numbness and tingling of the extremities (paresthesias), tinnitus, palpitations, dry mouth, sweating, chest pain, or nausea and vomiting. Late-stage signs and symptoms may include loss of consciousness or seizures. The most notable signs are rapid and deep respirations (Huether, 2010). The neurologic symptoms may be caused by a hypocalcemic state, which is commonly seen with a respiratory alkalosis. This acid–base disturbance can cause an increase in protein binding of ionized calcium (the amount of calcium not bound to protein and available for use by the body). Treatment is aimed at correcting the underlying cause.

Metabolic Alkalosis

Common causes of metabolic alkalosis in the postoperative cardiac surgery patient are presented in **Table 17-5**. Like respiratory alkalosis, metabolic alkalosis is usually seen later in the postoperative cardiac surgery patient.

It is likely related to citrate in banked blood (Kouchoukos, Blackstone, Hanley, & Kirklin, 2013). Patients often have concomitant hypokalemia and hypocalcemia; these underlying conditions must be simultaneously corrected. With a metabolic alkalosis, as the hydrogen ion concentration increases in the blood, potassium ions move into the cells to maintain neutrality. This results in a hypokalemic state. Signs and symptoms of metabolic alkalosis include poor skin turgor (from fluid loss). Treatment is aimed at restoring fluid balance and correcting the underlying disorder.

ELECTROLYTE IMBALANCES

Electrolyte imbalances are frequently seen in postoperative cardiac surgery patients. The ICU nurse should recognize normal values, signs, and symptoms associated with these imbalances, and implement appropriate interventions to correct the imbalances. **Table 17-6** lists the common electrolytes and their associated normal values.

Table 17-6 Electrolyte Reference Values	
Electrolyte	**Normal Value***
Potassium	3.5–5.0 mEq/L
Sodium	135–145 mEq/L
Magnesium	1.8–2.4 mg/dL†
Phosphorus	2.5–4.5 mg/dL
Calcium	8.5–10.5 mg/dL‡

*Normal value markers may vary according to facility. Always check with your local laboratory if unsure of the normal values for any laboratory finding.

†Serum magnesium may also be reported in millimoles per liter (mmol/L). In these cases, normal values would be in the range of 0.65–1.1 mmol/L.

‡Serum calcium can be reported as total calcium, ionized calcium, or non-ionized calcium. The value provided in the table is for the total calcium. A normal ionized calcium value is in the range of 4.4–5.3 mg/dL.

Potassium

Fluctuations in potassium levels are common following cardiac surgery and can affect cardiac automaticity and conduction (Khalpey et al., 2012). Potassium works with sodium to help maintain fluid balance within the body, with kidney regulation being the mechanism that governs the balance (Flanagan, Devereaux, Abdallah, & Remington, 2007). The potassium found in the extracellular fluid is responsible for neuromuscular function and plays a major role in myocardial contractility, function, and rhythm (Felver, 2010).

Hyperkalemia

Patients with progressive hyperkalemia will present with ventricular dysrhythmias and may develop nausea, intestinal cramping, diarrhea, paresthesias, muscle weakness, or paralysis (muscle weakness first appears in the larger muscles and the myocardium). These symptoms are directly related to the effect of the elevated potassium on the cellular membrane potential. Respiratory failure secondary to muscle weakness and paralysis may also occur as a result of hyperkalemia. Cardiac arrest will occur if left untreated (Felver, 2010; Lemmer & Vlahakes, 2010).

Treatment of moderately elevated serum potassium levels may include sodium polystyrene sulfonate (Kayexalate®). Kayexalate® acts by exchanging sodium ions for potassium ions in the gastrointestinal (GI) tract, thereby allowing for elimination of excess potassium in the stool. Before Kayexalate® is administered, however, it must be known if a patient can tolerate an increase in serum sodium (Shires, 2010).

Emergent renal replacement therapy (RRT) is an option to lower serum potassium levels in those patients who do not respond to conservative therapy. With severe hyperkalemia, 10 units of regular insulin with one ampule of $D_{50}W$, calcium gluconate (if no cardiac symptoms related to the hyperkalemic state are present), a beta agonist, or sodium bicarbonate may be administered. These interventions are temporary in nature but will provide almost immediate lowering of potassium levels and allow time for the patient to be prepared for dialysis therapy (Lemmer & Vlahakes, 2010; Shires, 2010).

The major causes of hyperkalemia in the postoperative cardiac surgery patient are decreased urinary output, cardioplegia, decreased insulin levels, metabolic acidosis, diabetes, and hemolysis of red blood cells (Felver, 2010; Khalpey et al., 2012). Acute kidney injury or failure to excrete and metabolize potassium through the kidneys may occur postoperatively as well (Parker, 2006). Many cardiac medications can cause hyperkalemia (e.g., angiotensin-converting enzyme [ACE] inhibitors, potassium-sparing diuretics, beta blockers, unfractionated heparin, and digoxin). Massive blood transfusions are also associated with higher levels of potassium. Age-related renal changes with distal renal tubular function decline and reduced renin-aldosterone response can exacerbate hyperkalemia in the elderly patient (El-Sharkawy, Sahota, Maughan, & Lobo, 2014).

Evidence of hyperkalemia may be noted in the electrocardiogram (ECG). Peaked T waves (see **Figure 17-1**), a widening QRS complex, a prolonged PR interval, and atrioventricular

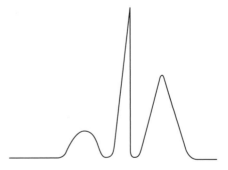

Figure 17-1   Hyperkalemia—peaked T wave.

Source: Illustrated by James R. Perron.

(AV) block may be noted (Lemmer & Vlahakes, 2010; Montague, Ouellette, & Buller, 2008). Cardiac arrest may occur at any point if potassium levels continue to increase. Treatment needs to begin at a level of 6.5 mEq/L even if there are no ECG changes (Lemmer & Vlahakes, 2010).

Hypokalemia

The major causes of hypokalemia in cardiac surgery patients include brisk diuresis, rapid correction of hyperglycemia with insulin, adrenal hyperreactivity, vomiting, alkalosis, and hypothermia (Lemmer & Vlahakes, 2010; Shires, 2010).

Hypokalemia is associated with increased dysrhythmias by delay in ventricular repolarization with a prolonged PR interval, prolonged QT interval, U-wave development as the T wave flattens, and ST-segment depression. Sinus bradycardia, AV blocks, premature atrial contractions, paroxysmal atrial tachycardia, ventricular ectopy, ventricular tachycardia (VT), and ventricular fibrillation may result. Depending on rapidity of potassium loss, skeletal muscle weakness, smooth muscle atony, and respiratory weakness that can lead to respiratory arrest may result if left untreated (Felver, 2010; Huether, 2010). **Figure 17-2** illustrates the development of U waves in the hypokalemic patient.

Hypokalemia can manifest as muscle weakness, fatigue, postural hypotension, absent or diminished bowel sounds, distended abdomen, constipation, and flaccid paralysis (Felver, 2010). Cardiac dysrhythmias that may develop include atrial ectopy, supraventricular tachycardias and atrial flutter, ventricular ectopy, VT, VF, and torsades de pointes. Patients may be more susceptible to digitalis toxicity (Felver, 2010; Lemmer & Vlahakes, 2010). Hypokalemia is frequently accompanied by metabolic alkalosis and hypomagnesemia.

Treatment of hypokalemia involves replacement of potassium, either orally or intravenously. If concomitant hypomagnesemia exists, correction of magnesium levels is required before or simultaneously with potassium correction (Sedlacek, Schoolwerth, & Remillard, 2006). In an adult, a decrease in the plasma potassium level of 1 mEq/L constitutes a total body loss of at least 100 mEq (Lemmer & Vlahakes, 2010). Replacement will need to reflect this.

Sodium

Sodium is the major extracellular ion found in the body; its concentration normally ranges between 135 and 145 mEq/L. Sodium is directly responsible for maintaining the fluid balance in the body, ensuring appropriate water distribution, and maintaining the ECF volume status. The serum sodium concentration parallels with the osmolality of the blood. Antidiuretic hormone is the primary regulator of osmolality (Felver, 2010).

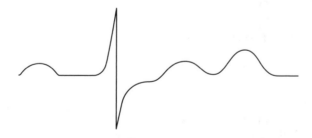

Figure 17-2   Hypokalemia—U wave.
Source: Illustrated by James R. Perron.

Hypernatremia

Hypernatremia is a relatively uncommon phenomenon but is associated with a 40% to 60% (or greater) mortality rate. This imbalance occurs when there is a gain of sodium in excess of water or a loss of water in excess of sodium. In the postoperative cardiac surgery patient, it is most commonly seen in conjunction with hyperventilation. Hypernatremia may also develop secondary to dehydration from fever, diabetes, or use of osmotic diuretics. Usually, the patient's blood urea nitrogen (BUN) and creatinine will be elevated as well (Lindner & Funk, 2013).

Signs and symptoms of hypernatremia may include thirst, fever, restlessness, irritability, ataxia, seizures, weakness, dry oral mucosa or tongue, poor skin turgor, and disorientation with possible progression to lethargy, stupor, or coma (Lemmer & Vlahakes, 2010; Shires, 2010). The majority of patients exhibiting this are also hypovolemic and hyperosmolar (Lindner & Funk, 2013). Depending on the cause, treatment will focus on either increasing water within the body or removing sodium from it (Lindner & Funk, 2013). Lemmer and Vlahakes recommend that if treating with free water, do so at a rate that corrects the serum sodium by less than 0.7 mEq/L/hr.

Postoperative cardiac surgery patients with a severe hypernatremia (greater than 150 mEq/L) may experience an acid–base imbalance that is difficult to correct. In this situation, use of tromethamine or tris(hydroxymethyl)aminomethane (Tham®) to treat metabolic acidosis is recommended instead of sodium bicarbonate because the latter therapy may increase sodium levels further, worsen intracellular acidosis, reduce ionized calcium, create hyperosmolality, and cause central nervous system effects. Tham® buffers without creating CO_2; patients will need intact kidneys, dialysis, or continuous renal replacement therapy (CRRT). Potassium and acid–base levels must be monitored regularly when using Tham® (Kraut & Madias, 2012).

Hyponatremia

Hyponatremia is the most common electrolyte abnormality in hospitalized patients and is associated with increased mortality, increased hospital length of stay (LOS), gait imbalance, falls, rhabdomyolysis, bone fractures, and increased healthcare costs (Crestanello et al., 2013; El-Sharkawy et al., 2014; Kovesdy et al., 2012; Stelfox, Ahmed, Zygun, Khandwala, & Laupland, 2010). Up to 21% of preoperative cardiac surgery patients are known to have hyponatremia (Crestanello et al., 2013). Hyponatremia commonly arises when cells swell as water enters them. This swelling can progress to the point that it eventually leads to cellular rupture. Common causes of hyponatremia include use of certain medications (e.g., thiazide diuretics, nonsteroidal anti-inflammatory drugs, ACE inhibitors), pneumonia, and acute respiratory failure. Excess fluid volume and the stressors from cardiac surgery (e.g., nausea, pain, anesthesia) can stimulate release of ADH, causing hyponatremia for the first few days after surgery. It also occurs in patients with congestive heart failure with diminished CO, stimulating release of ADH (Felver, 2010). Signs and symptoms may include headache, confusion, nausea and vomiting, generalized muscle weakness, fatigue, and seizures and coma if severe. Symptoms vary according to the severity of hyponatremia and how quickly it occurs (Felver, 2010; Shires, 2010). Cheyne-Stokes respirations and respiratory failure may accompany severe hyponatremia (Thomas, 2014). Hyponatremia and hyperglycemia are often noted together (El-Sharkawy et al., 2014). Common characteristics of patients with hyponatremia include lower left ventricular function, higher pulmonary artery pressures, lower glomerular filtration rates (GFRs), and higher rates of comorbidities such as diabetes, hypertension, previous myocardial infarction (MI), COPD, peripheral vascular disease, and previous cardiac surgical procedures (Crestanello et al., 2013).

Hyponatremia may be seen in patients who are either hypovolemic, normovolemic, or hypervolemic. Most often, this type of sodium imbalance is seen in patients with severe heart failure, in whom a decrease in CO triggers the release of ADH, which in turn causes hypervolemia. Patients who are hypovolemic may develop hyponatremia secondary to brisk diuresis, excess insensible loss from the skin or GI tract, or glucocorticoid deficiency. Those who are normovolemic may develop hyponatremia secondary to hypokalemia, medications, or hypothyroidism. Patients with hypervolemia may also develop hyponatremia secondary to renal failure or heart failure and increased total body water accumulation (Huether, 2010).

The patient with hypervolemia-associated hyponatremia will present with changes in mental status, restlessness, anxiety, decreased urinary output, weight gain, peripheral and dependent edema (including pitting edema; see **Figure 17-3**), hypertension, jugular vein distention, shortness of breath, diffuse crackles, and muffled heart sounds (Flanagan et al., 2007). Because of their fluid volume status, these patients also present with low hematocrit levels (Flanagan et al., 2007).

Treatment of hyponatremia includes replacement of fluid in patients with hypovolemic hyponatremia, water restriction in hypervolemic or normovolemic hyponatremia, and management of associated adrenal and ADH imbalances, as appropriate. For those patients with volume overload, treatment includes a loop diuretic agent and moderate fluid restriction (Lemmer & Vlahakes, 2010). During treatment, close monitoring and accurate intake and output records should be maintained, and the nurse should monitor the patient's vital signs closely to assess for rapid fluid changes (Flanagan et al., 2007). In case of severe hyponatremia (less than 120 mEq/L) or if the patient is symptomatic, infusions of 3% sodium may be indicated. Patients must be closely monitored while receiving this infusion. Rapid changes in level of consciousness indicate a worsening cerebral edema.

Magnesium

Magnesium is an electrolyte that plays a key role in cellular function and is a major intracellular cation. Magnesium helps maintain cellular permeability, promotes ion transport across the cellular membranes, and increases neuromuscular excitability. Magnesium is intrinsically involved with potassium, sodium, and adenosine triphosphatase (ATPase)—the enzyme that helps regulate potassium concentration, especially in the myocardium (Felver, 2010; Huether, 2010). Several studies have been done in the last few years looking at the efficacy of magnesium supplementation to control atrial and ventricular arrhythmias. Its use has been compared to amiodarone and sotalol and has been found to be of benefit in controlling and preventing both ventricular rate and rhythm and atrial arrhythmias (Shepherd et al., 2008; Tiryakioglu et al., 2009). Levels of this ion are regulated by GI absorption and renal excretion; the normal range is 1.8–2.4 mg/dL.

Hypermagnesemia

Hypermagnesemia (greater than 2.5 mEq/L) is rare and is most likely to occur in patients with decreased renal function. The patient

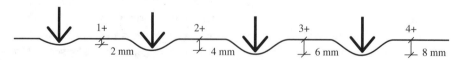

Figure 17-3   Pitting edema.
Source: Illustrated by James R. Perron.

with an elevated magnesium level will present with flushing, warmth, lethargy, muscle weakness, diminished deep tendon reflexes, dilated pupils, vomiting, diarrhea, anorexia, muscle weakness, decreased or absent bowel sounds, hypotension, and respiratory depression (Felver, 2010; Huether, 2010). Ventricular dysrhythmias, bradycardia, a prolonged PR interval, widened QRS, complete heart block, and cardiac arrest are not uncommon in patients whose magnesium levels exceed 2.5 mg/dL (Felver, 2010; Shires, 2010).

Magnesium levels greater than 10 mg/dL (particularly 15 mg/dL) are usually fatal. Treatment for symptomatic hypermagnesemia includes an infusion of insulin and glucose as well as intravenous calcium gluconate, which acts as a magnesium antagonist. Calcium gluconate rapidly reverses cardiac dysrhythmias or respiratory depression directly related to hypermagnesemia. The ICU nurse should prepare to administer 10–20 mEq of calcium gluconate over 10 minutes or follow facility policy in cases of life-threatening hypermagnesemia. Patients who develop this electrolyte imbalance will also require fluid resuscitation and loop diuretics. Mechanical ventilation may be required for those individuals with severe respiratory depression. A temporary pacemaker may be required in patients who experience severe bradycardia. Hemodialysis may be required if the patient's renal function is inadequate (Shires, 2010).

Hypomagnesemia

Hypomagnesemia is a common clinical problem in postoperative cardiac surgery patients, especially in those individuals who develop hemodilution following CPB or who receive diuretics (Felver, 2010; Shires, 2010). It is also a common problem associated with normal aging; it is commonly thought to arise from decreased dietary intake and worsens with elevated acids (El-Sharkawy et al., 2014). This electrolyte imbalance is associated with atrial

and ventricular dysrhythmias. Patients are more apt to develop atrial fibrillation (AF) in the postoperative phase with hypomagnesemia. A meta-analysis recently revealed that 2,988 patients receiving magnesium therapy had a 10% reduced chance of AF postoperatively (Tokmaji, McClure, Kaneko, & Aranki, 2013). In addition, affected patients may present with depression, muscle weakness, coronary spasm, confusion, irritability, hyperactive reflexes, positive Chvostek's sign, leg and foot cramping, twitches and tremors, tetany, delirium, and seizures (Felver, 2010). Vascular effects include an increased peripheral vascular resistance with hypertension resulting and potential for vasospasms.

Hypomagnesemia is often accompanied by hypophosphatemia, hypocalcemia, and hypokalemia. This can lead to osteoporosis, arrhythmias, and MI (El-Sharkawy et al., 2014). Changes will appear on the ECG tracing, including nonspecific T wave changes, appearance of U waves, prolonged QT intervals, widened QRS complex, ST-segment depression, peaked T waves, and torsades de pointes. Ventricular ectopy, paroxysmal supraventricular tachycardia, premature ventricular contractions, and AF and VF are likely to occur as well (Felver, 2010; Shires, 2010). Finally, insulin resistance may occur in patients with severe hypomagnesemia, making serum glucose levels hard to control (Chhabra, Chhabra, Chhabra, & Ramessur, 2012).

Treatment entails magnesium repletion. If magnesium is to be administered intravenously, the patient's renal function should be determined prior to its administration to help avoid hypermagnesemia (Sedlacek et al., 2006). Additionally, during infusions of magnesium, urinary output should be closely monitored. If urinary output decreases to less than 100 mL over 4 hours, the infusion of magnesium should be discontinued and the surgeon notified.

Protection of the patient's overall condition remains a high priority in a hypomagnesemic patient. Seizure precautions should be implemented, the airway and respiratory status should be continually monitored, and fall precautions should be implemented for those individuals who have an altered mental status.

Calcium

The majority (greater than 99%) of the body's calcium is found in the skeletal system. Most of the remaining calcium is found inside cells. The serum calcium is found bound to protein, bound or complexed with anions, and ionized (free) (Huether, 2010; Shire, 2010). A normal serum calcium level is in the range of 8.5–10.5 mg/dL in individuals with a normal pH and normal serum albumin levels. Assessment of total calcium level requires pH and serum albumin evaluation.

In cases of protein malnutrition or other issues affecting serum albumin, an ionized calcium level is a more accurate indicator of calcium status than total calcium level. Ionized calcium is the calcium that is not bound to protein; its normal range is from 4.4 to 5.3 mg/dL (Fukagawa, Kurokawa, & Papadakis, 2008). Adequate levels of ionized calcium are essential for cardiac performance (Khalpey et al., 2012).

Hypercalcemia

Three basic causes exist for hypercalcemia: increased intestinal absorption, increased bone resorption, and decreased elimination (Felver, 2010). Decreased elimination of calcium is seen generally with medication use, or when decreased availability of physiologic calcium is present (such as with acidosis). Medications that increase serum calcium levels include thiazide diuretics and lithium carbonate, both of which decrease renal calcium excretion. Some estrogens also increase calcium levels. Immobilization, rhabdomyolysis, and excess Vitamin D can also lead to this condition (Felver, 2010; Gurrado et al., 2012).

Patients with hypercalcemia will present with altered mental status, fatigue, muscle weakness, lethargy, anorexia, nausea, vomiting, constipation, abdominal pain, decreased renal function or AKI, polyuria, polydipsia, shortened QT segments, and depressed T waves. Nonspecific dysrhythmias, bradycardia, and first-, second-, or third-degree AV block may develop. Bundle branch blocks may also be seen. The patient with severe hypercalcemia may develop confusion, personality change, psychosis, or lethargy that can lead to coma (Clines, 2011; Felver, 2010).

Goals for treatment are to restore urinary calcium excretion and inhibit bone resorption. Prior to treating hypercalcemia, it is important to determine if serum albumin is low. Because calcium binds to albumin, it is important to correct an elevated calcium before treatment begins; once a corrected calcium is calculated, the patient may no longer have hypercalcemia. A corrected calcium can be calculated using the formula in **Box 17-1**.

Calcitonin is able to meet both goals and may be given intravenously as a treatment for hypercalcemia; it may also be given intramuscularly or subcutaneously (Clines, 2011). Hydration with saline to promote urine output can be utilized depending on the patient's age and comorbidities (congestive heart failure, renal failure). Glucocorticoids have also been used successfully in cases of hypercalcemia; however, results will not be seen for 5 to 7 days with this therapy; if no positive results are seen within 10 days, this treatment should be stopped. Patients may develop increased risks for hyperglycemia and sodium and water retention while being treated with

Box 17-1   Corrected Calcium Formula

Corrected calcium = (4 − serum albumin in g/dL) × 0.8 + serum calcium

Source: Data from Agraharkar, M. (2012). *Hypercalcemia*. Retrieved from http://emedicine.medscape.com/article/240681-overview

glucocorticoids such as methylprednisolone (Medrol®) or prednisone (Clines, 2011).

Hypocalcemia

Hypocalcemia occurs when serum calcium is less than 8.5 mg/dL. At a minimum, measurement of ionized calcium level is needed to confirm a diagnosis of hypocalcemia, and these data should always be reviewed in conjunction with the acid–base status of the patient. A patient with a low serum calcium but normal ionized calcium is typically asymptomatic, and is referred to as having pseudohypocalcemia.

Development of hypocalcemia is expected following CPB, hemodilution, low CO, or administration of citrated blood (Khalpey et al., 2012). Packed red blood cells, for example, are conditioned with citrate to prevent their coagulation. When citrate combines with calcium, hypocalcemia can occur. This effect generally does not occur during normal blood transfusions, because citrate has adequate time to metabolize in the liver; only in cases of faster than normal blood transfusions or cases of liver dysfunction does this citrate–calcium binding become a potential problem. Cardiac surgery patients who develop sepsis or rhabdomyolysis are also predisposed to hypocalcemia (Felver, 2010; Lemmer & Vlahakes, 2010). Vitamin D deficiency, malnourishment, renal failure, or hyperparathyroidism are other reasons that a patient may become hypocalcemic. Altered magnesium levels, elevated phosphorus, and alkalosis can lead to hypocalcemia. Hyperphosphatemia is noted with rhabdomyolysis as hypocalcemia is seen in early stages of this disease process (Grecian, Ainslie, Liliker, & Sarma, 2011).

Patients with hypocalcemia may report numbness or tingling of the fingers and toes. Muscle cramps, spasms, tremors, twitching, and abdominal and intestinal cramps are common. Bowel sounds are hyperactive. Because of the increased neuromuscular activity, hypocalcemic patients who are left untreated may develop tetany, seizures, laryngospasm, and bronchospasm. These spasms may lead to laryngeal stridor, which will eventually necessitate intubation if the calcium level is not adequately treated (Shires, 2010). Auscultation of breath sounds may reveal inspiratory and expiratory wheezing. In approximately 70% of patients with hypocalcemia, positive Trousseau's and Chvostek's signs are present. Trousseau's sign is considered positive when an inflated blood pressure cuff elicits a carpopedal spasm (see **Figure 17-4**). Chvostek's sign is considered positive when tapping of the facial nerve elicits facial muscle movement (Shires, 2010).

Cardiac complications associated with hypocalcemia include a decrease in myocardial contractility and CO. Symptoms of hypocalcemia will likely include hypotension, a prolonged QT interval, shortness of breath, and dysrhythmias ranging from bradycardia to asystole. Heart sounds may be muffled (Khalpey et al., 2012; Szymanski, Karpinski, Platek, Puchalski, & Filipiak, 2013).

Acute hypocalcemia should be promptly corrected with administration of 10% calcium gluconate. This medication may be given either as an intravenous push over 5 to 10 minutes or mixed in 0.9% normal saline (NS) for infusion according to facility policy.

Phosphorus

Phosphorus is located primarily in bone, with the rest located in intracellular and extracellular compartments. These ions play integral roles in the repair of cells and tissues, and are crucial ions in the production of adenosine triphosphate (ATP) (Huether, 2010). Phosphorus is excreted through the kidneys; as kidney function declines, phosphorus levels are likely to increase (Shires, 2010). As is the case with calcium, hormonal regulation is provided through the parathyroid gland (Weinman et al., 2007). A normal serum phosphorus is in the range of 2.5–4.5 mg/dL.

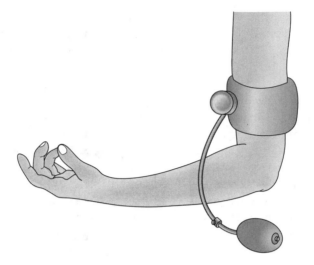

Figure 17-4 Test for hypocalcemia.
Source: Illustrated by James R. Perron.

Hyperphosphatemia

Hyperphosphatemia is defined as a serum phosphorus level greater than 4.5 mg/dL but becomes clinically significant when phosphorus levels exceed 5.0 mg/dL (Lederer, Ouseph, & Nayak, 2014). Almost all cases of hyperphosphatemia are a direct result of decreased renal function. When the glomerular filtration rate falls below 50 mL/min, the kidneys are no longer able to adequately metabolize phosphorus (Van Pottelbergh et al., 2012). Respiratory acidosis and DKA may also lead to hyperphosphatemia. It is suggested that the relationship between a respiratory acidosis and hyperphosphatemia is twofold. First, a sudden rise in carbon dioxide levels can lead to an elevation in phosphorus levels. Second, presence of a respiratory acidosis causes phosphorus to move from the intracellular to extracellular fluid compartment. Presence of a metabolic acidosis, as seen in DKA, is associated with hyperphosphatemia (Lederer et al., 2014).

Signs and symptoms of hyperphosphatemia may include altered mental status, delirium, seizures, paresthesias (especially around the mouth or in the fingers and toes), and tetany. Positive Trousseau's and Chvostek's signs, hypotension, and cardiac dysrhythmias may also be present. Heart sounds may be muffled, and a pericardial friction rub may be present, indicative of potential heart failure. The QT interval is often prolonged.

If kidney function is adequate, an NS infusion may help return the serum phosphorus levels to baseline. If the patient is symptomatic, emergent renal replacement therapy may be indicated (Lederer et al., 2014).

Hypophosphatemia

Patients with a serum phosphorus level less than 1.0 mg/dL are considered severely compromised. Because of the key role that phosphorus plays with ATP, a sharp decrease in phosphorus levels results in cell energy depletion (Moore & Rosh, 2012). Causes for hypophosphatemia include chronic alcoholism, hyperparathyroidism, excessive antacid use, malnutrition or malabsorptive conditions, intravenous glucose or bicarbonate infusions, emesis, dialysis, and respiratory alkalosis or hyperventilation (Felver, 2010; Moore & Rosh, 2012).

Signs and symptoms of severe hypophosphatemia include paresthesias; severe, profound, and progressive muscle weakness; tremors; muscle pain and tenderness; lethargy; confusion; anxiety; and apprehension. If this condition is left untreated, the patient will develop hypoxia and bradycardia. Hypotension will be present, and stroke volume will be decreased. Muscle weakness will eventually lead to acute respiratory failure from decreased contraction of the diaphragm. Seizures and coma may also be present. Hypophosphatemia may cause eventual rhabdomyolysis secondary to muscle cell's inability to maintain cell membrane integrity with the overall ATP depletion. Hemolytic anemia as well as leukocyte and platelet dysfunction will be noted. Respiratory rate decreases as phosphorus levels decrease. However, if the hypophosphatemia is related to presence of respiratory alkalosis, tachypnea will be present. Hypomagnesemia and hypercalcemia are oftentimes present in conjunction with hypophosphatemia (Moore & Rosh, 2012).

Treatment for severe hypophosphatemia requires intravenous replacement of phosphorus. The precise therapy employed depends on the patient's renal status because one phosphorus preparation is built on sodium and the other relies on potassium. For the patient with adequate renal function, potassium phosphate may be administered; sodium phosphate should be administered to those patients with decreased renal function.

Should a heart block or flaccid paralysis develop, the infusion of phosphorus should be immediately discontinued, as these symptoms indicate rebound hyperphosphatemia. A patient with severe hypophosphatemia may also be more prone to infection. Consequently, a complete blood count should be performed on the postoperative cardiac surgery patient to provide information about the presence of bleeding and possible infection.

FLUID BALANCE AND VOLUME MANAGEMENT

Fluids shift on an as-needed basis between compartments to maintain homeostasis. This fluid exchange is partly affected by osmolarity, and hence by electrolyte concentrations (Huether, 2010). Shifts between compartments occur as the body seeks to maintain an appropriate cation and anion distribution as well as optimal fluid levels in each compartment. Frequently, alterations in fluid volume status accompany electrolyte imbalances. For the nurse caring for the postoperative cardiac surgery patient, either hypovolemia or hypervolemia may represent worsening of a preexisting medical condition or may be related to the surgical procedure and associated interventions. In either case, it is important to recognize the implications of alterations in fluid volume status and to determine appropriate courses of treatment.

Hypovolemia

Hypovolemia, which is also known as fluid volume deficit (FVD), results when both water and electrolytes are lost together. This condition is not the same as dehydration, which results from water loss alone (and, therefore, leads to hypernatremia). An isotonic FVD indicates that electrolyte levels remain essentially unchanged (Huether, 2010). Common causes of fluid losses in the postoperative cardiac surgery patient include blood loss, fever, and third spacing of fluid. Hypovolemic shock results when circulating blood volume falls to such level that vital organs are not perfused adequately, causing potential damage to these organs (Wilkins & Wheeler, 2006).

Assessment

Hypovolemia is common postoperatively, but often proves difficult to assess. Fluid volume deficit is generally gauged as mild, moderate, or severe. Mild FVD represents a loss of approximately 2% of total body weight, moderate FVD entails an approximately 2% to 5% body weight loss, and severe FVD involves a greater than 8% body weight loss (Plumer & Cosentino, 2007). Signs and symptoms of FVD and hypovolemia include decreased capillary refill time, central venous pressure (CVP), and urinary output; dizziness; increased osmolality, specific gravity, thirst sensation in conscious patients, hematocrit, and BUN to serum creatinine ratio (usually greater than 30:1); postural or prolonged hypotension; tachycardia; weak and thready pulse; and decreased vein filling. A urinary output rate that is less than 0.5 mL/kg/hr is indicative of severe FVD and inadequate renal perfusion. Assessment of skin turgor reveals skin that does not "spring" back, but rather remains in the tented position; dry mucous membranes; reduced sweating in axillas (especially in elderly); and a tongue that appears shrunken, with fissures. Severe FVD is also accompanied by confusion, upper body weakness, and speech difficulties. Shock develops when FVD is left untreated. In such cases, hypotension becomes severe and perfusion to vital organs is compromised (Wilkins & Wheeler, 2006).

Treatment

Treatment of hypovolemia depends on the cause of the FVD. Hypoxia is likely to develop in cases of shock; oxygen should be administered to maintain adequate saturation (Wilkins & Wheeler, 2006). The goal of FVD treatment is to expand plasma volume until a desired MAP has been attained and sustained. When planning for delivery of replacement fluids, daily fluid losses and intraoperative fluid loss must also be accounted for and added into the replacement. A fever greater than 101 °F (38.3 °C) increases the daily fluid requirement by approximately 500 mL. If the patient is not severely hypotensive, the fluid replacement plan may be based on an assumption that 50% to 80% of the fluid loss will be replaced over 12 to 24 hours; in cases where severe hypotension or shock exists, volume repletion must take place much more quickly (Sue & Bongard, 2008). The vasodilation that occurs with rewarming following CPB may necessitate administration of additional fluid to maintain adequate CO (Royster, Thomas, & Davis, 2008).

Fluid Challenge

For the patient who has developed oliguria, has a urinary output of less than 0.5 mL/kg/hr with symptomatic hypotension, and has had fluid losses (blood, urine, preoperative fasting), a fluid challenge should be anticipated (Ricci, Romagnoli, & Ronco, 2012). The goal of a fluid challenge is to replenish the intravascular volume. A supplemental dose of fluid (e.g., 250 mL) is administered over a short period of time (e.g., 15 minutes). Using pulse contour systems to provide dynamic indices can reflect intravascular volume status when mechanical ventilation is used and the patient is in normal sinus rhythm. Measurements of stroke volume variation and pulse pressure variation can give a positive reflection of response to fluid challenges/treatment (Greilich & Johnston, 2011; Shaw, 2012). Parameters such as CVP, pulmonary artery occlusive pressure, MAP, and even urinary output are not as reliable in identifying response to fluid challenges in improving cardiac function (Shaw, 2012).

Instead of liberal use or restricted use of fluid therapy, many now prefer to use a goal-directed fluid therapy approach with a combination of inotropic therapy when needed (Corcoran, Rhodes, Clarke, Myles, & Ho, 2012; Doherty & Buggy, 2012; Prowle, Chua, Bagshaw, & Bellorno, 2012). Fluid needs will differ for patients based on their history, comorbidities, and the surgical procedure performed. In addition, patients' hemodynamic profiles and tolerance to fluid will vary. For example, postoperative patients who underwent valve repair for aortic stenosis will initially continue to have left ventricular hypertrophy following surgery. This condition may result in outflow obstruction and subsequent postoperative hemodynamic instability from preload reduction. Treatment will include volume repletion. Conversely, postoperative patients who underwent repair for aortic regurgitation will likely require vasodilator therapy. Patients who underwent repair for mitral stenosis will likely need prudent fluid administration in combination with inotropic support to augment CO. Finally, patients who underwent repair for mitral regurgitation may develop postoperative right ventricular failure and, therefore, require inotropic administration (Khalpey et al., 2012).

Crystalloid Therapy

Crystalloid solutions contain solutes that dissolve and crystallize easily such as dextrose and sodium. *Isotonic* refers to the osmolality (normal total body water is 295 mOsmol/kg) and helps control distribution of water across the cell membrane (endothelial glycocalyx layer) of the ICF and ECF with oncotic pressure from their solutes (Annane et al., 2013; Shaw, 2012).

Commonly used isotonic replacement fluids include 0.9% NS, lactated Ringer's (LR), Ringer's acetate (RA), and Plasma-Lyte. Normal saline is a non-buffered solution (a simple salt solution). Lactated Ringer's and Plasma-Lyte are buffered solutions because they are balanced with acids and bases similar to the balance in the body. Buffered solutions do not have the problem with hyperchloremic acidosis and, hence, metabolic acidosis (Burdett et al., 2012). Normal saline is excreted more slowly than LR, increasing the volume effect for a longer period of time (Hahn, 2011a). Lactated Ringer's and RA can increase blood sugar levels, which may affect diabetic patients, slightly increase oxygen consumption secondary to the lactate and acetate, and have vasodilator (lactate and acetate) properties with rapid administration (Hahn, 2011a). Patients who received RA versus hydroxyethyl starch (HES) had decreased risk of death and were less likely to require renal replacement therapy (Perner et al., 2012). Factors driving the use of crystalloid therapy include the solutions' ready availability in the ICU and their low cost. Other considerations with crystalloid administration for volume repletion include crystalloids' tendency to cause decreased blood viscosity, increased urinary output with associated sodium and potassium excretion, and increased peripheral blood flow, thereby improving tissue perfusion (Margereson, 2003).

A negative aspect of isotonic crystalloid administration is that approximately 75% of the volume moves out of the vascular space, with half being lost to the circulating volume shortly after crystalloid administration. Further, one of the components of crystalloids used for fluid repletion in postoperative cardiac surgery patients is sodium. If excessive amounts of sodium are administered, the patient's osmolarity may become elevated and water may be drawn from cells, resulting in cellular dehydration and reduction in renal blood flow secondary to accumulation of chloride (Ricci et al., 2012). In addition, infusion of 2 liters or more of NS can cause hyperchloremic metabolic acidosis because this fluid has chloride ions in it and is not buffered (Hahn, 2011a). Some providers prefer to alternate administration of 0.9% NS with administration of LR in an effort to avoid this excessive sodium load. Administration of LR, however, can result in hyperkalemia, especially in patients with renal dysfunction (Margereson, 2003).

Administration of hypotonic crystalloids may occasionally result in cerebral edema or seizures and can worsen cerebral damage in the event of cardiac arrest, acute stroke, or in cardiac surgery secondary to high risk of cerebral ischemia (Hahn, 2011a). Administration of glucose-containing solutions for volume repletion (e.g., D_5W) can cause dilutional hyponatremia or hyperglycemia with hyperosmolarity and osmotic diuresis because such solutions do not contain any electrolytes (Margereson, 2003).

Colloid Therapy

Following CPB, patients develop a low COP secondary to a systemic inflammatory response. Colloids such as albumin, plasma protein fraction, fresh frozen plasma, gelatins, HES, or dextran solutions can raise COP. Unlike crystalloids, colloids remain in the intravascular space for an extended period of time, allowing for the osmotic force to promote movement of water back into the intravascular space from the interstitium. They do, however, carry a risk for allergic reactions not seen with crystalloids (Hahn, 2011b; Haljamae, 2011).

Although they are more expensive than crystalloids, colloids may be preferred following cardiac surgery because crystalloid therapy may decrease COP and increase the risk of pulmonary edema. In some patients, colloid administration may improve the patient's hemodynamic profile and improve balance between oxygen supply and demand through enhancement of microvascular blood flow (Haljamae, 2011). The CRISTAL trial determined that those who received colloids had more days without mechanical ventilation, less use of inotropic agents, less use of RRT,

and decreased mortality at 90 days (Annane et al., 2013). The update of the Cochrane review (Mutter, Ruth, & Dart, 2013) after investigating 42 randomized clinical trials concluded that HES products compared to other fluid therapies increased the risk of AKI by 59% and had a 32% increased risk of needing dialysis. Their recommendation was to avoid use of HES products and use alternative therapies instead. Similar results were found in the CHEST trial when HES use was compared to NS (Myburgh et al., 2012). In another study, patients receiving a chloride-restrictive fluid strategy (Plasma-Lyte or chloride-poor albumin) had a reduced risk for developing AKI in comparison to other fluids with higher levels of chloride such as NS and 4% albumin, no change in LOS for ICU or hospital, or mortality (Yunos et al., 2012). Dextrans can be used as volume expanders and to prevent thromboemboli, decrease blood viscosity, and improve microcirculatory flow. They do have a risk for anaphylaxis in patients who have antibodies to dextran. There is a risk for bleeding if large doses are administered (Hahn, 2011b).

Healthcare providers should remember that colloids do not contain clotting factors or contribute to oxygen-carrying capacity (Margereson, 2003). In addition, some of the protein molecules do eventually leak into the interstitium when the endothelial glycocalyx layer has been disrupted secondary to systemic inflammatory states such as diabetes, hyperglycemia, surgery, trauma, and sepsis (Ricci et al., 2012). When this phenomenon occurs, the oncotic pull may promote third spacing of fluid as the COP equalizes in ICF and ECF (Ricci et al., 2012).

The efficacy of fluid challenges is traditionally assessed based on improvements in the patient's hemodynamic profile and physical assessment findings. Completing a passive leg raise maneuver is a quick assessment to see if the patient will respond to a fluid bolus before actually giving volume (Shaw, 2012).

Third Spacing

Third spacing refers to the movement of fluids from the vascular space to a part of the body where exchange with the rest of ECF is decreased, resulting in alterations of capillary membrane permeability (Khalpey et al., 2012). Symptoms of third spacing will mimic those associated with FVD, except that either weight gain may occur or weight may remain stable.

Third spacing occurs in two phases. The first phase mimics FVD (except for the weight loss), and the second (recovery) phase mimics hypervolemia. In the postoperative cardiac surgery patient, third spacing is most likely to arise as a result of vasodilation, hypothermia, or hyperemia (increased amount of blood) to the tissue bed (Khalpey et al., 2012). Treatment is aimed at moving the fluid from the third space to the cellular compartments as well as forcing diuresis. During the initial stage, treatment with LR is generally considered appropriate unless other alterations in electrolyte balance are present. The goal remains to provide adequate circulating volume to maintain an optimal blood pressure and urinary output until the recovery phase begins (Hammon & Hines, 2012).

Hypervolemia

Fluid weight gain with subsequent diuresis should be anticipated following CPB. Hypervolemia, which is also known as fluid volume excess (FVE), occurs when water and serum sodium are proportionately increased in the body. Common causes of FVE include excessive intake of fluids that cannot be removed (e.g., as occurs in renal failure or heart failure, or following administration of fluids at an excessive rate), excessive sodium intake, or inadequate sodium and water elimination (e.g., secondary to heart, renal, or liver failure). In the postoperative cardiac surgery patient, hypervolemia is most commonly related to excessive fluid administration intraoperatively, most notably in patients with either preexisting renal dysfunction, heart failure, or hypoalbuminemia (Shires, 2010).

Assessment

Patients with FVE will manifest weight gain, peripheral edema, distended peripheral veins, jugular venous distention, increased CVP, crackles, decreased dilutional BUN and hematocrit, and bounding pulses. Patients may also develop hypertension, cough, heart murmur, and dependent edema. In cases of severe FVE, pulmonary edema, ascites, or pleural effusion may develop (Felver, 2010; Huether, 2010; Shires, 2010).

Treatment

For patients who do not have preexisting renal dysfunction, diuresis is attempted to normalize volume status when hypervolemia occurs, usually with loop diuretics either through continuous infusion or intermittent boluses (Shaw, 2012). Electrolyte balance must be carefully monitored during this time to avoid potentially life-threatening complications of rapid diuretic therapy. For the patient with AKI, RRT (usually through hemodialysis or CRRT) will be necessary to maintain an appropriate fluid volume state. Fluid restriction to less than 1,000 mL/day is typically implemented as well.

Glycemic Issues

Postoperative cardiac surgery patients may have comorbidities that include either type 1 or 2 diabetes mellitus. During times of increased stress, serum glucose levels become more labile, and the patient with or without a history of diabetes is more likely to exhibit hyperglycemia (greater than 110 mg/dL) or hypoglycemia (Hargraves, 2014). Fluctuations in blood glucose levels will also result in alterations in fluid and electrolyte status. Insulin resistance may be noted with utilization of inotropic agents (epinephrine, norepinephrine), glucocorticoids, or both (Klinkner & Murray, 2014). Tight glycemic control (blood sugars less than 180 mg/dL) is essential to optimize patient outcomes (Breithaupt, 2010).

In 2009, the Society of Thoracic Surgery published blood glucose guidelines for cardiac surgery patients that recommended use of continuous insulin infusions during the perioperative phase, up to 24 hours after surgery to maintain blood glucoses at a target of less than 180 mg/dL (Lazar et al., 2009). In 2012, the Society of Critical Care Medicine published a glycemic control guideline recommending starting insulin infusion therapy for a blood glucose greater than 150 mg/dL to maintain a range of 110–150 mg/dL and keep below a target of 180 mg/dL for critically ill patients (Jacobi et al., 2012). As of January 2014, the Surgical Care Improvement Plan Inf-4 measure was changed to maintain blood glucose levels less than 180 mg/dL between 18 and 24 hours after anesthesia end time (Klinkner & Murray, 2014).

ACUTE KIDNEY INJURY AND RENAL INSUFFICIENCY

Unfortunately, some postoperative cardiac surgery patients may have sustained renal damage from ischemia or decreased blood flow. Cardiopulmonary bypass causes an increased secretion of catecholamines, renin, angiotensin II, aldosterone, vasopressin, atrial natriuretic peptide, and proinflammatory mediators. Release of these substances leads to decreases in renal blood flow and GFR (Khalpey et al., 2012). During CPB, attempts to protect the kidneys focus on ensuring hemodilution, returning

to a pulsatile flow as soon as possible, and reestablishing a normal body temperature as quickly as possible (Hammon & Hines, 2012; Mao et al., 2013). Monitoring of serum creatinine levels post-surgery usually conveys a 0.1–0.2 mg/dL decrease for most patients; when it does not, patients need close monitoring for potential in worsening kidney function (Shaw, 2012).

The incidence of AKI in patients undergoing cardiac surgery is approximately 25% to 30%. Of these patients, 1% to 5% may require dialysis therapy (Ricci et al., 2012). Patients who had a myocardial infarction may have resultant renal impairment or acute tubular necrosis (ATN) from the ischemia. Patients who are older, have diabetes mellitus, or who have a history of heart failure are more likely to develop AKI following a cardiovascular event (Ricci et al., 2012). Other individuals at higher risk include those with poor underlying cardiac performance, advanced atherosclerosis, and preexisting decreased GFR. The amount of time spent on CPB and intraoperative instability are also predictors of the development of postoperative renal impairment (Hammon & Hines, 2012).

Renal perfusion must be maintained in all patients. Urinary output should be at least 0.5 mL/kg/hr. For these goals to be met, satisfactory CO and blood pressure are essential. Maintaining them at appropriate levels can be accomplished by delivering volume repletion to keep up with urinary output, which is typically 200–300 mL/hr following CPB. If urinary output is maintained with use of diuretics, renal perfusion is considered adequate (Khalpey et al., 2012).

Azotemia

Azotemia is the buildup of nitrogenous waste products from protein metabolism; these wastes are normally eliminated by urination (Huether & Forshee, 2010; Remer et al., 2013).

The patient with azotemia will demonstrate increasing serum creatinine and BUN levels, and GFR will decrease. As GFR continues to decline, FVE will develop. Sodium retention with a urine sodium concentration less than 20 mEq/L is a common finding. In this state, a fluid challenge to correct hypovolemia will correct the early renal failure with the exceptions of heart failure or liver failure (Remer et al., 2013).

Acute Kidney Injury

Formerly known as acute renal failure (Shaw, 2012), AKI may be recognized by a sudden, rapid deterioration in renal function. Despite new treatment strategies and improved surveillance methods, the number of patients who develop AKI after cardiac surgery varies in studies from 8% to 39% (Mao et al., 2013). Incidence of requiring RRT is 1% to 5% with cardiac surgery AKI (Mao et al., 2013). This is dependent on preoperative renal function and the complexity of the surgical procedure (Shaw, 2012). An increase in serum creatinine of 0.3 mg/dL within 48 hours of surgery signifies Stage I injury according to the Acute Kidney Injury Network (Shaw, 2012).

Elderly patients (older than 70 years); African Americans; or those with diabetes mellitus, obesity, metabolic syndrome, peripheral vascular disease, preoperative hyperglycemia (greater than 300 mg/dL), preoperative serum creatinine in the range of 1.4–2.0 mg/dL, or heart failure prior to admission are at greater risk for development of AKI (Khalpey et al., 2012; Shaw, 2012). In addition, emergency, aortic, redo, or revision surgeries; prolonged bypass runs (greater than 3 hours); ventricular dysfunction; hypothermia; exposure to nephrotoxic agents such as contrast media and antibiotics; transfusions; and poor intraoperative blood pressure control contribute to development of AKI postoperatively (Ricci et al., 2012; Shaw, 2012).

Three types of AKI exist, and diagnosis is based on the point of initial renal insult:

- Prerenal: injury occurring before the kidney
- Intrarenal: intrinsic to the kidney
- Postrenal: injury occurring after the kidney

Acute kidney injury results in alterations in electrolyte balance, acid–base and fluid volume status, nitrogenous waste accumulation, and decreased production of erythropoietin. In the majority of cases, an insult occurs, resulting in multiple organ damage and affecting the ability of the kidneys to function appropriately. Management of AKI will vary based on the etiology and the degree of renal injury (MacKusick, 2007).

The predominant cause of AKI in postoperative cardiac surgery patients is ATN (Huether & Forshee, 2010). What leads to the cardiac surgery patient developing ATN? Decreased perfusion (MAP less than 50 mmHg), extremes in anemia, and use of transfusions when hemoglobin is greater than 8 g/dL have been identified as precursors to AKI with cardiac surgery patients (Haase et al., 2012). A drop in MAP greater than 26 mmHg from the patient's usual preoperative MAP has been associated with a 2.8 times greater risk of developing AKI (Kanji et al., 2010). A meta-analysis showed that timing of coronary angiography, if less than 1 day to time of surgery, significantly increased incidence of AKI postoperatively (Hu et al., 2013). A newly published study comparing a higher MAP (75–85 mmHg) while on normothermic CPB versus a control group with a MAP of 50–60 mmHg on normothermic CPB did not reduce the incidence of postoperative AKI (Azau et al., 2014). Though these do not answer the question specifically, they are helping to identify ways to prevent ATN and AKI and focus research questions for the future.

The majority of cases of ATN result in suppression of bone marrow, endocrine disturbance, coagulopathy, and cardiovascular dysfunction as normal homeostasis can no longer be maintained (MacKusick, 2007). Acute tubular necrosis can be post-ischemic, nephrotoxic, or a combination. Prolonged hypotension and hypovolemic shock are the most common causes of post-ischemic ATN. Renal cellular death begins to occur when MAP falls below 75 mmHg (Richard, 2001). The extent of the renal damage may be estimated by determining the length of time of renal ischemia, with ischemia of 25 minutes or less generally causing reversible mild injury, ischemia of 40-60 minutes causing damage that will take the kidneys 2 to 3 weeks to recover from, and ischemia lasting longer than 1-1.5 hours causing irreversible damage (Richard, 2001). As ischemia progresses, the renal tubular cells swell, become injured, and eventually become necrotic (MacKusick, 2007).

Assessment

The patient with ATN will present with oliguria or anuria, elevated BUN and serum creatinine, and isosthenuria (a condition in which urinary osmolality approximates plasma osmolality). Oliguria is generally defined as urinary output less than 500 mL over a period of 24 hours; anuria is defined as urinary output less than 50 mL in 24 hours. Patients should be closely monitored for life-threatening alterations in electrolyte levels. Frequent laboratory testing will be necessary to monitor serum electrolytes and complete blood count. Fluid volume excess will develop, and the patient will present with its associated signs and symptoms.

The patient with ATN will progress through the four stages of AKI in a relatively predictable pattern. Initiation is the first stage; it is followed by oliguria, diuresis, and then recovery. The last two stages will typically not be managed in the ICU and, therefore, are not within the scope of this chapter. The total length of time from onset of renal damage to recovery can last from months to 1 year.

Initiation Stage

The initiation stage of AKI begins when the renal insult occurs and lasts from a few hours to a few days. Initial signs and symptoms of renal impairment are noticed, and the cause of AKI is investigated. Initial signs and symptoms generally include a decrease in urinary output, crackles, muffled heart sounds, development of a new heart murmur or S_3 gallop, and an increase in body weight indicating FVE (MacKusick, 2007). There are three new biomarkers that can be measured through plasma or urine—neutrophil gelatinase-associated lipocalin, kidney injury molecule-1, and cystatin C—and that may be indicative of early kidney ischemia/injury in as little as 2-24 hours after surgery (Shaw, 2012). In addition, urine interleukin-18 is another promising biomarker being studied to identify early kidney injury (Mao et al., 2013). The earlier that injury can be identified, the earlier treatment can begin.

Oliguric Stage

Oliguria is a decrease in urinary volume to less than 500 mL/24 hours or less than 0.5 mL/kg/hr for more than 6 hours. The diminished urinary output seen with ATN occurs when shock or dehydration leads to inadequate perfusion of the kidneys. The oliguric stage generally lasts from 1 to 3 weeks (Dynamed, 2014; Huether & Forshee, 2010).

Laboratory data will indicate a decrease in GFR, an increase in serum creatinine and BUN, and an elevation in the electrolytes excreted by the renal system (potassium, sodium, and phosphorus). Laboratory data must be closely monitored because these patients are susceptible to developing hyperkalemia and hyperphosphatemia from apoptosis (cellular death and breakdown). A frequent cause of death during the oliguric stage is cardiac arrest secondary to hyperkalemia. Symptoms of heart failure may occur as FVE increases. Potential for infection, particularly pulmonary, and delay in incisional wound healing may occur (Huether & Forshee, 2010).

Approximately half of all patients with AKI do not present with oliguria (MacKusick, 2007). Anuria is rare in ATN and does involve injury to both kidneys. Nonoliguria is evidenced in 10% to 20% of cases and is less severe with fewer complications (Huether & Forshee, 2010).

During the oliguric or anuric phase, the patient needs to be closely monitored for alterations in electrolyte status and prepared for RRT to remove waste products and excess fluid, and to return electrolytes to near normal levels.

Treatment

Morbidity and mortality rates are significantly increased in postoperative cardiac surgery patients who develop renal dysfunction (Khalpey et al., 2012). The most essential prevention measure and treatment intervention for AKI is maintaining adequate renal perfusion. Normal autoregulation in healthy individuals maintains a MAP of 60–120 mmHg (Shaw, 2012). Nursing interventions focus on maintaining strict intake and output and monitoring oxygen saturation, vital signs, and fluid volume status. Prevention of further ischemia is necessary to prevent additional renal damage from occurring. Because third spacing and significant diuresis are common following CPB, a fluid challenge will likely be initiated. Urinary output should be maintained at a rate of at least 0.5 mL/kg/hr. The patient's hemodynamic profile must be optimized, and use of nephrotoxic agents should be avoided (Khalpey et al., 2012). If the patient progresses to oliguria or anuria, RRT will be required.

Both hemodialysis and CRRT act via the principles of osmosis, diffusion, and filtration. Continuous renal replacement therapy has the added advantage of being able to slowly and safely provide for ultrafiltration and thereby help remove excess fluid over a slower period of time. This gradual action is beneficial when cardiac performance is compromised and the patient cannot tolerate rapid fluctuations in fluid volume status. Cardiac failure intrinsically leads to hemodynamic instability, making CRRT an optimal choice for the postoperative cardiac surgery patient with AKI (Brownback, Fletcher, Pierce, & Klaus, 2014).

While receiving CRRT, the patient must be closely monitored for alterations in fluid and electrolyte status, as well as cardiac, respiratory, GI, and neurologic function. Successful CRRT results in removal of fluid and toxins, clearer breath sounds, improved CO, and stabilization in vital signs (Ash, 2009).

SUMMARY

Caring for postoperative cardiac surgery patients requires extensive knowledge, skill, and sound critical thinking that allow the critical care nurse to perform patient assessment and management in a rapidly changing environment. Life-threatening alterations in fluid and electrolyte balances may be present from previous surgery, previous comorbid conditions, or a combination of these factors. Nurses caring for postoperative cardiac surgery patients should also be aware of the manifestations of AKI and its treatment options. The primary methods of prevention and treatment of AKI for cardiac surgery patients entail interventions that optimize perfusion and oxygen delivery to all tissues. Patients usually receive diuretic therapy starting on the first postoperative day. This therapy typically continues until the patient's preoperative weight has been reestablished (Mullen-Fortino & O'Brien, 2008). The ICU nurse plays a pivotal role in attaining and maintaining fluid and electrolyte balance and optimizing patient outcomes.

CASE STUDY

A 72-year-old male patient with a history of angina, hypertension, hyperlipidemia, diet-controlled diabetes, and tobacco use is admitted to the emergency department with chest pain. An ECG revealed ST-segment elevation, echocardiogram revealed an ejection fraction of 25%, and cardiac catheterization revealed 3-vessel disease. He is taken to the operating room for an on-pump coronary artery bypass grafting (CABG) procedure. Cardiopulmonary bypass and aortic cross-clamp times are 180 minutes and 124 minutes, respectively. He is admitted to the ICU postoperatively.

Critical Thinking Questions

1. Based on this patient's clinical course, for which electrolyte abnormalities should the nurse observe?
2. What risk factors put the patient at risk for electrolyte disturbances postoperatively?
3. For which symptoms should the nurse assess?

Answers to Critical Thinking Questions

1. This patient is at particular risk for depleted levels of potassium, magnesium, and phosphorus.
2. Patients who receive CPB are at risk for electrolyte depletion. These depletions are likely related to intracellular ion shift and increased urinary elimination of electrolytes from the bypass circuitry and from intraoperative hypothermia.
3. Signs and symptoms of hypokalemia include muscle weakness, fatigue, postural hypotension, decreased or absent bowel sounds, distended abdomen, constipation, and flaccid paralysis. Cardiac manifestations may include atrial or ventricular ectopy, supraventricular tachycardia, atrial flutter, ventricular tachycardia, or ventricular fibrillation. Hypomagnesemia may be manifested with atrial fibrillation, depression, muscle weakness, coronary spasm, confusion, irritability, hyperactive reflexes, positive Chvostek's sign, tremors, tetany, delirium, or seizures. Patients with hypophosphatemia may present with paresthesias, progressive muscle weakness, tremors, muscle pain and tenderness, lethargy, confusion, anxiety, or apprehension.

SELF-ASSESSMENT QUESTIONS

1. Which of the following consequences affecting fluid exchange should the nurse anticipate following cardiac surgery?
   a. Increased hydrostatic pressure
   b. Increased colloid osmotic pressure
   c. Decreased hydrostatic pressure
   d. Decreased colloid osmotic pressure

2. Which of the following should the nurse anticipate following cardiopulmonary bypass?
   a. Sodium excretion
   b. Potassium retention
   c. Increased cortisol levels
   d. Decreased extracellular volume

3. A patient with a body mass index of 35 kg/m² immediately following cardiac surgery has pain and shivering and

develops dizziness, weakness, confusion, and tetany. Which of the following ABG results should the nurse expect?

pH	pCO$_2$	HCO$_3$
a. 7.30	50	25
b. 7.49	42	31
c. 7.51	31	22
d. 7.31	35	18

4. A postoperative cardiac surgery patient has the following ABG values: pH 7.24, pCO$_2$ 30, pO$_2$ 65, HCO$_3$ 16. For which of the following should the nurse assess?
   a. Hypercalcemia
   b. Hyperkalemia
   c. Hypocalcemia
   d. Hypokalemia

5. A postoperative cardiac surgery patient develops the following ABG values: pH 7.50, pCO$_2$ 30, pO$_2$ 68, HCO$_3$ 23. For which of the following should the nurse assess?
   a. Pain
   b. Hypothermia
   c. Atelectasis
   d. Hyperkalemia

6. A patient following cardiac surgery has the following ABG results: pH 7.51, pCO$_2$ 45, pO$_2$ 80, HCO$_3$ 30. For which of the following electrolyte abnormalities should the nurse observe?
   a. Hypocalcemia
   b. Hyperkalemia
   c. Hyponatremia
   d. Hyperphosphatemia

7. A postoperative cardiac surgery patient has the following laboratory results: Na 137 mEq/L, K 2.9 mEq/L, Mg 1.4 mg/dL, pH 7.50, pCO$_2$ 39, pO$_2$ 78, HCO$_3$ 30. For which of the following should the nurse observe?

   a. Shortened PR interval
   b. Peaked T waves
   c. ST-segment elevation
   d. U wave

8. A postoperative cardiac surgery patient presents with lethargy, muscle weakness, and dilated pupils. A magnesium level of 3.2 mg/dL is noted. For which of the following should the nurse observe?
   a. Shortened PR interval
   b. Tachycardia
   c. Atrial arrhythmias
   d. Complete heart block

9. A patient following CPB who received multiple transfusions intraoperatively and postoperatively develops tremors, muscle cramps, numbness of the fingers, and hyperactive bowel sounds. For which of the following should the nurse observe?
   a. Shortened QT interval
   b. Asystole
   c. Tachycardia
   d. Bundle branch block

10. A patient is receiving 0.45% NS. For which of the following should the nurse observe?
    a. Hyperosmolarity
    b. Hyponatremia
    c. Osmotic diuresis
    d. Cerebral edema

Answers to Self-Assessment Questions

1. d		6. a	
2. c		7. d	
3. a		8. d	
4. b		9. c	
5. a		10. d	

Clinical Inquiry Box

Question: Does postoperative fluid status predict risk of development of major complications following on-pump CABG procedures?

Reference: Morin, J., Mistry, B., Langlois, F., Ma, P., Chamoun, P., & Holcroft, C. (2011). Fluid overload after coronary artery bypass grafting surgery increases the incidence of post-operative complications. *World Journal of Cardiovascular Surgery, 1*(2), 18–23.

Objective: To determine if postoperative fluid status predicts risk of development of major complications following on-pump CABG procedures.

Method: Prospective trial over 5 months.

Results: One hundred nine patients underwent on-pump CABG surgery. The risk of major postoperative complications increased when patients had fluid overload levels with associated weight gain of more than 5 kg. This is compared to patients with fluid overload weight gain of 1–5 kg. The risk of major postoperative complications was not significantly different for patients with less than 1 kg weight gain from fluid overload when compared to patients with a 1–5 kg weight gain. The risk of major postoperative complications also increased when patients had fluid overload lasting for 5 days or more as compared to those who had fluid overload for 1 day or less.

Conclusion: Degree of fluid overload and amount of time fluid overload persists help predict if patients who had on-pump CABG will experience major postoperative complications.

REFERENCES

Agraharkar, M. (2012). *Hypercalcemia*. Retrieved from http://emedicine.medscape.com/article/240681-overview

Annane, D., Siami, S., Jaber, S., Martin, C., Elatrous S., Declere, A. D., . . . Chevret, S. (2013). Effects of fluid resuscitation with colloids vs crystalloids on mortality in critically ill patients presenting with hypovolemic shock: The CRISTAL randomized trial. *Journal of the American Medical Association, 310*(17), 1809–1817.

Ash, R. A. (2009). Indications, contraindications, and complications of peritoneal dialysis in acute renal failure. In C. Ronco, R. Bellomo, & J. A. Kellum (Eds.), *Critical care nephrology* (4th ed., pp. 1459–1466). Philadelphia, PA: Elsevier Saunders.

Azau, A., Markowicz, P., Corbeau, J. J., Cottineau, C., Moreau, X., Baufreton, C., & Beydon, L. (2014). Increasing mean arterial pressure during cardiac surgery does not reduce the rate of postoperative acute kidney injury. *Perfusion, 29*(6), 496–504.

Breithaupt, T. (2010). Postoperative glycemic control in cardiac surgery patients. *Baylor University Medical Center Proceedings, 23*(1), 79–82.

Brownback, C. A., Fletcher, P., Pierce, L. N., & Klaus, S. (2014). Early mobility activities during continuous renal replacement therapy. *American Journal of Critical Care, 23*(4), 348–351.

Burdett, E., Dushianthan, A., Bennett-Guerrero, E., Cro, S., Gan, T. J., Grocott, M. P. W., . . . Rowan, K. (2012). Perioperative buffered versus non-buffered fluid administration for surgery in adults. *Cochrane Database of Systematic Reviews, 12*, CD004089. doi: 10.1002/14651858.CD004089.pub2

Chhabra, N., Chhabra, S., Chhabra, S., & Ramessur, K. (2012). *Hypomagnesemia and its implications in type 2 diabetes mellitus—A review article.* Retrieved from https://www.webmedcentral.com/article_view/3878

Clines, G. A. (2011). Mechanisms and treatment of hypercalcemia of malignancy. *Current Opinion in Endocrinology, Diabetes and Obesity, 18*(6), 339–346.

Corcoran, T., Rhodes, J. E., Clarke, S., Myles, P. S., & Ho, K. M. (2012). Perioperative fluid management strategies in major surgery: A stratified meta-analysis. *Anesthesiology & Analgesia, 114*(3), 640–651.

Crestanello, J. A., Phillips, G., Firstenberg, M. S., Sai-Sudhakar, C., Sirak, J., Higgins, R., . . . Abraham, W. T. (2013). Postoperative hyponatremia predicts an increase in mortality and in-hospital complications after cardiac surgery. *Journal of the American College of Surgeons, 216*(6), 1135–1143.

Doherty, M., & Buggy, D. J. (2012). Intraoperative fluids: How much is too much? *British Journal of Anaesthesia, 109*(1), 69–79.

Dynamed. (2014). *Acute kidney injury.* Ipswich, MA: EBSCO Information Services.

El-Sharkawy, A. M., Sahota, O., Maughan, R. J., & Lobo, D. N. (2014). The pathophysiology of fluid and electrolyte balance in the older adult surgical patient. *Clinical Nutrition, 33*(1), 6–13.

Felver, L. (2010). Fluid and electrolyte and acid-base balance and imbalance. In S. Woods, E. S. Froelicher, S. Motzer, & E. Bridges (Eds.), *Cardiac nursing.* Seattle, WA: Lippincott Williams & Wilkins. Retrieved from http://www.r2library.com/Resource/Title/0781792800

Flanagan, J., Devereaux, K., Abdallah, L., & Remington, R. (2007). Interpreting laboratory values in the rehabilitation setting. *Rehabilitation Nursing, 32*(2), 77–84.

Forshee, B. A., Clayton, M. F., & McCance, K. L. (2010). Stress and disease. In K. L. McCance, S. E. Huether, V. L. Brashers, & N. S. Rote (Eds.), *Pathophysiology: The biologic basis for disease in adults and children* (6th ed., pp. 336–359). Maryland Heights, MO: Mosby Elsevier.

Fukagawa, M., Kurokawa, K., & Papadakis, M. A. (2008). Fluid and electrolyte disorders. In S. J. McPhee, M. A. Papadakis, & L. M. Tierney (Eds.), *Current medical diagnosis and treatment* (pp. 757–784). New York, NY: McGraw-Hill.

Gerhardt, M. A. (2007). Postoperative care of the cardiac surgical patient. In F. A. Hensley, D. E. Martin, & G. P. Gravlee (Eds.), *A practical approach to cardiac anesthesia* (pp. 261–288). Philadelphia, PA: Lippincott Williams & Wilkins.

Grecian, S., Ainslie, M., Liliker, J., & Sarma, J. (2011). Decompensated heart failure secondary to hypocalcaemia post coronary artery bypass grafting. *BMJ Case Reports*, 2011. Retrieved from http://casereports.bmj.com/content/2011/bcr.03.2011.4032.abstract

Greilich, P. E., & Johnston, W. E. (2011). Invasive hemodynamic monitoring. In R. G. Hahn (Ed.), *Clinical fluid therapy in the perioperative setting* (pp. 82–90). New York, NY: Cambridge University Press.

Gurrado, A., Piccinni, G., Lissidini, G., Di Fronzo, P., Vittore, F., & Testini, M. (2012). Hypercalcaemic crisis due to primary hyperparathyroidism—A systematic literature review and case report. *Endokrynologia Polska, 63*(6), 494–502.

Haase, M., Bellomo, R., Story, D., Letis, A., Klemz, K., Matalanis, G., . . . Haase-Fielitz, A. (2012). Effect of mean arterial pressure, haemoglobin and blood transfusion during cardiopulmonary bypass on post-operative acute kidney injury. *Nephrology Dialysis Transplantation, 27*(1), 153–160.

Hahn, R. G. (2011a). Crystalloid fluids. In R. G. Hahn (Ed.), *Clinical fluid therapy in the perioperative setting* (pp. 1–10). New York, NY: Cambridge University Press.

Hahn, R. G. (2011b). Colloid fluids. In R. G. Hahn (Ed.), *Clinical fluid therapy in the perioperative setting* (pp. 11–17). New York, NY: Cambridge University Press.

Haljamae, H. (2011). Rules of thumb. In R. G. Hahn (Ed.), *Clinical fluid therapy in the perioperative setting* (pp. 18–28). New York, NY: Cambridge University Press.

Hammon, J. W., & Hines, M. H. (2012). Extracorporeal circulation. In L. H. Cohn (Ed.), *Cardiac surgery in the adult* (4th ed.). Retrieved from http://accesssurgery.mhmedical.com/content.aspx?bookid=476&Sectionid=39679028

Hargraves, J. D. (2014). Glycemic control in cardiac surgery: Implementing an evidence-based insulin infusion protocol. *American Journal of Critical Care, 23*(3), 250–258.

Hu, Y., Zhiping, L., Chen, J., Shen, C., Song, Y., & Zhong, Q. (2013). The effect of the time interval between coronary angiography and on-pump cardiac surgery on risk of postoperative acute kidney injury: A meta-analysis. *Journal of Cardiothoracic Surgery, 8*, 178. Retrieved from http://www.cardiothoracicsurgery.org/content/8/1/178

Huether, S. E. (2010). The cellular environment: Fluids and electrolytes, acids and bases. In K. L. McCance, S. E. Huether, V. L. Brashers, & N. S. Rote (Eds.), *Pathophysiology: The biologic basis for disease in adults and children* (6th ed., pp. 96–125). Maryland Heights, MO: Mosby Elsevier.

Huether, S. E., & Forshee, B. A. (2010). Alterations of renal and urinary tract function. In K. L.

McCance, S. E. Huether, V. L. Brashers, & N. S. Rote (Eds.), *Pathophysiology: The biologic basis for disease in adults and children* (6th ed., pp. 1365–1401). Maryland Heights, MO: Mosby Elsevier.

Jacobi, J., Bircher, N., Krinsley, J., Agus, M., Braithwaite, S. S., Deutschman, C., . . . Schunemann, H. (2012). Guidelines for the use of an insulin infusion for the management of hyperglycemia in critically ill patients. *Critical Care Medicine, 40*(12), 3251–3276.

Kanji, H. D., Schulze, C. J., Hervas-Malo, M., Wang, P., Ross, D. B., Zibdawi, M., . . . Bagshaw, S. M. (2010). Difference between pre-operative and cardiopulmonary bypass mean arterial pressure is independently associated with early cardiac surgery-associated acute kidney injury. *Journal of Cardiothoracic Surgery, 5,* 71. Retrieved from http://www.cardiothoracicsurgery.org/content/5/1/71

Khalpey, Z. I., Schmitto, J. D., Rawn, J. D., Khalpey, Z. I., Schmitto, J. D., & Rawn, J. D. (2012). Postoperative care of cardiac surgery patients. In L. H. Cohn (Ed.), *Cardiac surgery in the adult* (4th ed.). Retrieved from http://accesssurgery.mhmedical.com/content.aspx?bookid=476&Sectionid=39679028

Klinkner, G., & Murray, M. (2014). Clinical nurse specialists lead teams to impact glycemic control after cardiac surgery. *Clinical Nurse Specialist, 28*(4), 240–246.

Kouchoukos, N. T., Blackstone, E. H., Hanley, F. L., & Kirklin, J. K. (2013). Postoperative care. In N. T. Kouchoukos, E. H. Blackstone, F. L. Hanley, & J. K. Kirklin (Eds.), *Kirklin/Barratt-Boyes cardiac surgery* (4th ed., pp. 189–250). Philadelphia, PA: Elsevier Saunders.

Kovesdy, C. P., Lott, E. H., Lu, J. L., Malakauskas, S. M., Ma, J. Z., Molnar, M. Z., & Kalantar-Zadeh, K. (2012). Hyponatremia, hypernatremia, and mortality in patients with chronic kidney disease with and without congestive heart failure. *Circulation, 125*(5), 677–684.

Kraut, J. A., & Madias, N. E. (2012). Treatment of acute metabolic acidosis: A pathophysiologic approach. *Nature Reviews: Nephrology, 8*(10), 589–601.

Lazar, H. L., McDonnell, M., Chipkin, S. R., Furnary, A. P., Engelman, R. M., Sadhu, A. R., . . . Shemin, R. J. (2009). The Society of Thoracic Surgeons practice guideline series: Blood glucose management during adult cardiac surgery. *Annals of Thoracic Surgery, 87,* 663–669.

Lederer, E., Ouseph, R., & Nayak, V. (2014). *Hyperphosphatemia.* eMedicine Update. Retrieved from http://emedicine.medscape.com/article/241185-overview

Lemmer, J., & Vlahakes, G. (2010). Postoperative management. In J. Lemmer & G. Vlahakes (Eds.), *Handbook of patient care in cardiac surgery* (7th ed.). Portland, OR: Lippincott Williams & Wilkins. Retrieved from http://www.r2library.com/Resource/Title/0781773857

Lindner, G., & Funk, G.-C. (2013). Hypernatremia in critically ill patients. *Journal of Critical Care, 28,* 216.e11–216.e20.

MacKusick, C. (2007). Acute renal failure. In R. Kaplow & S. R. Hardin (Eds.), *Critical care nursing: Synergy for optimal outcomes* (pp. 543–552). Sudbury, MA: Jones and Bartlett.

Margereson, C. (2003). Postoperative care following cardiothoracic surgery. In C. Margereson & J. Riley (Eds.), *Cardiothoracic surgical nursing trends in adult nursing* (pp. 129–204). Boston, MA: Blackwell.

Mao, H., Katz, N., Ariyanon, W., Blanca-Martos, L., Adybelli, Z., Giuliani, A., . . . Ronco, C. (2013). Cardiac surgery-associated acute kidney injury. *Cardiorenal Medicine, 3*(3), 178–199.

Montague, B. T., Ouellette, J. R., & Buller, G. K. (2008). Retrospective review of the frequency of ECG changes in hyperkalemia. *Clinical Journal of the American Society of Nephrology, 3*(2), 324–330.

Moore, D. J., & Rosh, A. J. (2012). *Hypophosphatemia.* eMedicine Update. Retrieved from http://emedicine.medscape.com/article/767955-overview

Mullen-Fortino, M., & O'Brien, N. (2008). Caring for a patient after coronary artery bypass graft surgery, *Nursing, 38*(3), 46–52.

Mutter, T. C., Ruth, C. A., & Dart, A. B. (2013). Hydroxyethyl starch (HES) versus other fluid therapies: Effects on kidney function. *Cochrane Database of Systematic Reviews, 7,* Art. No.:CD007594. doi: 10.1002/14651858.CD007594.pub3

Myburgh, J. A., Finfer, S., Bellomo, R., Billot, L., Cass, A., Gattas, D., . . . Webb, S. A. R. (2012). Hydroxyethyl starch or saline for fluid resuscitation in intensive care. *New England Journal of Medicine, 367*(20), 1901–1911.

Parker, K. P. (2006). Alterations in fluid, electrolyte, and acid–base balance. In A. Molzahn (Ed.), *Contemporary nephrology nursing: Principles and practice* (2nd ed., pp. 121–140). Pitman, NJ: American Nephrology Nurses' Association.

Perner, A., Haase, N., Guttormsen, A. B., Tenhunen, J., Klemenzson, G., Aneman, A., . . . Wetterslev, J. (2012). Hydroxyethyl starch 130/0.42 versus ringers acetate in severe sepsis. *New England Journal of Medicine, 367*(2), 124–134.

Plumer, A. L., & Cosentino, F. (2007). Evaluation of water and electrolyte balance. In A. L. Plumer & F. Cosentino (Eds.), *Plumer's principles and practice of intravenous therapy* (4th ed., pp. 139–151). Philadelphia, PA: Lippincott Williams & Wilkins.

Pollock, F., & Funk, D. C. (2013). Acute diabetes management: Adult patients with hyperglycemic crises and hypoglycemia. *AACN Advanced Critical Care, 24*(3), 314–324.

Prowle, J. R., Chua, H.-R., Bagshaw, S. M., & Bellorno, R. (2012). Clinical review: Volume of fluid resuscitation and the incidence of acute kidney injury—A systematic review. *Critical Care, 16*(4), 230–245.

Remer, E. M., Papanicolaou, N., Casalino, D. D., Bishoff, J. T., Blaufox, M. D., Coursey, C. A., . . . Weinfeld, R. M. (2013). *ACR Appropriateness Criteria®: Renal Failure.* Retrieved from http://www.guideline.gov/content.aspx?id=47681

Ricci, Z., Romagnoli, S., & Ronco, C. (2012). Perioperative intravascular volume replacement and kidney insufficiency. *Best Practice & Research Clinical Anaesthesiology, 26*, 463–474.

Richard, C. (2001). Renal disorders. In L. E. Lancaster (Ed.), *Core curriculum for nephrology nursing* (4th ed., pp. 83–115). Pitman, NJ: American Nephrology Nurses' Association.

Royster, R. L., Thomas, S. J., & Davis, R. F. (2008). Termination from cardiopulmonary bypass. In G. P. Gravlee, R. F. Davis, A. H. Summers, & R. M. Underleider (Eds.), *Cardiopulmonary bypass: Principles and practice* (3rd ed., pp. 614–632). Philadelphia, PA: Lippincott Williams & Wilkins.

Sedlacek, M., Schoolwerth, A. C., & Remillard, B. D. (2006). Electrolyte disturbances in the intensive care unit. *Critical Care Issues for the Nephrologist, 19*(6), 496–501.

Shaw, A. (2012). Update on acute kidney injury after cardiac surgery. *The Journal of Thoracic and Cardiovascular Surgery, 143*(3), 676–681.

Shepherd, J., Jones, J., Frampton, G. K., Tanajewski, L., Turner, D., & Price, A. (2008). Intravenous magnesium sulfate and sotalol for prevention of atrial fibrillation after coronary artery bypass surgery: A systematic review. *Health Technology Assessment, 12*(28), iii–iv, ix–95.

Shires, G. (2010). Fluid and electrolyte management of the surgical patient. In F. Brunicardi, D. K. Andersen, T. R. Billiar, D. L. Dunn, J. G. Hunter, J. B. Matthews, & R. E. Pollock (Eds.), *Schwartz's principles of surgery* (9th ed.). Retrieved from http://accesssurgery.mhmedical.com/content.aspx?bookid=352&Sectionid=40039744

Stelfox, H. T., Ahmed, S. B., Zygun, D., Khandwala, F., & Laupland, K. (2010). Characterization of intensive care unit acquired hyponatremia and hypernatremia following cardiac surgery. *Canadian Journal of Anaesthesia, 57*(7), 650–658.

Sue, D. Y., & Bongard, F. S. (2008). Fluid, electrolytes, and acid–base. In F. S. Bongard, D. Y. Sue, & J. R. Vintch (Eds.), *Current critical care diagnosis and treatment: Critical care* (3rd ed., pp. 14–70). New York, NY: McGraw-Hill.

Szymanski, F. M., Karpinski, G., Platek, A. E., Puchalski, B., & Filipiak, K. J. (2013). Long QT interval in a patient after out-of-hospital cardiac arrest with hypocalcaemia, undergoing therapeutic hypothermia. *American Journal of Emergency Medicine, 31*(12), 1722.e1–1722.e3.

Thomas, C. P. (2014). *Syndrome of inappropriate antidiuretic hormone secretion.* Retrieved from http://emedicine.medscape.com/article/246650-overview

Tiryakioglu, O., Demirtas, S., Ari, H., Tiryakioglu, S. K., Huysal, K., Selimoglu, O., & Ozyazicioglu, A. (2009). Magnesium sulphate and amiodarone prophylaxis for prevention of postoperative arrhythmia in coronary by-pass operations. *Journal of Cardiothoracic Surgery, 4*(8). doi:10.1186/1749-8090-4-8

Tokmaji, G., McClure, R. S., Kaneko, T., & Aranki, S. F. (2013). Management strategies in cardiac surgery for postoperative atrial fibrillation: Contemporary prophylaxis and futuristic anticoagulant possibilities. *Cardiology Research and Practice 2013*, article ID 637482, 1–16. http://dx.doi.org/10.1155/2013/637482

Van Pottelbergh, G., Vaes, B., Jadoul, M., Mathei, C., Wallemacq, P., & Degryse, J. M. (2012). The prevalence and detection of chronic kidney disease (CKD)-related metabolic complications as a function of estimated glomerular filtration rate in the oldest old. *Archives of Gerontology and Geriatrics, 54*(3), e419–e425.

Weinman, E. J., Biswas, R. S., Peng, Q., Shen, L., Turner, C. L., Xiaofei, E., . . . Cunningham, R. (2007). Parathyroid hormone inhibits renal phosphate transport by phosphorylation of serine 77 of sodium–hydrogen exchanger regulatory factor-1. *Journal of Clinical Investigation, 117*(11), 3412–3420.

Wilkins, I., & Wheeler, D. (2006). Recognizing and treating postoperative complications. *The Foundation Years, 2*(6), 244–250.

Yunos, N. M., Bellomo, R., Hegarty, C., Story, D., Ho, L., & Bailey, M. (2012). Association between a chloride-liberal vs chloride-restrictive intravenous fluid administration strategy and kidney injury in critically ill adults. *Journal of the American Medical Association, 308*(15), 1566–1572.

WEB RESOURCES

Fluid and Electrolytes Part 1: http://www.youtube.com/watch?v=vvGyHBWcQQU

Fluid and Electrolytes Part 2: https://www.youtube.com/watch?v=G7lDP6ygGBE

Fluid and Electrolytes Part 3: https://www.youtube.com/watch?v=FmIEvP_KDLw

Fluid and Electrolytes Part 4: https://www.youtube.com/watch?v=QANBPawIPpQ

Fluid and Electrolytes Part 5: https://www.youtube.com/watch?v=zhqV9dFfS8Y

Fluid and Electrolytes Part 6: https://www.youtube.com/watch?v=m5NN6Oct3bY

Fluid and Electrolytes Part 7: https://www.youtube.com/watch?v=cZwTOls9oEY

Fluid and Electrolytes Part 8: https://www.youtube.com/watch?v=ux4vmSMUkIM

Chapter 18

Wound Care

Vicki Morelock and Mary Zellinger

INTRODUCTION

Assessment and care of postoperative surgical sites will have a profound impact on patient outcomes after cardiac surgery. Surgical site infections (SSIs) of the sternum and underlying mediastinum occur in 0.25% to 5% of patients who undergo such procedures (Bryan & Yarbrough, 2013; Cove, Spelman, & MacLaren, 2012; Juhl, Koudahl, & Damsgaard, 2012). Infections can lead to significant morbidity, warranting an increased length of hospitalization and higher costs at best, and patient mortality at worst. Observant practitioners must routinely assess for factors that may potentially slow surgical wound healing, and follow strict and consistent protocols in caring for these incisions. This chapter describes the wound care that is required for the postoperative cardiac surgery patient and explores the pivotal role the intensive care unit (ICU) nurse plays in preventing potentially fatal complications associated with SSIs.

INCISION SITES

Surgical access options in cardiac surgery patients have greatly increased in the past several years. Midline sternotomy access is still the most common access and is used for patients who are operated on with or without the aid of cardiopulmonary bypass (CPB). The lengths of these incisions can range from 6 to 10 inches. Mini-thoracotomy incisions of approximately 2 inches are also used in cardiac surgery. Alternative approaches to the traditional midsternal incision include submammary incisions (can be full or partial sternotomies) and anterolateral or posterolateral thoracotomies. All of these have an improved cosmetic appeal. A right mini-thoracotomy approach may also be used to reach the aortic area to repair congenital heart defects, such as ventricular septal defects in adults (Ding et al., 2012; Jung et al., 2010). Right vertical infra-axillary and totally thorascopic approaches can be used for atrial septal defects in adults and children (Luo et al., 2014). Port-access and robotic surgeries approach the heart through the left chest wall in the case of coronary artery bypass and through the right chest wall for mitral valve repair or replacement.

In minimally invasive bypass, ports for the left internal thoracic artery (ITA) harvest are placed in the third, fifth, and seventh intercostal spaces (ICSs), with a fourth slightly larger working port (2 to 3 inches) for the anastomosis located in the fourth or fifth ICS. Minimally invasive valve procedures may utilize a mini-right thoracotomy (third ICS for aortic valve and fourth ICS for mitral valve) or a hemisternotomy (upper for aortic valve procedures and lower for mitral valve procedures) (Kaneda et al., 2013). Each of these procedures has the potential to result in the complication of infection.

CONDUITS

The ITA is an ideal conduit to use for bypass grafting, although other conduits may be used as well. The ITA does not have valves as the vein grafts do, so there is no obstruction to flow. In addition, arteries are more vasoresponsive than veins. The ITA is taken down from the chest wall during on-pump, off-pump, and minimally invasive surgery and does not require a separate incision for removal.

The radial artery is another frequently used conduit. It can be removed without fear of diminishing blood flow to the hand if the ulnar artery is functioning adequately. Removal of the radial artery typically requires a 2- to 4-inch incision. Because of its visibility, it may be easily monitored in the postoperative period.

The gastroepiploic artery is rarely used as a conduit during cardiac surgery because of the high chance of contamination that may occur when the abdominal cavity is open at the same time as the sternum.

The saphenous vein is often removed from the leg when the other arteries are not available or when additional grafts are needed. The saphenous vein may be removed by utilizing an open vein harvest procedure or through an endoscopic procedure using two or three small (1.5–3 cm) incisions via endoscope (Raja & Sarang, 2013). The saphenous vein is the most commonly used graft, even though within 1 year 10% to 20% fail, an additional 5% to 10% fail in 1–5 years, and an additional 20% to 25% fail in 6–10 years. At 10 years, only about half of saphenous vein grafts are patent, and of those only half are free of angiographic arteriosclerosis (Sabik, 2011). Patients who undergo endoscopic vein harvest may develop a myocardial infarction (MI) as there is an increased incidence of this complication with this process. Revascularization may need to be repeated. Increased mortality rates are also associated with endoscopic vein harvesting (Kiani & Poston, 2011).

Wound complication incidence with open vein harvest procedures ranges from 2% to 25%. It is well documented through multiple studies and meta-analyses that the endoscopic vein harvest has significantly reduced infection rates. In addition, with the increased use of endoscopic vein harvest, noninfective wound derangements have lessened (e.g., wound drainage, edema, erythema, dehiscence) (Raja & Sarang, 2013). Although wound complications are reduced, reported endoscopic harvested vein graft failure has heightened the need for further randomized clinical trials (Lopes et al., 2009). When comparing a preoperative microbial skin sealant on the skin versus bare skin in a randomized control study, Falk-Brynhildsen, Soderquist, Friberg, and Nilsson (2014) found no significant difference in infection or dehiscence rates. They observed a 16.8% infection rate, with *Staphylcoccus aureus* as the pathogen 62% of the time; this was thought to be contamination from the hands and nares of the patient, healthcare workers, environment, or any combination of these.

While saphenous veins are the most commonly utilized grafts, arterial grafts are the preferred conduits. Arterial grafts have better long-term patency, but are short in length, have a small diameter, and have limited availability, resulting in the need for multiple grafts.

RISK FACTORS FOR WOUND COMPLICATIONS

Several factors put patients at greater risk for developing postoperative wound complications. These risk factors can be categorized as preoperative, intraoperative, or postoperative.

Preoperative Risk Factors

Preoperative assessment of risk factors for wound complications is imperative. Early and sustained attention to these risk factors is mandatory. **Table 18-1** lists the most common preoperative risk factors.

The presence of diabetes may impede wound healing by leading to a compromised immune system. Both chemotaxis and phagocytosis play a role in the wound healing

Table 18-1   Preoperative Risk Factors for Wound Complications

Diabetes
Elevated HbA$_{1c}$
Advanced age
Obesity
Large breast size
COPD (i.e., emphysema)
Urgent or emergent CABG repeat operations
Steroids
Preoperative hospital stay of greater than
    5 days
Poor nutrition
Venous impairment
Renal failure
Certain medications
Jaundice
Decreased mobility/activity
Dehydration
Respiratory disease
Infection
Anemia
Smoking
Pain
Decreased immunity

CABG, coronary artery bypass grafting; COPD, chronic obstructive pulmonary disease; HbA$_{1c}$, hemoglobin A$_{1c}$

Sources: Data from Bryan, C. S., & Yarbrough, W. M. (2013). Preventing deep wound infections after coronary artery bypass grafting. *Texas Heart Institute Journal, 40*(2), 125–139; Buonocore, D. (2008). Treatment of hyperglycemia. *Critical Care Nurse, 28*(6), 72–73; Chen, L. F., Arduino, J. M., Sheng, S., Muhlbaier, L. H., Kanafani, Z. A., Harris, A. D., . . . Fowler, V. G., Jr. (2012). Epidemiology and outcome of major postoperative infections following cardiac surgery: Risk factors and impact of pathogen type. *American Journal of Infection Control, 40*(10), 963–968; Subramaniam, B., Lerner, A., Novack, V., Khabbaz, K., Paryente-Wiesmann, M., Hess, P., . . . Talmor, D. (2014). Increased glycemic variability in patients with elevated preoperative HbA1C predicts adverse outcomes following coronary artery bypass grafting surgery. *Anesthesia & Analgesia, 118*(2), 277–287.

process. If serum glucose levels remain elevated, both processes will be compromised (Koh & DiPietro, 2011). Chemotaxis is the oriented movement toward or away from a chemical stimulus—in this case, the process by which white cells are attracted to the site of an infection. Phagocytosis is the ingestion of bacteria by these white cells. Delayed macrophage introduction and diminished leukocyte migration, which cause a prolonged inflammatory phase, interfere in the wound healing process (Koh & DiPietro, 2011; Xuan et al., 2014). Unfortunately, a large number of patients presenting for surgery are unaware of their diabetic status and, therefore, may have an uncontrolled serum glucose level preoperatively. It is becoming common practice for HbA$_{1c}$ to be tested preoperatively because it is a high predictor of adverse outcomes (Subramaniam et al., 2014). Faritous and colleagues (2014) found that patients with elevated HbA$_{1c}$ and elevated fasting blood sugars had significantly higher rates of wound infection, sepsis, and postoperative reintubation.

Advanced age may also diminish wound healing. There are age-related changes affecting all aspects of wound healing (Guo & DiPietro, 2010). Evidence suggests that inherent diminished phagocytic activity may impair tissue repair and regeneration in older patients (Sen, 2009). Comorbidities are more common among the elderly (e.g., peripheral vascular disease, pneumonia, and heart disease); any of these may affect wound healing (Sen, 2009). Osteoporosis, decreased bone tissue, and increased fragility of bone tissue can cause poorly healing sternums, sternal dehiscence, and increased potential for mediastinitis (Schimmer et al., 2008). Mortality is five times higher in elderly surgical patients who develop an SSI (Lipke & Hyott, 2010).

Obesity is a risk for sternal infections because of the increased force applied to the line of closure in these patients, which affects the quantity, aggregation, and orientation of collagen fibers. This may be the result of ischemia or possible relative hypoperfusion that may occur in the subcutaneous adipose tissue (Guo & DiPietro, 2010). In addition, undue pressure on the wound, venous insufficiency, chronic inflammation with release of inflammatory mediators, and edema contribute to poor oxygenation that may lead to ischemia of the surrounding tissues (Pierpont et al., 2014). Increased tension on wound edges contributes to wound dehiscence. Wound tension increases pressure on tissues. Perfusion to the microcirculation is reduced, thereby decreasing oxygen delivery to the wound (Guo & DiPietro, 2010). Antibiotics may be inadequately distributed in the adipose tissue secondary to the impaired vascularity. Obesity along with poor nutrition and osteoporosis may exacerbate poor bone healing, increasing the likelihood of sternal dehiscence (Pierpont et al., 2014). Skin folds make it more difficult to maintain sterility intraoperatively. There is difficulty in suturing, whether the patient is in the sitting position (skin edges forced apart in an inframammary fold) or in the supine position (the weight of the mammaries tends to pull apart skin edges) (Grauhan et al., 2013). Pharmacokinetics of drugs can be altered in the obese, requiring dosage adjustments based on body weight and a need for redosing intraoperatively (Bratzler et al., 2013; Chen et al., 2012).

Chronic obstructive pulmonary disease, pneumonia, and anemia may present problems because effective wound healing requires adequate oxygenation, hemoglobin for oxygen transport, and adequate tissue perfusion (Guo & DiPietro, 2010; Sen, 2009). Oxygen supply must meet the increased tissue demand for wound healing to occur. Protein-calorie malnutrition and the resultant body composition changes are additional considerations that may delay wound healing. The local ability to supply oxygen to the healing wound process is inhibited by peripheral vascular disease, previous radiation, chronic inflammation with elevated inflammatory mediators, chronic edema states, or any combination of these conditions (Pierpont et al., 2014). Carbohydrates, fats, protein, and vitamins all provide energy needed for wound healing; iron deficiency may impair collagen production (Guo & DiPietro, 2010).

Prior ventricular assist device insertion and preoperative inotropic support have been identified as risk factors for orthotopic heart transplants (Filsoufi et al., 2007). In a retrospective, non-randomized study, Kim and colleagues (2013) found a 2% deep sternal wound infection (SWI) rate for the 239 adult patients enrolled undergoing heart transplantation between 1999 and 2011.

Intraoperative Risk Factors

Intraoperative risk factors also affect the potential for postoperative problems related to wound healing (see **Table 18-2**). Use of both ITAs is associated with increased chance of infection because these arteries provide the major source of blood supply to the sternum (Nakano et al., 2008). The removal of the ITA significantly devascularizes the sternal half from which it is taken. Surgical technique and adherence to sterile technique certainly have critical implications for incision and mediastinum status (Bilgin et al., 2011; Bryan & Yarbrough, 2013; Nakano et al., 2008).

An increase in the number of coronary artery grafts, which can prolong surgical time, increases the likelihood of infection. Long CPB pump runs, long surgical procedure times (greater than 4 hours), and any infractions in sterile technique are all known to increase the risk for infection (Bryan & Yarbrough, 2013; Nakano et al., 2008). Hypothermia, which is used for cardiac protection during surgery, needs to be corrected quickly in the immediate postoperative period because prolonged hypothermia increases the risk for infection. Hypothermia impairs neutrophil function and indirectly may cause tissue hypoxia through vasoconstriction of

Table 18-2   Intraoperative Risk Factors

Use of both internal thoracic arteries
Surgical technique and adherence
Number of grafts
Electrocautery use
Bone wax
Prolonged operative time
Blood transfusions
Long cardiopulmonary pump runs
Infractions in sterile technique
Hypothermia
Periods of ischemia

Sources: Data from Anderson, D. J., Podgorny, K., Berrios-Torres, S. I., Bratzler, D. W., Dellinger E. P., Greene, L., . . . Kaye, K. S. (2014). Strategies to prevent surgical site infections in acute care hospitals: 2014 update. *Infection Control & Hospital Epidemiology, 35*(6), 605–627; Athanassiadi, K., Theakos, N., Benakis, G., Kakaris, S., & Skottis, I. (2007). Omental transposition: The final solution for major sternal wound infection. *Asian Cardiovascular Thoracic Annals, 15*(3), 200–203; Bryan, C. S., & Yarbrough, W. M. (2013). Preventing deep wound infections after coronary artery bypass grafting. *Texas Heart Institute Journal, 40*(2), 125–139; Buonocore, D. (2008). Treatment of hyperglycemia. *Critical Care Nurse, 28*(6), 72–73.

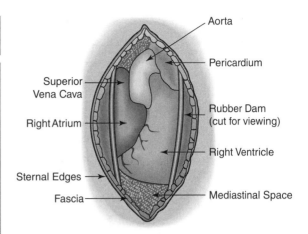

Figure 18-1   Rubber dam.

Source: Data from Zellinger, M., & Lienberger, T. (1991). Use of the rubber dam after open heart surgery. *Critical Care Nurse, 11*(8), 24–27.

the subcutaneous tissue layer. Maintaining warmth preoperatively and intraoperatively helps minimize the effects (Anderson et al., 2014). Rewarming immediately postoperatively can be carried out using warming blankets, fluid warmers, and radiant heat lamps. Occasionally, patients have periods of ischemia leading to the development of myocardial or pulmonary edema, hemodynamic instability, recurrent dysrhythmias, a pressure tamponade, or any combination of these (Pye & McDonnell, 2010). A pressure tamponade may result from an edematous organ possibly prohibiting closure of the chest wall and subsequently resulting in a significant decrease in the cardiac index (the amount of blood ejected by the heart in relation to the body surface area). This complication may warrant leaving the chest cavity open after the procedure for a period of several days to allow for cardiac recovery. During this time, the sternal opening is covered by a variety of methods including a plastic film, a silicone membrane, a sterile drape, or an impermeable piece of rubber latex called a "rubber dam" (Pye & McDonnell, 2010; Yasa et al., 2010; Zellinger & Lienberger, 1991) (see **Figure 18-1**).

While the mediastinum is left open in such cases, it does not remain exposed. The rubber dam is securely sutured to the skin edges, covered with gauze that has been soaked in povidone-iodine, and then covered with a sterile dressing. The initial dressing change should be performed with the surgeon in attendance so that the site can be assessed and evaluated together with the ICU nurse, thereby preventing unnecessary additional site exposures. All dressing changes are done with strict aseptic technique using full barrier precautions. The use of delayed sternal closure does not increase the risk of sternal infection (Boeken et al., 2011; Yasa et al., 2010).

Postoperative Risk Factors

In the immediate postoperative period, risk factors for wound infection (see **Table 18-3**) include early chest re-exploration, need for

Table 18-3   Postoperative Risk Factors
Chest re-exploration
Blood transfusions
Hypothermia ($< 36.0\ °C$)
Prolonged ventilation time
Impaired oxygenation
Impaired perfusion
Prolonged cardiopulmonary resuscitation
Autotransfusions
Low cardiac output
Sternal instability
Infections from other sites or sources (e.g., central line–associated bloodstream infections, pneumonia)

Sources: Data from Bilgin, Y. M., Van de Watering, L. M., Versteegh, M. I., Van Oers, M. H., Vamvakas, E. C., & Brand, A. (2011). Postoperative complications associated with transfusion of platelets and plasma in cardiac surgery. *Transfusion, 51*(12), 2603–2610; Bryan, C. S., & Yarbrough, W. M. (2013). Preventing deep wound infections after coronary artery bypass grafting. *Texas Heart Institute Journal, 40*(2), 125–139; Buonocore, D. (2008). Treatment of hyperglycemia. *Critical Care Nurse, 28*(6), 72–73; Cove, M. E., Spelman, D. W., & MacLaren, G. (2012). Infectious complications of cardiac surgery: A clinical review. *Journal of Cardiothoracic Anesthesiology, 26*(6), 1094–1100; Hartsell, T. L. (2008). Postoperative infection in cardiac surgery. In J. V. Conte, W. A. Baumgartner, S. G. Owens, & T. Dorman (Eds.), *The Johns Hopkins manual of cardiac surgical care* (2nd ed., 361–388). Philadelphia, PA: Mosby Elsevier.

transfusion of multiple units of blood (Bilgin et al., 2011), hypothermia, periods of impaired oxygenation and/or tissue perfusion, and prolonged mechanical ventilation time (Hartsell, 2008). Other postoperative risk factors include autotransfusion of mediastinal blood, low cardiac output (CO; the amount of blood ejected by the heart each minute), prolonged periods of cardiopulmonary resuscitation, sternal instability, and infections arising from sites other than the sternal incision. For example, a patient with a tracheostomy is at greater risk for poor wound healing because of the close proximity of the surgical incision to the tracheal stoma, which is colonized by bacteria. In such a case, the sternal wound should be protected from the tracheostomy

by dressings. Another example is if a patient develops a central line–associated bloodstream infection, the risk for an SSI increases fivefold (Cove et al., 2012).

WOUND INFECTIONS CLASSIFICATION

An infection that occurs within 30 days of a surgical procedure is considered an SSI, according to the definition established by the Centers for Disease Control and Prevention's (CDC) National Healthcare Safety Network (NHSN) (Anderson et al., 2014; CDC, 2014) (see **Box 18-1**). Numerous classifications of SSIs have been developed. Most often, they are classified as either superficial, deep, or organ/space, although a more structured approach utilizing numerous classification types has been proposed in the literature (Vlajcic, Zic, Stanec, & Stanec, 2007).

Superficial Wound Infections

Superficial wound infections are classified as Type 1. These wound infections involve only the skin or subcutaneous tissue around the incision and occur within 30 days of surgery. They may be identified by purulent drainage; isolated organisms upon culture; signs and symptoms of purulent infection such as pain, tenderness, swelling, redness or heat, or purulent drainage; diagnosis of an SSI by the healthcare provider; or any combination of these. These are usually identified and treated in an outpatient setting (Anderson et al., 2014).

Sternal Wound Dehiscence

Sternal wound dehiscence is associated with a Type 2 infection. A Type 2 infection is further classified into one of three subcategories:

- Type 2A: a sterile viable bone
- Type 2B: a nonviable bone in the presence of sternal osteitis (inflammation) in the upper two-thirds of the sternum

Box 18-1   Criteria for Defining Surgical Site Infections

Superficial Incisional SSI

- Infection occurs within 30 days after surgery
- Involvement of only the skin and subcutaneous tissue of the incision
- Dehiscence of superficial incision
- Stable sternum
- At least one of the following:
  - Purulent drainage from the incision
  - Organisms isolated from an aseptically obtained culture of superficial incision's tissue or fluid
  - Presence of signs and symptoms of infection of incision (e.g., pain, tenderness, localized swelling, redness, heat) *and* superficial incision deliberately opened by surgeon or affiliate and is culture positive or not cultured (negative culture is not an SSI)
  - Diagnosis of superficial SSI made by a healthcare provider
- Please note that there are two specific types of superficial SSIs:
  1. *Superficial incisional primary*—infection identified in the primary or chest incision
  2. *Superficial incisional secondary*—infection identified in the secondary or donor site such as leg (saphenous vein grafts) or arm incision (radial grafts)

Deep Incisional SSI

- Infection occurs within 30 days after surgery (if no implant was left in place) or within 1 year (if an implant was left in place and infection appears to be related to surgery)
- Involves fascia and muscle layers of incision
- Presence of at least one of the following:
  - Purulent drainage from the deep incision (e.g., mediastinum)
  - Dehiscence of deep incision, spontaneous or opened by surgeon, and culture positive or not cultured when the patient has at least one of the following symptoms: fever ($> 38.0°$ C), localized pain, or tenderness
  - Presence of an abscess or other signs of deep incision infection found on direct exam, reoperation, or via radiography/histology
  - Diagnosis of deep SSI made by a healthcare provider
- Please note that there are two specific types of deep SSIs:
  1. *Deep incisional primary*—infection identified in the primary or chest incision
  2. *Deep incisional secondary*—infection identified in the secondary or donor site such as leg (saphenous vein grafts) or arm incision (radial grafts)

Notes:

1. If there is presence of both superficial and deep SSIs, it should be reported as a deep incisional SSI.
2. If there is an infection with drainage to an organ/space related to the surgery, it should be reported as a deep incisional SSI.

Organ/Space SSI

- Infection occurs within 30 days after surgery (if no implant was left in place) or 1 year (if an implant was left in place and infection appears to be related to surgery)
- Infection entails any anatomical structure (e.g., organ, space) aside from the skin incision, fascia, or muscle layers

(Continued)

Box 18-1   Criteria for Defining Surgical Site Infections (*Continued*)

- Presence of at least one of the following:
  - Purulent drainage from a drain placed through a stab wound or incision in the organ/space
  - Organisms isolated from an aseptically obtained culture of issue or fluid from the organ/space
  - Abscess or other evidence of infection in organ/space found on direct exam, reoperation, or via radiology/histology
  - Diagnosis of organ/space SSI made by a healthcare provider

Note: Report mediastinitis following cardiac surgery that is accompanied by osteomyelitis as SSI-MED rather than SSI-BONE.

Sources: Data from Anderson, D. J., Podgorny, K., Berrios-Torres, S. I., Bratzler, D. W., Dellinger, E. P., Greene, L., . . . Kaye, K. S. (2014). Strategies to prevent surgical site infections in acute care hospitals: 2014 update. *Infection Control & Hospital Epidemiology, 35*(6), 605–627; Athanassiadi, K., Theakos, N., Benakis, G., Kakaris, S., & Skottis, I. (2007). Omental transposition: The final solution for major sternal wound infection. *Asian Cardiovascular Thoracic Annals, 15*(3), 200–203; Centers for Disease Control and Prevention. (2014). CDC/NHSN Surveillance Definitions for Specific Types of Infections. Retrieved from http://www.cdc.gov/nhsn/PDFs/pscManual/17pscNosInfDef_current.pdf; Chen, Y., Almeida, A. A., Mitnovetski, S., Goldstein, J., Lowe, C., & Smith, J. A. (2008). Managing deep sternal wound infections with vacuum-assisted closure. *AustraliAsian Journal of Surgery, 78*(5), 333–336.

- Type 2C: a nonviable bone in the presence of sternal osteitis in the lower third of the sternum

A Type 2 sternal wound infection could require any number of interventions, ranging from debridement and rewiring to flap surgery (Vlajcic et al., 2007).

Mediastinitis

Deep wound infections that occur within 30 days of a procedure and involve the deep soft tissue (i.e., the fascia and muscle) warrant a diagnosis of mediastinitis, which is considered a Type 3 sternal wound infection. Typically, purulent drainage, dehiscence of the surgical site, fever, pain, tenderness at the site, possible sternal instability, and evidence of infection will be noted. A diagnosis of a deep incisional infection will be made (Anderson et al., 2014). Treatment of a Type 3 sternal wound infection, deep or organ space, may require a sternectomy and a muscle flap(s). There may be a single advanced flap of the pectoralis major, the latissimus dorsi, or the rectus abdominis, or these can be used in combination (Berg & Jaakkola, 2013; Hillis et al., 2012; Juhl et al., 2012; Vlajcic et al., 2007).

Septicemia

A Type 4 infection is characterized by the presence of a Type 2 or 3 wound infection along with septicemia. Treatment of such an infection involves radical debridement, delayed closure, and aggressive intravenous antibiotic therapy (Vlajcic et al., 2007).

PREVENTION OF SURGICAL SITE INFECTION

Appropriate incisional care must be initiated in the preoperative phase and includes a variety of necessary interventions. The CDC and Healthcare Infection Control Practices Advisory Committee are currently updating the 1999 guidelines for prevention of SSIs (Anderson et al., 2014). Preoperative prevention of SSIs begins with meticulous handwashing of all of the surgical team members and preparation of the operative site (Anderson et al., 2014; Yavuz et al., 2013). In addition, a multitude of preventive strategies (listed in **Box 18-2**) are incorporated into any cardiac surgical program to decrease the risk of postoperative complications.

Box 18-2   Strategies for Preventing Surgical Site Infections

- Identify and treat infections before the patient undergoes an elective operation.
- Minimize hair removal at or around the incision site. Use clipping instead of shaving when hair removal is needed.
- Bathe the patient with an antiseptic solution at least the night before surgery.
- Clean the incision site of any gross contaminants and then prep the skin with chlorhexidine gluconate, povidone-iodine, or alcohol-containing products prior to making the incision.
- Use local collagen-gentamicin.
- Use additional fixation wires at the lower sternum.
- Use the vertical interrupted mattress suture technique with cyanoacrylate sealant in high-risk groups (e.g., obese patients).

Sources: Data from Bryan, C. S., & Yarbrough, W. M. (2013). Preventing deep wound infections after coronary artery bypass grafting. *Texas Heart Institute Journal, 40*(2), 125–139; Buonocore, D. (2008). Treatment of hyperglycemia. *Critical Care Nurse, 28*(6), 72–73; Grauhan, O., Navasardyan, A., Hofmann, M., Muller, P., Stein, J., & Hetzer, R. (2013). Prevention of poststernotomy wound infections in obese patients by negative pressure wound therapy. *The Journal of Thoracic and Cardiovascular Surgery, 145*(5), 1387–1392; Hartsell, T. L. (2008). Postoperative infection in cardiac surgery. In J. V. Conte, W. A. Baumgartner, S. G. Owens, & T. Dorman, T. (Eds.), *The Johns Hopkins manual of cardiac surgical care* (2nd ed., 361–388). Philadelphia, PA: Mosby Elsevier; Mishra, P. K., Ashoub, A., Sallayeh, K., Aktuerk, D., Ohri, S., Raja, S. G., . . . Luckraz, H. (2014). Role of topical application of gentamicin containing collagen implants in cardiac surgery. *Journal of Cardiothoracic Surgery, 9*(122), 1–20.

Local Collagen-Gentamicin

The use of local collagen-gentamicin sponges has been found to reduce the incidence of SWIs caused by all major clinically important microbiological agents, including coagulase-negative *Staphylococcus* (CoNS) (Friberg et al., 2009; Godbole, Pai, Kolvekar, & Wilson, 2012; Mishra et al., 2014). Godbole and colleagues noted that two of four randomized controlled trials (RCTs) showed benefits when used in both routine and emergent surgeries. One RCT showed sternal rebleeding occurring when gentamicin sponges were used in double layers. Another RCT showed that there was no significant difference between the gentamicin arm and the control arm when treating patients at high risk for SWIs (diabetics, obesity of body mass index [BMI] > 30, or both). This study did have a few patients with methicillin-resistant *Staphylococcus aureus* (MRSA), which gentamicin does not affect (Bennett-Guerrero et al., 2010). Friberg and colleagues (2009) found that aminoglycoside resistance

did not increase during a long-term study lasting more than 2 years. If a patient has a suspected infection prior to an elective operation, the infection source and site need to be identified and treated before the patient undergoes surgery. Elective surgery should be postponed until the infection has resolved.

Hair Removal

It is recommended not to remove hair preoperatively unless the hair at or around the incision site might interfere with the surgical procedure. If hair removal is necessary, hair should be removed with electrical clippers or a depilatory agent rather than the traditional shaving method. Clipping is recommended to be performed immediately prior to the operation—but completed outside of the operating room (OR) (Anderson et al., 2014).

Preoperative Skin Cleansing

Cleansing the patient's skin at least the night before surgery is imperative. In particular, removing gross contaminants by showering or bathing, and then cleansing the skin with a preparation that lowers microbial skin burden, has been shown to be effective in lowering the incidence of SSIs (Anderson et al., 2014; Edmiston et al., 2013; Edmiston, Okoli, Graham, Sinski, & Seabrook, 2010; Graling & Vasaly, 2013).

Several antimicrobial preparations are currently available: chlorhexidine gluconate (CHG), povidone-iodine, alcohol, and triclosan (an antibacterial chemical). Reports suggest that CHG is the superior product in terms of its ability to remove the microbial burden on the skin and to maintain a greater residual activity hours after the skin is prepared (Anderson et al., 2014; Chien, Lin, & Hsu, 2014; Edmiston et al., 2013; Eiselt, 2009; Lipke & Hyott, 2010). In addition, CHG no rinse reduces MRSA and vancomycin-resistant *Enterococcus* (VRE) counts and reduces risk for central line infections. *Acinetobacter* counts did not decrease (Karki & Cheng, 2012).

Two methods are currently used to prepare patients' skin:

- The rinse-off method, which uses a CHG 4% solution or presoaked scrub packets
- The no-rinse method, which uses CHG 2% presoaked preparation cloths, allowing a residual barrier layer once skin dries

To lower the microbial count, it is recommended to apply the antiseptic several times. Studies comparing these two methods have shown some positive results with the no-rinse method (Edmiston et al., 2013; Edmiston et al., 2010; Eiselt, 2009; Lipke & Hyott, 2010). With this method, the patient takes an initial shower to wash any gross contaminants off the skin and to enhance comfort. After a minimum of 1 hour, the no-rinse method cloth is used to prepare the skin. It is recommended that the no-rinse method be used at least once the evening before and again the morning of surgery. It is then followed by the skin preparation in the OR (Darouiche et al., 2010).

Skin preparation in the OR before surgery begins is standard practice. An ideal surgical skin antiseptic has the ability to significantly reduce microorganisms, has a rapid and persistent effect, has broad spectrum activity, and is easy to use. Darouiche and colleagues (2010) compared use of CHG to use of povidone-iodine as preoperative skin preparation. Chlorhexidine gluconate was significantly more protective against both superficial and deep incisional infections; no difference was noted in organ/space infections. The effects are most likely related to CHG's more rapid and prolonged action, continued activity with exposure to body fluids, and its residual effect (Darouiche et al., 2010).

MRSA Prophylaxis

Staphylococcus aureus is a frequent offender in sternal wound infections. The nares are known to be colonized with *S. aureus* in approximately 20% of the healthy population (Cove et al., 2012). Infections post coronary artery bypass surgery are due to *S. aureus*, including resistant strains, 40% to 80% of the time (Bryan & Yarbrough, 2013; Chen et al., 2012; Cove et al., 2012). Mupirocin (Bactroban®) ointment, a topical antibiotic, is effective in treating nasal colonization, including some resistant strains of this pathogen (Bode et al., 2010). Mupirocin, given intranasally, is recommended preoperatively for all cardiac surgical patients in the absence of documented *S. aureus* colonization testing (Bryan & Yarbrough, 2013). It is administered by the patient for a period up to 5 days to reduce any nasal colonization involving *S. aureus*. Treatment should begin at least 1 day preoperatively and may extend into the postoperative period until the treatment is complete (Walsh, Greene, & Kirshner, 2011).

Phillips and colleagues (2014) conducted an investigator-initiated, open-label randomized study comparing use of mupirocin for 5 days twice daily versus two applications of povidone-iodine solution in each nostril 2 hours prior to incision. Both treatments were found effective. The povidone-iodine may be a viable alternative treatment, and it is slated for future studies in multiple centers. This is worth considering in light of the potential for mupirocin resistance and costs (povidone-iodine treatment is less expensive).

Preoperative Antibiotic Administration

Preoperative antibiotic administration should be performed for all cardiac surgical patients to reduce their risk of postoperative infection (Bryan & Yarbrough, 2013; Hillis et al., 2012). This measure reduces the incidence of infection fivefold; *S. aureus* has been identified as the infective organism in more than 50% of all SSIs (Chen et al., 2012). A cephalosporin is the preferred prophylactic agent of choice for cardiac surgery procedures in populations who do not have a high incidence of MRSA (Hillis et al., 2012). Data suggest that prophylaxis with glycopeptides, such as vancomycin (Vancocin®), is more effective in preventing infection by methicillin-resistant organisms, but is less effective in countering methicillin-sensitive organisms (Hillis et al., 2012). One or two doses of a glycopeptide in combination with a cephalosporin are reasonable when a healthcare facility has a "high incidence" of MRSA, the patient is especially susceptible to colonization, or the patient is having a prosthetic valve or vascular graft inserted (Chen et al., 2012).

If a patient is allergic to cephalosporins, a glycopeptide should not be used as a sole agent because it does not provide any coverage for Gram-negative organisms. In such a case, it is recommended that an aminoglycoside be used in addition to the glycopeptide.

Prophylaxis is accomplished by administering one preoperative dose and one postoperative dose (Bratzler et al., 2013). Correctly timing the preoperative antibiotic dose is essential so that a bactericidal concentration of the drug is present in the patient's serum and tissues by the time the skin incision is made (Bratzler et al., 2013; Cove et al., 2012). With the cephalosporins, the dose needs to be administered within 30–60 minutes of the time the incision is made. It is best accomplished by the anesthesiologist after induction of anesthesia and may be included in the call to order and OR checklist processes. The surgeon should confirm that the antibiotic dosing has occurred prior to the scalpel being in hand. If the length of the operative procedure exceeds 3 hours, redosing is mandated based on cephalosporin pharmacokinetics. Redosing should occur at intervals of 2 half-lives (measured from time the preoperative dose was administered) (Anderson et al., 2014). If the combination of a glycopeptide and an aminoglycoside is used, the medications are usually administered over a 60- to 90-minute period (dependent on dosage) to avoid red-man syndrome and impairing renal function. There is no associated benefit to administering prophylactic antibiotics beyond 48 hours (Anderson et al., 2014; Bratzler et al., 2013; Cove et al., 2012).

Glycemic Control

According to a 2009 consensus statement by the American Association of Clinical Endocrinologists and American Diabetes Association, for patients who are not critically ill (e.g., cardiac surgery patients who are preparing for discharge and are healing at home), it is recommended that preprandial serum glucose should be 110 mg/dL, up to a maximum of 180 mg/dL (Moghissi et al., 2009). Attaining these goals reduces mortality, reduces length of stay (LOS) in hospital, improves healing potential, and lessens the risk of mediastinitis (Hillis et al., 2012; Lazar et al., 2009). As of January 2014, the Surgical Care Improvement

Project (SCIP)—Infection Prevention 4 (SCIP-Inf 4) measure changed. Blood glucose levels must be maintained less than 180 mg/dL between 18 and 24 hours after anesthesia end time (Klinkner & Murray, 2014). Pezzella, Holmes, Pritchard, Speir, and Ad (2014) compared a tight target (90–120 mg/dL) versus a liberal target (121–180 mg/dL) in diabetic and nondiabetic patients and found that the liberal target was easier to maintain and stay within the target levels, avoiding hypoglycemic events. These patients were contacted at 6 months and 40 ($\pm$4.4) months after surgery; the survival rate was the same in both groups (diabetics included), and physical health-related quality of life was improved in the liberal group.

Appropriate glycemic control is accomplished by assessing the patient preoperatively for elevated HbA_{1c} levels, noting any history of diabetes, and checking for any elevated serum glucose. If a patient's HbA_{1c} level is greater than 7%, the risk for morbidity and mortality is known to be significantly increased. The patient should begin insulin therapy at least 1 day before surgery (Lazar et al., 2009; McDonnell, Alexanian, White, & Lazar, 2012). Ideally, achieving adequate glycemic control before the patient's admission for surgery will lower the risk for infection (Lazar et al., 2009).

If patients have elevated serum glucose levels, they should be treated with a continuous intravenous insulin infusion immediately prior to, during, and immediately following surgery in the postanesthesia care unit and the ICU. Hargraves (2014) describes use of an insulin infusion protocol post cardiac surgery. She found that educating the nursing team on glycemic control and implementing an insulin infusion protocol developed by an interdisciplinary team improved overall glycemic control and minimized hypoglycemic episodes. Klinkner and Murray (2014) found that improving access of insulin orders, using an insulin infusion protocol, developing a nursing protocol to initiate the insulin infusions, and increasing frequency/regularity of glucose monitoring improved postoperative glycemic protocol in cardiac surgery patients. It is suggested that published protocols in the literature be reviewed, and that one be selected that is appropriate for the respective facility. Regardless of which protocol is followed, serum glucose levels should be checked frequently (e.g., every 1 to 2 hours during this timeframe) to adjust the insulin infusion.

Once the patient is being advanced on a diet, serum glucose targets should be adjusted to 150 mg/dL as a mean target (100–140 mg/dL preprandial; 180 mg/dL maximum serum glucose) (McDonnell et al., 2012). The patient is then transitioned from the intravenous insulin to a combination of subcutaneous injections: basal, nutritional, and a supplemental corrective dosing (McDonnell et al., 2012; Moghissi et al., 2009). Noninsulin agents have limited use in the hospital secondary to irregular meal intake. Caution must be used with the oral agents to prevent complications (Moghissi et al., 2009). Sulfonylureas can be started slowly based on patient's dietary intake. Patients must have a documented return to normal or baseline renal function before restarting metformin (McDonnell et al., 2012). If serum glucose levels remain elevated, consultation with an endocrinologist to attain tighter glycemic control is advisable.

Avoiding Potentially Contaminated Sources

Reestablishing the skin barrier can prevent the onset of superficial infections. Diabetes, obesity, and renal failure are all conditions that can delay wound closure. Dressings are not the only way to protect the incision site. Electrocardiogram wires are known to be a source of infection; disposable lead wires are now available and should be considered for SSI prevention (Brown, 2011). Reusable blood pressure cuffs have also been noted to be infection sources; disposable cuffs are now available. Individual stethoscopes should be cleansed with alcohol after each individual patient assessment. It is imperative that the nurse assess the incision regularly and protect the incision as it heals.

Postoperative Dressings

Postoperative incisional dressing assessment should be performed upon admission and every 4 hours thereafter until the patient is transferred out of the ICU. To minimize the risk of infection, most cardiac surgical centers opt to keep the initial dressing on the incision for 24 to 48 hours, as per CDC recommendations.

If the patient is experiencing a coagulopathy, a small amount of blood or blood-tinged fluid may drain from the incisional site. The dressing should be changed when it becomes saturated using sterile technique. Dumville, Gray, Walter, Sharp, and Page (2014) reviewed 16 RCTs comparing use of different types of dressings or no dressing and found they showed no difference in healing, degree of infection, comfort, or amount of scarring. Silver-impregnated dressings (Huckfeldt et al., 2008) need a large controlled study to determine effects on wound healing, infection prevention, and a cost–benefit analysis. Negative pressure incision management systems have been utilized in some centers over closed incisions for the first 6–10 days on high-risk patients (e.g., obese or diabetic patients) with good success (Colli, 2011; Grauhan et al., 2013). Optimal dressing characteristics are permeable to allow for gas exchange, impermeable to prevent microorganism and exogenous sources of contamination, and the ability to provide an insulating effect. Dressing decisions should be based on cost and managing specific conditions, such as drainage absorption (Dumville et al., 2014).

Evaluation of the Incision Site: Phases of Incision Healing

An incision goes through three major phases as it heals. During the inflammatory phase, after the incision is made, a cascade of clotting and immune responses produces inflammation at the incision site. After incisional closure, neutrophils migrate toward the fibrin clot at the margins of the incision and fill in the incisional space. During the proliferative phase, new capillaries are formed, and fibrin, collagen, and growth factors spread across the wound bed. Basophils (white blood cells) migrate to the incision borders and multiply. During the maturation phase, collagen matrix development furthers wound closure. As keratinization occurs, the skin thickness returns to normal (Rote & Huether, 2010). Recent studies have found that placement of additional fixation wires at the lower sternum, along with prophylaxis with a local collagen-gentamicin, decreases the incidence of deep sternal wound infections (Friberg et al., 2009; Godbole et al., 2012).

After waiting the designated time stated in the institution's protocol, performing appropriate hand hygiene, and donning clean gloves, the nurse should remove and discard the dressing. Initially, the incision site may appear slightly red around the edges. The edges should be well approximated, with minimal tension evident. The surrounding tissue should display no inflammation, hematoma, swelling, erythema, skin discoloration, or warmth, and it should not cause pain when palpated. Several variables, if present, need to be documented and brought to the attention of the surgeon; the variables indicative of an infection are listed in **Table 18-4**.

Saphenous vein graft infections occur more frequently in patients with obesity, diabetes, extracardiac arteriopathy, decreased glomerular filtration rate, or any combination of these. Staples versus suture closure of leg wounds after vein harvest have no

Table 18-4   Variables Indicative of Infection
A nonapproximated incision Excessive pain and tenderness Redness, odor, or swelling Wound breakdown Exudate (Note the amount—none, minimal, moderate, heavy leakage through the bandage—and type—serous/straw-colored fluid or serosanguineous/red fluid, as well as any frank blood or pus [creamy yellow or green].) Sternal instability Fever ($> 38.0°$ C)

statistically significant difference in complications based on three trial reviews (Biancari & Tiozzo, 2010). Drainage of noninfected serosanguineous fluid from leg incisions is common. Oftentimes, the drainage results from an underlying hematoma that has liquefied and is draining out of the neighboring skin incision. The presence of erythema, induration, and undue tenderness to palpation indicates infection. In such cases, the patient may require a dilation and curettage procedure, followed by open packing of the wound and administration of antibiotics.

If unresolved, these infections, late lower limb ischemia, or both can lead to the need for further interventions, including skin grafts, vascular procedures, or even amputations (Biancari, Kangasniemi, Mahar, & Ylonen, 2008).

NURSING RESPONSIBILITIES TO ENHANCE WOUND HEALING

The radial artery site is easy to assess because of its visibility. Regular assessments (minimum every 2 hours) should always include color, capillary refill time, temperature, and presence of an ulnar artery pulse. Assessment for an underlying incision hematoma is imperative because its presence may impede

blood flow to the hand and lead to loss of function. Elevation of the arm and affected hand on pillows will help decrease any edema.

The multitude of factors that may potentially affect wound healing should be examined for each individual patient. Providing for optimal wound healing, eliminating any underlying causative or contributory factors, and stimulating positive physiologic factors required for the healing process are essential ICU nursing interventions. Optimizing the patient's nutritional status, including assuring that the patient is consuming a diet with adequate protein and caloric intake, trace metals, and vitamins, is equally essential. Collaboration with a dietitian is recommended.

The ICU nurse should also assess the patient's emotional and psychosocial status. Depression makes it difficult for a patient to be fully compliant with treatment regimens, which may potentially inhibit wound healing. Ensuring adequate pain control helps enhance the patient's willingness to be active and ability to adhere to treatment regimens. If the patient has an elevated serum glucose level, close monitoring to maintain tight glycemic control to promote wound healing is required. Renal or liver insufficiency also requires correction because both of these conditions will impede healing. Finally, ICU nurses must implement measures to optimize perfusion and oxygenation and promote early ambulation, as soon as feasible. Early goal-directed mobilization helps minimize complications of immobility and delirium and decreases LOS both in ICU and hospital (Barr et al., 2013; Meyer et al., 2013).

WOUND INFECTION SEQUELAE

When wound infections occur, they can be devastating. Most SSIs are identified on a post-hospitalization basis. They can require frequent outpatient and emergency department (ED) visits, radiology services, lab work, home health services, hospital readmissions for treatment, and possibly, further surgery. In addition, the patient and family will deal with the consequences of a loss in the patient's productivity. In particular, the patient may be out of work for an extended period of time. The patient's functional status may be decreased, such that the individual requires assistance to complete activities of daily living, including transportation to and from the many visits for health care.

Impact of Postoperative Infection

There are more than 230 million operations worldwide annually. Infections are estimated to occur in approximately 5% of the patients. This is a significant healthcare issue both economically and as a potential detriment to patient morbidity/mortality (Chen et al., 2012; Walter, Dumville, Sharp, & Page, 2012). Surgical site infections can add an additional 10 hospital days to a patient's LOS (Chen et al., 2012). Hospital costs can range from $40,000–$53,000 higher with SSIs, particularly MRSA (Lipke & Hyott, 2010).

Reducing the potential for any SSI to occur is a paramount concern with any surgical procedure. Approximately 300,000–400,000 SSIs occur in conjunction with the estimated 45 million surgical procedures performed in the United States annually (Lobdell, Stamou, & Sanchez, 2012). The Deficit Reduction Act, passed in 2005, allows the Centers for Medicare & Medicaid Services (CMS) to adjust payments downward for patients experiencing hospital-acquired infections; this provision took effect in October 2008. As of October 1, 2008, the CMS no longer reimburses for hospital-acquired conditions such as SSIs—specifically, mediastinitis after coronary artery bypass grafting (CABG) surgery (Richter, Jarrett, & LaBresh, 2014) or flap surgery due to an SSI. Hospitals are now paid at the "without complications rate" when such SSI-related events occur, instead of the "with complications" higher rate that

they had been receiving in the past (Richter et al., 2014). The impact of this change in billing practice on hospitals' financial status can be considerable.

Surgical site infections affect numerous parties: the patient, insurance companies, medical caregivers, and hospitals. There has been increasing focus on preventing SSIs as one element of the Institute for Healthcare Improvement's initiatives in the "Protect 5 Million Lives from Harm" campaign (McCannon, Hackbarth, & Griffin, 2007).

The general trend is toward surgical patients who are increasingly sicker and have more complex comorbidities. Many of these patients are elderly (older than 80 years). When these patients get SSIs, increasing numbers of them are infected with resistant strains of microbes (e.g., MRSA and VRE).

WOUND INFECTION PREDICTION

The CDC's NHSN, formerly the National Nosocomial Infection Surveillance System, predicts the risk of SSI based on three factors: length of surgery, wound class, and the patient's American Society of Anesthesiology score (Maragakis et al., 2009). This system has not been adapted specifically for cardiac surgery.

The first scale to predict surgical wound infections in CABG patients was developed in 1998 (Hussey, Leeper, & Hynan, 1998; Troutman, Hussey, Hynan, & Lucisano, 2001). This scale, which is known as the Sternal Wound Infection Predictor Scale (SWIPS), consists of weighted predictors related to the preoperative, intraoperative, and postoperative phases of care (see **Table 18-5**).

In 1986, the Society of Thoracic Surgeons developed its first risk scoring system for CABGs. This has been updated several times with the latest update published in 2009 (Shahian et al., 2009a). The society has created two additional scoring systems

Table 18-5 Sternal Wound Infection Predictor Scale (SWIPS)	
Variable	**Weight**
Preoperative	
Smoking	9
Diabetes mellitus	
IDDM	7
NIDDM	5
COPD	8
Preoperative ICU stay	4
Obesity (> 30 kg/m^2)	4
Advanced age (> 70 years)	3
Sex (male)	1
Impaired immune response	8
Intraoperative	
Bilateral ITA	6
Single ITA	3
Long operative time (> 4 hr)	7
Reexploration for bleeding	6
Long cardiopulmonary bypass time (> 2 hr)	6
Postoperative	
Hypoperfusion/hypotension	8
Ventilator support (> 48 hr)	6
Pharmacologic support	
Dopamine/dobutamine only	2
All others	6
Postoperative CPR	7
Hypoxemia	5
Banked blood transfusions	3

COPD, chronic obstructive pulmonary disease; CPR, cardiopulmonary resuscitation; ICU, intensive care unit; IDDM, insulin-dependent diabetes mellitus; ITA, internal thoracic artery; NIDDM, non-insulin-dependent diabetes mellitus.

Source: Reprinted from *Heart & Lung, 27*(5), Hussey, LC., Leeper, B., & Hynan, L. S. (1998). Development of the Sternal Wound Infection Prediction Scale, Pages 326–336, Copyright 1998, with permission from Elsevier.

predicting risk for infection following valve surgery (O'Brien et al., 2009) and one for combination valve surgery plus CABG (Shahian et al., 2009b), which includes both preoperative and intraoperative scores and takes several variables into account.

Currently, mediastinitis occurs in 0.25% to 4.0% of cardiac surgical patients, with more than 50% of these infections involving *S. aureus* and *S. epidermidis*. Those with a major infection had higher mortality than those without an infection (17% vs. 3%) and were more likely to have a prolonged hospital LOS, often exceeding 14 days (Bryan & Yarbrough, 2013).

MANAGEMENT OF WOUND INFECTIONS

Sternal Wound Infections

Sternal wound infections may be superficial, involving only the skin and subcutaneous fat, or they may be deep, involving the sternum and underlying structures. Superficial infections are characterized by drainage from the wound and local inflammation, even as the underlying sternum remains stable (see Box 18-1). In this instance, removal of the overlying skin sutures, culture of the drainage, administration of antibiotics, and local dressings are often effective interventions. Reconstructive surgery can be avoided in clinically stable patients with the use of vacuum-assisted closure (Deniz et al., 2012).

Mediastinitis

Bacterial mediastinitis starts when the invasion of a pathogen causes an inflammatory response. The invading bacteria proliferate, and the body forms a thick layer of fibrin in an attempt to encapsulate the foreign agents. An area of dead space forms underneath the sternum as the infection expands through sinus tracts that have formed. The patient develops fever, and the systemic inflammatory response causes production of leukocytes and pro-inflammatory mediators. Staphylococci, including CoNS (usually *S. epidermidis* or *S. aureus*), have been identified as the most common causative agents of SWIs (Mishra et al., 2014).

Mediastinitis can develop as early as 7 to 10 days following a cardiac surgical procedure. Patients have often been discharged home before any sign of this infection occurs. Oftentimes, the first sign is significant serous drainage that appears 4 to 5 days postoperatively. Patients experience fever, chills, pain, and leukocytosis within 2 to 5 days after the onset of infection. Erythema may form on the outside borders of the incision and is often first seen at the xiphoid process. Occasionally, a section of the incision may dehisce and purulent drainage will exude from the site.

More commonly, mediastinitis becomes evident later in the postoperative course, usually within 30 days after surgery. Patients often develop sternal pain, become lethargic, and demonstrate unwillingness to do many activities that they were doing previously. The incision then begins to drain purulent fluid and will separate. Upon assessment, the nurse often finds that the sternum is unstable, with the borders rubbing against each other. Pain will be worse with respiration. Fever, chills, and leukocytosis are evident.

Treatment of mediastinitis depends on the stage of the infectious process at the time of diagnosis. If identified early, the sternum is not destroyed—success may be achieved with prompt surgical intervention, debridement of the sternal edges, copious irrigation of the mediastinum, placement of retrosternal irrigation and drainage catheters, rewiring of the sternum, and closure of the fascia and skin. Appropriate intravenous antibiotic therapy is given for a minimum of 7 days. The results of a Gram stain are utilized to identify the appropriate antibiotic to infuse through an irrigating catheter, with the fluid being directed to exit via drainage catheters. The irrigation

continues for 3 to 5 days, until the drainage is sterile as confirmed by culture. Although frequently successful, this treatment method can have serious complications—for example, erosion of the catheters into mediastinal structures and systemic toxicity from absorption of the irrigating antibiotic. For these reasons, this procedure is reserved for specific groups of patients (Lemmer & Vlahakes, 2010; Shi, Qi, & Zhang, 2014).

More longstanding, advanced infections are associated with large amounts of suppurative fluid in the mediastinum, loss of integrity of the sternum, and diffuse cellulitis of the skin and subcutaneous tissue. Patients with such infections may require opening of the sternum and debridement of necrotic tissue, exposure and draining of the mediastinum, and packing of the wound with moist gauze. Vacuum-assisted closure therapy can be used as a bridge between debridement and closure of the wound. It can assist in decreasing overall wound edema, reduce bacterial counts in the wound, and reduce the time to closing the wound (Deniz et al., 2012; Hillis et al., 2012; Shi et al., 2014). After control of the infection is achieved and a healthy-appearing bed of granulation tissue forms, secondary closure is performed with or without a muscle flap. The treatment plan depends on severity of the infection and may involve a combination of debridement, packing, closure delay, reconstruction, rewiring, and irrigation with antibiotics (Deniz et al., 2012).

The most frequently used approach to treating serious mediastinitis is a single-stage procedure in which radical debridement of the sternum and cartilage is performed with advanced muscle flaps, using the pectoralis major and/or rectus muscles (Deniz et al., 2012). Depending on the degree of sternal resection required, the remaining bone tissue may or may not be approximated. Soft silastic drains are placed beneath the muscle flaps and connected to gentle suction. Often performed by a plastic surgeon, this procedure may be associated with decreased morbidity and mortality and a decreased LOS. The patient may be discharged home with the drains in place. The drains remain in place until the daily drainage volume becomes small; they may then be removed in the healthcare provider's office. Early aggressive use of debridement and muscle flaps in serious mediastinitis is considered the optimal approach (Hillis et al., 2012; Vlajcic et al., 2007).

Several long-term complications are associated with mediastinitis. Notably, patients have a significant increase in mortality during the first year and subsequent 4 years. The potential for other nosocomial infections, including systemic infections, is increased as well. Patients may develop sepsis and organ system failure. Identifying mediastinitis early allows for earlier treatment and is associated with a better prognosis (Vlajcic et al., 2007).

For patients who have a relatively uneventful postoperative course, discharge may occur on the third or fourth postoperative day. Many infections do not become evident until after the patient has been discharged, which makes early diagnosis of sternal infection and mediastinitis after cardiac surgery difficult. In some patients, fever, leukocytosis, and a positive blood culture will be the first manifestations of a hidden infection that will become obvious only later. The most common early sign is fluid drainage from the wound; sternal instability usually develops subsequently.

Clear and thorough patient education reviewing the appearance of a normally healing incision is of utmost importance in recognizing postoperative wound infections. The patient and family members must be instructed to frequently observe the incision for any changes in status and to call the surgeon's office if changes or questions arise (see **Box 18-3**). Given the trend toward earlier hospital discharge following cardiac surgery, fewer SSIs will be detected prior to patient discharge. Without careful supervision and intervention, the physical and financial costs of these infections will increase.

Effective wound infection prevention strategies and opportunities for group review of data are essential for all cardiac surgical programs. Members of the interdisciplinary team must continuously review the literature and revise practices and guidelines based on the latest evidence. Process measures and compliance must be assessed, and education must be initiated whenever deviations are noted.

Box 18-3   Patient/Family Discharge Education Regarding Incision Care

Emphasize the following points when explaining wound care at home:
- Shower daily with soap and water.
- Avoid sitting in bathtub.
- A dressing is needed only if drainage is present.
- Remove any dressings applied during hospitalization on the day after going home.
- Inspect the wound daily using a mirror. If you see any redness, irritation, swelling, tenderness, or unusual drainage, contact the surgeon or surgeon on call.

Optimal Patient Outcomes
- Patient can perform appropriate incision care.
- Patient has no signs and symptoms of infection.
- Patient can list signs and symptoms of infection.
- Patient modifies lifestyle to reduce risk factors that may impede wound healing.

SUMMARY

Sternal wound infections occur in a small percentage of patients who undergo cardiac surgery. There is a high associated cost in terms of morbidity, mortality, LOS, time away from work, and financial costs if an infection develops. Infected patients have increased potential for pain and delirium, often seen as complications of immobility and prolonged ICU and hospital stays. Delirium can have deleterious long-term effects post hospitalization (Barr et al., 2013; Jenks, Laurent, McQuarry, & Watkins, 2014).

A number of predictive variables have been identified that put the patient at greater risk for development of an SWI, and a number of preventive strategies must be implemented to avoid development of this potentially catastrophic complication. A strong team approach utilizing evidenced-based practices is statistically significant in minimizing sternal infections (Travis et al., 2009). Although an SWI is not likely to develop while the patient is in the ICU postoperatively, initiation of preventive measures must begin while the patient is in the early phase of recovery. The ICU nurse has a pivotal role in preventing SWIs and beginning the essential patient and family education that must be accomplished to help ensure optimal postoperative outcomes are attained.

CASE STUDY

A 77-year-old obese male patient who underwent CABG surgery for left main stenosis has a history of diabetes and mild COPD. The patient had excessive postoperative bleeding from the chest tube necessitating a return to the OR. His postoperative course was otherwise uncomplicated. He was successfully discharged home. Two weeks postoperatively, he returned to the ED with fever, chills, tachycardia, shortness of breath, and chest wall tenderness adjacent to the median sternotomy wound. The symptoms have been present for the past 2 days.

Critical Thinking Questions

1. What should the nurse suspect as being the underlying cause of this patient's condition?
2. What risk factors did the patient have for this complication?
3. What are the nursing implications for this situation?

Answers to Critical Thinking Questions

1. This patient is manifesting signs and symptoms of mediastinitis.
2. Patient's age, gender (male), left main stenosis, obesity, COPD, diabetes, and increased blood transfusion requirements.
3. Before discharge, the nurse should have reviewed normal healing and symptoms of complications that should be observed for. Given the patient's risk factors, the patient should have been told why he is at risk for mediastinitis. The patient should have been taught any appropriate wound care. When this patient presented with mediastinitis, verification that all of this discharge teaching occurred should take place. Efforts to prevent such complications in the future can be enhanced with root cause analyses being performed to identify deficits in care.

SELF-ASSESSMENT QUESTIONS

1. Which of the following patients is at greatest risk for wound complications following cardiac surgery?
   a. A 68-year-old with BMI 24 kg/m^2
   b. A 65-year-old with chronic bronchitis
   c. A 50-year-old with HbA$_{1c}$ 5.5%
   d. A 60-year-old with albumin level 2.5 mg/dL

2. Use of which of the following vessels for grafts puts the patient at increased risk of postoperative infection?
   a. Internal thoracic artery
   b. Radial artery
   c. Saphenous vein
   d. Gastroepiploic artery

3. Which of the following intraoperative conditions puts the patient at increased risk for postoperative infections?
   a. Need for fewer coronary artery grafts
   b. Shorter pump runs
   c. Shortened hypothermia time
   d. Decreased cardiac index

4. Which of the following patients is at greatest risk for a postoperative wound infection following cardiac surgery? A patient:
   a. with a rubber dam
   b. needing autotransfusion of mediastinal blood
   c. with peripheral edema
   d. with an elevated cardiac output

5. Which of the following patients should be suspected as having a deep incisional surgical site infection? A patient with:
   a. an infection and drainage to an organ related to surgery
   b. dehiscence of a superficial incision
   c. organisms aseptically obtained from tissue of an incision
   d. purulent drainage from an incision of a sterile sternum

6. Which of the following is suggested to help ensure adequate glycemic control for postoperative cardiac surgery patients?
   a. Begin an insulin infusion if blood glucose > 180 mg/dL
   b. Monitor blood glucose levels every 2 hours
   c. Target blood glucose level range 80–110 mg/dL if on an insulin infusion
   d. Use the recommended protocol published in the literature

7. Which of the following is a target blood glucose level for a postoperative cardiac surgery patient who is advancing on a diet?
   a. 80 mg/dL preprandial
   b. 110 mg/dL preprandial
   c. 140 mg/dL maximum
   d. 150 mg/dL maximum

8. Presence of which of the following should cause the nurse to suspect presence of an infection?
   a. Approximated wound
   b. Hematoma
   c. Minimal wound tension
   d. Incision site slightly red at edges

9. A patient with a BMI of 31 kg/m^2 has a saphenous vein graft. Erythema and induration are noted. For which of the following should the nurse anticipate preparing the patient?
   a. Wound irrigation and closure with packing
   b. Dilation and curettage
   c. Open sternotomy and evacuation of any hematomas
   d. Use of no-rinse CHG 2% twice daily

10. Nursing responsibilities to enhance wound healing following cardiac surgery may include:
    a. limiting ambulation until the wound is approximated.
    b. encouraging consumption of a high-carbohydrate diet for energy.
    c. discouraging resuming use of antidepressants until discharge.
    d. administering pain medication as needed.

Answers to Self-Assessment Questions

1. b
2. a
3. d
4. b
5. a
6. c
7. b
8. b
9. b
10. d

Clinical Inquiry Box

Question: What is the incidence of mediastinitis, its risk factors, and its effect on early and long-term survival?

Reference: Risnes, I., Abdelnoor, M., Almdahl, S. M., & Svennerig, J. L. (2010). Mediastinitis after coronary artery bypass grafting: Risk factors and long-term survival. *Annals of Thoracic Surgery, 89,* 1502–1510.

Objective: To determine the incidence of mediastinitis, its risk factors, and its effect on early and long-term survival.

Method: Dual design; case-control and retrospective cohort of 18,532 consecutive patients who underwent CABG procedures over a 12-year period.

Results: 0.6% of patients developed mediastinitis. The diagnosis was made during days 9 and 19 postoperatively. The identified risk factors in these patients were advanced age, male gender, left main stenosis, BMI 30 kg/m^2 or higher, COPD, diabetes, and increased blood transfusion requirements. There was no increase in early mortality. There was an increased risk of need for intra-aortic balloon pump therapy, ventricular tachycardia, supraventricular tachycardia, stroke, need for inotrope therapy, and myocardial infarction. Survival rates were 49.5% versus 71% in patients who developed mediastinitis and those who did not, respectively. There were more cardiac-related deaths in the patients who developed mediastinitis.

Conclusion: There was a low incidence of mediastinitis in these patients.

REFERENCES

Anderson, D. J., Podgorny, K., Berrios-Torres, S. I., Bratzler, D. W., Dellinger, E. P., Greene, L., . . . Kaye, K. S. (2014). Strategies to prevent surgical site infections in acute care hospitals: 2014 update. *Infection Control & Hospital Epidemiology, 35*(6), 605–627.

Barr, J., Fraser, G. L., Puntillo, K., Ely, E. W., Gélinas, C., Dasta, J. F., . . . Jaeschke, R. (2013). Clinical practice guidelines for the management of pain, agitation, and delirium in adult patients in the intensive care unit. *Critical Care Medicine, 41*(1), 263–306.

Bennett-Guerrero, E., Ferguson, T. B., Lin, M., Garg, J., Mark, D. B., Scavo, V. A., Jr., . . . Corey, G. R. (2010). Effect of an implantable gentamicin-collagen sponge on sternal wound infections following cardiac surgery: A randomized trial. *Journal of the American Medical Association, 304*(7), 755–762.

Berg, L. T., & Jaakkola, P. (2013). Kuopio treatment strategy after deep sternal wound infection. *Scandinavian Journal of Surgery, 102*(1), 3–8.

Biancari, F., Kangasniemi, O. P., Mahar, M. A., & Ylonen, K. (2008). Need for late lower limb revascularization and major amputation after coronary artery bypass surgery. *European Journal of Vascular & Endovascular Surgery, 35*(5), 596–602.

Biancari, F., & Tiozzo, V. (2010). Staples versus sutures for closing leg wounds after vein graft harvesting for coronary artery bypass surgery. *Cochrane Database of Systematic Reviews, 5:* CD008057. doi: 10.1002/14651858. CD008057.pub2

Bilgin, Y. M., Van de Watering, L. M., Versteegh, M. I., Van Oers, M. H., Vamvakas, E. C., & Brand, A. (2011). Postoperative complications associated with transfusion of platelets and plasma in cardiac surgery. *Transfusion, 51*(12), 2603–2610.

Bode, L. G., Kluytmans, J. A., Wertheim, H. F., Bogaers, D., Vandenbroucke-Grauls, C., Roosendaal, R., . . . Ves, M. C. (2010). Preventing surgical-site infections in nasal carriers of *Staphylococcus aureus. New England Journal of Medicine, 362*(1), 9–17.

Boeken, U., Feindt, P., Schurr, P., Assmann, A., Akhyari, P., & Lichtenberg, A. (2011). Delayed sternal closure (dsc) after cardiac surgery: Outcome and prognostic markers. *Journal of Cardiac Surgery, 26*(1), 22–27.

Bratzler, D., Dellinger, E. P., Olsen, K., Perl, T., Auwaerter, P., Bolon, M., . . . Weinstein, R. A. (2013). Clinical practice guidelines for antimicrobial prophylaxis in surgery. *American Journal of Health-System Pharmacy, 70*(3), 195–283.

Brown, D. (2011). Disposable vs reusable electrocardiography leads in development of and cross-contamination by resistant bacteria. *Critical Care Nurse, 31*(3), 62–69.

Bryan, C. S., & Yarbrough, W. M. (2013). Preventing deep wound infections after coronary artery bypass grafting. *Texas Heart Institute Journal, 40*(2), 125–139.

Centers for Disease Control and Prevention. (2014). *CDC/NHSN Surveillance Definitions for Specific Types of Infections.* Retrieved from http://www.cdc.gov/nhsn/PDFs/pscManual/17pscNosInfDef_current.pdf

Chen, L. F., Arduino, J. M., Sheng, S., Muhlbaier, L. H., Kanafani, Z. A., Harris, A. D., . . . Fowler, V. G., Jr. (2012). Epidemiology and outcome of major postoperative infections following cardiac surgery: Risk factors and impact of pathogen type. *American Journal of Infection Control, 40*(10), 963–968.

Chien, C. Y., Lin, C. H., & Hsu, R. B. (2014). Care bundle to prevent methicillin-resistant *Staphylococcus aureus* sternal wound infection after off-pump coronary artery bypass. *American Journal of Infection Control, 42*(5), 562–564.

Colli, A. (2011). First experience with a new negative pressure incision management system on surgical incisions after cardiac surgery in high risk patients. *Journal of Cardiothoracic Surgery, 6*(160), 1–6.

Cove, M. E., Spelman, D. W., & MacLaren, G. (2012). Infectious complications of cardiac surgery: A clinical review. *Journal of Cardiothoracic Anesthesiology, 26*(6), 1094–1100.

Darouiche, R. O., Wall, M. J., Itani, K. M., Otterson, M. F., Webb, A. L., Carrick, M. M., . . . Berger, D. H. (2010). Chlorhexidine–alcohol versus povidone–iodine for surgical site antisepsis. *New England Journal of Medicine, 362*(1), 18–26.

Deniz, H., Gokaslan, G., Arslanoglu, Y., Ozcaliskan, O., Guzel, G., Yasim, A., . . . Ustunsoy, H. (2012). Treatment outcomes of postoperative mediastinitis in cardiac surgery; negative pressure wound therapy versus conventional treatment. *Journal of Cardiothoracic Surgery, 7.* Retrieved from http://www.cardiothoracicsurgery.org/content/7/1/67

Ding, C., Wang, C., Dong, A., Kong, M., Jiang, D., Tao, K., . . . Shen, Z. (2012). Anterolateral minithoracotomy versus median sternotomy for the treatment of congenital heart defects: A meta-analysis and systematic review. *Journal of Cardiothoracic Surgery, 7.* Retrieved from http://www.ncbi.nlm.nih.gov/pubmedhealth/PMH0054652/

Dumville, J. C., Gray, T. A., Walter, C. J., Sharp, C. A., & Page, T. (2014). Dressings for the prevention of surgical site infection. *Cochrane Database of Systematic Reviews, 9* CD003091.

Edmiston, C. E., Bruden, B., Rucinski, M. C., Henen, C., Graham, M. B., & Lewis, B. L. (2013). Reducing the risk of surgical site infections: Does chlorhexidine gluconate provide a risk reduction benefit? *American Journal of Infection Control, 41*(5), S49–S55.

Edmiston, C. E., Okoli, O., Graham, M. B., Sinski, S., & Seabrook, G. R. (2010). Evidence for using chlorhexidine gluconate preoperative cleansing to reduce the risk of surgical site infection. *AORN Journal, 92*(5), 509–518.

Eiselt, D. (2009). Presurgical skin preparation with a novel 2% chlorhexidine gluconate cloth reduces rates of surgical site infection in orthopedic surgical patients. *Orthopaedic Nursing, 28*(3), 141–145.

Falk-Brynhildsen, K., Soderquist, B., Friberg, O., & Nilsson, U. (2014). Bacterial growth and wound infection following saphenous vein harvesting in cardiac surgery: A randomized control trial of the impact of microbial skin sealant. *European Journal of Clinical Microbiology & Infectious Diseases, 33*(11), 1981–1987.

Faritous, Z., Ardeshiri, M., Yazdanian, F., Jalali, A., Totonchi, Z., & Azarfarin, R. (2014). Hyperglycemia or high hemoglobin a1c: Which one is more associated with morbidity and mortality after coronary artery bypass graft surgery? *Annals of Thoracic and Cardiovascular Surgery, 20*(3), 223–228.

Filsoufi, F., Rahmanian, P. B., Castillo, J. G., Pinney, S., Broumand, S. R., & Adams, D. H. (2007). Incidence, treatment strategies and outcome of deep sternal wound infection after orthotopic heart transplant. *Journal of Heart and Lung Transplantation, 26*(11), 1084–1090.

Friberg, O., Dahlin, L.-G., Kallman, J., Kihlstrom, E., Soderquist, B., & Svedjeholm, R. (2009). Collagen-gentamicin implant for prevention of sternal wound infection; long-term follow-up of effectiveness. *Interactive Cardiovascular and Thoracic Surgery, 9*(3), 454–458.

Godbole, G., Pai, V., Kolvekar, S., & Wilson, A. (2012). Use of gentamicin-collagen sponges in closure of sternal wounds in cardiothoracic surgery to reduce wound infection. *Interactive Cardiovascular and Thoracic Surgery, 14*(4), 390–394.

Graling, P. R., & Vasaly, F. W. (2013). Effectiveness of 2% CHG cloth bathing for reducing surgical site infections. *AORN Journal, 97*(5), 547–551.

Grauhan, O., Navasardyan, A., Hofmann, M., Muller, P., Stein, J., & Hetzer, R. (2013). Prevention of poststernotomy wound infections in obese patients by negative pressure wound therapy. *The Journal of Thoracic and Cardiovascular Surgery, 145*(5), 1387–1392.

Guo, S., & DiPietro, L. A. (2010). Factors affecting wound healing. *Journal of Dental Research, 89*(3), 219–229.

Hargraves, J. D. (2014). Glycemic control in cardiac surgery: Implementing an evidence-based insulin infusion protocol. *American Journal of Critical Care, 23*(3), 250–258.

Hartsell, T. L. (2008). Postoperative infection in cardiac surgery. In J. V. Conte, W. A. Baumgartner, S. G. Owens, & T. Dorman (Eds.), *The Johns Hopkins manual of cardiac surgical care* (2nd ed., 361–388). Philadelphia, PA: Mosby Elsevier.

Hillis, L. D., Smith, P., Anderson, J., Bittl, J., Bridges, C., Byrne, J., . . . Winniford, M. D. (2012). 2011 ACCF/AHA guideline for coronary artery bypass graft surgery: Executive summary. A report of the American College of Cardiology Foundation/American Heart Association Task Force on Practice Guidelines. *Anesthesia & Analgesia, 114*(1), 11–45.

Huckfeldt, R., Redmond, C., Mikkelson, D., Finley, P. J., Lowe, C., & Robertson, J. (2008). A clinical trial to investigate the effect of silver nylon dressings on mediastinitis rates in postoperative cardiac sternotomy. *Ostomy Wound Management, 54*(10), 36–41.

Hussey, L. C., Leeper, B., & Hynan, L. S. (1998). Development of the Sternal Wound Infection Prediction Scale. *Heart & Lung, 27*(5), 326–336.

Jenks, P. J., Laurent, M., McQuarry, S., & Watkins, R. (2014). Clinical and economic burden of surgical site infection (SSI) and predicted financial consequences of elimination of SSI from an English hospital. *Journal of Hospital Infection, 86*(1), 24–33.

Juhl, A. A., Koudahl, V., & Damsgaard, T. E. (2012). Deep sternal wound infection after open heart surgery—Reconstructive options. *Scandinavian Cardiovascular Journal, 46*(5), 254–261.

Jung, S. H., Je, H. G., Choo, S. J., Yun, T. J., Chung, C. H., & Lee, J. W. (2010). Institutional report—Congenital right or left anterolateral minithoracotomy for repair of congenital ventricular septal defects in adult patients. *Interactive Cardiovascular and Thoracic Surgery, 10*(1), 22–26.

Kaneda, T., Nishino, T., Saga, T., Nakamoto, S., Ogawa, T., & Satsu, T. (2013). Small right vertical infra-axillary incision for minimally invasive port-access cardiac surgery: A moving window method. *Interactive Cardiovascular and Thoracic Surgery, 16*(4), 544–546.

Karki, S., & Cheng, A. C. (2012). Impact of non-rinse skin cleansing with chlorhexidine gluconate on prevention of healthcare-associated infections and colonization with multi-resistant organisms: A systematic review. *Journal of Hospital Infection, 82*(2), 71–84.

Kiani, S., & Poston, R. (2011). Is endoscopic harvesting bad for saphenous vein graft patency in coronary surgery? *Current Opinion in Cardiology, 26*(6), 518–522.

Kim, H. J., Jung, S. H., Kim, J. B., Choo, S. J., Yun, T. J., Chung, C. H., . . . Lee, J. W. (2013). Early postoperative complications after heart transplantation in adult recipients: Asan Medical Center experience. *The Korean Journal of Thoracic and Cardiovascular Surgery*, *46*(6), 426–432.

Klinkner, G., & Murray, M. (2014). Clinical nurse specialists lead teams to impact glycemic control after cardiac surgery. *Clinical Nurse Specialist*, *28*(4), 240–246.

Koh, T. J., & DiPietro, L. A. (2011). Inflammation and wound healing: The role of the macrophage. *Expert Reviews in Molecular Medicine*, *13*, e23. doi: 10.1017/S1462399411001943

Lazar, H., McDonnell, M., Chipkin, S., Furnary, A., Engelman, R., Sadhu, A., . . . Shemin, R. J. (2009). The Society of Thoracic Surgeons practice guideline series: Blood glucose management during adult cardiac surgery. *Annals of Thoracic Surgery*, *87*(2), 663–669.

Lemmer, J., & Vlahakes, G. (2010). Postoperative management. In J. Lemmer & G. Vlahakes, (Eds.), *Handbook of patient care in cardiac surgery* (7th ed.). Portland, OR: Lippincott Williams & Wilkins. Retrieved from http://www.r2library .com/Resource/Title/0781773857

Lipke, V. L., & Hyott, A. S. (2010). Reducing surgical site infections by bundling multiple risk reduction strategies and active surveillance. *AORN Journal*, *92*(3), 288–296.

Lobdell, K. W., Stamou, S., & Sanchez, J. A. (2012). Hospital-acquired infections. *The Surgical Clinics of North America*, *92*(1), 65–77.

Lopes, R., Hafley, G., Allen, K., Ferguson, T., Peterson, E., Harrington, R., . . . Alexander, J. H. (2009). Endoscopic versus open vein-graft harvesting in coronary-artery bypass surgery. *New England Journal of Medicine*, *361*(3), 235–244.

Luo, H., Wang, J., Qiao, C., Zhang, X., Zhang, W., & Song, L. (2014). Evaluation of different minimally invasive techniques in the surgical treatment of atrial septal defect. *The Journal of Thoracic and Cardiovascular Surgery*, *148*(1), 188–193.

Maragakis, L. L., Cosgrove, S. E., Martinez, E. A., Tucker, M. G., Cohen, D. B., & Perl, T. M. (2009). Intraoperative fraction of inspired oxygen is a modifiable risk factor for surgical site infection after spinal surgery. *Anesthesiology*, *110*(3), 556–562.

McCannon, C. J., Hackbarth, A. D., & Griffin, F. A. (2007). Miles to go: An introduction to the 5 Million Lives campaign. *The Joint Commission Journal on Quality and Patient Safety*, *33*(8), 477–484.

McDonnell, M., Alexanian, S., White, L., & Lazar, H. (2012). A primer for achieving glycemic control in the cardiac surgical patient. *Journal of Cardiac Surgery*, *27*(4), 470–477.

Meyer, M. J., Stanislaus, A. B., Lee, J., Waak, K., Ryan, C., Saxena, R., . . . Eikermann, M. (2013). Surgical Intensive care unit Mobilisation Score (SOMS) trial: A protocol for an international, multicentre, randomised controlled trial focused on goal-directed early mobilization of surgical ICU patients. *British Medical Journal*, *3*(8). Retrieved from http://bmjopen.bmj.com/ content/3/8/e003262.full

Mishra, P. K., Ashoub, A., Sallayeh, K., Aktuerk, D., Ohri, S., Raja, S. G., . . . Luckraz, H. (2014). Role of topical application of gentamicin containing collagen implants in cardiac surgery. *Journal of Cardiothoracic Surgery*, *9*(122), 1–20.

Moghissi, E. S., Korytkowski, M. T., DiNardo, M., Einhorn, D., Hellman, R., Hirsch, I. B., . . . Umpierrez, G. E. (2009). American Association of Clinical Endocrinologists and American Diabetes Association consensus statement on inpatient glycemic control. *Diabetes Care*, *32*(6), 1119–1131.

Nakano, J., Okabayashi, H., Hanyu, M., Soga, Y., Nomoto, T., Arai, Y., . . . Kawatou, M. (2008). Risk factors for wound infection after off-pump coronary artery bypass grafting: Should bilateral internal thoracic arteries be harvested in patients with diabetes? *The Journal of Thoracic and Cardiovascular Surgery*, *135*(3), 540–545.

O'Brien, S. M., Shahian, D. M., Filardo, G., Ferraris, V. A., Haan, C. K., Rich, J. B., . . . Anderson, R. P. (2009). The Society of Thoracic Surgeons 2008 cardiac surgery risk models: Part 2–Isolated valve surgery. *Annals of Thoracic Surgery*, *94*(6), 2166–2171.

Pezzella, A. T., Holmes, S. D., Pritchard, G., Speir, A. M., & Ad, N. (2014). Impact of perioperative glycemic control strategy on patient survival after coronary bypass surgery. *Annals of Thoracic Surgery*, *98*(4), 1281–1285.

Phillips, M., Rosenberg, A., Shopsin, B., Cuff, G., Skeete, F., Foti, A., . . . Bosco, J. (2014). Preventing surgical site infections: A randomized, open-label trial of nasal mupiro-cin ointment and nasal povidone-iodine solution. *Infection Control & Hospital Epidemiology*, *35*(7), 826–832.

Pierpont, Y. N., Dinh, T. P., Salas, R. E., Johnson, E. L., Wright, T. G., Robson, M. C., . . . Payne, W. G. (2014). Obesity and surgical wound healing: A current review. *International Scholar Research Notices: Obesity*, *2014*. Article ID 638936. Retrieved from http://www.hindawi.com/journals/isrn/2014/638936/

Pye, S., & McDonnell, M. (2010). Nursing considerations for children undergoing delayed sternal closure after surgery for congenital heart disease. *Critical Care Nurse*, *30*(3), 50–61.

Raja, S. G., & Sarang, Z. (2013). Endoscopic vein harvesting: Technique, outcomes, concerns & controversies. *Journal of Thoracic Disease*, *5*(Suppl. 6), S630–637.

Richter, J. H., Jarrett, N. M., & LaBresh, K. A. (2014). *Evidence-based guidelines for selected, candidate, and previously considered hospital acquired conditions, Final report*. Retrieved from http://www.cms.gov/Medicare/Medicare-Fee-for-Service-Payment/HospitalAcqCond/Downloads/Evidence-Based-Guidelines.pdf

Rote, N. S., & Huether, S. E. (2010). Innate immunity: Inflammation. In K. L. McCance, S. E. Huether, V. L. Brashers, & N. S. Rote (Eds.), *Pathophysiology: The biologic basis for disease in adults and children* (6th ed., pp. 183–213). Maryland Heights, MO: Mosby Elsevier.

Sabik, J. F. (2011). Understanding saphenous vein graft patency. *Circulation*, *124*(3), 273–275.

Schimmer, C., Sommer, S. P., Bensch, M., Bohrer, T., Aleksic, I., & Leyh, R. (2008). Sternal closure techniques and postoperative sternal wound complications in elderly patients. *European Journal of Cardio-Thoracic Surgery*, *34*(1), 132–138.

Sen, C. K. (2009). Wound healing essentials: Let there be oxygen. *Wound Repair and Regeneration*, *17*(1), 1–18.

Shahian, D. M., O'Brien, S. M., Filardo, G., Ferraris, V. A., Haan, C. K., Rich, J. B., . . . Anderson, R. P. (2009a). The Society of Thoracic Surgeons 2008 cardiac surgery risk models: Part 1—Coronary artery bypass grafting surgery. *Annals of Thoracic Surgery*, *88*(Suppl. 1), S2–22.

Shahian, D. M., O'Brien, S. M., Filardo, G., Ferraris, V. A., Haan, C. K., Rich, J. B., . . . Anderson, R. P. (2009b). The Society of Thoracic Surgeons 2008 cardiac surgery risk models: Part 3—Valve plus coronary artery bypass grafting surgery. *Annals of Thoracic Surgery*, *88*(Suppl. 1), S43–62.

Shi, Y. D., Qi, F. Z., & Zhang, Y. (2014). Treatment of sternal wound infections after open-heart surgery. *Asian Journal of Surgery*, *37*(1), 24–29.

Subramaniam, B., Lerner, A., Novack, V., Khabbaz, K., Paryente-Wiesmann, M., Hess, P., . . . Talmor, D. (2014). Increased glycemic variability in patients with elevated preoperative HbA1C predicts adverse outcomes following coronary artery bypass grafting surgery. *Anesthesia & Analgesia*, *118*(2), 277–287.

Travis, J., Carr, J. B., Saylor, D., King, A., Bence, W., Key, S., . . . Trienski, T. (2009). Coronary artery bypass graft surgery: Surgical site infection prevention. *Journal for Healthcare Quality*, *31*(4), 16–23.

Troutman, S., Hussey, L. C., Hynan, L., & Lucisano, K. (2001). Sternal Wound Infection Prediction Scale: A test of the reliability and validity. *Nursing & Health Sciences*, *3*(1), 1–8.

Vlajcic, Z., Zic, R., Stanec, S., & Stanec, Z. (2007). Algorithm for classification and treatment of poststernotomy wound infections. *Scandinavian Journal of Plastic and Reconstructive Surgery and Hand Surgery*, *41*(3), 114–119.

Walsh, E. E., Greene, L., & Kirshner, R. (2011). Sustained reduction in methicillin-resistant *Staphylococcus aureus* wound infections after cardiothoracic surgery. *Archives of Internal Medicine*, *171*(1), 68–73.

Walter, C., Dumville, J., Sharp, C., & Page, T. (2012). Systematic review and meta-analysis of wound dressings in the prevention of surgical-site infections in surgical wounds healing by primary intention. *British Journal of Surgery*, *99*(9), 1185–1194.

Xuan, Y., Huang, B., Tian, H., Chi, L., Duan, Y., Wang, X., & Jin, L. T. (2014). High-glucose inhibits human fibroblast cell migration in wound healing via repression of bFGF-regulating JNK phosphorylation. *PLOS ONE*, *9*(9), e108182. doi:10.1371/journal.pone.0108182

Yasa, H., Lafci, B., Yilik, L., Bademci, M., Sahin, A., Kestelli, M., . . . Gürbüz, A. (2010). Delayed sternal closure: An effective procedure for life-saving in open heart surgery. *Anadolu Kardiyoloji Dergisi, 10*(2), 163–167.

Yavuz, S. S., Tarcin, O., Ada, S., Dincer, F., Toraman, S., Birbudak, S., . . . Yekeler, I. (2013). Incidence, aetiology, and control of sternal surgical site infections. *Journal of Hospital Infection, 85*(3), 206–212.

Zellinger, M., & Lienberger, T. (1991). Use of the rubber dam after open heart surgery. *Critical Care Nurse, 11*(8), 24–27.

WEB RESOURCES

Medicare Program; Changes to the hospital inpatient prospective payment systems and fiscal year 2008 rates: https://www.cms.gov/Medicare/Medicare-Fee-for-Service-Payment/AcuteInpatientPPS/downloads/CMS-1533-FC.pdf

Centers for Disease Control and Prevention, National Healthcare Safety Network (NHSN): Surveillance for Surgical Site Infection (SSI) Events: http://www.cdc.gov/nhsn/acute-care-hospital/ssi/index.html

Guideline for the Prevention of Surgical Site Infection, 1999: http://www.cdc.gov/HAI/ssi/ssi.html

The Society of Thoracic Surgeons: http://www.sts.org/

Chapter 19

Bridge to Transplant and Cardiac Transplantation

Tracy D. Andrews and Roberta Kaplow

INTRODUCTION

According to the American Heart Association's (AHA) 2013 cardiology update, 5.1 million Americans in 2006 had a diagnosis of heart failure (HF). In 2009, one in nine U.S. deaths included HF as a contributing cause (Go et al., 2013). Of those people who develop HF, approximately 50% will die within 5 years of diagnosis. There are approximately 400,000 to 700,000 new cases being diagnosed in the United States each year (Heart Failure Society of America, 2014). Total inclusive HF costs (including medications, hospitalizations, missed work days) in the United States are estimated to be $32 billion (Go et al., 2013).

Since the early 2000s, medical advances have greatly increased treatment options for people living with HF. In particular, mechanical circulatory support (MCS) technology has emerged as a life-saving option for patients with acute and chronic HF not amenable to maximal therapy.

In the United States, 273 facilities currently have the ability to perform cardiac transplantation. In 2013, 2,531 heart transplants were performed in this country. To date, 58,528 heart transplants have been performed in the United States. As of October 24, 2014, there were 4,053 waitlisted candidates for a heart transplant (Organ Procurement and Transplantation Network [OPTN], 2014a). An estimated 10% to 15% of these patients will die each year while awaiting a heart transplant

(McCalmont & Ohler, 2008). The mortality rate of those waiting for heart transplant has decreased over time due to changes in an allocation algorithm that allow more wide-ranging sharing of organs (Singh, Almond, Taylor, & Graham, 2012). Stringent cardiac transplantation screening tools exist with considerable variations in inclusion criteria between transplant centers. Not all patients are deemed transplant candidates regardless of the degree of decompensation.

This chapter reviews the management of HF as the patient moves through the trajectory of illness toward consideration for MCS, transplantation, or both. The role of the critical care nurse is discussed during the various phases of illness, including the special decision regarding mechanical assistance devices and transplantation.

MANAGEMENT OF HEART FAILURE

Prior to initiating a discussion regarding HF management, the critical care nurse must be cognizant of the fact that there are two types of HF: systolic and diastolic. Diastolic failure is a result of poor left ventricular relaxation. This causes the left ventricle (LV) to become stiff. The stiff ventricle then struggles to contract appropriately. After prolonged or poorly managed diastolic dysfunction, systolic failure can ensue. Systolic failure is the classic and most well-known "heart failure." Systolic failure is a result of poor left ventricular pump function. As a result, over time, the LV will remodel and dilate. Patients become volume overloaded as a result of the LV failing to effectively pump out the blood volume accumulated between ejection phases. As a result, the volume accumulates in the LV and then backflows throughout the heart, even into the pulmonary system at advanced stages. When patients are diagnosed with systolic HF, a regimen of diuretics and neurohormonal agents is started. The gold standard of HF management includes diuretic therapy for meticulous volume management, beta blockade, and angiotensin-converting enzyme (ACE) inhibitors. A third tier of management includes spironolactone (Aldactone®). As patients' HF progresses, some may require advanced therapies for volume management, including thoracentesis for accumulative pleural effusions or ultrafiltration for overall volume reduction. When their clinical status declines and these measures begin to lose efficacy, end-organ perfusion is compromised. Patients may appear to an intensive care unit (ICU) with either a "warm and wet" profile, which means that they are volume overloaded but still have compensatory perfusion, or they will present with a "cold and wet" profile, which means that they are either in or nearing cardiogenic shock. When patients reach this point, advancement in therapy will typically include inotropic agents (e.g., dobutamine [Dobutrex®], dopamine [Intropin®], milrinone [Primacor®], inamrinone [Inocor®]), or intra-aortic balloon pump (IABP) insertion. Intra-aortic balloon pump placement assists the LV to unload some of the redundant accumulating volume. Intra-aortic balloon pump placement is not feasible in all patients though. Those patients with severe aortic insufficiency, peripheral artery disease, or major aortopathies (e.g., dissection, large untreated aortic aneurysms) would not be suitable candidates for IABP placement. Some patients require even more advanced therapies, including ventricular assist device (VAD) implantation. Multidisciplinary teams have become an integral part of HF management. Critical care nurses play a major role in this management if the patient requires ongoing hospitalizations for HF and management strategies are not beneficial (McCalmont & Ohler, 2008). Intra-aortic balloon pump therapy and pharmacologic interventions for HF are discussed in Chapters 10 and 12, respectively.

CRITERIA FOR HEART TRANSPLANTATION

A patient may become a candidate for a heart transplant based on specific criteria. The patient may have terminal HF that has not responded to medical therapy or cardiomyopathy (ischemic, nonischemic, idiopathic, or valvular). In addition, the predicted 1-year survival rate for the patient should be 50%. The American College of Cardiology/AHA has guidelines for indications for heart transplantation. Absolute indications for transplant for patients with HF-related hemodynamic compromise include refractory cardiogenic shock, intravenous inotrope dependence to maintain adequate organ perfusion, peak oxygen consumption at less than 10 mL/kg/min with achievement of anaerobic metabolism. Indications also include severe ischemia that consistently limits activity that cannot be corrected with coronary artery bypass surgery or percutaneous coronary intervention as well as recurrent symptomatic and refractory ventricular dysrhythmias. Relative indications for heart transplant include a peak oxygen consumption of 11 to 14 mL/kg/min (or 55% predicted) and major limitations to activities of daily living, recurrent unstable ischemia that is not amenable to other interventions, and recurrent fluid balance/renal function instability that is not related to patient nonadherence to a medical regimen (Hunt et al., 2009; Mancini, 2014).

Patients are excluded from heart transplantation if they meet any absolute contraindications. A number of relative contraindications for transplant must also be considered. These relative contraindications include increased pulmonary vascular resistance (PVR) higher than 6 Wood units (or 320–480 dynes/sec/cm^{-5}). These patients have an increased risk of right ventricular (RV) failure immediately following heart transplantation. The donor heart will not be able to pump effectively. Patients currently being treated for cancer are not considered candidates for heart transplant. These patients are at risk for their condition to be worsened from the required immunotherapy to prevent graft rejection. Similarly, patients with an active infection cannot receive a heart transplant. The immunosuppressive therapy can increase the severity of the infection. Age has been considered a relative contraindication for heart transplant. Patients over age 60 to 65 have been excluded in the past. However, physiologic versus chronological age is now being considered; heart transplants have now been performed on patients up to age 72 if certain added criteria are met. Patients with diabetes mellitus who have significant end-organ damage are typically not considered candidates for heart transplant. Similarly, patients with obstructive or restrictive lung disease, or both, are often excluded from receiving a heart transplant because of the increased risk of postoperative pulmonary complications. Other relative exclusion criteria for heart transplant include advanced liver disease, renal dysfunction (serum creatinine higher than 2 mg/dL or creatinine clearance below 40 mL/min), advanced peripheral vascular disease, morbid obesity (body mass index greater than 35 kg/m^2), active peptic ulcer disease, cholelithiasis, and diverticulosis. These latter criteria are related to the effects of immunosuppressants, cyclosporine A (CsA, Sandimmune®), and other anti-rejection medications (especially calcineurin inhibitors [CNIs]). These agents are discussed later in this chapter. Finally, patients must have a psychosocial evaluation to help determine ability to cope with a transplant, including waiting for a donor organ and recovery, and to help predict long-term adherence to immunosuppressive therapy. Included in the psychosocial evaluation is determining use of alcohol, tobacco, recreational drugs, or any combination of these (Botta, 2014a; Mancini, 2014).

While absolute and relative exclusion criteria are delineated in the literature, institutional contraindications may also be noted. Therefore, the critical care nurse should be cognizant of those contraindications as well.

MECHANICAL CIRCULATORY SUPPORT

Counterpulsatile IABP therapy was initially thought to be an effective mechanical support mechanism for patients with cardiogenic shock and acute myocardial infarction (AMI); however, in the IABP-Shock II trial, this was shown not to be true. Development of more powerful means of hemodynamic support has been required to manage advanced HF. Therefore, the implementation of implantable continuous-flow left ventricular assist devices (LVADs) has highlighted the meeting of this requirement. Furthermore, because the number of transplant candidates exceeds the number of available organs, many patients awaiting transplantation endure protracted waiting list status. During this wait time, these patients often have rapid clinical deterioration with notable lack of medication/treatment efficacy. Patients may then be evaluated for MCS as the wait continues; this care is termed "bridge to transplant." (See **Table 19-1.**)

Mechanical circulatory support has three primary functions: bridge to transplant, bridge to recovery, and destination therapy (DT). For those patients who meet heart transplantation criteria, have New York Heart

Table 19-1 Short-Term MCS Device Comparisons

	HeartMate II	HeartMate XVE	Thoratec PVAD	NOVACOR	Total Artificial Heart	ABIOMED (AB5000)	TandemHeart
Type of blood flow	Pulsatile flow	Continuous flow (axial)	Pulsatile flow	Pulsatile flow	Pulsatile flow	Pulsatile flow	Continuous flow (axial)
BSA limitation (m^2)	1.5	1.3	Smallest used on 0.73	1.5	1.7	1.2	1.2
Anticoagulation	ASA only	Antiplatelet therapy and initial heparin followed by warfarin	Initial heparin followed by warfarin or ASA	Antiplatelet therapy and initial heparin followed by warfarin	Antiplatelet therapy and initial heparin followed by warfarin	Antiplatelet therapy and initial heparin followed by warfarin	Antiplatelet therapy and heparin
Indications for use	Destination and bridge to transplant	Destination and bridge to transplant	Bridge to transplant	Bridge to transplant	Bridge to transplant	Temporary support and bridge to recovery	Temporary support and bridge to recovery
Positive aspects	Permits non-tethered ambulation Approved for patient discharge No warfarin required	Permits non-tethered ambulation Approved for patient discharge Quiet operation Small percutaneous lead	Permits discharge home Wide range of flow capacities	Three-year durability	Biventricular support	Flexible design for biventricular support	Percutaneous placement by cardiology
Negative aspects	Limited durability Large device Potential for infection and discomfort	Fixed motor speed with risk of LV suction events	Potential for infection due to being paracorporeal	Large size limits application to small people	Large console limits mobility System not designed for hospital discharge	Cannot be discharged Extracorporeal design limits mobility	Patients must remain in bed with no mobility Partial support
Support design	LVAD	LVAD	LVAD, RVAD, or BiVAD	LVAD	Total orthotopic heart	LVAD, RVAD, or BiVAD	LVAD
Internal or Paracorporeal (external)	Internal	Internal	Paracorporeal	Internal	Paracorporeal	Internal	Paracorporeal

	HeartWare	Jarvic 2000 Flowmaker	CentriMag	HeartWare HVAD	Thoratec IVAD
Type of blood flow	Continuous flow (axial)	Continuous flow (axial)	Continuous flow (axial)	Continuous flow (axial)	Pulsatile flow
BSA limitation (m^2)	1.2	2.3	> 1.4	> 1.2	> 1.5
Anticoagulation	ASA or ASA + low dose heparin or ASA + warfarin or ASA + Aggrenox⁻ + extended-release dipyridamole or ASA + clopidogrel	Heparin (some proceed without anticoagulation)	Heparin	ASA	Initially heparin, then warfarin
Indications for use	Refractory advanced HF	CHF, bridge to transplant, destination therapy	Cardiogenic Shock	Bridge to transplant	Bridge to transplant
Positive aspects	Designed for in-hospital and out-of-hospital settings, including fixed-wing aircraft and helicopter	Avoids extracorporeal circulation and decreased transfusion requirements Silent Lightweight and small size	Delivers high flows Minimal complications Less hemolysis	Small size May be placed in the pericardial space In-hospital and out-of-hospital use May be taken on fixed-wing aircraft or helicopter	In-hospital and out of hospital use May be taken on fixed-wing aircraft or helicopter
Negative aspects	Life-threatening adverse events, including stroke	Not for patients in cardiogenic shock Risk of thrombus formation	Approved for up to 6 hours of support No rechargeable battery	Several associated risks but these risks are reportedly outweighed by the benefits	Risk of clot formation if blood is not ejected with each beat
Support design	LVAD	LVAD	RVAD	LVAD	LVAD, RVAD, or BiVAD
Internal or Paracorporeal (external)	Internal	Internal	Internal	Internal	Internal

ASA, aspirin; BiVAD, biventricular assist device; BSA, body surface area; CHF, congestive heart failure; HF, heart failure; LV, left ventricular; LVAD, left ventricular assist device; RVAD, right ventricular assist device; TAH, total artificial heart

Association Stage 4 HF, and have deterioration of their clinical status to the point they can no longer live without mechanical support, bridge to transplantation is explored. Intermediate- to long-term VAD placement is utilized to provide these patients support until heart transplantation can occur. Patients who may have short-term contraindications to heart transplantation, end-organ compromise secondary to advanced HF, or lack of approval for heart transplantation listing are selected for bridge to decision.

Between June 2006 and June 2010, 42% of VADs listed in the Interagency Registry for Mechanically Assisted Circulatory Support (INTERMACS) database were implanted in patients deemed as bridge to decision (Kirklin et al., 2012). For those patients who are ineligible for heart transplantation but meet MCS criteria, DT is explored. As of July 2014, there are 101 centers in the United States that have been deemed DT centers by the Centers for Medicare & Medicaid (Kirklin et al., 2012). Bridge to recovery therapy is sought for those patients who have had an AMI or cardiogenic shock that has been deemed to be reversible. By LV unloading, these patients have the benefit of most or all of their native heart function. Just as is seen with heart transplantation, centers that provide MCS also have algorithms that help decide appropriateness of treatment. Contraindications for MCS may include septic shock, prolonged cardiopulmonary resuscitation, predicted extremely short-term life expectancy due to comorbidities, patient/family declination of MCS, or clinical judgment against MCS by primary medical team (Takayama, Takeda, Doshi, & Jorde, 2014).

Ventricular Assist Devices (VADs)

Ventricular assist devices can provide left, right, or biventricular support. The most common scenario involves the use of an LVAD to counteract left ventricular dysfunction.

Mechanisms for movement of blood vary among the different types of pumps. In general, blood is drained from the apex of the LV to the pump via the inflow cannula. It is returned to the body via an outflow cannula, which is attached to the aorta. The pump is housed in the pre-peritoneal space of the abdomen, near the stomach. A percutaneous driveline that is tunneled across the pre-peritoneal space to the left side of the body carries the electrical cable and air vent to the electrical controller outside the patient's body. The risk of pump infection is reduced by tunneling the cable across the abdomen, thereby increasing the distance from the pump to the exit site and allowing the body to form a natural seal around the driveline.

Research supports the use of VADs as DT. In 2001, the Randomization Evaluation of Mechanical Assistance for the Treatment of Congestive Heart Failure (REMATCH) trial compared the outcomes with LVAD devices for DT and the outcomes with medical therapy. Rose and colleagues (2001) noted that survival rates at 1 year were better in the LVAD patients than in the medical therapy patients (52% versus 25%, respectively). In addition to realizing a survival benefit, patients on LVAD therapy gained energy and vitality as a result of improved organ perfusion, and they reported overall increased quality of life.

VAD Selection Criteria

Selection criteria for patients requiring VAD, any MCS therapy, or both are rigorous. As part of patient evaluation, a battery of lab and diagnostic tests is performed to determine eligibility for a device. This process can also help decide which device, if any, is most appropriate for the patient. A VAD medical service is typically comprised of advanced HF-certified cardiologists, social workers, nurses, VAD coordinators, and cardiac surgeons who collaborate to determine the appropriateness of the device for the patient and decide on the plan of care. The surgeon and cardiologist determine the type of support required (i.e., LVAD, right ventricular assist device [RVAD], or biventricular assist device [BiVAD]). Left ventricular assist device recipients must have adequate RV function to achieve a successful outcome because the LVAD is dependent on blood flow from the right ventricle. If RV failure is present, patients' length of stay, post-implantation morbidity/mortality, and costs are increased. In such cases, RV failure must be treated with inotropics, decreasing PVR, and adjusting the flow of the LVAD. Insertion of an RVAD should be considered only a last resort if RV failure persists with medical therapy (Meineri, Van Rensburg, & Vegas, 2012).

Types of Short-Term Assist Devices

There are two types of short-term assist devices currently used to treat decompensated advanced HF: percutaneous and surgically implantable devices. Mechanical assist devices have greatly improved since the first generation of VADs that required pulsatile flow. An example of a VAD that has pulsatile flow is an ABIOMED, Inc. BVS 5000 (Danvers, MA). As of 2014, current percutaneous ventricular assist devices (pVADs) available include the TandemHeart system (CardiacAssist, Inc., Pittsburgh, PA) and the Impella® System (ABIOMED, Inc.). According to Takayama and colleagues (2014), there are two additional pVADs currently under investigation: the Reitan Catheter Pump (CardioBridge GmbH, Hechingen, Germany) and the Percutaneous Heart Pump (Thoratec, Pleasanton, CA). Percutaneous ventricular assist devices are advantageous in management of acutely decompensated HF patients because of their ability to be quickly inserted via a less invasive procedure for the already unstable patient (Bunch, Mahapatra, Reddy, & Lakkireddy, 2012). All of the short-term devices require anticoagulation, generally with heparin.

Figures 19-1, 19-2, and 19-3 show an LVAD, RVAD, and BiVAD, respectively.

TANDEMHEART PTVA

The TandemHeart PTVA® system is a continuous flow pump that can provide up to 4 L/min of flow at 7,500 grams (Takayama et al., 2014). The system is inserted via the femoral vein into the left atrium through a transseptal puncture. An added feature of the TandemHeart is that the positioning of the cannulae in the main pulmonary artery and right atrium allows for RVAD configuration (Bunch et al., 2012). The pump withdraws oxygenated blood from the left atrium, propels it via a magnetically driven, six-bladed impeller through the outflow port, and returns it to the femoral artery via an arterial cannula. A disadvantage of the Tandem-Heart is the technical complexity of transseptal puncture and occasional dislodgement of left atrial cannulae into the right atrium (Agarwal, Cascade, & Pagani, 2009). The TandemHeart is illustrated in **Figure 19-4.**

IMPELLA SYSTEM

The Impella VAD system uses rotary pump technology in a miniaturized form. Hemodynamic support is achieved secondary to decreasing workload of the LV while simultaneously improving cardiac output (CO) by augmenting forward flow. Pump sizes are as small as 12-Fr, which makes this device amenable to percutaneous insertion. Under both fluoroscopic and echocardiographic guidance, an experienced cardiothoracic surgeon or interventional cardiologist places a catheter-mounted continuous-flow axial pump across the aortic valve with the inflow in the LV and the outflow in the ascending aorta. Because of this positioning, the Impella device provides active flow and systemic pressure improvement. Inflow of the device draws blood directly from the LV, resulting in decreased LV workload and myocardial oxygen demand. Impella devices include Impella 2.5 (12-Fr, 2.5 L/min of

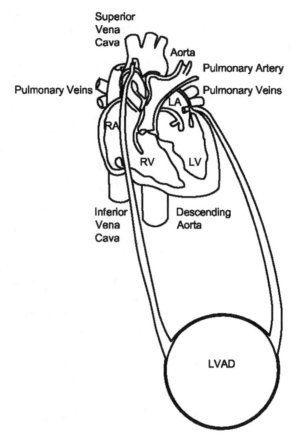

Figure 19-1   Left ventricular assist device.
Source: Illustrated by James R. Perron.

flow; most widely used model), Continuous Power (14-Fr, 3.5 L/min flow), 5.0 (21-Fr, 5 L/min flow), and a right VAD (23-Fr, 5 L/min flow). All pumps are operated through an 11-Fr catheter (Agarwal et al., 2009). In addition to improving access time, use of smaller cannulae also helps reduce the risk of limb ischemia frequently seen in devices that require larger cannula insertion (i.e., TandemHeart and extracorporeal membrane oxygenation [ECMO], discussed later in the chapter). Contraindications to Impella use include LV thrombus, moderate to severe aortic stenosis or insufficiency, and moderate to severe peripheral arterial disease (McCulloch, 2011).

SURGICAL SHORT-TERM, CONTINUOUS-FLOW VADS

Although pVADs are popular, surgical implantation of a VAD may be advantageous. Surgically implanted VADs have notable durability, stability, and generation of excellent forward flow. The CentriMag® VAD (Thoratec Corp., Pleasanton, CA) is the most commonly surgically implanted short-term, continuous-flow VAD. CentriMag can generate up to 10 L/min of flow at 5,500 grams. The system utilizes a magnetic levitation, bearingless centrifugal pump, which greatly improves cardiac output and reduces myocardial oxygen demand.

CentriMag implantation requires surgical cut-down. Traditionally, a sternotomy

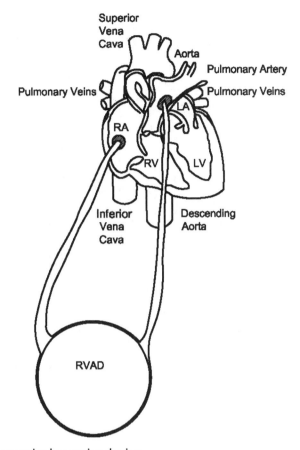

Figure 19-2   Right ventricular assist device.

Source: Illustrated by James R. Perron.

has been required; however, there have recently been developments to allow for mini-thoracotomy implantation. Postoperative management of CentriMag VADs is often easier for critical care nurses than that seen with pVADs. CentriMag has extracorporeal tubing that facilitates the bedside nurse's ability to quickly identify the need for additional fluid resuscitation. This can be noted when the VAD tubing begins to shake, which is called "chatter." Also, cannula stability facilitates ambulatory rehabilitation, whereas patients with pVADs require bed rest, which can alone have serious consequences (Gregoric et al., 2008).

Extracorporeal Membrane Oxygenation

Extracorporeal membrane oxygenation is a technique of partial cardiopulmonary bypass (CPB) that was initially developed to treat reversible neonatal respiratory failure. There are three types of ECMO: venous-arterial (VA), veno-venous (VV), and arterial-arterial (AA). Veno-venous ECMO is primarily used in respiratory failure, whereas VA ECMO is used in cardiac collapse. The equipment typically used for standard CPB in open-heart surgery has been modified to reduce hemolysis, thrombus formation, and risk of air embolus. Extracorporeal

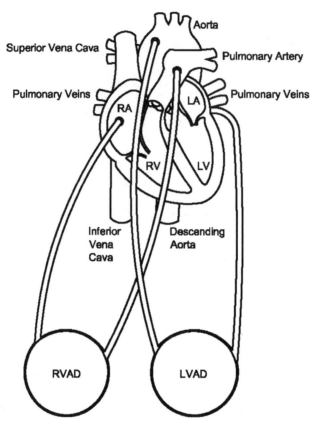

Figure 19-3   Biventricular assist device.

Source: Illustrated by James R. Perron.

membrane oxygenation can provide support for days or weeks. With this technique, blood is continuously withdrawn from any large central vein and pumped into a gas exchanger that oxygenates hemoglobin and removes carbon dioxide. The oxygenated blood is then pumped into any large artery (see **Figure 19-5**). The heart and lungs are bypassed, providing both hemodynamic and respiratory support. The blood oxygenation provided by this method is a distinct advantage of ECMO (Rodriguez-Cruz, 2013).

Short-Term Mechanical Circulatory Support

Following placement of a short-term circulatory assist device (e.g., VAD) and a period of hemodynamic stability, the patient's heart function and need for continued support are assessed. Some patients will regain some or most of their previous cardiac function, thus allowing for the removal of the assist device. Patients with acute viral myocarditis, for example, often experience improved cardiac function once the initial inflammatory processes within the cardiac muscle have resolved. Many patients, however, have chronic irreversible HF such that long-term mechanical support, transplant, or both will be necessary.

Recovery of heart function is assessed by briefly decreasing the amount of support provided by the device (e.g., decreasing device blood flow to 2 L/min) and monitoring the

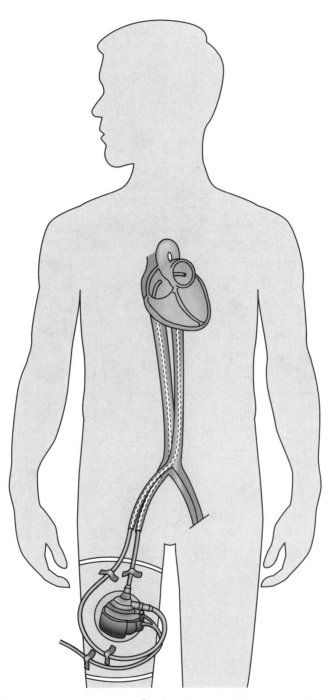

Figure 19-4   The TandemHeart PTVA®—this device utilizes a centrifugal pump and is inserted percutaneously.

Source: Illustrated by James R. Perron.

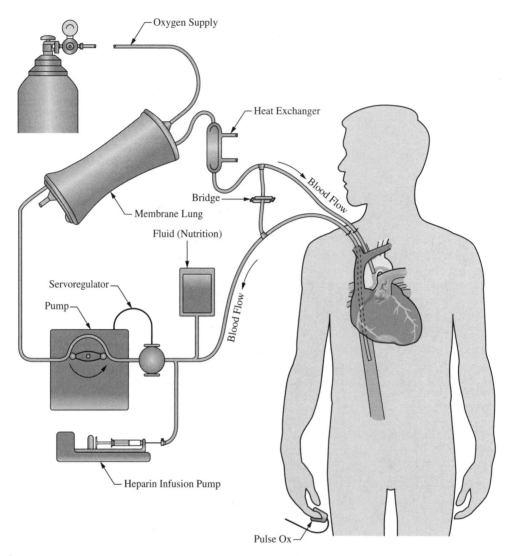

Figure 19-5   ECMO.
Source: Illustrated by James R. Perron.

patient's hemodynamic parameters. If this brief trial is well tolerated, a surface echocardiogram is obtained during a trial of decreased support to more accurately assess valve and ventricular function. Depending on the results of these trials, plans are made for device removal followed by appropriate medical therapy if there has been adequate recovery

of cardiac function, or for transition to a longer term implanted device, heart transplant, or both if poor cardiac function persists.

Long-Term Mechanical Circulatory Support

As previously mentioned, patients who are deemed bridge to transplant, bridge to decision, or DT candidates require longer MCS. For those who are deemed bridge to transplant, intermediate to long-term VAD use provides hemodynamic support until a suitable organ can be located. Ventricular assist device selection is determined by the patient's hemodynamic needs. Ventricular assist device technology has greatly improved since the mid-1990s.

First-generation VADs employed pulsatile positive displacement pumps. HeartMate I® and PVAD™ (paracorporeal ventricular assist device; both from Thoratec) are examples of first-generation VADs. Because of improved technology, these types of VADs are rarely used; however, HeartMate I use in the REMATCH trial is the basis for the concept of DT. Second-generation VADs use non-pulsatile (continuous) axial or centrifugal flow pumps.

Second-generation VADs are more durable than first-generation VADs because they have only one moving part, the rotor. They are also smaller, quieter, and require a less traumatic surgical implantation. They also have smaller driveline circumferences, which has been shown to decrease driveline infection rates. Because of these vast improvements, second generations have predominantly overtaken VAD implantation. Upon review of the INTERMACS database, second-generation VAD implantation increased from zero in 2007 to 1,145 in 2010, while use of first-generation VADs decreased from 219 in 2007 to six in 2010 (Kirklin et al., 2012). Examples of second-generation VADs include HeartMate II (Thoratec), Jarvik 2000 (Jarvik Heart, Inc.), MicroMed DeBakey (MicroMed), and INCOR (Berlin Heart).

As VAD technology has improved, there have still been challenges with VAD durability. Ventricular assist device exchange is not uncommon; therefore, a third generation of VAD development has begun. Third-generation VADs are being developed for longer durability, compact size, and optimization of forward flow to reduce risk of thrombosis and hemolysis

(Alba & Delgado, 2009). Examples of third-generation VADs include HeartWare® (HeartWare, Inc.) and DuraHeart" (Terumo Heart, Inc.). Both are available in the United States.

Biventricular Support

In patients with biventricular failure, biventricular support is often required. This support can be provided through a single unit like the Thoratec BiVAD or through use of more temporary support like the Tandem-Heart or CentriMag. Biventricular support can be provided until transplantation or can be slowly weaned off to ascertain return of native function (Adler & Enciso, 2013). Right ventricular assistance is typically weaned first. This weaning can be done either at the bedside or in the operating room (OR).

HeartMate XVE

The HeartMate XVE is another type of implanted, long-term pump with pulsatile blood flow. It is used for left ventricular support and is U.S. Food and Drug Administration (FDA) approved for both destination therapy and bridge to transplant. Because this model is a larger pump, patient selection criteria include the requirement that the patient's body surface area (BSA) be greater than 1.5 m². As a consequence, the HeartMate XVE device is used more frequently in males. The surface of the device is coated with a unique texture, allowing antiplatelet therapy to consist of aspirin alone. This is an important advantage because it means there is a decreased risk of thromboembolism with this device (Bojar, 2011). Bleeding risks are also minimized because warfarin therapy is not required.

HeartMate II

The HeartMate II is an axial (continuous) flow LVAD device that is more compact than the HeartMate XVE, so it can be used in patients who have smaller frames (BSA of 1.3–2.3 m^2). This device is FDA approved for use as a bridge to transplant; approval for DT is expected. Clinical trials of this device by the manufacturer have demonstrated its superior durability in comparison with pulsatile pumps (Haft et al., 2007). In addition, the HeartMate II generates less noise and has a smaller percutaneous lead than the HeartMate XVE. These features are appreciated by patients. Because the HeartMate II pump requires anticoagulation with heparin/warfarin and antiplatelet therapy, the risk of postoperative bleeding is increased with this device.

Total Artificial Heart

A total artificial heart (TAH) is a treatment alternative for patients with biventricular failure who are hospitalized candidates for heart transplant. Examples of a TAH are the CardioWest™ (SynCardia) and AbioCor® (ABIOMED). The TAH replaces the function of both ventricles and the four heart valves. The TAH is implanted in the patient's chest and attached to the atria. Tubes from the CardioWest ventricles continue from the patient's chest to outside the body through holes in the patient's abdomen to a power-generating console. The AbioCor does not have an outside power source; this is the main difference between these two devices. The AbioCor TAH is powered through a battery that is charged through the skin with a magnetic charger (National Heart, Lung, and Blood Institute, 2012).

The TAH can deliver CO as high as 9.5 L/min. It reportedly augments renal and hepatic blood flow and improves survival of heart transplant patients with preoperative biventricular failure (McCalmont & Ohler, 2008). In one report, the most frequent adverse events with a TAH included infection (either respiratory, urinary tract, or device; 77%), bleeding (62%), hepatic dysfunction (37%), respiratory dysfunction (36%), renal dysfunction (31%), neurologic event (27%), and device malfunction (17%). Most patients (79%) survived with a TAH until a donor heart was available (Friedline & Hassinger, 2012).

Postoperative Complications

Ventricular assist device placement is a major surgical procedure with significant risk for postoperative complications. The most common complications in the immediate postoperative period are bleeding, arrhythmias, RV failure, and infection. Later postoperative complications include bleeding, thrombosis, venous thrombotic event, device failure, and psychological problems. Infusion of fluids and inotropes may be required until the patient becomes hemodynamically stable following insertion of the device (Allen & Sidebotham, 2012).

Infection control guidelines for VADs are provided in **Table 19-2**. Bleeding in the immediate post-insertion period is common owing to the frequent use of aspirin and warfarin in HF patients preoperatively for severely depressed LV function, coronary artery disease (CAD), dysrhythmias, or any combination of these conditions.

Because LVAD function depends on adequate flow from the right ventricle, patients are monitored closely for signs of right HF. Pulmonary artery catheters are inserted preoperatively for close monitoring of right-sided function (right atrial pressure, central venous pressure [CVP]).

Nitric oxide (NO) has been shown to improve RV function by selective pulmonary vasodilation, which in turn improves LV filling, CO, and systemic arterial pressure (Idrees et al., 2008). Nitric oxide delivered postoperatively can be continued until the chest is closed and RV stability is achieved (McCalmont & Ohler, 2008).

Respiratory therapy can help promote pulmonary vasodilation by making ventilator adjustments that allow for permissive

Table 19-2   General Infection Control Guidelines

- Dressings over driveline exit sites must be kept clean and dry at all times.

- Sterile dressing changes to the driveline exit site must be performed at least daily. Dressing should be changed more frequently when increased drainage is observed.

- Immobilize the driveline or exit cannulas with abdominal binders continuously. This prevents trauma to the exit site and helps to develop tissue ingrowth around the driveline, which promotes formation of a skin barrier. Trauma to exit sites significantly increases the risk of infection.

- Remove monitoring lines as soon as possible to decrease the risk of infection.

- Notify the physician of a change in the patient's temperature ($< 36\ °C$ [96.9 °F] or $> 38.5\ °C$ [101.4 °F]) or other signs and symptoms of driveline infection (e.g., redness, increase in drainage, foul odor, or skin separation from driveline).

- Ensure adequate nutrition (maintain albumin > 2.5 g/dL). This is essential for the healing process to occur.

hypercarbia. Prevention of hypoxia is also important to avoid pulmonary vasoconstriction (Kollef & Isakov, 2012).

The patient who has undergone LVAD placement may have baseline renal dysfunction. This may be due to renal hypoperfusion. It has been suggested that renal function may improve following implantation of an LVAD (Hasin et al., 2012). Conflicting data exist as some data suggest a decline in renal function following LVAD implantation (Patel et al., 2012). Because renal failure or severe renal insufficiency is generally a contraindication to heart

transplant, care must be taken to minimize injury to the kidneys in this patient population. Diligent intake and output surveillance and medication administration are necessary so that the kidneys can recover for the impending heart transplant. The ICU nurse should monitor for improvement in renal function during LVAD therapy.

Transient hepatic dysfunction may occur following LVAD implantation (Nishi et al., 2013). An inflammatory response from LVAD placement may be an etiologic factor (Toda et al., 2011). The hepatic dysfunction may compound a preexisting condition due to congestion associated with HF. Supportive care, including maintenance of appropriate fluid balance and optimizing CVP, is essential to help overcome this complication.

Requirements for Being Discharged with an LVAD

Patients who return home with an LVAD require extra education to ensure the safety of this therapy. A grounded, three-pronged plug outlet near the patient's sleeping site will be required for the patient to switch to the power source during sleep. In the event of battery or generator failure, ongoing functioning of the device can be ensured through hand pumping, switching power sources, emergency interventions, or a combination of these. Extra batteries should always be available (Mason & Konicki, 2003). Routine care and provisions for emergencies must be addressed. Education should include troubleshooting of alarms, exit site infection prevention, immobilization of the percutaneous lead, and maintaining fluid volume status/dehydration prevention. Outcomes of patients who have been discharged home with an LVAD have been exceptional (Slaughter et al., 2010). **Table 19-3** lists the safety precautions required of the patient who is discharged to home with an LVAD.

Table 19-3   Safety Precautions at Discharge

- Maintain a method to obtain a backup generator in case of power failure.
- Notify the local electricity provider of the use of life support equipment.
- Use a transport power base unit to and from the hospital.
- Avoid immersion in water (e.g., do not sit in a tub of water).
- Avoid static electricity (e.g., touching a computer screen).
- Never disconnect both batteries simultaneously.
- Protect the vent filter from water.
- Cardiopulmonary resuscitation varies depending on the model of LVAD used.
- Do not engage in excessive jumping or contact sports.
- Do not let children sit on the patient's chest.
- No exposure to MRI is allowed.
- Pregnancy is not permitted.

LVAD, left ventricular assist device; MRI, magnetic resonance imaging.

Sources: Data from Ashikhmina, E. A., Schaff, H. V., Sinak, L. J., Li, Z., Dearani, J. A., Suri, R. M., . . . Sundt III, T. M. (2010). Pericardial effusions after cardiac surgery: Risk factors, patient profiles, and contemporary management. *Annals of Thoracic Surgery, 89,* 112–118; Kaplow, R. (2013). Cardiac tamponade. Retrieved from http://www.inpractice. com/Textbooks/Oncology-Nursing/Oncologic-Emergencies/Cardiac-Tamponade.aspx; Simsch, O., Gromann, T., Knosalla, C., Hübler, M., Hetzer, R., & Lehmkuhl, H. (2011). The intensive care management of patients following heart transplantation at the Deutsches Herzzentrum Berlin. *Applied Cardiopulmonary Pathophysiology, 15,* 230–240; Yarlagadda, C. (2014). *Cardiac tamponade clinical presentation.* Retrieved from http://emedicine.medscape.com/article/152083-clinical

HEART TRANSPLANTATION

Although many patients can be supported with either medical management or a VAD, another cohort of patients would benefit from receiving a heart transplant. There are two approaches to performing a heart transplant. The orthotopic approach is most commonly performed. With the orthotopic approach, the recipient's heart is replaced with a donor heart. With the heterotopic approach, the recipient's heart is left in place and the donor heart is "piggybacked" to the right side of the recipient's heart. The latter approach is rarely used.

Donor hearts are typically placed either with the Lower and Shumway method (the donor heart is anastomosed to the left atrium, right atrium, pulmonary artery, and aorta), atrial cuff technique (anastomoses are made at the inferior and superior venae cavae), or the heterotopic method (end-to-end anastomoses of the donor superior vena cava, pulmonary artery, and aorta) (Botta, 2014b). Regardless of

which technique is employed, denervation of the donor heart results in a higher heart rate because of loss of vagus nerve input (Eisen & Kusmirek, 2012), orthostatic hypotension, and the inability to experience angina in the transplant recipient. The patient has a median sternotomy incision and is placed on CPB during the transplant procedure (National Heart, Lung, and Blood Institute, 2014).

Once the transplant procedure is completed, pacing wires are secured. The patient may require inotropic support to be removed from CPB. Once the patient is successfully removed from CPB and the donor heart is functioning, the patient is transferred to the ICU for recovery (Simsch et al., 2011).

Care in the Immediate Postoperative Period

Factors Influencing Patient Recovery

After the transplantation procedure is complete, the heart recipient's postoperative care and course will vary depending on many factors. Comorbidities such as renal or pulmonary dysfunction will affect patient progress.

Donor and harvest factors may influence the postoperative course. For example, mismatch of heart size (i.e., a smaller heart being implanted into a larger recipient), older age, left ventricular dysfunction, and longer ischemic time of the donor may result in graft dysfunction (Anderson et al., 2010). Duration of the cold ischemia of the donated heart will also be relevant to the recipient's recovery. Cold ischemic time refers to the amount of time from cross-clamping of the donor with subsequent removal and immersion of the heart in iced saline until removal of the cross-clamp after it has been implanted into the patient (Anderson, 2008). The maximum cold ischemic time is 6 hours and preferably should be less than 4 hours. Younger organs tolerate relatively longer ischemic times; older organs tolerate shorter ischemic times (Costanzo et al., 2010; Pham, 2014a).

Postoperative Complications

Once admitted to the ICU, heart transplant patients typically remain on mechanical ventilation for 12–48 hours and remain in the ICU for 2–3 days. The overall reported ICU mortality is less than 5% in this population. One common complication is neurologic in nature (e.g., delirium or encephalopathy). Other complications may include bleeding, hyperacute rejection, infection, steroid-induced psychiatric disturbances, rejection, and allograft vascular disease (Botta, 2014a). Other common causes of mortality include infection, graft vascular disease, acute graft failure, and acute rejection (Alejaldre, Delgado-Mederos, Santos, & Martí-Fàbregas, 2010).

The immediate postoperative period can be quite challenging for both patients and nurses. While the immediate postoperative recovery after a heart transplant generally progresses without complication, patients may demonstrate high levels of vulnerability and low levels of stability. Clinical issues and implications specific to the recovery from anesthesia and CPB are discussed in detail in Chapter 8. Hemodynamic monitoring and care for the patient on mechanical ventilation, including weaning and extubation, are described in Chapters 9 and 11, respectively. Postoperative complications related to CPB are discussed in detail in Chapter 13; those specific to heart transplantation are discussed next.

Neurologic Complications

In the perioperative period, delirium and encephalopathy are the most common neurologic complications. They occur in 5% to 11% of cases. Etiologic factors include history of prior stroke, atrial fibrillation (AF), endocarditis-related septic emboli, cardiac catheterization, and perioperative hemodynamic instability (Alejaldre et al., 2010).

Other neurologic complications that can occur include stroke, seizures, infection, and peripheral neuropathy. One class of anti-rejection medications, CNIs (discussed later in this chapter), may cause headaches, tremor, and insomnia. These symptoms typically decrease with dose reduction of the causative agent. While these complications are associated with significant morbidity and can result in decreased quality of life, they are usually self-limiting and are not a primary cause of death in heart transplant recipients (Bhat et al., 2010).

Seizures occur in approximately 15% of patients and are usually related to focal ischemic injury, anoxic encephalopathy, toxicity from CNIs, or metabolic imbalances. Use of long-term anti-seizure medications is usually not required. Encephalopathy that occurs in the immediate postoperative period is multi-factorial in etiology. Some data suggest reducing the dose of CNIs (if felt to be the cause) while considering the risk of potentially ineffective immunosuppression. Treatment of hypomagnesemia is also recommended (Costanzo et al., 2010).

Peripheral neuropathy in the immediate postoperative period is often due to brachial plexopathy from intraoperative positioning or perineal injury from IABP (Bhat et al., 2010). Neurologic complications are discussed in more detail in Chapter 16.

Bleeding

Postoperative bleeding is a common problem in all cardiac surgery patients, including those who have undergone heart transplant. Postoperative bleeding may be related to preoperative use of a VAD that required anticoagulation or mediastinal scarring from previous procedures (Simsch et al., 2011). Other causes of postoperative bleeding may include hypothermia, administration of heparin for CPB, preexisting hepatic dysfunction from HF and associated low CO, surgical-site tissue trauma, and platelet destruction from CPB (Granton & Cheng, 2011; Simsch et al., 2011). While protamine sulfate is often given in the OR to reverse the heparin effects, an additional dose may be required in the immediate postoperative period. Heart transplant recipients, however, are at greater risk for bleeding than other cardiac surgery patients. Many of these patients have prior sternotomies. For this reason, the current sternotomy wound is often left open, covered with a sterile, occlusive, transparent dressing to permit visualization of accumulating blood and rapid mediastinal exploration, should it be required. In addition, the pericardial sac is larger than normal in order to accommodate an enlarged heart. Patients may also have preoperative liver dysfunction from long-standing HF.

The ICU nurse should observe the patient for signs of bleeding (e.g., tachycardia), chest tube drainage greater than 100 mL/hr, cardiac index (CI) less than 3 L/min/m², falling hemoglobin and hematocrit levels, decreased mixed venous saturation (SvO_2),

and increasing oxygen requirements. Results of coagulation profiles and platelet count should be evaluated as well. Hypotension and decreasing pulmonary artery and central venous pressures are late signs of bleeding. If the patient is to be transfused with blood or blood products, cytomegalovirus (CMV)-negative patients must receive CMV-negative products (Jahan, Tabassum, Aziz, Ahmed, & Islam, 2010).

Strategies employed for bleeding are the same as those used in other cardiac surgery patients. These interventions include eradicating the underlying cause of bleeding, aggressive transfusion of blood products (e.g., fresh frozen plasma, cryoprecipitate) as indicated; use of plasminogen inhibitors (e.g., aminocaproic acid [Amicar®], aprotinin [Trasylol®]) and factor VII; administration of additional protamine sulfate; and re-exploration based on the amount of chest tube output and the patient's coagulation status. While institutional guidelines may vary, a general guideline of 400 mL of blood via the chest tube in the first postoperative hour or 200 mL/hour for the first 4 postoperative hours typically warrants re-exploration if the patient has a normal coagulation profile (Simsch et al., 2011). Due to lack of efficacy data in large randomized controlled trials, use of desmopressin (DDAVP®) is not recommended (Achneck et al., 2010; Raja & Shahbaz, 2006). Gentle milking of chest tubes may be required to dislodge clots and maintain the patency of the chest tubes, if permitted based on institutional policy. Of note, stripping of chest tubes can create large amounts of negative pressure, which can hasten bleeding.

Hypovolemia

Post-transplant hypovolemia has the same etiology in heart transplant recipients as it does in other cardiac surgery patients who have undergone CPB. Cardiopulmonary bypass causes increased capillary permeability, with resultant third spacing of fluid. Intraoperative use of diuretics and initial high post-CPB urinary output further contribute to the postoperative heart transplant patient's hypovolemic state. Hypovolemia, in turn, results in a decrease in preload and cardiac function (Sidebotham & Gillham, 2007).

The ICU nurse must observe heart transplant recipients for hypotension; decreased pulmonary artery, pulmonary artery occlusive, and central venous pressures; decreased urinary output; and decreased cardiac output/index. Hematocrit levels may be elevated as a consequence of hemoconcentration (Sidebotham & Gillham, 2007). Treatment of hypovolemia focuses on volume repletion. This goal may be accomplished through administration of either a crystalloid or a colloid, depending on facility protocol. As discussed in Chapter 17, the debate over the efficacy of crystalloid versus colloid therapy continues. The ICU nurse must carefully monitor the patient's vital signs, urinary output, and hemodynamic profile both during and following volume resuscitation. Development of fluid overload can cause dilation of the right ventricle and pulmonary edema, which can be life threatening (Schumacher & Gajarski, 2011). Fluid resuscitation is discussed in detail in Chapter 17.

Right Heart Failure

Right HF is a major cause of morbidity and mortality in the post-heart transplant period. Right HF is the most common reason for patients not being able to wean from CPB following heart transplant. Chronically high pressure on the left side of the heart resulting in increased PVR contributes to the development of right HF following transplant (Shanewise, 2004). One factor identified to contribute to the development of dysfunction of the right ventricle following a heart transplant is ischemia-reperfusion injury. This can occur during harvesting and procurement of the organ and

the reperfusion that follows. A number of factors during the transplantation can make the right ventricle vulnerable to damage from ischemia. These include hypothermic cardioplegia, which has been found to be less effective on the right ventricle as compared to the LV; trauma to the organ during harvesting and the transplant procedure, intraoperative warm ischemia, air embolism in the right coronary artery, mechanical ventilation with positive end-expiratory pressure, and high PVR (Klima et al., 2005). A fragile donor heart (from ischemia-reperfusion injury) may not be accustomed to an elevated PVR, which can result in right HF (Wagner, 2011). The LV is generally able to tolerate increased afterload (the amount of work the heart must do to eject blood). However, the implanted right ventricle is not physiologically adapted to overcome high afterload as would be encountered with pulmonary hypertension, which develops frequently in HF patients. Opposed by high pulmonary pressures or PVR, the implanted right ventricle dilates readily and fails. This chain of events is difficult to reverse once it begins (Wagner, 2011). Further, right heart dilation alters septal position and function, which in turn interferes with LV function (Haddad, Hunt, Rosenthal, & Murphy, 2011). High preoperative pulmonary artery pressure (PAP) may predict increased risk for development of this syndrome; however, normal PAP does not preclude it. Right HF is characterized by an elevated CVP, edema, and hepatomegaly (Taegtmeyer, 2006).

Treatment of right HF depends on the severity of the condition. Goals of therapy include optimizing RV filling pressures, augmenting contractility, decreasing afterload of the right ventricle, and increasing coronary perfusion. Interventions include avoiding fluid overload; a maximum CVP of 10 mmHg should be achieved. Inotropic support with dobutamine is indicated in patients with a low CI. Decreased oxygen and elevated carbon dioxide levels should be avoided as these contribute to pulmonary vasoconstriction (Wagner, 2011).

Hypertension

Differences in the physiology between the recipient's original heart and the transplanted heart are related primarily to the fact that the transplanted heart is denervated (afferent and efferent). This means that the nerve supply has been severed; this results in absence of autonomic nervous system innervation of the donor heart. This mechanism is not restored during the transplant process. Efferent denervation has implications for heart rate; afferent denervation has implications for blood pressure. As a result of afferent denervation, there will be impairment of the renin-angiotensin aldosterone system and impairment of normal vasoregulatory responses to changes in cardiac filling pressures. Both of these can result in hypertension.

Up to 95% of patients report hypertension within 5 years of heart transplant. It is thought to be due to CNIs. The treatment of hypertension is the same as it is for non-heart transplant patients. Interventions include lifestyle modification (e.g., sodium restriction, weight loss, exercise). Patient and family education should begin as early as feasible in the postoperative period. Medication selection depends on patient response. Calcium channel blockers, ACE inhibitors, or angiotensin receptor blockers may be used. The latter two classes of agents may be preferred in patients with diabetes. Modification of risk factors may also include management of diabetes and elevated lipids. Modification of immunosuppressive therapy may be indicated as well (Bhat et al., 2010). Prevention and prompt detection and management of hypertension following heart transplantation are essential to prevent surgical site dehiscence.

Pulmonary Hypertension

Preemptive protective maneuvers are frequently successful in avoiding right HF. Pulmonary artery catheters are placed in all heart transplant patients. Nitric oxide is frequently utilized to selectively dilate the pulmonary vasculature without decreasing systemic blood pressure (Ichinose & Zapol, 2010); its administration has been shown to decrease the incidence of RV dysfunction in patients with pulmonary hypertension (Matthews & McLaughlin, 2008). Other agents that dilate the pulmonary vasculature (e.g., nitroglycerin [Tridil®], sodium nitroprusside [Nipride®], prostaglandin E-1 [PGE1], and prostacyclin [PGH2]) may cause hypotension and, therefore, are used less often in post-heart transplant patients.

Patients are generally weaned from NO on the first postoperative day or later, depending on the overall clinical picture and their degree of hemodynamic stability. Nitric oxide has a very short half-life, and patients are weaned from it very slowly (over hours). Rebound pulmonary hypertension and acute RV dysfunction are likely if use of NO is abruptly discontinued or weaning proceeds too quickly. Acidosis, hypercarbia, and hypoxemia increase PVR. Patients are, therefore, hyperventilated to achieve a pH in the range of 7.45–7.49 and a pCO_2 in the range of 30–35 mmHg. Hypoxemia must be avoided (Ichinose, Roberts, & Zapol, 2004).

Chronotropy (Rate) Issues

Bradycardia following a heart transplant may be due to denervation, sinoatrial (SA) node ischemic injury, or effects of some drugs (Thajudeen et al., 2012). Sinus node dysfunction may also occur due to injury of the donor heart during removal or preservation. Preoperative administration of amiodarone (Cordarone®) has also been implicated. If the latter is the case, the postoperative patient may manifest rhythms originating from the atrioventricular (AV) node. Sinus node dysfunction may last for up to several weeks following transplant. In the immediate postoperative period, bradycardia should be managed with a temporary pacemaker.

Medications such as theophylline (Theo-Dur®), terbutaline (Brethine®), or isoproterenol (Isuprel®) may be used to keep the heart rate at 90-110 beats/minute (Anderson et al., 2010). Isoproterenol administration should be used cautiously because of associated high myocardial oxygen demand, which has been known to cause acute ischemia. Implantation of a permanent pacemaker may be considered if bradycardia does not resolve. Typically, this will occur after 3 weeks following transplant. Few patients (less than 10%) will require a permanent pacemaker. Some data suggest that more than 20% may require this intervention (Thajudeen et al., 2012). Management of bradycardia is discussed in detail in Chapter 15.

Tachycardia, which decreases ventricular filling time, and hence the risk of RV dilation, is achieved with an atrial pacer set to the AAI (atria paced, atria sensed, inhibited) mode and a rate of 100-120 beats per minute via epicardial pacing wires. The AAI mode is selected because transplanted hearts generally have intact conduction systems (unlike in valve surgery patients, who are susceptible to temporary heart blocks). Utilization of the heart's intrinsic conduction system promotes ventricular synchrony, which stabilizes the septum in a manner that facilitates LV and RV function. Tachycardia is also achieved pharmacologically with isoproterenol, which also dilates pulmonary vasculature; dobutamine; and dopamine. Specific tachyarrhythmias following cardiac surgery, including heart transplant, are discussed in detail in Chapter 15.

Contractility (Inotropy) Issues

Inotropic agents such as dopamine, dobutamine, and milrinone are used to support RV and LV function. Milrinone is frequently given at a dose of 0.125-0.375 mcg/kg/min and has the added benefit of promoting pulmonary vascular dilation. If these pharmacologic interventions (which are described

in detail in Chapter 12) are not successful in preventing or ameliorating right HF, insertion of an IABP (see Chapter 10) or RVAD may be necessary. Patients often need support with inotropes following heart transplantation. Therapy may be required for a few days; weaning from these meds can take place when hemodynamic stability has been attained (Shanewise, 2004).

Hypotension

As in other cardiac surgery populations, blood pressure variability is common in patients who have received heart transplants. Hypotension decreases coronary artery perfusion, which is undesirable in all cardiac surgery patients and may contribute to right HF in the heart transplant patient. Treatment is directed at the underlying mechanism.

Vasodilation may be exacerbated by medications such as milrinone. Decreasing the dose of vasodilator medications, if feasible, may mitigate hypotension. Vasopressors such as norepinephrine (Levophed®) and vasopressin (antidiuretic hormone) are often required to maintain a mean arterial pressure greater than 65 mmHg. Vasopressin is thought to cause less constriction of the pulmonary vasculature, is associated with lower arrhythmogenicity, and increases glomerular filtration rate (GFR) (Yimin, Xiaoyu, Yuping, Weiyan, & Ning, 2013).

Allograft Dysfunction

Primary graft failure is the most common cause of death in the first 30 days after a heart transplant. The incidence of graft dysfunction following heart transplant is variable but is reported to range from 2.3% to 26%. One reason cited for the development of this complication is the use of "marginal donors" in response to the limited supply of donated organs.

Graft failure is manifested with symptoms of acute ventricular dysfunction. One or both ventricles may be affected and circulatory demands of the patient cannot be met. Symptoms include hypotension and decreased CO despite filling pressures being adequate. Etiologic factors may be related to the transplant process, patient, or donor (Iyer et al., 2011). Hormonal effects of brain death in the donor may contribute to graft failure. Massive amounts of catecholamines are released and may lead to systemic hypertension and possibly direct myocardial injury. Age of the donor, cause of donor death, degree of cardiac dysfunction on the part of the donor, and level of inotropic support required prior to procurement may be other causes. Higher levels of support may lead to myocardial depression. During organ procurement, prolonged ischemic time may contribute to graft failure. Ischemic times of more than 4 hours may result in graft dysfunction. Mismatches between donor and recipient in relation to weight and female donor to a male patient have also been implicated in the development of graft failure. Effects of hypothermic preservation may be another cause of graft failure. Although hypothermia remains the preferred method for preservation, there is thought that there may be injury to the microcirculation of the heart, which may result in decreased contractility upon reperfusion. Injury during implantation or reperfusion may also cause graft failure (Iyer et al., 2011). Patient factors have also been identified. These include age; need for inotropic, mechanical, or ventilator support; presence of pulmonary hypertension; diabetes; or being overweight. Most forms of early graft dysfunction are reversible, resulting in normal donor heart function if the heart is properly supported during its recovery phase. Less than 3% of patients die from early graft failure.

Left ventricular systolic dysfunction is categorized as either early or late. Early left ventricular dysfunction occurs either intraoperatively or in the immediate postoperative period. Late left ventricular dysfunction develops weeks to years following a heart transplant. The most common cause of both early and late left ventricular dysfunction is allograft rejection. If left ventricular dysfunction develops within days of the transplant, it typically occurs secondary to one of three etiologies: hyperacute rejection, reperfusion injury, or a suboptimal donor heart (Anderson, 2008).

REPERFUSION INJURY DURING SURGERY

Allograft dysfunction may be caused by reperfusion ischemia, prolonged cold ischemic time (greater than 5 hours), or both. This condition may be only a temporary complication (myocardial stunning), and resolve within 12 to 24 hours after heart transplant. The heart does sustain ischemic injury when such dysfunction occurs, despite the short duration (Anderson, 2008).

SUBOPTIMAL DONOR HEART

As the number of heart transplant candidates far exceeds the number of donor hearts available, some transplant programs have been accepting "suboptimal" donors (e.g., patients older than 63 years of age, hearts with mild left ventricular hypertrophy [LVH]). These hearts have typically been treated with higher doses of inotropic agents or vasopressors or have left ventricular dysfunction (Anderson, 2008).

Left ventricular systolic dysfunction is treated with inotropic support and appropriate fluid administration. Dopamine, dobutamine, or milrinone may be used to increase CO without associated increases in systemic vascular resistance (SVR). Each of these inotropic agents is discussed in detail in Chapter 12. Intra-aortic balloon pump therapy may be initiated if high doses of inotropes are required to maintain LV function; IABP therapy is discussed in detail in Chapter 10. Monitoring of the patient's vital signs and hemodynamic profile is essential while any of these therapies is being used.

If the patient's SVR is elevated, an associated decrease in CO may ensue. An elevated SVR may be managed with administration of a vasodilator such as nitroglycerin or nitroprusside.

On rare occasions, a patient's SVR may be low following heart transplant. This condition is believed to be related to use of ACE inhibitors for HF, release of pro-inflammatory mediators as occurs with CPB, or decreased levels of vasopressin. Low SVR may be treated with a vasopressor such as nor-epinephrine or epinephrine (Adrenaline®). If neither of these medications is effective in reversing the deficit, vasopressin may be given (Sudarshan, Kreisel, & Rosengard, 2008). All of these agents are discussed in detail in Chapter 12.

Right ventricular dysfunction following heart transplantation is likely due to pulmonary hypertension and can be difficult to manage. Patients with HF have chronic high left atrial pressure. Following the transplant, pulmonary hypertension and RV failure can occur because the donor heart may not be accustomed to pumping against such a high PAP. Management of pulmonary hypertension may include administration of a vasodilator (e.g., nitroglycerin) with an inotrope (e.g., dobutamine or milrinone). If the patient's pulmonary artery systolic pressure exceeds 50 mmHg, administration of intravenous prostaglandin E_1 and prostacyclin may be considered (Ruan, Dixon, Willerson, & Ruan, 2010). Inhaled NO is another agent that may be used to decrease PVR without diminishing SVR (Ichinose & Zapol, 2010).

The condition of the donor's heart is one of the factors that can impact early outcomes of the recipient. For example, the presence of LVH in the donor heart can result in less optimal outcomes when compared to a heart without LVH. If the donor had elevated troponin levels, indicating myocardial damage, there is an increased risk of the recipient developing HF early in the postoperative course. Age of the heart itself is reported not to affect long-term survival of the recipient; however, there is an increased chance of CAD being present in hearts over age 40 (Eisen, 2014a).

Rhythm Disturbance and Electrocardiograph Changes

Development of cardiac dysrhythmias is common following heart transplant. For patients who undergo transplants, the likelihood of such abnormalities in heart rhythm is higher in the immediate postoperative period. Such dysrhythmias may result from surgical trauma to the SA and AV nodes, ischemia, suture lines, rejection, and cardiac allograft vasculopathy (CAV) (Eisen & Kusmirek, 2012).

BRADYCARDIA
Bradycardia may occur in the immediate postoperative period. This complication affects as many as 50% of orthotopic heart transplant patients, typically taking the form of SA node dysfunction. Sinoatrial node dysfunction occurs as a result of ischemia during hypothermic preservation, intraoperative trauma to the SA node, perinodal atrial tissue, SA artery trauma, or pre-transplant use of amiodarone (Eisen & Kusmirek, 2012). Bradycardia immediately following surgery has little prognostic significance, but it may affect morbidity secondary to an associated decrease in CO. Permanent pacemaker insertion may be indicated (Eisen & Kusmirek, 2012).

Atropine sulfate is not effective in denervation of the sympathetic and parasympathetic nerves. Bradycardia may be treated with administration of a beta$_1$-receptor agonist (e.g., dobutamine or isoproterenol). It has also been suggested that administration of theophylline or terbutaline may increase heart rate in heart transplant patients who develop bradycardia. These agents are typically used only in cases of mild to moderate SA node dysfunction because the underlying SA node abnormality is only partially corrected with their use (Eisen & Kusmirek, 2012).

Clinically significant bradycardia will typically be treated with epicardial pacing. Dual-chamber pacing is preferred so that the patient's CO can be augmented from the atrial kick (Eisen & Kusmirek, 2012).

ATRIAL DYSRHYTHMIAS

The incidence of AF in heart transplant patients ranges from 10% to 24%; incidence of atrial flutter is reported at 12% to 15% (Eisen & Kusmirek, 2012). Atrial fibrillation usually occurs within the first 1–2 months (Eisen & Kusmirek, 2012). It has been suggested that AF is attributable to surgical isolation of the pulmonary vein and denervation of the heart. When AF develops later, it is typically associated with loss of function of the transplanted heart; the overall mortality is higher in this instance (Eisen & Kusmirek, 2012).

Treatment of atrial dysrhythmias entails controlling ventricular response rate. Immunosuppression is indicated if the cause is thought to be rejection. Atrial flutter may be managed with overdrive pacing; success of greater than 90% has been reported (Eisen & Kusmirek, 2012). Radiofrequency ablation has also been used to treat atrial flutter in heart transplant patients (Eisen & Kusmirek, 2012).

SUPRAVENTRICULAR TACHYCARDIA (SVT)

Types of supraventricular dysrhythmias that have been reported in orthotopic transplant patients include AV reentrant tachycardia, Wolff-Parkinson-White syndrome, and non-paroxysmal atrial tachycardia. Supraventricular tachycardia has been treated successfully with radiofrequency ablation (Eisen & Kusmirek, 2012).

VENTRICULAR DYSRHYTHMIAS

Premature ventricular contractions may occur in as many as 100% of orthotopic heart transplant patients early in the postoperative period (Eisen & Kusmirek, 2012).

Paroxysmal ventricular tachycardia (VT) decreases in incidence after the initial postoperative period. There may be a correlation between VT, rejection, and transplant vasculopathy. Non-paroxysmal ventricular dysrhythmias are rare in the postoperative heart transplant patient. Development is usually related to severe CAV or allograft rejection (Eisen & Kusmirek, 2012).

CONDUCTION DELAYS

Right bundle branch block (RBBB) is a common electrocardiogram (ECG) finding posttransplant, occurring in up to 70% of patients. This conduction delay was not present on the ECG of the donor. Development of an RBBB may be associated with prolonged donor ischemic time and several rejection episodes. Etiologic factors may include RV hypertrophy from elevated PAPs or right bundle damage during endomyocardial biopsy procedures (Eisen & Kusmirek, 2012).

Atrioventricular node function remains intact following a heart transplant. As a consequence, high-degree AV block is rare in posttransplant patients, especially in the early postoperative period. Late development carries an increased mortality rate (Eisen & Kusmirek, 2012). There is no associated increase in mortality. However, when patients have progressive bundle branch blocks, there is an increase in mortality rate (Thajudeen et al., 2012).

Cardiac Tamponade

While pericardial effusions may develop in over 20% of patients who undergo a heart transplant, few lead to development of hemodynamic instability/cardiac tamponade (Anderson et al., 2010). Cardiac tamponade may develop either gradually or suddenly in patients who have undergone heart transplantation. It results from fluid accumulating in the pericardial sac, which causes compression of the atria, restriction of venous return to the heart and ventricular filling, and results in a decrease or cessation of preload and a potential precipitous decline in CO (Ashikhmina et al., 2010). Early tamponade may also result from persistent mediastinal bleeding not being evacuated by chest tubes or clot formation. Cardiac tamponade may also develop following removal of pacing wires or endomyocardial biopsy.

The diagnosis of cardiac tamponade may be difficult in heart transplant recipients because hypotension and tachycardia are common scenarios in the immediate postoperative period. When caring for these patients, the ICU nurse should maintain patency of chest tubes, monitor vital signs and hemodynamic profiles, and observe for signs and symptoms including those listed in **Table 19-4** (Simsch et al., 2011).

If cardiac tamponade develops, initial management should include volume resuscitation to optimize filling pressures (being careful not to overload the right ventricle) and initiation and titration of inotropes (if blood pressure is not responsive to fluid resuscitation). Diagnosis is made by echocardiogram. Definitive treatment entails surgical intervention or emergent bedside sternotomy (Kaplow, 2013). The required equipment and nursing care for the latter procedure are discussed in Chapter 13.

Renal Dysfunction

In the immediate post-transplant period and following CPB, the patient's urinary output will be increased. Once these effects have worn off, it is important that urinary output be maintained at a rate of at least 0.5 mL/kg/hr. Renal function requires preservation because of the nephrotoxic immunosuppression agents that will be administered to prevent rejection of the donated heart. The ICU nurse must maintain adequate renal perfusion with fluids, vasoactive agents, or combinations of these to maintain a mean arterial pressure in the range of 60–80 mmHg. Monitoring of hourly urinary output and all renal

Table 19-4   Signs and Symptoms of Cardiac Tamponade

- Sudden decrease or cessation of chest tube drainage
- Dyspnea
- Chest pain
- Abdominal pain
- Decreasing cardiac index
- Narrowing pulse pressure
- Inappropriately fluctuating mean arterial pressure
- Systolic blood pressure < 90 mmHg
- Heart rate > 100 beats/min
- Paradoxical pulse
- Increased central venous pressure
- Altered mental status
- Fatigue
- Malaise
- Diaphoresis
- Dysrhythmias, including tachycardia
- Cyanosis or pallor
- Increasing metabolic acidosis
- Anxiety
- Restlessness
- Low-voltage QRS on ECG
- Electrical alternans on ECG
- Cardiac arrest
- "Water bottle heart" and cardiac silhouette enlargement on chest radiograph
- Hepatomegaly
- Decreased urinary output

ECG, electrocardiogram.

Sources: Data from Ashikhmina, E. A., Schaff, H. V., Sinak, L. J., Li, Z., Dearani, J. A., Suri, R. M., . . . Sundt III, T. M. (2010). Pericardial effusions after cardiac surgery: Risk factors, patient profiles, and contemporary management. *Annals of Thoracic Surgery, 89,* 112–118; Kaplow, R. (2013). *Cardiac tamponade.* Retrieved from http://www.inpractice.com/Textbooks/Oncology-Nursing/Oncologic-Emergencies/Cardiac-Tamponade.aspx; Simsch, O., Gromann, T., Knosalla, C., Hübler, M., Hetzer, R., & Lehmkuhl, H. (2011). The intensive care management of patients following heart transplantation at the Deutsches Herzzentrum Berlin. *Applied Cardiopulmonary Pathophysiology, 15,* 230–240; Yarlagadda, C. (2014). *Cardiac tamponade clinical presentation.* Retrieved from http://emedicine.medscape.com/article/152083-clinical

function tests should be performed by the ICU nurse as well.

Anti-rejection medications, specifically tacrolimus (Prograf®), are known nephrotoxic agents that will require monitoring of both renal function (creatinine) as well as medication levels. Tacrolimus and CsA toxicity are two of the main causes of acute kidney injury in heart transplant patients. This is felt to be due to vasoconstriction of the afferent and efferent arterioles causing a decrease in renal blood flow and GFR (Bennett, 2014).

Pre-existing renal insufficiency from prolonged low CO states and administration of chronic high-dose diuretics may also predispose the patient to post-transplant acute kidney injury. Patients who have been receiving high-dose diuretic therapy pre-transplant may manifest relative oliguria if the diuretic therapy is stopped abruptly. Combining this diuretic use with abnormal renal perfusion during CPB places the patient at greater risk for renal impairment post-transplant. Diuretics may be used to maintain adequate urinary output in these patients. The ICU nurse must be mindful of intravascular volume status in these (and all) post-transplant patients. The main determinant of adequate renal function early post-transplant is adequate cardiac performance. As such, optimizing hemodynamics in the immediate postoperative period is essential. When early renal dysfunction is reversed, there typically is no long-term effect following transplant. If renal function is inadequate and refractory to other measures, hemodialysis or continuous renal replacement therapies may be initiated. These therapies are typically well tolerated in patients with strong cardiac performance.

Psychosocial Conditions

In addition to all of the physiologic stressors associated with heart transplantation, a variety of psychosocial conditions may surface in the postoperative period. Patients are typically and predictably euphoric and relieved that they were recipients of a long-awaited organ. However, depression, anxiety, confusion, and delirium may develop in a few postoperative days. It is common for the patient to inquire about the donor and to experience difficulty coping with the knowledge that a death was associated with the organ procurement. Patients may manifest violent outbursts, attempt to climb out of bed, inappropriately yell at staff, or have hallucinations. Maintaining patient safety during this time is essential. The etiology and specific management of these neurocognitive disorders are discussed in detail in Chapter 16. Maintaining a calm, reassuring environment and demonstrating a high level of caring practices are essential for optimal psychological patient outcomes.

PROGRESSION OF CARE

Transfer to a progressive care unit occurs after the patient is extubated, hemodynamically stable, and no longer receiving any vasoactive medications. The expectation throughout the hospitalization period and beyond is that patients will participate actively and fully in their own recovery.

Pain Management

Transplant patients' requirements for pain medications vary. Back, shoulder, and chest discomfort are common. While the patient is intubated, a continuous infusion of either morphine or fentanyl is typically administered. The narcotic should be titrated so that the patient is easily arousable to verbal stimuli and able to follow simple commands. Once the patient has been extubated, use of acetaminophen and oral narcotics (e.g., oxycodone) is preferred. Nonsteroidal anti-inflammatory drugs (NSAIDs) are avoided given the compounded risk of nephrotoxicity when these medications are utilized in conjunction with CNIs (e.g., tacrolimus, CsA) to prevent rejection (Bennett, 2014).

Nutrition

Nutritional implications exist for the heart transplant recipient. Adequate nutrition is essential to prevent infection, augment wound healing, carry metabolic demand, and mediate an immune response (Posada-Moreno et al., 2012). Nutritional counseling is provided as patient education.

A number of recommendations regarding food intake following heart transplant have been published. Patients should be instructed not to consume raw food for the first 6 months following transplant. Casseroles should be cooked at home and eaten immediately after cooking, should be kept in the refrigerator covered, and eaten within 24 hours. Sauces should be kept separate (Posada-Moreno et al., 2012). Patients should consume a diet low in sodium and potassium.

Patients should avoid excessive weight gain after undergoing heart transplantation. This is essential to help avoid development of hypertension, diabetes, or hyperlipidemia. Patients who are obese or underweight 1 year after transplant are at increased risk for rejection than those patients of normal weight or overweight (Posada-Moreno et al., 2012).

Hyperlipidemia is common following heart transplant. Etiologic factors include poor diet, decreased physical activity, immunosuppressant therapy with CsA or steroids, antihypertensive medications, male gender, age, obesity, and diabetes. To prevent hyperlipidemia, it is recommended to maintain daily total cholesterol intake of less than 300 mg, limit fat intake to less than 30% of total caloric intake, limit saturated fat to less than 10% of total calories, and increase mono- and polyunsaturated fats; the latter should be kept to 7% of total calories (Posada-Moreno et al., 2012).

If the patient had preoperative cachexia, improvements in nutritional status have implications for early and late postoperative morbidity and mortality. Patients should be monitored for development of diabetes and metabolic syndrome as changes in immunosuppression may be indicated (Amarelli, Buonocore, Romano, Maiello, & De Santo, 2012).

A clear liquid diet is initiated at the time of extubation and advanced as tolerated. Because many heart transplant recipients are malnourished preoperatively with little nutritional reserve, caloric intake is followed closely and enteral feeding is initiated readily for patients who are not meeting caloric requirements.

Adequate intake of calcium and vitamin D is essential for patients with osteoporosis. Magnesium depletion has been documented in patients who have undergone heart transplantation. This may be related to diuretic therapy. Similarly, folate and vitamin B_6 deficiencies are common, especially in older patients and those with renal insufficiency. Intake of 5 mg of folic acid is recommended daily. L-arginine supplementation results in increased NO. This improves endothelial function and exercise tolerance following transplant. Each of these dietary interventions may augment quality of life when combined with other therapies (Posada-Moreno et al., 2012).

Data suggest that enteral nutrition is safe following cardiac surgery, even in patients with hemodynamic compromise (Lasierra et al., 2013). All transplant patients should be followed by a registered dietitian. When providing nutritional education, factors such as ethnicity, culture, and social issues need to be considered.

The nurse should be aware of food–drug interactions. A well-known interaction is that of grapefruit juice, a potent CYP3A4 inhibitor (Posada-Moreno et al., 2012).

Patients should be instructed to avoid nutritional and herbal supplements except as directed by their transplant team. Herbal supplements are increasing in popularity in the United States (Rispler & Sara, 2011). Because herbal supplements are not regulated by the FDA, a great deal is not known about these products. However, over time, knowledge has been gained about these agents regarding interactions and side effects that can impact recovery of the heart transplant patient. For example, decreased CsA levels have been shown with St. John's wort; this can potentially result in rejection. St. John's wort also interacts with CNIs, mammalian target of rapamycin (mTOR) inhibitors, and warfarin (Coumadin®). Increased CsA levels have been reported in patients who have consumed grapefruit juice and chamomile. Feverfew, ginger, cranberry, St. John's wort, and ginseng can interact with warfarin. Ginseng should be avoided in patients taking immunosuppressants. Feverfew, ginger, and ginkgo biloba can interact with aspirin. Ginger and melatonin may increase insulin levels. Melatonin has immunostimulant properties; therefore, it should be avoided in patients receiving immunosuppressant therapy. Garlic interferes with CsA and anticoagulants; increased bleeding times and clotting time can result. Glucosamine chondroitin and cat's claw can affect clotting agents. Astragalus is contraindicated with immunosuppressants. Black cohosh and Echinacea may cause hepatotoxicity. Kava interacts with sedatives. It may affect the CYP3A4 enzyme system. As such, it should be avoided in patients receiving CNIs and mTOR inhibitors (Colombo, Lunardon, & Bellia, 2014; Gellatly, 2012).

Activity and Exercise

Coughing, deep breathing, and early ambulation are important in heart transplant recipients, as in all postoperative patients. Physical and occupational therapy services are consulted for all transplant patients, and a program of progressive activity is undertaken as soon as the patient's status permits. This program is implemented during hospitalization and continued upon discharge. Patients are also referred for cardiac rehabilitation. Patients are encouraged to assume gradually increasing responsibility for their self-care needs.

The transplanted heart responds differently to exercise than does a native heart. For instance, the resting heart rate is higher because of the lack of vagal innervation. Heart rate is slower to increase with exercise, and slower to return to baseline following physical exertion. In addition, the maximal heart rate is lower in a transplanted heart. Long-term physical activity is important to ensure favorable results following heart transplantation.

Data support progressive early mobility following cardiac surgery. The type and duration of therapy remains unclear and there are great variations in implementation that exist. There are concerns about weight bearing and exercising in patients with a documented sternotomy. General guidelines reported not using arms to push up from a lying to a sitting position, arms to push from a sitting to a standing position, arms and shoulders for full active movement, lifting with weights, or using a walker or crutches (Westerdahl & Möller, 2010).

Following a heart transplant, patients should participate in regular weight-bearing exercise as well as muscle strengthening. These are important to help mitigate falls and fractures and side effects of CNIs and CsA, and to increase bone density. Participation in cardiac rehabilitation and aerobic exercising is further recommended (Costanzo et al., 2010).

Exercise ability decreases after a heart transplant. This is thought to be related to preoperative and postoperative factors. Patients with severe, protracted HF who are awaiting transplantation have exercise intolerance for a number of reasons. These include development of skeletal muscle atrophy, fatigue, and deconditioning from being hospitalized while awaiting transplant and decreased physical ability if a VAD is in place.

Denervation of the heart also impacts the ability to participate in aerobic activities.

Corticosteroids and CNIs may decrease skeletal muscle function. There is some improvement in exercise tolerance following heart transplantation, but skeletal muscle atrophy does not resolve immediately following heart transplantation. As such, exercise intolerance persists to some degree postoperatively.

Some data suggest that exercise training may increase exercise tolerance. Oxygen consumption increased by 27% to 33%. Methodological flaws are noted in these studies. The improvements in exercise tolerance are thought to be due to improved endothelial function and skeletal muscle oxidative capacity. Exercise training may mitigate some side effects of immunosuppressant therapy and decrease risk factors for cardiovascular disease (e.g., insulin resistance, obesity, diabetes, dyslipidemia) (Hunt et al., 2009).

As part of patient teaching, the nurse must review the anticipated schedule of return visits. Clearance to return to work or school or to resume driving will depend on each individual's progress. Physical restrictions include no lifting, pulling, or pushing of any item weighing more than 10 pounds for the first 6 weeks post-transplant. This is followed by orders not to lift, pull, or push anything weighing more than 25 pounds for at least 12 weeks. Patients should also be provided with a MedicAlert® bracelet.

Rejection

Rejection occurs when T cells recognize the implanted heart tissue as foreign and mount an immune response targeted at eliminating it. The immune response leads to inflammation, cell damage, and death. If left unchecked, progressive decline in organ function ensues.

Three types of rejection are distinguished: hyperacute, acute, and chronic. Hyperacute rejection is rare but is caused by an antigen–antibody reaction. It may occur within minutes to hours after a transplant and is often fatal. Acute rejection occurs when surface cell antigens of the donor heart are recognized as being "non-self." This type of rejection usually occurs within the first few weeks after a transplant, but may occur years later. Chronic rejection is manifested by accelerated graft vasculopathy and typically does not occur within the first year of a transplant (Anderson, 2008).

Despite use of immunosuppressive medications, rejection is a relatively common occurrence. Risk factors for rejection include race (African American), age (older than 45 years), history of hypertension, mismatched donor, use of tacrolimus (versus CsA), and male gender (Yusabai et al., 2013). Gender data are not consistent. Other data suggest female donor and recipient is a risk factor for rejection (Aggarwal & Pagani, 2011; Eisen & Jessup, 2013a). Patients at risk for lethal rejection include those who are younger, are African American, had a high number of human leukocyte antigen (HLA) mismatches, or were on a VAD and had high levels of preformed antibodies (Pham, 2014b).

Patients experiencing rejection may be asymptomatic, or they may demonstrate symptoms consistent with left ventricular failure (e.g., dyspnea on exertion or at rest, paroxysmal nocturnal dyspnea, orthopnea, palpitation, or syncope). However, most patients are diagnosed during routine surveillance (Eisen & Jessup, 2013a). A myocardial biopsy is needed for definitive diagnosis. Complications of myocardial biopsy include pneumothorax, cardiac perforation, and tricuspid valve injury. Surveillance is discussed later in this chapter.

Rejection is prevented by ongoing administration of immunosuppressive agents. Protocols for immunosuppression are facility specific. The components of standard immunosuppression may include a corticosteroid, an antithymocyte globulin (ATG), or a murine monoclonal antibody OKT3 (Eisen & Jessup, 2013b).

Corticosteroids inhibit the synthesis of cytokines. By suppressing interleukin-1 by macrophages, decreased T-cell production of interleukin-2 by activated T cells results; this decreases the cellular immune response. It is not completely clear how they reverse acute rejection (Eisen & Jessup, 2013b). Antithymocyte globulin is derived from rabbits (thymoglobulin) or horses (lymphocyte immune globulin [ATGAM®]) with lymphoid cells from humans. A number of mechanisms are involved in reversing rejection with these agents. Side effects of these agents include allergic and immune reactions, fever, chills, and arthralgias. Patients are typically premedicated to prevent these reactions (Eisen & Jessup, 2013b).

Muromonab-CD3 is a murine monoclonal antibody. It binds to the CD3 antigen near the surface of T cells. It inhibits T-cell function in a number of ways. Side effects include a cytokine-mediated reaction (to the first dose). Patients with this reaction may manifest fever, rigors, nausea, vomiting, diarrhea, hypotension, chest pain, dyspnea, or wheezing. As with ATG, patients are typically premedicated to prevent these reactions. Increased risk of infection and lymphoproliferative disease are also possible (Eisen & Jessup, 2013b).

The treatment of rejection depends on the histologic grade, degree of hemodynamic compromise, patient symptoms, and the number of rejections that have occurred in the past. Mild rejections (grade R [formerly 1A, grade 1B, or low grade 2]) are typically not treated unless the patient is experiencing hemodynamic compromise. Corticosteroids will not resolve hemodynamic compromise. Moderate rejections (grade 2R [formerly grade 3A]) without hemodynamic compromise are usually treated with a temporary increase in dose of corticosteroids, either orally or intravenously. Patients usually undergo endomyocardial biopsy to determine resolution. Once resolved, the patient returns to the original plan for surveillance biopsies. Post-transplant surveillance is discussed in more detail later in this chapter. Severe rejection is understood to be grade 2R with hemodynamic compromise or grade 3R (formerly grades 3B and 4) or patients who develop rejection that does not respond to corticosteroids. These patients are typically treated with ATG or OKT3; the former is preferred because the cytokine reaction is less severe with this agent. Calcineurin inhibitors and mycophenolate mofetil (MMF, CellCept®) or azathioprine (AZA, Imuran®) therapy will continue at the prescribed dose if therapeutic blood levels have been attained. Alternatively, tacrolimus can replace CsA. Treatment for rejection should be stopped on confirmed resolution by endomyocardial biopsy (Eisen & Jessup, 2013b).

Immunosuppression

The term *immunosuppression* is used in the organ transplant setting to describe methods by which the transplant recipient's immune system is prevented from "attacking" the newly implanted organ. Given that rejection is mediated almost entirely by T cells, with B cells playing a lesser role, immunosuppressants target T-cell function in a variety of ways (Pham, 2014b). Immunosuppression regimens generally consist of two phases—induction and maintenance—with intensification of treatment or addition of new agents for episodes of rejection. Induction therapy offers strong suppression of the immune system in the immediate postoperative period. Use of induction agents also delays the use of immunosuppressants that are nephrotoxic. This is especially important in patients with impaired renal function. The maintenance regimen is lifelong. The goals of immunosuppression are to prevent acute and chronic rejection and mitigate toxicities and complications associated with the agents (Pham, 2014b). The particular strategy employed varies by surgeon preference, facility practice, and patient factors, but is uniformly initiated at the time of transplant. A discussion of the most commonly used immunosuppressant medications follows.

Induction Therapy

Classes of immunosuppressants used during the induction phase are the interleukin-2 receptor antagonist (IL-2Ra), polyclonal antithrombocyte antibodies, and monoclonal antibodies.

INTERLEUKIN-2 RECEPTOR AGONIST

The one IL-2Ra that is available in the United States at present is basiliximab (Simulect®). As its name connotes, basiliximab is a chimeric (a combination of mouse and human cells) monoclonal antibody. It is used to suppress the immune system. It works by stopping IL-2 from binding to a surface receptor of activated T cells, rather than all T cells. As such, basiliximab prevents T-cell proliferation, which is responsible for the cellular immune response of rejection. Basiliximab has fewer side effects than OKT3 and anti-thrombocyte antibodies. The side effects are primarily gastrointestinal (GI) in nature (Pham, 2014b).

A Cochrane review of randomized trials revealed a decreased incidence of acute rejection in patients who received an IL-2Ra as compared to those patients who received no induction therapy. There was also a lower incidence of acute rejection with IL-2Ras than in patients who received polyclonal antibodies (Pham, 2014b).

POLYCLONAL ANTIBODIES

Polyclonal antibodies originate from immunized horses (ATGAM®, lymphocyte immune globulin) or rabbits (Thymoglobulin®) with human lymphocytes. These agents have antibodies that work against a number of T lymphocytes. Compared with monoclonal antibodies (discussed in the next section), which act on a specific protein found on T cells, Thymoglobulin® contains antibodies

that bind to multiple T-cell antigens (i.e., CD2, 3, 4, 8, 11a, and 18). Side effects include serum sickness (e.g., fever, chills, tachycardia, hypotension, myalgia, and rash). The side effects typically occur with the first or second infusion. Stopping the infusion and then restarting it at a slower rate is suggested. Patients are usually premedicated with an intravenous glucocorticoid, antihistamine, antipyretic, and H_2 blocker to mitigate or prevent reactions. Some patients develop leukopenia and thrombocytopenia, which respond to dose reduction or discontinuation of the agent. Life-threatening side effects include being at risk for CMV and other opportunistic infections and malignancies (Pham, 2014b).

MONOCLONAL ANTIBODIES

Muromonab-CD3 (OKT3) is a murine (mouse-derived) monoclonal antibody that binds to the CD3 site on T lymphocytes. This 1) transiently activates and eliminates nearly all T cells from peripheral circulation, and 2) renders remaining or subsequent T cells incapable of activation. As a result, T cells cannot perform their immunologic function. Muromonab-CD3 may be used as induction therapy, particularly in patients with renal dysfunction who would not tolerate CNIs. Response to therapy can be assessed by measurement of CD3-expressing lymphocytes.

Because OKT3 initially activates T cells through binding of the monoclonal antibody with the CD3 surface protein, side effects are those associated with cytokine release. These side effects may range from common, minor flu-like symptoms (e.g., fever, chills, and minor pulmonary or GI symptoms) to life-threatening symptoms (e.g., bronchospasm, tachycardia, bradycardia, encephalopathy, seizures, renal insufficiency, and graft thrombosis). Symptoms from a first or second dose response are termed cytokine release syndrome (CRS), which is manifested with fever, rigors, nausea, vomiting, diarrhea, hypotension, chest pain, dyspnea, wheezing, increased capillary permeability, myalgias, and arthralgias. Cytokine release syndrome is caused by activation of T cells with release of cytokines. Patients are premedicated to prevent CRS. A life-threatening infection (especially CMV), an Epstein–Barr virus (EBV)-related lymphoproliferative disorder, and other opportunistic infections may also develop in some patients. Muromonab-CD3 significantly decreases the patient's lymphocyte count, so there is an increased risk of lymphoma and vascular rejection when this medication is given to heart transplant patients (Sánchez-Lázaro et al., 2010). Because of these side effects, use of OKT3 has dramatically decreased. Less than 1% of heart transplant patients receive this agent (Pham, 2014b).

In a comparison of basiliximab and OKT3 as induction agents after heart transplant, researchers found that both agents had similar efficacy. However, basiliximab was associated with shorter ICU length of stay post-transplant, a better safety profile, and easier patient management during the initial hospitalization (Delgado et al., 2011; Pham, 2014b).

Maintenance Therapy

Most of the regimens used for maintenance therapy are comprised of three agents—a CNI (e.g., CsA or tacrolimus), an antiproliferative agent (mycophenolate mofetil, sirolimus [Rapamune®], or AZA—the latter agent is used less often), and glucocorticoids (administered with tapered dosing) (Pham, 2014b).

CALCINEURIN INHIBITORS

The CNI category of anti-rejection agents includes tacrolimus and CsA. As the name connotes, CNIs inhibit calcineurin. Calcineurin transcribes interleukin-2 (IL-2). The end result is diminishing of T-lymphocyte activation and proliferation in response to antigens (something "other than self," such as a transplanted heart). Each of the available agents

forms complexes with different proteins. The drug–protein complexes bind to and inhibit calcineurin. Calcineurin inhibitors block this pathway, thereby inhibiting clonal expansion of T cells (Pham, 2014b).

This type of immunosuppression is highly effective, but significant toxicities—most notably nephrotoxicity—limit their use in the post-transplant setting. Cyclosporine A causes kidney injury in 75% of patients (Lehne, 2013). Other significant toxicities include new-onset diabetes mellitus, hyperkalemia, hypomagnesemia, hypertension, dyslipidemia, increased risk for opportunistic infection, and malignancy. The incidence of hypertension and hyperlipidemia is reportedly lower with tacrolimus than with CsA; a higher incidence of diabetes is noted with tacrolimus, however (Fitzsimmons, 2012; Pham, 2014b).

Because a significant proportion of heart transplant patients have baseline renal dysfunction (and possibly additional insult following CPB), CNIs are more often included in maintenance therapy rather than being used as induction therapy. The nurse should monitor renal function tests and intake and output. Levels (troughs) are followed daily until stable, and then periodically. Because CNIs are metabolized by the cytochrome P450 3A (CYP3A4) enzyme system, drug interactions are common and can significantly alter drug levels (Ashavaid, Raje, Shalia, & Shah, 2010). When administered concomitantly, CYP3A4 inhibitors will increase CsA levels; CYP3A4 inducers will decrease CsA levels (Lehne, 2013).

Tacrolimus is available in oral and intravenous formulations. It can lead to kidney injury. As such, it is suggested that tacrolimus not be administered with other nephrotoxic agents (Lehne, 2013).

Cyclosporine A is also available in oral and intravenous formulations. When administered intravenously, it should be administered as two infusions, given 12 hours apart.

Cyclosporine A is titrated according to blood levels. The dose should be based on renal function, side effects, infection, and according to the patient's risk of developing rejection. Side effects specific to CsA include CAD, elevated uric acid levels, dyslipidemia, neurotoxicity, and liver toxicity. Gingival hyperplasia and hirsutism have also been reported and are specific to CsA (Pham, 2014b).

Antiproliferative Agents

MYCOPHENOLATE MOFETIL

Mycophenolate mofetil is an antiproliferative agent that inhibits an enzyme that is necessary for deoxyribonucleic acid (DNA) synthesis. It inhibits proliferation of T cells and B cells (Pham, 2014b). It is available in oral and intravenous formulations; the dose is the same for both. Mycophenolate mofetil is used concomitantly with CNIs, corticosteroids, or both. Side effects are largely GI in nature, although leukopenia may occur as well. A connection between MMF and progressive multifocal leukoencephalopathy is suggested (Pham, 2014b). There is an increased risk of the patient developing CMV. Patients who receive immunosuppressants are also at risk for developing cancer, especially lymphoma (Seo, 2014). A rare case of pulmonary hemorrhage has also been reported with MMF (Gorgan, Bockorny, Lawlor, Volpe, & Fiel-Gan, 2013). Because it causes less bone marrow suppression and is not nephrotoxic, MMF is used more often than AZA. Titration of MMF is based on leukopenia and GI intolerance (Pham, 2014b).

SIROLIMUS

Sirolimus (Rapamune®), a proliferation inhibitor or mTOR inhibitor, is a relatively new agent that blocks T-cell proliferation through a mechanism similar to, but distinct from, the mechanism underlying CNIs' activity. It binds to the same protein and acts similar to tacrolimus. The complex that forms between the agent and protein it binds to inhibits mTOR. Mammalian target of rapamycin interferes with two phases of the cell cycle. The end result is T and B cell proliferation. Sirolimus blocks the signaling necessary for T-cell growth (Pham, 2014b).

The ultimate role of mTOR inhibitors in the immunosuppressant armamentarium and their impact on long-term outcomes remain to be determined. It has been suggested that sirolimus might be administered early in the post-transplant period as a means to delay initiation of CNIs, thereby avoiding the nephrotoxicity concerns associated with the latter medications. While fluid retention is clinically demanding when mTOR inhibitors are given, renal and cardiac function may be maintained using this approach (Dy & Adjei, 2013; Pham, 2014b).

Other side effects of sirolimus include dyslipidemia, impaired wound healing, edema, hypertension, headache, progressive multifocal encephalopathy, pancytopenia, venous thrombotic events, dyspnea, interstitial pneumonitis, alveolar hemorrhage, elevated triglycerides, hyperglycemia, new-onset diabetes, acneiform rash, extremity lymphedema, GI upset, proteinuria, urinary tract infections, and infertility (Kaplan, Qazi, & Wellen, 2014). Pericardial and pleural effusions have been reported. Pulmonary toxicity is rare (Pham, 2014b).

Sirolimus is an oral agent. Dosage is based on serum drug levels. Sirolimus does not cause nephrotoxicity, but when used with a CNI, it can augment the nephrotoxic effects of CNIs. It is therefore suggested that CNI dosage be decreased by 25% if given together. Nursing monitoring of patients receiving mTOR inhibitors includes assessment of complete blood count data to evaluate for development of myelosuppression and to monitor sirolimus levels (Pham, 2014b).

Glucocorticoids

Glucocorticoids (e.g., methylprednisolone [Medrol®], prednisone) are useful in all phases of immunosuppression (induction, maintenance, and management of acute rejection), as these agents suppress nearly all mechanisms of the immune system. They act directly on cell DNA to influence transcriptional regulation, which alters the expression of genes involved in immune and inflammatory responses (Pham, 2014b). Through this mechanism, corticosteroids affect the number and distribution of leukocytes, their ability to signal other immune cells, and their functional ability (e.g., decreased phagocytosis, inhibition of secretion of inflammatory substances). Glucocorticoids are typically part of a three-drug regimen. Patients are usually weaned to a lower dose or off after the first 6 to 12 months following transplant (Pham, 2014b).

Long-term use of glucocorticoids is associated with hyperglycemia, diabetes, hyperlipidemia, hypertension, fluid retention, myopathy, osteoporosis, and vulnerability for opportunistic infections (Pham, 2014b). Other reported side effects include emotional instability, headache, peptic ulcers, esophagitis, pancreatitis, pathological fractures, loss of muscle mass, hypokalemia, pituitary-adrenal insufficiency, herpes zoster, increased intraocular pressure, glaucoma, cataracts, euphoria, dysphoria, depression, mania, and insomnia (Saag & Furst, 2014).

Azathioprine (Imuran®)

Azathioprine is another antiproliferative agent that may be used to prevent rejection following a heart transplant. It inhibits DNA, thereby preventing cellular mitosis and proliferation of activated B and T lymphocytes. It inhibits most T-cell function (Pham, 2014b).

Azathioprine is typically administered in combination with a glucocorticoid or CNI. Oral and intravenous formulations are available. Side effects include myelosuppression (especially leukopenia), hepatotoxicity, and pancreatitis. Azathioprine should temporarily

be discontinued if the patient's white blood cell count decreases by 50% or is less than 3,000 m³ (Pham, 2014b). As AZA may be more carcinogenic, patients have been switched to other agents (Dhiantravan et al., 2013). Regardless of which antiproliferative agent is used, the nurse should monitor complete blood counts to evaluate for presence of associated myelosuppression.

Infectious Disease Following Heart Transplant

Infection is a primary complication following a heart transplant and is a common cause of morbidity and mortality in the first year in this patient population. Bacteria are the most frequent cause in the first postoperative week (Anderson et al., 2010; Eisen, 2014a). Interventions to prevent development of infection are essential. Prophylactic antibiotic administration based on institutional guidelines is recommended. Strict aseptic technique is required for surgical wound care as well as for management of all invasive lines, catheters, and devices. Once the surgical dressing is removed, usually after 48 hours, cleaning with an antimicrobial solution should be performed until wound healing has taken place (Anderson et al., 2010). Mediastinitis is discussed in detail in Chapter 18.

Heart transplant patients are at increased risk for development of infection for a number of reasons. For example, anti-rejection medications, especially when used in combination, uniformly increase the risk of infection. Transplant recipients are also at risk for common hospital-acquired infections as well as opportunistic infections (e.g., *Pneumocystis jiroveci* pneumonia [PJP], formerly *Pneumocystis carinii*; yeast; fungus). *Pneumocystis jiroveci* pneumonia can lead to the development of life-threatening pneumonitis. This complication is seen in heart–lung transplant recipients and others with impaired cellular immunity (Jana, 2012). Reactivation of old infections, such as CMV, toxoplasmosis, herpes simplex virus (HSV), varicella zoster virus (VZV), or EBV poses another threat: Primary infection by these organisms is not "cured," but rather is controlled by a competent immune system. Reactivation of infection does not occur in the immunocompetent patient because T and B cells are constantly circulating and immediately respond to any renewed activity of these latent organisms. T- and B-cell function in the immunocompromised patient, however, is diminished; thus reactivation of these infections will not be curtailed by a weakened immune system (Eisen, 2014a).

Other common sources of nosocomial infection include invasive lines, catheters, and devices; surgical incisions; and mechanical ventilation equipment. An infectious organism may also be present in the allograft (Alexander & Fishman, 2014).

Meticulous nursing care is essential to prevent this potentially lethal complication. Preventive measures are crucial in this regard; they include meticulous handwashing, administration of antimicrobial agents (the choices will be facility-specific), and discouraging visitation by persons with colds or flu or by persons who recently received a live vaccine. Invasive lines, catheters, and devices should be managed using evidence-based guidelines and removed as early as possible. When feasible, early ambulation should be encouraged.

As discussed in Chapter 18, strict glycemic control decreases the risk of deep sternal wound infection. While the patient is intubated and on mechanical ventilation, evidence-based interventions should be implemented to prevent ventilator-associated conditions (VACs). Guidelines to prevent VACs may be found on the American Association of Critical-Care Nursing's website in the "Practice Alerts" section.

Donor-derived infections are now being recognized as potential etiologic factors for post-transplant infections. For the first month following transplant, patients are at increased risk for antibiotic-resistant bacterial infections (e.g., methicillin-resistant *Staphylococcus aureus*, vancomycin-resistant *Enterobacter*, *Clostridium difficile*, and Gram-negative organisms). These patients are also at risk for multidrug-resistant *Pseudomonas aeruginosa*. Tuberculosis may become reactivated in the transplant recipient (Jana, 2012). The most common sites of bacterial infections in heart transplant recipients are lung, urinary tract, bloodstream, and abdomen. *Escherichia coli* and *Staphylococcus aureus* are the two most common organisms. *Klebsiella* is common as well (DeNofrio & Snydman, 2010).

Parasites can be transmitted from the donor. For example, *Toxoplasma gondii* persists in myocardial tissue; this puts recipients at risk for the development of toxoplasmosis. Prophylaxis with trimethoprim-sulfamethoxazole (Bactrim®) has decreased the incidence of toxoplasmosis (DeNofrio & Snydman, 2010).

Gastrointestinal toxicities secondary to immunosuppressive agents may result in the development of viruses. Examples of viruses that heart transplant patients are at increased risk for include CMV and EBV. More than 50% of patients who receive a solid organ transplant develop CMV within the first 90 days following transplant (Jana, 2012). Cytomegalovirus is an important predictor of patient outcome (DeNofrio & Snydman, 2010). Mycophenolate mofetil and mTOR inhibitors put the patient at risk for hepatitis E development and progression (Jana, 2012).

Candida, Aspergillus, and *Cryptococcus* are the most common fungal infections. Prophylactic measures have lowered the incidence of these infections. Cryptococcal infections are thought to be observed because older patients are being transplanted and from use of tacrolimus in the anti-rejection regimen (Jana, 2012).

Assessment for and prompt recognition of presence of signs and symptoms are equally important. These may include fever, chills, rigors, mental status changes, shortness of breath, elevated white blood cell count, fatigue, malaise, nausea, and vomiting (Kalil, 2014).

Infection Prophylaxis

Several well-established procedures to minimize infectious risks exist. First, the heart donor is screened for human immunodeficiency virus (HIV), hepatitis B virus (HBV), hepatitis C virus (HCV), CMV, syphilis, EBV, and *T. gondii*. Likewise, the heart recipient is screened before transplant for antibodies to CMV, toxoplasmosis, HIV, HSV, VZV, HBV, HCV, *T. gondii*, endemic fungi, and EBV. Presence of antibodies indicates previous infection and confirms the risk for reactivation of these infections in the setting of immunosuppression. The patient also receives a tuberculin skin test (Centers for Disease Control and Prevention, 2013; OPTN, 2014b). Prophylactic medications are used to prevent reactivation of a latent infection when appropriate.

To prevent de novo (new infection in recipient) infections with PJP, patients receive trimethoprim-sulfamethoxazole. Antifungal prophylaxis is facility based. *Candida* and *Aspergillus* are the primary fungal organisms seen in heart transplant recipients. Drug interactions with azole drugs and CNIs and rapamycin need to be considered when deciding on appropriate preventive measures. Data further suggest that neither ketoconazole (Nizoral®) nor clotrimazole (Mycelex® Troche) decreased the incidence of invasive fungal infections. Patients who should be considered for antifungal prophylaxis include those with kidney or liver dysfunction, large packed red blood cell requirements, prolonged ICU stay, need for additional surgery following transplant, known preoperative colonization with fungus, prior broad-spectrum antibiotic use, or prolonged use of total parenteral nutrition (Alexander & Fishman, 2014).

Cytomegalovirus is the most common opportunistic organism following solid organ transplant. It may be acquired from the donor, blood products, or reactivated in the recipient. Acyclovir (Zovirax®), ganciclovir (Cytovene®), or valacyclovir (Valtrex®) may be used for prevention (Alexander & Fishman, 2014).

Hepatitis B can be reactivated following heart transplantation due to anti-rejection medications. Vaccine administration is recommended prior to transplant. In order to prevent influenza, vaccine administration is recommended. The live, attenuated intranasal vaccine is contraindicated. Patients with a history of HSV or VZV infection should receive antiviral therapy for 3 to 6 months following transplant and during high-dose anti-rejection therapy (Alexander & Fishman, 2014).

Although these regimens are highly effective in preventing infectious complications, infection remains a significant cause of mortality through the 1-year mark following transplant (Eisen, 2014a).

Cardiac Allograft Vasculopathy

Cardiac allograft vasculopathy refers to allograft CAD in the transplanted heart. It is the leading cause of death in patients after the first 5 years following a heart transplant (Eisen & Jessup, 2013a). Cardiac allograft vasculopathy in transplant recipients is distinguished from CAD in other populations in that it results in diffuse luminal narrowing rather than discrete lesions. Therefore, it is often not amenable to percutaneous or surgical intervention. Another difference is the absence of collateral circulation. Cardiac allograft vasculopathy remains the predominant barrier to long-term survival following a heart transplant (Eisen, 2014a). The incidence of CAV is reported at up to 28% the first year after heart transplant and 40% to 70% after 5 years of transplant (Eisen, 2014b).

Some of the etiologic factors associated with CAV include older age of the donor,

donor history of hypertension, younger age of the recipient, number of HLA mismatches, and the recipient's pre-transplant history of ischemic heart disease (Gustafsson, 2013).

Diagnosis of CAV may be difficult based on symptomatology. Because of afferent and efferent denervation, patients rarely develop angina. As such, silent myocardial infarction, progressive HF, and sudden cardiac death may be how the patient presents with CAV. Possible manifestations include chest pain, dyspnea, diaphoresis, GI upset, syncope, or near syncope, but these are typically absent (Gustafsson, 2013).

Patients may have changes found on echocardiogram or changes in allograft function found on echocardiogram or right cardiac catheterization. Other invasive options are available. Coronary angiography will reveal vessel narrowing and filling of the coronary arteries. Thrombolysis in Myocardial Infarction frame count is the "number of cine frames required for dye to reach distal coronary landmarks during coronary angiography" (Gustafsson, 2013). Thrombolysis in Myocardial Infarction frame count reveals a decrease in coronary blood flow in patients with transplant atherosclerosis in some studies. Coronary flow reserve may be used to measure the speed of coronary blood flow and coronary flow reserve (increase in blood flow following administration of a vasodilator [e.g., adenosine [Adenocard®]). Patients with CAV are more likely to have decreased reserve than patients without CAV. Intravascular ultrasound may be performed with coronary angiography. Ultrasound will detect thickening of the intimal layer of coronary arteries (Gustafsson, 2013).

Noninvasive diagnostic studies are not sensitive enough to be performed in lieu of coronary angiography. Select low-risk patients may be followed with noninvasive methods. If abnormalities are noted, coronary angiography can then be performed. Invasive methods include dobutamine stress echocardiography, computed tomography (CT) coronary angiography, and biomarkers (e.g., C-reactive protein, N-terminal pro-brain natriuretic peptide [NT-pro BNP], and von Willebrand factor). Neither C-reactive protein nor NT-pro BNP are predictive of CAV; patients with high levels of these biomarkers are at greater risk of developing CAV. Endomyocardial biopsy is performed as part of surveillance for rejection (Gustafsson, 2013).

Prevention of CAV is essential because of poor outcomes associated with this complication. Preventive strategies that are reported include administration of statins. Patients who are transplant recipients have a high incidence of hyperlipidemia. Statin administration decreases the risk of CAV and improves mortality rates. One concern about this therapy is the associated development of myopathy. This is especially true when statins are administered with CsA or tacrolimus. Both of these anti-rejection medications inhibit the CYP3A4 enzyme system; the CYP3A4 enzyme system metabolizes most of the statin medications. One statin, pravastatin (Pravachol®), is not metabolized by the CYP3A4 enzyme, so the risk of myopathy is less with this statin (Eisen, 2014b).

Administration of sirolimus, an mTOR inhibitor and another anti-rejection medication, has been shown to decrease the incidence of CAV. Sirolimus decreases cell production. Its use in the prevention of CAV, however, may be concerning because of reports of poor wound healing with this agent (Eisen, 2014b).

Because oxidative stress has been implicated in the development of CAV, it is logical that antioxidants be considered to help prevent this condition. More data are needed. Administration of antioxidants (vitamins C and E), when given with pravastatin, has been shown to decrease the progression of atherosclerosis. This effect is thought to be due to decreased oxidative stress effects with antioxidants (Eisen, 2014b).

Administration of diltiazem (Cardizem®), if started shortly after heart transplant, has been shown to prevent development of CAV. The data are not definitive to support diltiazem's contribution regarding CAV prevention. However, it is suggested that it may be considered in patients early after transplant if hypertension is present. The need for a prudent lifestyle and preventive measures is emphasized to include smoking cessation, control of hypertension, and cholesterol reduction (with diet and medications) (Eisen, 2014b).

At present, the only definitive treatment for CAV is retransplantation. Ethical issues surround this treatment option given the limited number of organs available for transplant. Some question why a person should get a second heart while so many are awaiting transplantation of a first (Eisen, 2014b). Other treatment options that are described in the literature include altering the immunosuppression regimen by either increasing the dosage of the agents or changing them and revascularization (percutaneous or surgical). Increasing the dose of immunosuppressants is not recommended because of the increased risk of infection and malignancy. Percutaneous coronary intervention has been used as a palliative procedure in patients with single-vessel disease. Its efficacy remains unsupported in the literature. Only a small number of patients have been treated and no data are available yet on graft survival. There are limited data to suggest that angioplasty with stenting can lead to a decreased incidence of restenosis when compared to angioplasty alone. The efficacy of drug-eluting stents with CAV needs to be evaluated (Eisen, 2014b).

Coronary artery bypass grafting has been performed on a small number of patients. The efficacy data are inconsistent (Bhama et al., 2009; Eisen, 2014a; Fujita et al., 2014).

Prophylactic insertion of an implantable cardioverter defibrillator is also reported. Limited data are available regarding prevention of sudden cardiac death in patients with CAV (Eisen, 2014b).

Sirolimus has been shown to decrease the incidence of CAV. A study entailed substituting a CNI for sirolimus. While there was more plaque buildup in patients receiving CNIs, concern about the potential for acute rejection has been raised. In a subsequent study to address this concern, heart transplant patients initially received CNIs. After 12 weeks, patients were randomized to receive either sirolimus or continue with CNI therapy. The study was closed early because four of the seven patients who received sirolimus developed a grade IIIA (now grade 2R) rejection (Eisen, 2014b).

Post-Transplant Surveillance

Patients who undergo heart transplantation receive lifetime follow up for rejection, drug toxicity from immunosuppressive therapy, infection, malignancy, and other complications of therapy. The frequency of the monitoring is based on the amount of time since transplantation and the patient's postoperative course. In general, patients receive follow up every 7 to 10 days for the first month after transplant; this is followed by every 2 weeks for 1 month, every month for the remainder of the first year, and then every 3 to 6 months thereafter. Frequency of follow up is increased if problems develop (International Society for Heart & Lung Transplantation, 2010).

Monitoring levels of immunosuppressive agents and for complications of these agents is essential. Assessment of bone density while the patient continues on bisphosphonate therapy continues for at least 1 year (Costanzo et al., 2010).

Because the transplanted heart is denervated, the transplanted heart will not receive autonomic nervous system or vagal nerve stimulation. As a result, the patient's heart rate will be higher than normal. Transplant recipients will also have physiologically altered responses to stress; the denervated heart is unable to compensate with an increase in heart rate to maintain CO. This lack of response makes orthostatic hypotension difficult to manage. Further, angina is not experienced in response to ischemia. Dyspnea on exertion may increase, although early signs of rejection or CAV may be absent.

An ECG, biomarkers, cardiac imaging, and endomyocardial biopsies are performed at regular intervals to monitor for development of rejection (Eisen & Jessup, 2013a).

A number of resources and opportunities for collaboration among disciplines are available for patients following heart transplantation. These include home health nurses, assistance with cardiac rehabilitation, psychological support, nutritional planning, and support groups (Costanzo et al., 2010). The latter is important for both the patient and caregiver.

OUTCOMES AFTER HEART TRANSPLANT

The 1-year survival rate following heart transplant is reported to be as high as 81.8%; the overall 5-year survival rate is 69.8%. Patients with preexisting comorbidities such as hypertension, diabetes, and obesity are subject to higher mortality rates. A higher mortality rate of 63% is reported in patients with these three comorbidities when compared to patients with none of the comorbidities (Botta, 2014a).

The Registry of the International Society for Heart & Lung Transplantation's 31st Official Adult Heart Transplantation Report provided detailed data on outcomes following transplant. These data are summarized in **Table 19-5**.

Kaplan-Meier curves continue to show a steep decline in survival during the first

Table 19-5 Cumulative Morbidity Rates in Survivors of Adult Heart Transplant Recipients, 1995–2013			
	Within 1 Year (%)	Within 5 Years (%)	Within 10 Years (%)
Hypertension	72	92	—
Renal Dysfunction			
All	26	52	68
Abnormal creatinine < 2.5 mg/dL	18	33	39
Creatinine > 2.5 mg/dL	6.3	15	20
Long-term dialysis	1.5	2.9	6
Renal transplant	0.3	1.1	3.6
Hyperlipidemia	60	88	—
Diabetes	25	38	—
Coronary artery vasculopathy	7.8	30	50

Source: Data from Lund, L. H., Edwards, L. B., Kucheryavaya, A. Y., Benden, C., Christie, J. D., Dipchand, A. I., . . . Stehlik, J. (2014). The registry of the International Society for Heart & Lung Transplantation: Thirty-first official adult heart transplant report—2014; Focus them: Retransplantation. *Journal of Heart and Lung Transplantation, 33*(10), 996–1008.

6 months following heart transplant, then a linear decline. Survival during the first 6 to 12 months after transplant has improved from 2006 to June 2012. The adjusted survival at 1 year is 84% to 85%. Causes of death include myopathy, CAV, acute rejection, malignancy, graft failure, multiple organ failure, acute kidney injury, and non-CMV infection (Lund et al., 2014).

PATIENT TEACHING

The complexity of transplant care and the consequences of noncompliance make effective patient teaching critically important. Adherence to mandated care regimens is more likely if patients understand why these practices are important. For this reason, several educational strategies are used to relay information and confirm understanding. Methods of teaching include provision of printed information, verbal instruction from multidisciplinary team members, opportunities to practice skills, demonstration, and return demonstration. Patients are also provided with contact information so they can call with questions.

Infection Avoidance

Because infection poses one of the greatest threats to the transplant patient, avoidance and recognition of infection constitute a major focus of teaching. Common signs of infection are reviewed and patients are instructed to call if they develop any of these signs. Response to infection will be blunted in the immunosuppressed patient, so signs of infection may be nonspecific (e.g., malaise, "don't feel right"). Patients are advised to avoid people who have received live vaccines, and to check with their transplant provider before receiving any immunization. Other routine practices include proper handwashing; avoiding contact with people who are ill; observing standard food hygiene procedures;

and avoiding stagnant water, gardening, and digging. Patients frequently assume that the risk of gardening can be avoided if their hands are protected with gloves; in reality, the risk with gardening relates to inhalation of spores mobilized by manipulation of dirt. Finally, patients are encouraged to avoid any unnecessary medical procedures in the first 6 months after transplant.

Sexual Activity

Issues related to sexuality are also included in discharge teaching; specific instructions are provided, as well as opportunity to discuss concerns. Sexual activity may be resumed as soon as the patient feels ready. For 6 weeks, patients should avoid putting weight on their arms and chest. Sexual activity may be aerobic and should be approached as such, with appropriate warm-up (e.g., foreplay) and cooldown (e.g., cuddling) periods being employed.

Patients should be given the opportunity to discuss other sexuality-related issues, such as anxiety, lack of desire, and body image concerns, and should be reassured that these concerns are not unusual. They should be invited to speak openly about their concerns and ask questions as they arise. Finally, all patients are strongly encouraged to avoid pregnancy due to the theoretical and documented risk to the fetus prenatally and later in life (Subramaniam & Robson, 2008).

Other Instructions

Other instructions included in discharge teaching include recommendations regarding pet care, travel, and procedure for contacting the donor family. Sunscreen use is encouraged due to risk of photosensitivity and increased risk of skin cancer associated with immunosuppressive medications. Skin squamous cell carcinoma is a significant cause of morbidity and mortality in organ transplant patients (Ulrich, Degen, Patel, & Stockfleth, 2008).

Medications

Transplant patients are prescribed multiple medications that must be taken exactly as prescribed. The consequences of noncompliance (whether intentional or inadvertent) may be devastating. Every effort is made to ensure that the patient understands the dosing and administration regimen for all medications to be taken. Printed information should be provided to patients listing each medication prescribed along with its mechanism of action, side effects, interactions, dosing schedule, and procedures to be followed for missed doses. Due to the risk of interactions or compounded toxicities, patients are instructed not to take any over-the-counter medication without clearance from the transplant provider. Exceptions to this rule include acetaminophen, acetylsalicylic acid, docusate sodium (Colace®), senna, loperamide (Imodium®), and bismuth subsalicylate (Kaopectate®).

New prescriptions from non-transplant care providers should also be cleared by the transplant team. Patients are instructed to avoid all NSAIDs. Herbal teas, medications, and other nutritional supplements should also be cleared with the transplant team.

SUMMARY

The ICU nurse plays a pivotal role in optimizing outcomes of patients and families during HF exacerbations and the wait for a heart transplant. High levels of critical thinking are required to care for the patient on inotropic or mechanical support. Evaluating the patient's candidacy for transplant and supporting the patient and family as they await availability of a suitable donor heart require high levels of clinical inquiry and caring practices. The ICU nurse also has a role as a facilitator of learning as the patient and family learn about management strategies for HF and about the transplant process. Bridge to transplant therapy requires the nurse to provide realistic information to both patients and families about the percentage of patients (20% to 40%) (Leeper, 2006) who may die while receiving VAD therapy either due to complications or while awaiting a heart transplant.

Post-transplant patients have a high degree of vulnerability in the immediate postoperative period. The ICU nurse must monitor for, promptly recognize, and treat the significant complications that can affect short-, intermediate-, and long-term survival following heart transplantation.

CASE STUDY

A 46-year-old man with a 5-year history of HF has been diagnosed with end-stage HF. He originally had viral myocarditis that resulted in a dilated cardiomyopathy. He has slowly deteriorated even though he has had medical intervention of a biventricular pacemaker and home-delivered inotropic medication. He has been on the transplant list for a heart for 3 months. It was recommended that he undergo evaluation for heart transplantation, with LVAD therapy serving as a bridge to heart transplant.

Critical Thinking Questions

1. What are the general indications for VAD implementation?
2. What are potential complications when using an LVAD?
3. What are key restrictions to living with an LVAD in the home after discharge?

Answers to Critical Thinking Questions

1. A medical evaluation is conducted to ensure that the VAD is the best option. The device is typically utilized for:

   a. *Bridge to transplant*: A patient's medical condition can be stabilized while waiting for a donor heart.

   b. *Bridge to recovery*: Patients who have had a heart attack or heart surgery and require the use of a pump while their heart recovers.

   c. *Destination therapy*: Patients who are not eligible to receive a heart transplant may be supported on a VAD indefinitely.

2. Left ventricular assist device placement is a major surgical procedure that carries a significant risk for postoperative complications. The most common complications are bleeding, thromboembolism, device failure, GI bleeding, epistaxis, pleural effusions, and driveline infection (Pepper, 2012). Bleeding in the immediate postoperative period is common due to the frequent use of aspirin and warfarin in HF patients preoperatively for severely depressed left ventricular function, CAD, or dysrhythmias.

3. The following information should be shared with the patient:

   a. The VAD is implanted near the stomach, which can make a patient feel full faster. Therefore, patients may need to eat more frequent, smaller portions throughout the day.

   b. The patient will be on an anticoagulant and will need dietary consult to review foods that may affect blood-thinning medications.

   c. The VAD depends on adequate blood volume to function properly. Therefore, patients are encouraged to drink plenty of fluids.

   d. Weight loss is recommended for patients who are overweight.

   e. Patients should avoid being active in very hot or very cold temperatures.

   f. Patients are not allowed to swim or take a bath, as water can get inside of the pump and cause it to stop.

   g. Showering is allowed after the VAD site has healed. Education is required to learn how to use a shower kit that protects the external components of the system from water.

   h. Patients are not allowed to drive or operate heavy machinery.

   i. Patients should not engage in strenuous activity or play contact sports.

   j. Patients must stop smoking due to constriction of vessels, which reduces blood flow to vital organs.

   k. Alcohol should be avoided due to impacting a patient's ability to respond to alarms in a timely manner.

   l. All dental procedures will require a prophylactic antibiotic.

   m. Magnetic resonance imaging can damage the pump or cause the pump to stop.

   n. Static electricity may damage the electrical components of the pump.

   o. Travel is limited and should be discussed with a primary care provider.

SELF-ASSESSMENT QUESTIONS

1. Which of the following heart failure patients may be a candidate for heart transplantation? A patient with heart failure who:
   a. is receiving ultrafiltration
   b. has a predicated 1-year survival rate of at least 35%
   c. has a maximum oxygen consumption of < 12 mL/kg/min who is receiving beta blockers
   d. is requiring high-dose inotropic support

2. Which of the following patients has an absolute contraindication for a heart transplantation? A patient with:
   a. bilirubin 2.0 mg/dL
   b. creatinine clearance less than 50 mL/min
   c. diabetes with a HgbA$_{1c}$ 8.0%
   d. body mass index 28 kg/m^2

3. Which of the following patients is a candidate for a heart transplant? A patient with a history of:
   a. peptic ulcer disease
   b. cirrhosis
   c. end-stage renal disease
   d. mild depression

4. Which of the following statements is true regarding extracorporeal membrane oxygenation?
   a. It can provide support to the patient awaiting heart transplant for months.
   b. It uses a centrifugal pump to propel blood from the LV to the systemic circulation.
   c. A sternotomy is required for direct access and cannulation of the heart and great vessels.
   d. Blood is withdrawn via a central vein to a gas exchanger so that the heart and lungs are bypassed.

5. Following ventricular assist device placement, the nurse should anticipate administration of which of the following?
   a. Anticoagulants
   b. Broad-spectrum antibiotics
   c. Judicious fluid administration
   d. Inotropic support

6. Which of the following arterial blood gas results will likely promote pulmonary vasodilation?

	pH	pCO$_2$	pO$_2$	HCO$_3$
a.	7.49	30	73	19
b.	7.30	38	79	18
c.	7.51	31	65	25
d.	7.29	50	68	28

7. Which of the following should the nurse include in teaching patients being discharged home with a left ventricular assist device?
   a. Wipe dust from a computer screen before use.
   b. Rinse the ventricular filter with water weekly.
   c. Avoid extreme temperatures when tub bathing.
   d. Obtain a backup generator.

8. Which of the following should the nurse anticipate to be ordered for a patient following heart transplantation?
   a. Monitor for orthostatic hypotension
   b. Atropine 0.5 mg IV for symptomatic bradycardia
   c. Nitroglycerin 0.4 mg SL for angina
   d. Nitric oxide administration based on systemic vascular resistance

9. Which of the following is an early sign of bleeding in a postoperative heart transplant patient?
   a. Pulmonary artery pressures of 13/9 mmHg
   b. Blood pressure of 80/40 mmHg
   c. SvO$_2$ of 58%
   d. Heart rate of 130 beats/minute

10. Which of the following hemodynamic parameters should be of greatest

concern to the nurse following heart transplantation of a patient with heart failure?

a. Pulmonary artery pressures 64/40 mmHg
b. Central venous pressure 2 mmHg
c. Heart rate 120 beats/minute
d. Blood pressure 80/60 mmHg

Answers to Self-Assessment Questions

1. c
2. c
3. d
4. d
5. d
6. d
7. d
8. a
9. d
10. a

Clinical Inquiry Box

Question: What is the experience of nurses caring for patients with a ventricular assist device?

Reference: Gibson, J. A., Henderson, A., Jillings, C., & Kaan, A. (2013). Nursing patients with ventricular assist devices: An interpretative description. *Progress in Transplantation, 23*(2), 147–153.

Objective: To investigate the experience of nursing patients with a ventricular assist device.

Method: A qualitative study was conducted with six registered nurses who provided care to VAD therapy patients. Data were collected through semi-structured interviews. The data were transcribed and analyzed.

Results: Four themes emerged from the data through inductive analysis. These themes were exclusive knowledge, human connection, ethics, and interdisciplinary stress and technology. The nurses spoke about specialized knowledge that was gained through the experience of working with VAD patients. The nurses discussed the human connection as a witnessing of human suffering and struggle. The ethic of "keeping a patient alive" was expressed as a form of distress for the nurses.

Conclusion: The nurse–patient relationship resulted in intensified emotions due to their exposure to the unpredictable dying trajectory. Counseling should be considered for nurses in this specialized field, especially when deaths occur.

REFERENCES

Achneck, H. E., Sileshi, B., Parikh, A., Milano, C. A., Welsby, I. J., & Lawson, J. H. (2010). Pathophysiology of bleeding and clotting in the cardiac surgery patient. *Circulation, 122,* 2068–2077.

Adler, E., & Enciso, J. S. (2013). Functional improvement after ventricular assist device implantation: Is ventricular recovery more common than we thought? *Journal of the American College of Cardiology, 61*(19), 1995–1997.

Agarwal, P. P., Cascade, P. N., & Pagani, F. (2009). Novel treatment options for chronic heart failure: A radiologist's perspective. *American Journal of Roentgenology, 193*(1), W14–W24.

Aggarwal, S., & Pagani, P. D. (2011). Complications following heart transplantation. In M. W. Mulholland & G. M. Doherty (Eds.), *Complications in surgery* (2nd ed., pp. 674–700). Philadelphia, PA: Lippincott Williams & Wilkins.

Alba, A. C., & Delgado, D. H. (2009). The future is here: Ventricular assist devices for the failing heart. *Expert Review of Cardiovascular Therapy, 7*(9), 1067–1077.

Alejaldre, A., Delgado-Mederos, R., Santos, M. A., & Martí-Fàbregas, J. (2010). Cerebrovascular complications after heart transplantation. *Current Cardiology Reviews, 6*(3), 214–217.

Alexander, B. D., & Fishman, A. A. (2014). *Prophylaxis of infection in solid organ transplantation.* Retrieved from http://uptodate.com/contents/prophylaxis-of-infection-in-solid-organ-transplantation

Allen, S. J., & Sidebotham, D. (2012). Postoperative care and complications after ventricular assist device implantation. *Best Practice and Research. Clinical Anaesthesiology, 26*(2), 231–246.

Amarelli, C., Buonocore, M., Romano, G., Maiello, C., & De Santo, L. S. (2012). Nutritional issues in heart transplant candidates and recipients. *Frontiers in Bioscience, 4*, 662–668.

Anderson, A. S. (2008). *Left ventricular dysfunction after orthotopic cardiac transplantation.* Retrieved from http://www.utdol.com/online/content/topic.do?topicKey=hrt_tran/5916&selectedTitle=2~150&source=search

Anderson, A., Chan, M., Desai, S., Fedson, S., Fischer, P., Gonzales-Stawinski, G., . . . Smith, J. (2010). *The International Society for Heart & Lung Transplantation guidelines for the care of heart transplant recipients. Task Force 1: Peri-operative care of the heart transplant recipient.* Retrieved from https://www.ishlt.org/ContentDocuments/ISHLT_GL_TaskForce1_080410.pdf

Ashavaid, T., Raje, H., Shalia, K., & Shah, B. (2010). Effect of gene polymorphisms on the levels of calcineurin inhibitors in Indian renal transplant recipients. *Indian Journal of Nephrology, 20*(3), 146–151.

Ashikhmina, E. A., Schaff, H. V., Sinak, L. J., Li, Z., Dearani, J. A., Suri, R. M., . . . Sundt, T. M., III. (2010). Pericardial effusions after cardiac surgery: Risk factors, patient profiles, and contemporary management. *Annals of Thoracic Surgery, 89*, 112–118.

Bennett, W. M. (2014). *Cyclosporine and tacrolimus nephrotoxicity.* Retrieved from http://www.uptodate.com/contents/cyclosporine-and-tacrolimus-nephrotoxicity

Bhama, J. K., Nguyen, D. Q., Scolier, S., Teuteberg, J. J., Toyoda, Y., Dormos, R. L., . . . Bermudez, C. A. (2009). Surgical revascularization for cardiac allograft vasculopathy: Is it still an option? *The Journal of Thoracic and Cardiovascular Surgery, 137*(6), 1488–1492.

Bhat, G., Canter, C., Chinnock, R., Crespo-Leiro, M., Delgado, R., Dobbels, F., . . . Wolfel, G. (2010). *The International Society for Heart & Lung Transplantation guidelines for the care of heart transplant recipients. Task Force 3: Long-term care of heart transplant recipients.* Retrieved from https://www.ishlt.org/ContentDocuments/ISHLT_GL_TaskForce3_080610.pdf

Bojar, R. (2011). Cardiovascular management. In *Manual of perioperative care in adult cardiac surgery* (5th ed., pp. 437–580). Boston, MA: Wiley-Blackwell.

Botta, D. M., Jr. (2014a). *Heart transplantation.* Retrieved from http://emedicine.medscape.com/article/429816-overview#aw2aab6b2b7

Botta, D. M., Jr. (2014b). *Heart transplantation technique.* Retrieved from http://emedicine.medscape.com/article/429816-technique#aw2aab6b4b2

Bunch, J., Mahapatra, S., Reddy, Y. M., & Lakkireddy, D. (2012). The role of percutaneous left ventricular assist devices during ventricular tachycardia ablation. *Eurospace, 14*(Suppl. 2), ii26–ii32.

Centers for Disease Control and Prevention. (2013). *Transplant safety: Donor screening and testing.* Retrieved from http://cdc.gov/transplant-safety/screening_testing.html

Colombo, D., Lunardon, L., & Bellia, G. (2014). Cyclosporine and herbal supplement interactions. *Journal of Toxicology, 2014.* Article ID 145325. Retrieved from http://www.hindawi.com/journals/jt/2014/145325/

Costanzo, M. R., Dipchand, A., Starling, R., Anderson, A., Chan, M., Desai, S., . . . Vanhaecke, J. (2010). The International Society for Heart & Lung Transplantation guidelines for the care of heart transplant recipients. *Journal of Heart and Lung Transplantation, 29*(8), 914–956.

Delgado, J. F., Vaqueriza, D., Sánchez, V., Escribano, P., Ruiz-Cano, M. J., Renes, E., . . . de la Calzada, C. (2011). Induction treatment with monoclonal antibodies for heart transplantation. *Transplantation Reviews, 25*, 21–26.

DeNofrio, D., & Snydman, D. R. (2010). Risks and epidemiology of infection after heart transplantation. In R. A. Bowden, P. Ljungman, & D. R. Snydman (Eds.), *Transplant infections* (3rd ed., pp. 104–113). Philadelphia, PA: Lippincott Williams & Wilkins.

Dhiantravan, V., Patel, J., Kittleson, M., Rafiei, M., Osborne, A., Chang, D., . . . Kobashigawa, J. (2013). Mycophenolate not azathioprine with increased risk for skin cancer after heart transplant. *Journal of the American College of Cardiology, 61*(10_S). doi: 10.1016/S0735-1097(13)60797-4

Dy, G. K., & Adjei, A. A. (2013). Understanding, recognizing, and managing toxicities of targeted anticancer therapies. *CA: A Cancer Journal for Clinicians, 63*(4), 249–279.

Eisen, H. (2014a). *Heart transplantation (Beyond the basics)*. Retrieved from http://www.uptodate.com/contents/heart-transplantation-beyond-the-basics

Eisen, H. (2014b). *Prevention and treatment of cardiac allograft vasculopathy*. Retrieved from http://www.uptodate.com/contents/prevention-and-treatment-of-cardiac-allograft-vasculopathy?source=see_link

Eisen, H. J., & Jessup, M. (2013a). *Acute cardiac allograft rejection: Diagnosis*. Retrieved from http://www.uptodate.com/contents/acute-cardiac-allograft-rejection-diagnosis?source=related_link

Eisen, H. J., & Jessup, M. (2013b). *Acute cardiac allograft rejection: Treatment*. Retrieved from http://www.uptodate.com/contents/acute-cardiac-allograft-rejection-treatment

Eisen, H. J., & Kusmirek, L. S. (2012). Arrhythmias following cardiac transplantation. Retrieved from http://www.uptodate.com/contents/arrhythmias-following-cardiac-transplantation

Fitzsimmons, W. E. (2012). Tacrolimus. In B. Kaplan, G. J. Burkhart, & F. G. Lakkis (Eds.), *Immunotherapy in transplantation: Principles and practice* (pp. 224–240). Hoboken, NJ: Wiley-Blackwell.

Friedline, K., & Hassinger, P. (2012). Total artificial heart freedom driver in a patient with end-stage biventricular heart failure. *AANA Journal, 80*(2), 105–112.

Fujita, T., Kobayashi, J., Hata, H., Murata, Y., Suguchi, O., Yanese, M., . . . Nakatani, T. (2014). Off-pump coronary artery bypass grafting for a left main lesion due to cardiac allograft vasculopathy in Japan: First report of a case. *Surgery Today, 44*(10), 1949–1952.

Gellatly, R. M. (2012). Complementary and alternative medicine use in the transplant patient. *International Society for Heart & Lung Transplantation* Links, 4(3). Retrieved from http://www.ishlt.org/ContentDocuments/2012JulLinks_Gellatly.html

Go, A., Mozaffarian, D., Roger, V., Benjamin, E., Berry, J., Borden, W., . . . Turner, M. B. (2013). Heart disease and stroke statistics—2013 update. *Circulation, 127*, e6–e245.

Gorgan, M., Bockorny, B., Lawlor, M., Volpe, J., & Fiel-Gan, M. (2013). Pulmonary hemorrhage with capillaritis secondary to mycophenolate mofetil in a heart-transplant patient. *Archives of Pathology & Laboratory Medicine, 137*(11), 1684–1687.

Granton, J. T., & Cheng, D. C. H. (2011). Heart transplantation and subsequent noncardiac surgery. In F.-S. F. Yao, V. Malhotra, & M. L. Fontes (Eds.), *Yao's & Artusio's anesthesiology: Problem-oriented patient management* (7th ed.). Philadelphia, PA: Lippincott Williams & Wilkins.

Gregoric, I. D., Cohn, W. E., Akay, M. H., La Francesca, S., Myers, T., & Frazier, O. H. (2008). CentriMag left ventricular assist system. *Texas Heart Institute Journal, 35*(2), 184–185.

Gustafsson, F. (2013). *Natural history and diagnosis of cardiac allograft vasculopathy*. Retrieved from http://www.uptodate.com/contents/natural-history-and-diagnosis-of-cardiac-allograft-vasculopathy?source=related_link

Haddad, F., Hunt, S., Rosenthal, D. N., & Murphy, D. J. (2011). Right ventricular function in cardiovascular disease: Part I. *Circulation, 117*, 1436–1448.

Haft, J. W., Suzuki, Y., Aaronson, K. D., Dyke, D. B., Wright, S., Poirier, V. L., & Pagani, F. D. (2007). Identification of device malfunction in patients supported with the HeartMate XVE left ventricular assist system. *ASAIO Journal, 53*(3), 298–303.

Hasin, T., Topilsky, Y., Schirger, J. A., Li, Z., Zhao, Y., Boilson, B. A., . . . Kushwaha, S. S. (2012). Changes in renal function after implantation of continuous-flow left ventricular assist devices. *Journal of the American College of Cardiology, 59*(1), 26–36.

Heart Failure Society of America. (2014). *Quick facts and questions about heart failure*. Retrieved from http://www.hfsa.org/hfsa-wp/wp/patient/questions-about-heart-failure/

Hunt, S. A., Abraham, W. T., Chink, M. H., Feldman, A. M., Francis, G. S., Ganiats, T. G., . . . Yancy, C. W. (2009). 2009 focused update incorporated into the ACC/AHA 2005 Guidelines for the Diagnosis and Management of Heart Failure in Adults: A report of the American College of Cardiology Foundation/American Heart Association Task Force on Practice Guidelines: Developed in collaboration with the International Society for Heart and Lung Transplantation. *Circulation, 119*(14), e391.

Ichinose, F., Roberts, J. D., Jr., & Zapol, W. M. (2004). Review: Cardiovascular drugs. Inhaled nitric oxide. *Circulation, 109,* 3106–3111.

Ichinose, F., & Zapol, W. M. (2010). Nitric oxide and inhaled pulmonary vasodilators. In R. D. Miller, L. I. Eriksson, L. A. Fleisher, J. P. Wiener-Kronish, & W. L. Young (Eds.), *Miller's anesthesia* (7th ed., pp. 941–956). Philadelphia, PA: Elsevier Churchill Livingstone.

Idrees, M. M., Al-Hajjaj, M., Khan, J., Al-Hazmi, M., Alanezi, M., Saleemi, S., . . . Barst, R. (2008). Saudi guidelines on diagnosis and treatment of pulmonary arterial hypertension. *Annals of Thoracic Medicine, 3*(5), 1–57.

International Society for Heart & Lung Transplantation. (2010). *The International Society for Heart and Lung Transplantation guidelines for the care of heart transplant recipients. Task force 2: Immunosuppression and rejection.* Retrieved from https://www.ishlt.org/ContentDocuments/ISHLT_GL_TaskForce2_110810.pdf

Iyer, A., Kumarasinghe, G., Hicks, M., Watson, A., Gao, L., Doyle, A., . . . MacDonald, P. S. (2011). Primary graft failure after heart transplantation. *Journal of Transplantation, 2011.* Retrieved from http://www.hindawi.com/journals/jtrans/2011/175768/

Jahan, M., Tabassum, S., Aziz, A., Ahmed, M., & Islam, N. (2010). Transfusion associated CMV infection: Transfusion strategies for high risk patients. *Bangladesh Journal of Medical Microbiology, 4*(2), 24–27.

Jana, A. A. (2012). *Infections after solid organ transplant.* Retrieved from http://emedicine.medscape.com/article/430550-overview

Kalil, A. (2014). *Septic shock clinical presentation.* Retrieved from http://emedicine.medscape.com/content/article/168402-clinical

Kaplan, B., Qazi, Y., & Wellen, J. R. (2014). Strategies for the management of adverse events associated with mTOR inhibitors. *Transplantation Reviews, 28*(3), 126–133.

Kaplow, R. (2013). *Cardiac tamponade.* Retrieved from http://www.inpractice.com/Textbooks/Oncology-Nursing/Oncologic-Emergencies/Cardiac-Tamponade.aspx

Kaplow, R., & Hardin, S. R. (2007). *Critical care nursing: Synergy for optimal outcomes.* Sudbury, MA: Jones and Bartlett.

Kirklin, J., Naftel, D., Kormos, R., Stevenson, L., Pagani, F., Miller, M., . . . Young, J. (2012). The fourth INTERMACS annual report: 4000 implants and counting. *Journal of Heart and Lung Transplantation, 31*(2), 117–126.

Klima, U., Ringes-Lichtenberg, S., Warnecke, G., Lichtenberg, A., Strüber, M., & Haverich, A. (2005). Severe right heart failure after heart transplantation: A single-center experience. *Transplant International, 18,* 326–332.

Kollef, M., & Isakov, W. (2012). Pulmonary hypertension and right ventricular failure in the intensive care unit. In M. Kollef & W. Isakov (Eds.), *The Washington manual of critical care* (2nd ed., pp. 87–96). Philadelphia, PA: Lippincott Williams & Wilkins.

Lasierra, J. L. F., Pérez-Vela, J. L., Makikado, L. D. U., Sánchez, E. T., Gómez, L. C., Rodriguez, B. M., . . . González, J. C. M. (2013). Early enteral nutrition in patients with hemodynamic failure following cardiac surgery. *Journal of Parenteral & Enteral Nutrition.* doi: 10.1177/0148607113504219

Leeper, B. (2006). Advanced cardiovascular concepts. In M. Chulay & S. M. Burns (Eds.), *AACN essentials of critical care nursing* (pp. 431–461). New York, NY: McGraw-Hill.

Lehne, R. A. (2013). Immunosuppressants. In R. A. Lehne (Ed.), *Pharmacology for nursing care* (8th ed., pp. 874–880). St. Louis, MO: Elsevier Saunders.

Lund, L. H., Edwards, L. B., Kucheryavaya, A. Y., Benden, C., Christie, J. D., Dipchand, A. I., . . . Stehlik, J. (2014). The registry of the International Society for Heart & Lung Transplantation: Thirty-first official adult heart transplant report-2014; Focus them: Retransplantation. *Journal of Heart and Lung Transplantation, 33*(10), 996–1008.

Mancini, D. (2014). *Indications and contraindications for cardiac transplantation.* Retrieved from http://www.uptodate.com/contents/indications-and-contraindications-for-cardiac-transplantation

Mason, V. F., & Konicki, A. J. (2003). Left ventricular assist devices as destination therapy. *AACN Clinical Issues: Advanced Practice in Acute and Critical Care, 14*(4), 488–497.

Matthews, J. C., & McLaughlin, V. (2008). Acute right ventricular failure in the setting of acute pulmonary embolism or chronic pulmonary hypertension: A detailed review of the patho-physiology, diagnosis, and management. *Current Cardiology Reviews, 4*(1), 49–59.

McCalmont, V., & Ohler, L. (2008). Cardiac transplantation: Candidate identification, evaluation, and management. *Critical Care Nursing Quarterly, 31*(3), 216–229.

McCulloch, B. (2011). Use of the Impella 2.5 in high-risk percutaneous coronary intervention. *Critical Care Nurse, 31,* e1–e16. Retrieved from http://ccn.aacnjournals.org/content/31/1/e1.full.pdf

Meineri, M., Van Rensburg, A. E., & Vegas, A. (2012). Right ventricular failure after LVAD implantation: Prevention and treatment. *Best Practice & Research. Clinical Anaesthesiology, 26*(2), 217–229.

National Heart, Lung, and Blood Institute. (2012). *What is a total artificial heart?* Retrieved from http://www.nhlbi.nih.gov/health/health-topics/topics/tah/

National Heart, Lung, and Blood Institute. (2014). *What to expect during a heart transplant.* Retrieved from https://www.nhlbi.nih.gov/health/health-topics/topics/ht/during.html

Nishi, H., Toda, K., Miyagawa, S., Yoshikawa, Y., Fukushima, S., Yoshioka, D., . . . Sawa, Y. (2013). Prediction of outcomes in patients with liver dysfunction after left ventricular assist device implantation. *Journal of Artificial Organs, 16*(4), 404–410.

Organ Procurement and Transplantation Network. (2014a). *Transplants in the U.S. by recipient ABO.* Retrieved from http://optn.transplant.hrsa.gov/PublicComment/pubcommentPropSub_281.pdf

Organ Procurement and Transplantation Network. (2014b). *Proposal to modify disease donor testing requirements. Toxoplasma screening by Toxoplasma gondii.* Retrieved from http://optn.transplant.hrsa.gov/PublicComment/pubcommentPropSub_323.pdf

Patel, A. M., Adeseun, G. A., Ahmet, I., Mitter, N., Rame, J. E., & Rudnick, M. R. (2012). Renal failure in patients with left ventricular assist devices. *Clinical Journal of the American Society of Nephrology.* doi: 10.2215/CJN.06210612. Retrieved from http://cjasn.asnjournals.org/content/early/2012/10/10/CJN.06210612.full.pdf+html

Pepper, J. R. (2012). Update on mechanical circulatory support in heart failure. *Heart, 98*(8), 663–669.

Pham, M. X. (2014a). *Prognosis after cardiac transplantation.* Retrieved from http://www.uptodate.com/contents/prognosis-after-cardiac-transplantation

Pham, M. X. (2014b). *Induction and maintenance of immunosuppressive therapy in cardiac transplantation.* Retrieved from http://www.uptodate.com/contents/induction-and-maintenance-of-immunosuppressive-therapy-in-cardiac-transplantation

Posada-Moreno, P., Ortuño-Soriano, I., Zaragoza-García, I., Rodríguez-Martinez, D., Pacheco-del-Cerro, J., Martínez-Rincón, C., . . . Villarino-Marín, L. (2012). Nutritional intervention in heart transplant recipients—Dietary recommendations. In S. Moffatt-Bruce (Ed.), *Cardiac transplantation.* Retrieved from http://www.intechopen.com/books/cardiac-transplantation/nutritional-intervention-in-people-with-heart-transplant-dietary-recommendations-

Raja, S. G., & Shahbaz, Y. (2006). Desmopressin for haemostasis in cardiac surgery: When to use? *Annals of Cardiac Anaesthesia, 9,* 102–107.

Rispler, D. T., & Sara, J. (2011). The impact of complementary and alternative modalities on the care of orthopaedic patients. *Journal of the American Academy of Orthopaedic Surgeons, 19*(10), 634–643.

Rodriguez-Cruz, E. (2013). *Extracorporeal membrane oxygenation.* Retrieved from http://emedicine.medscape.com/article/1818617-overview

Rose, E. A., Gelijns, A. C., Moskowitz, A. J., Heitjan, D. F., Stevenson, L. W., Dembitsky, W., . . . Meier, P. (2001). Long-term use of a left ventricular assist device for end-stage heart failure. *New England Journal of Medicine, 345*(20), 1435–1443.

Ruan, C.-H., Dixon, R. A. F., Willerson, J. T., & Ruan, K.-H. (2010). Prostacyclin therapy for pulmonary artery hypertension. *Texas Heart Institute Journal, 37*(4), 391–399.

Saag, K. G., & Furst, D. E. (2014). *Major side effects of corticosteroids.* Retrieved from http://www.uptodate.com/contents/major-side-effects-of-corticosteroids

Sánchez-Lázaro, I. J., Almenar, L., Martínez-Dolz, L., Agüeru, J., Buendia, F., Navarro, J., . . .

Salvador, A. (2010). Lymphomas in heart transplant recipients: Do antivirals protect against the neoplastic effect of anti-CD3 monoclonal antibody? *Transplantation Proceedings, 42*(8), 3206–3207.

Schumacher, K. R., & Gajarski, R. J. (2011). Postoperative care of the transplant patient. *Current Reviews in Cardiology, 7*(2), 110–122.

Seo, P. (2014). *Mycophenolate mofetil. Pharmacology and adverse events when used in the treatment of rheumatic diseases.* Retrieved from http://www.uptodate.com/contents/mycophenolate-mofetil-pharmacology-and-adverse-effects-when-used-in-the-treatment-of-rheumatic-diseases

Shanewise, J. (2004). Cardiac transplantation. *Anesthesiology Clinics of North America, 22,* 753–765.

Sidebotham, D., & Gillham, M. (2007). Hemodynamic instability and resuscitation. In D. Sidbotham, A. McKee, M. Gillham, & J. H. Levy (Eds.), *Cardiothoracic critical care* (pp. 295–315). Philadelphia, PA: Butterworth-Heinemann, Elsevier.

Simsch, O., Gromann, T., Knosalla, C., Hübler, M., Hetzer, R., & Lehmkuhl, H. (2011). The intensive care management of patients following heart transplantation at the Deutsches Herzzentrum Berlin. *Applied Cardiopulmonary Pathophysiology, 15,* 230–240.

Singh, T. P., Almond, C. S., Taylor, D. O., & Graham, D. A. (2012). Decline in heart transplant wait list mortality in the United States following broader regional sharing of donor hearts. *Circulation: Heart Failure, 5*(2), 249–258.

Slaughter, M. S., Pagani, F. D., Rogers, J. G., Miller, L. W., Sun, B., Russell, S. D., . . . Farrar, D. J. (2010). Clinical management of continuous-flow left ventricular assist devices in advanced heart failure. *Journal of Heart and Lung Transplantation, 29*(4S), S1–39. Retrieved from http://www.mc.vanderbilt.edu/documents/heart/files/Slaughter%20et%20al%20Clinical%20Management%20of%20LVADs.pdf

Subramanian, P., & Robson, S. (2008). Heart transplant and pregnancy. *O & G Magazine, 10*(3), 32–35.

Sudarshan, C., Kreisel, D., & Rosengard, B. R. (2008). Heart transplantation. In J. Norton, P. S. Barie, R. R. Bollinger, A. E. Cheng, S. Lowry, S. J. Mulvihill, . . . R. W. Thompson (Eds.), *Surgery: Basic science and clinical evidence* (2nd ed., pp. 1861–1888). New York, NY: Springer.

Taegtmeyer, H. (2006). Heart failure. In T. A. Miller (Ed.), *Modern surgical care: Physiologic foundations and clinical applications* (3rd ed., pp. 663–670). Boca Raton, FL: CRC Press.

Takayama, H., Takeda, K., Doshi, D., & Jorde, U. (2014). Short-term continuous-flow ventricular assist devices. *Current Opinion in Cardiology, 29*(3), 266–274.

Thajudeen, A., Stecker, E. C., Shehata, M., Patel, J., Wang, X., McAnulty, J. H., . . . Chugh, S. S. (2012). Arrhythmias after heart transplantation: Mechanisms and management. *Circulation, 1,* e001461. Retrieved from http://jaha.ahajournals.org/content/1/2/e001461.full

Toda, K., Fujita, T., Kobayashi, J., Shimahara, Y., Kitamura, S., Kitamura, S., . . . Nakatani, T. (2011). Impact of preoperative percutaneous cardiopulmonary support on outcomes following left ventricular assist device implantation. *Circulation Journal.* Retrieved from https://www.jstage.jst.go.jp/article/circj/advpub/0/advpub_CJ-11-0339/_pdf

Ulrich, C., Degen, A., Patel, M. J., & Stockfleth, E. (2008). Sunscreens in organ transplant patients. *Nephrology Dialysis Transplantation, 23*(6), 1805–1808.

Wagner, F. (2011). Monitoring and management of right ventricular function following cardiac transplantation. *Applied Cardiopulmonary Pathophysiology, 15,* 220–229.

Westerdahl, E., & Möller, M. (2010). Physiotherapy-supervised mobilization and exercise following cardiac surgery: A national questionnaire survey in Sweden. *Journal of Cardiothoracic Surgery, 5.* Retrieved from http://www.cardiothoracicsurgery.org/content/5/1/67

Yarlagadda, C. (2014). *Cardiac tamponade clinical presentation.* Retrieved from http://emedicine.medscape.com/article/152083-clinical

Yimin, H., Xiaoyu, L., Yuping, H., Weiyan, L., & Ning, L. (2013). The effect of vasopressin on the hemodynamics of CABG patients. *Journal of Cardiothoracic Surgery, 8.* Retrieved from http://www.cardiothoracicsurgery.org/content/8/1/49

Yusabai, A., Mehrnia, A., Kamgar, M., Sampaio, M., Huang, E., & Bunnapradist, S. (2013). Risk factors for acute rejection in heart transplanted recipients. *American Transplant Congress Meeting Abstracts.* Retrieved from http://www.atcmeetingabstracts.com/abstract/risk-factors-for-acute-rejection-in-heart-transplanted-recipients/

WEB RESOURCES

Cardiac surgery: http://www.youtube.com/watch?v=qVYiGdQKP4s

Ventricular assist device: http://www.youtube.com/watch?v=DLV6kIfvSDA

Life on the transplant list: http://www.youtube.com/watch?v=xS7v4M-VmGw

Heart-lung transplantation: http://www.youtube.com/watch?v=zuG3mJQ3p40

Deciding whether to have transplant surgery: http://www.youtube.com/watch?v=Q0qQX6Ps79c

Orthotopic heart transplant: http://www.youtube.com/watch?v=N7etGEtdCCk

ECMO cannulation technique: https://www.youtube.com/watch?v=ntBiTpwnKK4

ECMO: http://www.youtube.com/watch?v=Psci-wZKN_s

Chapter 20

Implications of Obesity of the Cardiac Surgery Patient

Roberta Kaplow and Sonya R. Hardin

INTRODUCTION

According to the Centers for Disease Control and Prevention (CDC), approximately 35% of adults in the United States are obese. Comorbidities associated with obesity result in annual medical costs that are $1,429 higher for people who are obese as compared to those of normal weight. The annual costs of medical care in the United States were approximately $147 billion in 2008 (CDC, 2014).

Obesity does not affect all racial groups equally. The group with the highest age-adjusted rate of obesity is non-Hispanic blacks (47.8%). This is followed by Hispanics (42.5%), non-Hispanic whites (32.6%), and non-Hispanic Asians (10.8%). Further, the highest rate of obesity occurs in adults 40–59 years of age (39.5%). This is compared to adults 20–39 years of age (30.3%) and those age 60 and older (35.4%) (CDC, 2014).

Obesity is defined based on body mass index (BMI). A person's BMI can be calculated using a calculator that is available free of charge online on any of several websites. It is based on the ratio of weight (in kilograms) and height (in centimeters). Many of the online BMI calculators allow one to enter his or her weight in pounds and height in inches. The World Health Organization (WHO) classifies obesity based on BMI. A person is classified as overweight with a BMI of 25–29.9 kg/m^2; obesity is defined as a BMI greater than 30 kg/m^2. Obese class I corresponds with a BMI of 30–34.99 kg/m^2, class II is a BMI of 35–39.99 kg/m^2, and class III is a BMI of 40 kg/m^2 or higher (WHO, 2015). Waist circumference is another way to classify presence of obesity. This method has not yet been uniformly adapted into clinical practice.

A number of comorbidities are associated with obesity. These include angina, hypertension, stroke, type 2 diabetes, hypercholesterolemia, and some types of cancer (Lamvu, Zolnoun, Boggess, & Steege, 2004). As the number of persons with obesity increases, so too will the number requiring cardiac surgery. Nurses caring for these patients require an understanding of the physiologic changes that are associated with obesity and must modify their care to meet the individual needs of this patient population. This chapter describes the physiologic changes that occur as a result of obesity and issues surrounding the patient with obesity who is undergoing cardiac surgery. Implications of care during the preoperative, intraoperative, and postoperative phases are also described.

PHYSIOLOGIC CHANGES ASSOCIATED WITH OBESITY

A number of physiologic changes occur in patients with obesity. The changes are typically due to an increase in body mass or adiposity.

Changes in the cardiovascular, respiratory, gastrointestinal (GI), and renal systems are addressed in the sections that follow.

Cardiovascular Changes

A number of cardiovascular and hemodynamic changes occur as a result of increased body mass. There is an increase in cardiac output (CO) in order to meet the increase in metabolic demands. Dilation of the left ventricle occurs due to the increase in venous return; this results in left ventricular hypertrophy (LVH). Heart failure can occur in patients with obesity as a result of increases in circulating volume and CO, LVH, and left ventricular diastolic dysfunction (Mathew, Francis, Kayalar, & Cone, 2008). Other cardiovascular changes include increases in stroke volume, myocardial workload, myocardial oxygen demand, and decreased vascular resistance. Hypertension and cardiomegaly result from increases in CO and stroke volume (Lamvu et al., 2004). Data suggest an increased risk of death associated with obesity-related dilation of cardiac chambers, ventricular hypertrophy, heart failure, and arrhythmias (Bauml, 2010; Koplan & Stevenson, 2007).

Respiratory Changes

There are changes in the respiratory system related to obesity. Obesity causes an increase in carbon dioxide (CO_2) production and oxygen consumption. There is a decrease in chest wall compliance due to the extra weight around the ribs, below the diaphragm, and in the abdominal area. Decreased lung compliance results from hindered expansion of the chest wall and increases in oxygen demand and pulmonary blood volume (Salome, King, & Berend, 2010). The decrease in lung compliance results in decreases in lung volumes (Littleton, 2012) such as expiratory reserve volume (the maximum amount of air that can be exhaled from the lungs following a normal exhalation) (White, 2013) and functional residual capacity

(FRC, the amount of air left in the lungs at the end of exhalation) (Ranu, Wilde, & Madden, 2011). Patients with obesity often have lower tidal volume with an associated increase in respiratory rate. Decreases in lung volumes and chest wall movement may result in increased work of breathing and oxygen consumption. Restrictive lung disease may develop in patients with obesity from increases in intra-abdominal pressure and decreased compliance of the chest wall (Pedoto, 2012). Mild hypoxia may exist due to ventilation-perfusion mismatch from basilar atelectasis (Littleton, 2012). An increase in intrapulmonary shunting from 2% to 5% in normal weight adults to up to 25% in obese adults has been reported (Lamvu et al., 2004; Poirier et al., 2009).

Patients with obesity may also develop obstructive sleep apnea (OSA). Obstructive sleep apnea has been reported in 5% of obese patients. It results in chronically low oxygen levels, elevated CO_2 levels, and pulmonary and systemic vasoconstriction. These put the patient at increased risk for intrapulmonary shunting and ischemia (cardiac and cerebral) (Pedoto, 2012).

Gastrointestinal Changes

Obesity is associated with a number of GI changes. For example, incidence of gastroesophageal reflux is higher because of increased intra-abdominal pressure. Patients also have increased gastric volume, lower gastric pH, and decreased gastric motility (Pedoto, 2012).

Renal Changes

Presence of obesity puts the patient at greater risk for developing hypertension and diabetes; both of these are implicated in the development of end-stage renal disease. Obesity also has effects on hemodynamics in the kidney; patients with fewer nephrons are more likely to develop these hemodynamic effects. Etiology factors of obesity-related kidney disease include hyperfiltration and increased wall tension on the glomerular capillaries (Wickman & Kramer, 2013).

DRUG PHARMACOKINETICS AND PHARMACODYNAMICS

The pharmacokinetics and pharmacodynamics of drugs are altered in patients with obesity. The distribution and elimination of drugs will be affected as a result of obesity-related decreased total body water and increased CO, volume of distribution, adiposity, and renal blood flow. It has been suggested that patients be dosed for medications based on ideal body weight (Pedoto, 2012).

THE PREOPERATIVE PHASE OF CARDIAC SURGERY

As described in Chapter 4, the nurse plays a pivotal role in performing a preoperative evaluation prior to cardiac surgery. During this time, a comprehensive history and physical may reveal pivotal information that can impact the patient's intraoperative and postoperative trajectory. The nurse should inquire about and assess for symptoms of OSA, obesity hypoventilation syndrome (OHS), and obesity-associated comorbidities (e.g., hypertension, angina, diabetes, and impaired renal function). Appropriate diagnostic tests should also be obtained (e.g., chest radiograph, electrocardiogram, and labs). Because OSA is often undiagnosed, it is suggested that a tool to screen patients should be used. An example of an OSA screen is the STOP-Bang questionnaire. This eight-question screening tool assesses for presence of snoring, feeling tired, and observed apnea. Neck size, gender, BMI, and age are all considered in determining the probability of presence of OSA (Chung et al., 2012; Chung et al., 2008).

Obesity hypoventilation syndrome is present when a person with obesity has a CO_2 level greater than 45 mmHg while awake. It is reported to be present in up to 20% of patients with OSA. Obesity hypoventilation syndrome is reported to be more common in patients with severe obesity and those with dyspnea on exertion. For patients deemed to be at risk for having OHS, the nurse performing the preoperative evaluation should obtain an order for an arterial blood gas to determine if hypercarbia is present. If a patient is found to have CO_2 retention, referral for sleep studies or to a pulmonologist is recommended prior to the patient having surgery, if possible (Sheen & Sheu, 2011).

During the preoperative evaluation, baseline vital signs should be obtained. If the patient has poorly controlled hypertension (systolic pressure greater than 170 mmHg or diastolic pressure greater than 110 mmHg), it should be determined if surgery can be delayed so that blood pressure control can be attempted (Sheen & Sheu, 2011).

Evaluation of the patient's management of diabetes should also occur during the preoperative evaluation. Data including degree of glycemic control and blood glucose range will be helpful during the perioperative period. Presence of metabolic syndrome, defined as the coexistence of type 2 diabetes and cardiovascular disease risk factors (e.g., hyperglycemia, dyslipidemia, hypertension, and abdominal obesity), is associated with an increased risk of postoperative complications. Optimization of any of these components prior to surgery is recommended. Baseline data will also help with perioperative management (Sheen & Sheu, 2011).

PREPARATION OF THE OPERATING ROOM AND STAFF

In order to best prepare the patient with obesity for cardiac surgery, the operating room (OR) staff and anesthesia provider must be aware of the patient's weight. The surgical table must be able to accommodate the patient's weight; two tables pushed together may be required. Need for additional padding, linen, and lifting equipment should be anticipated. Additional staff may be required to assist with patient transfer and proper positioning. Appropriately sized monitoring and safety equipment (e.g., blood pressure cuff and sequential compression sleeves) should be procured. Because of the conical shape of the upper arm that may exist in patients with obesity, it may not be possible to place the blood pressure cuff in that location; alternative sites may need to be considered (e.g., lower arm or lower leg) (Schumann et al., 2009).

Additional equipment may be needed to administer anesthesia to a patient with obesity. Needles with extra length may be required for administration of any epidural anesthesia or nerve blocks (Schumann et al., 2009). Because of the increased amount of adipose tissue in the pharyngeal walls, upper airway collapse may result; difficulty with bag-valve-mask ventilation, intubation, or both may be realized (Pedoto, 2012).

Supine positioning during cardiac surgery may further decrease FRC. Compliance of the chest wall and lungs also decreases when the patient with obesity is in supine position. This may result in hypoventilation and barotrauma while on mechanical ventilation (Pedoto, 2012).

Patients with OSA will have further decreases in lung volume and compliance when they receive anesthesia. This places them at greater risk for development of atelectasis during induction of anesthesia. An increase in intrapulmonary shunting can result. During induction, these patients are also at increased risk for aspiration due to the aforementioned GI changes associated with obesity.

POSTOPERATIVE CARE

Patients typically remain intubated for a period of time following cardiac surgery. It is common for lung volumes to remain low and for atelectasis to be present following open heart surgery. There remains a dilemma as to which mode of ventilation to use (pressure or volume controlled) because of the risk of ventilation-induced injury. No differences between these two modes of ventilation are reported (Aldenkortt, Lysakowski, Elia, Brochard, & Tramèr, 2012). It is suggested that the goal of mechanical ventilation focus on using peak inspiratory pressures and positive end-expiratory pressure that are adequate to open and keep open collapsed alveoli. Extubation failure is not uncommon in the immediate postoperative period for patients with obesity. This is especially true of patients with chronic obstructive pulmonary disease.

The incidence of atelectasis is reported to be more common following cardiopulmonary bypass procedures than in other surgical procedures. Atelectasis correlates well with intrapulmonary shunt (Magnusson & Spahn, 2003).

Use of noninvasive ventilation methods such as continuous positive airway pressure and bilevel positive airway pressure (BiPAP) is reported to decrease the incidence of reintubation in patients with obesity (Pedoto, 2012). Because of the increased work of breathing that is typically present in postoperative patients with obesity (Pedoto, 2012), the positive pressure associated with BiPAP may be beneficial. Because of the changes in lung volumes and the enhancement of these effects when placed in a supine position, patients with obesity should be positioned in a semi-sitting position unless contraindicated (Lemyze et al., 2013; Pedoto, 2012).

During handoff from the OR, the intensive care unit (ICU) nurse should inquire about any difficulties encountered during intubation. If these were present, diligence should be exercised when determining readiness for extubation. Once successfully extubated, strategies should be implemented to prevent postoperative respiratory complications. In one study, pain associated with decreased postoperative lung volumes was evaluated. Patients with a BMI greater than 25 kg/m² had lower inspiratory capacity. Higher pain levels during mobilization correlated with decreases in postoperative lung volumes (Urell, Westerdahl, Hedenström, Janson, & Emtner, 2012).

In an older meta-analysis, postoperative patients with obesity who used an incentive spirometer or who underwent chest physiotherapy had improved lung function and fewer complications. In this study, patients had a BMI of 30–40 kg/m² and performed coughing every 10 to 15 minutes for the first 2 hours following extubation (Thomas & McIntosh, 1994).

Patients with obesity, OSA, or both may be more sensitive to respiratory depression associated with the administration of sedatives and opioids (Adams & Murphy, 2000). There is a potential for airway obstruction to occur when sedated. Patients should be monitored with pulse oximetry and an end-tidal CO_2 detector.

Complications of cardiac surgery reported in the literature include increased length of stay (Curiel-Balsera et al., 2013; Sartini, Winfield, & Bizzarri, 2012; Wigfield et al., 2006), increased mortality rates (Bakaeen & Chu, 2011; Barnett, Martin, Halpin, & Ad, 2010; Curiel-Balsera et al., 2013; Del Prete et al., 2010; Demir et al., 2012; Rahmanian et al., 2007; Wagner et al., 2007; Wang, Yang, Wu, Cao, & Yang, 2013), sternal wound dehiscence (Santapino, Pfeiffer, Concistré, & Fischlein, 2013), wound infection (Grauhan et al., 2013; Rahmanian et al., 2007; Sartini et al., 2012), mediastinitis (Diez et al., 2007; Risnes, Abdelnoor, Almdahl, & Svennevig, 2010), readmission to the ICU (Sartini et al., 2012), acute kidney injury (Billings et al., 2012; Sartini et al., 2012; Virani et al., 2009; Wigfield et al., 2006), atrial fibrillation (Bramer et al., 2011; Hernandez et al., 2013; Sartini et al., 2012; Zacharias et al., 2005), increased prothrombotic state (Kindo et al., 2014), and increased ventilator time (Wigfield et al., 2006).

There are conflicting data on the incidence of complications and mortality rates following cardiac surgery when comparing obese patients with those who are not. Some data suggest no difference in the incidence of these complications or mortality rates in patients with obesity, while other data suggest statistically significant increased incidence of these outcome variables. The former has been called the "obesity paradox" (Stamou et al., 2011).

SUMMARY

Nurses caring for patients with obesity who underwent cardiac surgery procedures should anticipate the presence of and observe for signs and symptoms of these complications and promptly intervene if they manifest. Early recognition and prompt intervention are essential to optimize patient outcomes.

CASE STUDY

A 48-year-old male with a history of obesity, hypertension, diabetes, OSA, and hyperlipidemia was admitted to the ICU following coronary artery bypass grafting. His intraoperative course was uncomplicated. He is intubated and on mechanical ventilation. He is receiving a continuous infusion of morphine and a benzodiazepine to prevent inadvertent extubation and promote comfort.

Critical Thinking Questions

1. How should the ICU nurse position this patient?
2. For which complications should the ICU observe?
3. What changes in respiratory physiology should the ICU nurse anticipate?

Answers to Critical Thinking Questions

1. The patient should be positioned in a semi-sitting position to mitigate intrapulmonary shunting that is associated with a supine position in patients with obesity.
2. The nurse should observe for early signs of wound infection, acute renal failure, atrial fibrillation, and increased ventilator time.
3. Respiratory parameters the ICU nurse should anticipate include hypercarbia, increased oxygen consumption, decreased chest wall and lung compliance, decreased chest wall expansion, decreased tidal volume, increased respiratory rate, increased work of breathing, mild hypoxia, increased shunt, and signs and symptoms of OSA.

SELF-ASSESSMENT QUESTIONS

1. Which of the following is a cardiovascular change associated with obesity?
   a. Decreased CO
   b. Decreased metabolic demand
   c. Increased vascular resistance
   d. Increased stroke volume

2. Which of the following is an etiologic factor of hypertension and cardiomegaly associated with obesity?
   a. Increased CO
   b. Decreased stroke volume
   c. Increased myocardial workload
   d. Decreased vascular resistance

3. Which of the following is a respiratory change associated with obesity?
   a. Decreased respiratory rate
   b. Increased oxygen consumption
   c. Increased pulmonary compliance
   d. Decreased pulmonary blood volume

4. Which of the following is an etiologic factor associated with restrictive lung disease associated with obesity?
   a. Increased intra-abdominal pressure
   b. Increased chest wall compliance
   c. Decreased intrapulmonary shunting
   d. Decreased expiratory reserve volume

5. Which of the following is a sequela of OSA?
   a. Vasodilation of the pulmonary vasculature
   b. Low oxygen tension
   c. Low CO_2 levels
   d. Vasodilation of the systemic vasculature

6. Which of the following should the nurse anticipate affecting the pharmacokinetics of drugs administered to patients with obesity?
   a. Increased total body water
   b. Decreased volume of distribution

c. Decreased renal blood flow

d. Increased CO

7. Which of the following should be anticipated to occur upon induction of anesthesia in the patient with obesity undergoing cardiac surgery?

a. Decreased FRC

b. Increased chest wall compliance

c. Decreased aspiration risk

d. Increased lung compliance

8. Which of the following complications is a patient with obesity likely to experience in the immediate postoperative period following cardiac surgery?

a. Ventilator-associated barotrauma

b. Atelectasis

c. Wound infection

d. Atrial fibrillation

9. Which of the following occurs as a result of increased CO and LVH associated with obesity?

a. Ventilation/perfusion mismatch

b. Ventricular tachycardia

c. Heart failure

d. Decreased myocardial oxygen demand

10. Which of the following is a GI change associated with obesity?

a. Decreased gastric pH

b. Increased gastric motility

c. Decreased gastric volume

d. Increased gastric emptying

Answers to Self-Assessment Questions

1. d	6. d
2. a	7. a
3. b	8. b
4. a	9. c
5. b	10. a

Clinical Inquiry Box

Question: Does obesity predict acute kidney injury after cardiac surgery?

Reference: Billings, F. T., Pretorius, M., Schildcrout, J. S., Mercaldo, N. D., Byrne, J. G., Ikizler, T. A., . . . Brown, N. J. (2012). Obesity and oxidative stress predict AKI after cardiac surgery. *Journal of the American Society of Nephrology, 23*(7), 1221–1228.

Objective: To determine if obesity-related oxidative stress, endothelial dysfunction, and inflammation predict the development of acute kidney injury following cardiac surgery.

Method: A retrospective review of 445 patients who underwent cardiac surgery was performed. Markers for oxidative stress and inflammation were evaluated.

Results: Overall, 25% of the patients developed acute kidney injury following cardiac surgery. The inflammatory markers did not reveal an association between high BMI and development of acute kidney injury. However, increased BMI independently predicted development of acute kidney injury.

Conclusion: Obesity was an independent predictor of acute kidney injury following cardiac surgery. Oxidative stress might be implicated in its development.

REFERENCES

Adams, J. P., & Murphy, P. G. (2000). Obesity in anaesthesia and intensive care. *British Journal of Anaesthesia, 85*(1), 91–108.

Aldenkortt, M., Lysakowski, C., Elia, N., Brochard, L., & Tramèr, M. R. (2012). Ventilation strategies in obese patients undergoing surgery: A quantitative systematic review and meta-analysis. *British Journal of Anaesthesia, 109*(4), 493–502.

Bakaeen, F. G., & Chu, D. (2011). The obesity paradox and cardiac surgery: Are we sending the wrong message? *Annals of Thoracic Surgery*, *92*(3), 1153.

Barnett, S. D., Martin, L. M., Halpin, L. S., & Ad, N. (2010). Impact of body mass index on clinical outcome and health-related quality of life following open heart surgery. *Journal of Nursing Care Quality*, *25*(1), 65–72.

Bauml, M. A. (2010). Left ventricular hypertrophy: An overlooked cardiovascular risk factor. *Cleveland Clinic Journal of Medicine*, *77*(6), 381–387.

Billings, F. T., Pretorius, M., Schildcrout, J. S., Mercaldo, N. D., Byrne, J. G., Ikizler, T. A., . . . Brown, N. J. (2012). Obesity and oxidative stress predict AKI after cardiac surgery. *Journal of the American Society of Nephrology*, *23*(7), 1221–1228.

Bramer, S., van Straten, A. H., Albert, H. M., Hamad, M. A. S., Berreklouw, E., van den Broek, K. C., . . . Maessen, J. G. (2011). Body mass index predicts new-onset atrial fibrillation after cardiac surgery. *European Journal of Cardio-Thoracic Surgery*, *40*(5), 1185–1190.

Centers for Disease Control and Prevention. (2014). *Overweight and obesity*. Retrieved from http://www.cdc.gov/obesity/data/adult.html

Chung, F., Subramanyam, R., Liao, P., Sasaki, E., Shapiro, C., & Sun, Y. (2012). STOP-Bang score indicates a high probability of obstructive sleep apnea. *British Journal of Anaesthesia*, *108*(5), 768–775.

Chung, F., Yegneswaran, B., Liao, P., Chung, S. A., Vairavanathan, S., Islam, S., . . . Shapiro, C. M. (2008). STOP questionnaire: A tool to screen patients for obstructive sleep apnea. *Anesthesiology*, *108*(5), 812–821.

Curiel-Balsera, E., Muñoz-Bono, J., Rivera-Fernández, R., Benitez-Parejo, N., Hinojosa-Pérez, R., & Reina-Toral, A. (2013). Consequences of obesity in outcomes after cardiac surgery. Analysis of ARIAM registry. *Medical Clinics (Barcelona)*, *141*(3), 100–105. (Abstract).

Del Prete, J. C., Bakaeen, F. G., Dao, T. K., Huh, J., LeMaire, S. A., Coselli, J. S., . . . Chu, D. (2010). The impact of obesity on long-term survival after coronary artery bypass grafting. *Journal of Surgical Research*, *163*, 7–11.

Demir, A., Sydinh, B., Güçlü, Ç. Y., Yazicio lu, H., Saraç, A., Elhan, A. H., . . . Erdemli, Ö. (2012). Obesity and postoperative early complications in open heart surgery. *Journal of Anesthesia*, *26*, 701–710.

Diez, C., Koch, D., Kuss, O., Silber, R.-E., Friedrich, I., & Boergermann, J. (2007). Risk factors for mediastinitis after cardiac surgery—A retrospective analysis of 1700 patients. *Journal of Cardiothoracic Surgery*, *2*. Retrieved from http://www.cardiothoracicsurgery.org/content/2/1/23

Grauhan, O., Navasardyan, A., Hofmann, M., Muller, P., Stein, J., & Hetzer, R. (2013). Prevention of poststernotomy wound infections in obese patients by negative pressure wound therapy. *Journal of Thoracic and Cardiovascular Surgery*, *145*(5), 1387–1392.

Hernandez, A. V., Kaw, R., Pasupuleti, V., Bina, P., Ioannidis, J. P., Bueno, H., . . . Gillinov, M. (2013). Association between obesity and postoperative atrial fibrillation in patients undergoing cardiac operations: A systematic review and meta-analysis. *Annals of Thoracic Surgery*, *96*(3), 1104–1116.

Kindo, M., Minh, T. H., Gereli, S., Meyer, N., Schaeffer, M., Perrier, S., . . . Mazzucotelli, P. (2014). The prothrombotic paradox of severe obesity after cardiac surgery under cardiopulmonary bypass. *Thrombosis Research*, *134*(2), 346–353.

Koplan, B. A., & Stevenson, W. G. (2007). Sudden arrhythmic death syndrome. *Heart*, *93*(5), 547–548.

Lamvu, G., Zolnoun, D., Boggess, J., & Steege, J. F. (2004). Obesity: Physiologic changes and challenges during laparoscopy. *American Journal of Obstetrics & Gynecology*, *191*, 669–674.

Lemyze, M., Mallat, J., Duhamel, A., Pepy, F., Gasan, G., Barrailler, S., . . . Thevenin, D. (2013). Effects of sitting position and applied positive end-expiratory pressure on respiratory mechanics of critically ill obese patients receiving mechanical ventilation. *Critical Care Medicine*, *41*(11), 2592–2599.

Littleton, S. W. (2012). Impact of obesity on respiratory function. *Respirology*, *17*(1), 43–49.

Magnusson, L., & Spahn, D. R. (2003). New concepts of atelectasis during general anaesthesia. *British Journal of Anaesthesia*, *91*(1), 61–72.

Mathew, B., Francis, L., Kayalar, A., & Cone, J. (2008). Obesity: Effects on cardiovascular disease and its diagnosis. *Journal of the American Board of Family Medicine, 21*(6), 562–568.

Pedoto, A. (2012). Lung physiology and obesity: Anesthetic implications for thoracic procedures. *Anesthesiology Research and Practice, 2012* (Article ID 154208). Retrieved from http://www.hindawi.com/journals/arp/2012/154208/cta/

Poirier, P., Alpert, M. A., Fleisher, L. A., Thompson, P. D., Sugerman, H. J., Burke, L. E., . . . Franklin, B. A. (2009). Cardiovascular evaluation and management of severely obese patients undergoing surgery: A science advisory from the American Heart Association. *Circulation, 120*(1), 86–95.

Rahmanian, P. B., Adams, D. H., Castillo, J., Chikwe, J., Bodian, C. A., & Filsoufi, F. (2007). Impact of body mass index on early outcome and slate survival in patients undergoing coronary artery bypass grafting or valve surgery or both. *American Journal of Cardiology, 100,* 1702–1708.

Ranu, H., Wilde, M., & Madden, B. (2011). Pulmonary function tests. *Ulster Medical Journal, 80*(2), 84–90.

Risnes, I., Abdelnoor, M., Almdahl, S. M., & Svennevig, J. L. (2010). Mediastinitis after coronary artery bypass grafting risk factors and long-term survival. *Annals of Thoracic Surgery, 89*(5), 1502–1509.

Salome, C. M., King, G. G., & Berend, N. (2010). Physiology of obesity and effects on lung function. *Journal of Applied Physiology, 108*(1), 206–211.

Santapino, G., Pfeiffer, S., Concistré, G., & Fischlein, T. (2013). Sternal wound dehiscence from intense coughing in a cardiac surgery patient: Could it be prevented? *Il Giornale di Chirurgia, 34*(4), 112. (Abstract).

Sartini, P., Winfield, A., & Bizzarri, F. (2012). The successful introduction of an adapted form of the mini extra corporeal circulation used for cardiac surgery in an obese patient. *Journal of Cardiothoracic Surgery, 7,* 20.

Schumann, R., Jones, S. B., Cooper, B., Kelley, S. D., Bosch, M. V., Ortiz, V. E., . . . Carr, D. B. (2009). Update on best practice recommendations for anesthetic perioperative care and pain management in weight loss surgery, 2004–2007. *Obesity (Silver Spring), 17*(5), 889–894.

Sheen, Y. J., & Sheu, W. H. (2011). Metabolic syndrome and renal injury. *Cardiology Research and Practice, 2011* (Article ID 567389). doi: 10.4061/2011/567389

Stamou, S. C., Nussbaum, M., Stiegel, R. M., Reames, M. K., Skipper, E. R., Robicsek, F., . . . Lobdell, K. W. (2011). Effect of body mass index on outcomes after cardiac surgery: Is there an obesity paradox? *Annals of Thoracic Surgery, 91*(1), 42–47.

Thomas, J. A., & McIntosh, J. M. (1994). Are incentive spirometry, intermittent positive pressure breathing, and deep breathing exercises effective in the prevention of postoperative pulmonary complications after upper abdominal surgery? A systematic overview and meta-analysis. *Physical Therapy, 74*(1), 3–10.

Urell, C., Westerdahl, E., Hedenström, H., Janson, C., & Emtner, M. (2012). Lung function before and two days after open-heart surgery. *Critical Care Research and Practice, 2012* (Article ID 291628). Retrieved from http://www.hindawi.com/journals/ccrp/2012/291628/

Virani, S. S., Nambi, V., Lee, V. V., MacArthur, A. E., Pan, W., Petersen, L. A., . . . Ballantyne, C. M. (2009). Obesity. An independent predictor of in-hospital postoperative renal insufficiency among patients undergoing cardiac surgery. *Texas Heart Journal, 36*(6), 540–545.

Wagner, B. D., Grunwald, G. K., Rusfeld, J. S., Hill, J. O., Ho, P. M., Wyatt, H. R., . . . Shroyer, A. L. (2007). Relationship of body mass index with outcomes after coronary artery bypass graft surgery. *Annals of Thoracic Surgery, 84*(1), 10–16.

Wang, B., Yang, H., Wu, S., Cao, G., & Yang, H. (2013). Obesity and the risk of late mortality after aortic valve replacement with small prosthesis. *Journal of Cardiothoracic Surgery, 8,* 174.

White, G. C. (2013). Pulmonary function testing. In G. C. White (Ed.), *Basic clinical lab competencies for respiratory care: An integrated approach* (5th ed., pp. 75–108). Clifton Park, NY: Delmar.

Wickman, C., & Kramer, H. (2013). Obesity and kidney disease: Potential mechanisms. *Seminars in Nephrology, 33*(1), 14–22.

Wigfield, C. H., Lindsey, J. D., Muñoz, A., Chopra, P. S., Edwards, N. M., & Love, R. B. (2006). Is extreme obesity a risk factor for cardiac surgery? An analysis of patients with BMI ≥ 40. *European Journal of Cardio-Thoracic Surgery, 29,* 434–440.

World Health Organization. (2015). *Obesity.* Retrieved from http://www.who.int/topics/obesity/en/

Zacharias, A., Schwann, T. A., Riordan, C. J., Durham, S. J., Shah, A. S., & Habib, R. H. (2005). Obesity and risk of new-onset atrial fibrillation after cardiac surgery. *Circulation, 112,* 3247–3255.

WEB RESOURCES

Centers for Disease Control and Prevention, *Overweight and Obesity*; contains several obesity facts, including obesity statistics by state: http://www.cdc.gov/obesity/data/adult.html

National Heart, Lung, and Blood Institute. *Calculate Your Body Mass Index* (BMI Calculator; uses standard and metric for entries): http://www.nhlbi.nih.gov/health/educational/lose_wt/BMI/bmicalc.htm

Chapter 21

Cardiogenetics

Tracy D. Andrews and Sonya R. Hardin

INTRODUCTION

Typically, intensive care unit (ICU) nurses do not consider genetics an important part of their requisite knowledge base to care for critically ill patients. Many nurses have not been afforded genetic education in their nursing programs. Furthermore, continuing education opportunities in the United States regarding genetics, specifically cardiogenetics, is sparse. Although nurses are diligent to review family history with patients and their families, the usefulness of this information has not fully been utilized in nursing practice. This chapter is intended to give the ICU nurse a broad, generalized overview of genetic/genomic considerations that may be an integral part of their patient management. Management strategies are briefly discussed. An exhaustive review of management strategies for conditions with cardiogenetic basis exceeds the scope of this chapter.

HISTORY

Genetics has been a cornerstone of medicine for many years; however, it has only been within the past 20 years that genetics has taken a more central role in patient management. Where did genetics begin? Strangely enough, an Austrian monk who was observing changes in his pea plants has been named the father of modern genetics. Gregor Mendel found that when a yellow pea and a green pea were bred together, the offspring pea was always yellow. However, in the next generation, green peas reappeared at a ratio of 1:3. Thus, the terms *dominant* and *recessive* were coined. Although this information was remarkable, Mendel's work did not become famous until the 20th century. In 1871, Friedrich Miescher discovered "nuclein." Through various experiments, Dr. Miescher found that he could isolate components of the cytoplasm that only contained phosphorus and nitrogen and not sulfur. "Nuclein" was later referred to as deoxyribonucleic acid (DNA), which is now known to be the carrier of inheritance (Dahm, 2008). More famously, James Watson and Francis Crick discovered the double helix structure of DNA. Through these discoveries, the groundwork was laid to begin understanding how genetic instructions are encoded into all living organisms' cells.

In 1984, the U.S. government solicited and sanctioned the Human Genome Project. The project had dual goals: to determine the sequence of chemical base pairs that makes up human DNA and to identify/map all of the genes found in humans from both a physical and functional standpoint. The project was declared complete in 2003. Twenty universities and research centers within the United States, United Kingdom, France, Germany, Japan, and China were used for genetic sequencing. Although the initial plan was to study all DNA, this was not done. About 8% of the human genome was not sequenced secondary to DNA complexity within heterochromatic areas (Harmon, 2010). Around the same time that the Human Genome Project was in the planning phase, forensic science was beginning the use of DNA profiling to assist with criminal investigations, paternity testing, and immigration disputes (Newton, 2004). Several subspecialty fields have developed within the genetic community.

Cardiogenetics is the specialized focus on genetics related to the cardiovascular system within humans. This field focuses on any condition that can have cardiovascular impact, including conduction disorders, structural abnormalities, and syndromes. This chapter focuses on the most commonly seen disorders within the cardiac surgery practice area, specifically cardiothoracic surgery ICUs.

GENETICS TERMINOLOGY

In order to be able to discuss genetics, the reader should be familiar with basic genetic terms. The intent of this chapter is not to provide exhaustive genetic information; rather, it is to encourage further research into genetic information that is pertinent to the nurse's own practice. **Table 21-1** provides commonly used genetic terms that should be reviewed prior to proceeding with this chapter.

FAMILY HISTORY

Pedigrees (also known as genograms) are schematic renderings of family history. Family pedigrees provide a wealth of information about possible genetic links to diseases. Given that nurses are the frontline healthcare providers, nurse completion of patient pedigrees is highly encouraged. Pedigree construction is relatively easy to complete and can be done as the nurse asks family history. At least three generations of both paternal and maternal family history should be included. Some

clinicians focus only on practice-specific pedigrees; this should be discouraged. Many times, syndromes that would not normally contribute to disease processes can be key to uncovering important genetic causal factors in disease diagnosis, severity, and prognosis. An example of this is Duchenne muscular dystrophy (DMD), which is an X-linked genetic disorder where the mother passes on a genetic mutation to her son. It is highlighted by profound muscular weakness that progresses to death. Because of the X-link inheritance pattern, only males can be diagnosed with DMD; however, females can be carriers and can also have manifestations of this gene mutation. With regard to cardiogenetics, females with the DMD gene mutation can have dilated cardiomyopathy (DCM). Therefore, gleaning as much information as possible is extremely important. The following is another example: A nurse is taking a family history. The patient reveals that her brother died in a single-vehicle accident at the age of 23. During further discussion, the nurse notes that several of the patient's family members have required internal cardioverter-defibrillator (ICD) implantation or have died from "heart attacks." How does the young man fit into this? There is a high suspicion for a possible arrhythmogenic basis for this young man's death. Even if disorders of family members uncovered during this interview process do not seem to be important to the overall cause of a patient's condition, making note of those disorders may actually provide invaluable insight into the patient's condition.

The 2009 Heart Failure Society of America (HFSA) guideline recommends a careful family history for three or more generations for all patients with cardiomyopathy (Hershberger et al., 2009). The initial discussion with the patient should include family history and pedigree analysis for unexplained heart failure before age 60 or sudden cardiac death in the absence of ischemic disease. Referral to a center with expertise in genetic cardiomyopathies should be considered because these

Table 21-1	Common Genetic Nomenclature

Term	Definition
Pedigree	A diagram showing genetic relationships and medical history of a family using standardized symbols and terminology.
Chromosome	Organized packet of DNA found in the nucleus of cells.
Gene	Functional and physical heredity unit passed from parent to offspring. Genes are located on chromosomes.
Locus	The site or location of a specific gene on a chromosome.
Allele	One of the alternative versions of a gene at a given location.
Autosomal	Refers to any of the chromosomes other than sex-determining chromosomes.
Autosomal dominant	Inheritance pattern whereby there is a 50% chance of having a mutated gene passed onto offspring.
Autosomal recessive	Inheritance pattern where offspring must receive a copy of a mutated gene from both parents.
Phenotype	Observable characteristics of gene expression; clinical presentation.
Genotype	An individual's collection of genes.
X-linked	Inheritance pattern where a mother passes on a genetic mutation to her son.
Mitochondrial inheritance	Inheritance pattern passed on by mothers because sperm do not contain mitochondria, whereas ova do.
Heritability	Degree at which information contained within genes can be transmitted from parent to offspring.
Proband	Affected individual through whom a family with a genetic disorder is determined.
Consultant	The individual who presents for genetic counseling; not necessarily the proband.
Heterozygous	An individual who has inherited two different alleles; usually one is normal and one is abnormal.
Homozygous	Where an individual inherits the same alleles for a particular gene from both parents.

Source: Data from U.S. National Library of Medicine. (2014). *Genetics Home Reference*. Bethesda, MD The Library. Retrieved from http://ghr.nlm.nih.gov/

centers can provide comprehensive genetic counseling and testing. This is especially true when dealing with syndrome-related disease. Finally, these centers often maintain a comprehensive database that assists in research and treatment advances.

When completing family histories, there are cardiogenetic red flags to watch for during the interview process, including:

- "Heart attack" in a person younger than 50 years old (could be cardiomyopathy, aortic dissection, or arrhythmias)
- Two or more closely related family members on the same side of the family with the same or related condition (e.g., heart disease, arrhythmia, stroke)
- Unexplained sudden death (could be indicative of myocardial infarction [MI],

cardiomyopathy, arrhythmia, aortic dissection)

- An individual who has been diagnosed with a specific type of hereditary disease (e.g., hypertrophic cardiomyopathy [HCM], Marfan syndrome)
- Coronary heart disease (CHD) at an early age (males younger than 55; women younger than 65)
- Two or more family members with congenital heart defects/disease
- Family history of symptoms and procedures suspicious for hereditary arrhythmia syndrome: syncope, seizures, multiple family members with pacemaker/ICD, sudden death, or sudden infant death syndrome

CLINICAL SCREENING

Screening is an important consideration when dealing with cardiomyopathies. Dilated cardiomyopathy, HCM, arrhythmogenic right ventricular cardiomyopathy (ARVC), and other cardiomyopathies often are present in asymptomatic people. Progressive disease may occur within a relatively short period of time in those asymptomatic people; however, they may already have begun to have electrocardiographic or echocardiographic findings consistent with cardiomyopathy. As such, clinical screening protocols have been developed.

The 2009 HFSA genetic evaluation of cardiomyopathy guideline recommends the following screening for first-degree relatives of patients with DCM. This screening should include history (with special focus on heart failure symptoms, arrhythmias, presyncope, syncope), physical examination (special attention to cardiac/skeletal muscle systems), electrocardiogram (ECG), echocardiogram, and serum CK-MM. Even though initial screening may not reveal any problems, asymptomatic patients should be re-screened at 3- to 5-year intervals beginning in childhood or at any time symptoms begin to appear. Repeat clinical screening at 1 year is suggested in first-degree relatives with any abnormal clinical screening tests (Hershberger et al., 2009).

GENETIC COUNSELING/TESTING

Genetic and family counseling is recommended for all patients with cardiac-related genetic disorders. Because of the complexity of genetic testing/counseling, referral to specialized genetic cardiomyopathy/aortopathy centers should take place. All patients who are offered genetic testing should receive genetic counseling, including the explanation of genetic disease and risk, test sensitivities, heritability, and possible test outcomes, including the possibility of inconclusive or false-positive/-negative results. Genetic testing should be considered for the one most clearly affected person in a family to facilitate family screening and management.

Counseling and explanation of the Genetic Information Nondiscrimination Act, a U.S. Act of Congress, was passed in 2008 to prevent the use of genetic information in health insurance and employment for all U.S. citizens, except for those employed by the U.S. Armed Forces. Screening the most affected person in the family increases the likelihood of detecting a relevant mutation. This premise is held with all conditions involving cardiogenetics as well. For those patients with DCM and prominent conduction system disease, a family history of premature unexpected sudden death, or both, the European Heart Rhythm Association recommended through its consensus statement that comprehensive or targeted (LMNA and SCN5A) gene testing be performed (Ackerman et al., 2011).

CARDIAC GENERALIZATIONS

Most inherited cardiovascular diseases (CVDs) have an autosomal dominant pattern. This means that there is a 50% chance of a person passing a disorder on to offspring. Characteristically, a "traditional" inheritance pattern is seen with genetic disorders. This, however, is not true in CVD genetics. A lack of traditional inheritance pattern often makes prognosis difficult. This does not mean that diagnosis will be difficult, except some healthcare providers may overlook family history and be dismissive about its importance in those who typically do not have high cardiovascular risk (e.g., young women, non-obese patients). As defined in the genetics terminology table, penetrance refers to the frequency with which a heritable trait is manifested in people carrying the identified gene/genes conditioning it. Specifically, in medical genetics, penetrance refers to the proportion of people with a genetic mutation who exhibit clinical symptoms. Consider the following example. If a disorder is passed through an autosomal dominant mode of inheritance, this means that there is a 50% chance of passing on the disorder. Some genes have different penetrance levels; these levels are measured in percentages. If the autosomal dominant gene mutation has 95% penetrance, then 95% of those with gene mutation will develop the disease. In many genetic disorders, this is a relatively clear-cut view of penetrance. Unfortunately, cardiovascular genetics does not fit that pattern. Incomplete penetrance is often seen. This means that people who carry the genetic mutation do not always follow the normal penetrance patterns. The basis for this variation has been found to be multifactorial; environment, diet, gender, socioeconomic status, and other factors have all been found to be contributory to this incomplete penetrance. Variability in disease expression as well as small family size make additional diagnoses difficult.

CARDIOMYOPATHIES

According to the 2006 American Heart Association (AHA) scientific statement proposal for definition and classification of cardiomyopathies, cardiomyopathies include a "heterogeneous group of diseases of the myocardium associated with mechanical and/or electrical dysfunction that usually (but not invariably) exhibit inappropriate ventricular hypertrophy or dilatation and are due to a variety of causes that are frequently genetic" (Maron, 2006, p. 1807). There are two categories of cardiomyopathies: primary and secondary. Primary cardiomyopathy means that the heart is predominantly the main organ affected; secondary cardiomyopathy refers to other organ involvement besides the heart. Primary cardiomyopathies are then subdivided into those that are genetic, mixed (predominantly nongenetic or less commonly genetic), or acquired. The most commonly known cardiomyopathies include DCM, HCM, left ventricular non-compaction cardiomyopathy (LVNCC), ARVC, and restrictive cardiomyopathy (RCM). Hypertrophic cardiomyopathy, LVNCC, and ARVC are classified as genetic cardiomyopathies. Other common genetic cardiomyopathies include the 5'-AMP-activated protein kinase subunit gamma-2 gene, Danon glycogen storage diseases, conduction defects, mitochondrial myopathies, and ion channel disorders. Dilated cardiomyopathy and RCM are classified as mixed cardiomyopathies. Acquired cardiomyopathies include myocarditis, Takotsubo, peripartum, and tachycardia-induced cardiomyopathies. In 2013, the MOGE(S) classification of phenotype-/genotype-based cardiomyopathy was endorsed by the World Heart Federation. Because this cardiomyopathy classification system is new, clinical applicability of its use is still being researched. The system uses the following attributes to identify cardiomyopathies:

1) *Morphofunctional notation*: Indicates a descriptive phenotypic diagnosis (e.g., M_D = DCM)
2) *Organ involvement*: Indicates if heart and/or extracardiac involvement is present (e.g., O_{H+K} = heart and kidney involvement)

3) *Genetic/familial inheritance*: Nature of genetic transmission (e.g., G_{AD} = autosomal dominant)

4) *Etiology*: Description of specific cause (e.g., E_{G-MYH7})

5) *(S)taging*: Provides NYHA information (e.g., S_{C-II} = Stage C/NYHA Functional Status II) (Elliott, 2013)

Dilated Cardiomyopathy

Dilated cardiomyopathy is one of the main causative factors for congestive heart failure (CHF). It is also the main common diagnosis in patients referred for cardiac transplantation. Dilated cardiomyopathy is characterized by dilatation and systolic dysfunction of one or both ventricles, with specific detriment to left ventricular (LV) function. Causes may include infection, toxic exposure, metabolic derangements, ischemia, or genetic. Dilated cardiomyopathy often does not have a clear-cut disease process and is classified as idiopathic until the cause has been determined. Dilated cardiomyopathy is most commonly identified between the ages of 20 and 60 years and has an ethnic bias where African Americans are plagued with DCM more so than other ethnicities. Higher prevalence of DCM is also seen in men than in women. The genetic type of DCM is called familial cardiomyopathy. Through first-degree relative studies involving family screening, it has been established that familial DCM can be identified in 20% to over 50% of patients diagnosed with idiopathic DCM. Thus far, more than 30 genes have been shown to be associated with DCM.

Most familial DCM is transmitted in an autosomal dominant inheritance pattern; other inheritance patterns have been identified (autosomal recessive, X-linked, and mitochondrial). Mestroni and colleagues (1999) demonstrated the spectrum of familial DCM in a study that evaluated 350 patients with DCM and 281 of their relatives from 60 families. This study identified subtypes of DCM. These subtypes include autosomal dominant DCM with normal skeletal muscle examination/histology, autosomal recessive DCM (16%) with younger age of onset and rapid progression to death or transplant, X-linked (10%) in males with severe progressive heart failure associated with mutations of the dystrophin gene, a form of autosomal dominant DCM (7.7%) associated with subclinical skeletal muscle disease with variable levels of serum CK-MM and with dystrophic changes on skeletal muscle biopsy, familial DCM associated with conduction disorders (2.6%), and unclassified forms (7.7%) (Ackerman et al., 2011).

DCM Genes

Thirty percent of familial DCM cases are caused by abnormalities involving sarcomere protein. Sarcomere genes play a role in muscular development and function. The most common mutations have been identified in the beta myosin heavy chain (MYH7), alpha myosin heavy chain, cardiac troponin T (TNNT2), titin, alpha-tropomyosin, and cardiac troponin C genes. Different mutations in these genes can also cause HCM, which is discussed later in this chapter. Other genes beyond sarcomeric involvement are also documented. The most common mutations have been found in laminin-alpha 4, vinculin, ABCC9, delta-sarcoglycan, and the presenilins. Dilated cardiomyopathy that has associated conduction disorders has also been shown to have a familial tendency. Mutations in the gene that encodes lamin A and C (LMNA) have been the most commonly identified causes of genetic DCM with prevalence ranging from 5% to 8%. LMNA cardiomyopathy usually occurs with heart block (first degree that progresses to second then third degree), supraventricular arrhythmias (atrial fibrillation [AF]/flutter), and sick sinus syndrome, with progressively worsening ventricular arrhythmias including ventricular tachycardia and fibrillation. Dilated cardiomyopathy can occur at any point in the development of conduction system disease. Sudden cardiac death is prominent with LMNA mutations, which means that most patients with this mutation will require pacemaker insertion. SCN5A mutations include conduction disorders and ventricular dysfunction. Sinoatrial node dysfunction and atrial arrhythmias are common. In a report from Olson and colleagues (2005), 27% of patients with SCN5A mutations had early features of DCM (mean age of diagnosis: 20), 38% had DCM (mean age of diagnosis: 48), and 43% had AF (mean age of diagnosis: 28).

X-linked DCM transmission is also documented. Familial DCM that is transmitted as an X-linked trait most often results from mutations in Xp21, the dystrophin gene. Most dystrophin mutations produce either Duchenne or Becker muscular dystrophy, both of which are associated with cardiac involvement. Autosomal recessive transition is rare but still occurs. Mutations in the ALMS1 gene on chromosome 2p13 produce the most common autosomal recessive disorder with cardiac involvement: Alström syndrome. Alström syndrome is characterized by DCM (Olson et al., 2005).

Treatment of DCM

Medical therapy is recommended based on the cardiac phenotype outlined in general guidelines provided by heart failure experts. It is not generally governed by finding a specific genetic mutation. Exclusion to this would be in the event of DCM with associated conduction disorders. Those patients who have idiopathic DCM or those with known desmin or LMNA mutations should be considered for prophylactic pacemaker insertion. Early treatment with angiotensin-converting enzyme (ACE) inhibitors has been shown to slow progression of LV enlargement in patients who have not shown evidence of decreased LV function; the greatest efficacy has only been shown with those patients with LV ejection fraction of less than 35% to 40%. Some experts have recommended initiation of ACE inhibitor or beta blocker therapy with early signs of familial DCM; however, this approach has not been adopted in major society guidelines.

Hypertrophic Cardiomyopathy

Hypertrophic cardiomyopathy is the most common inherited cardiac disorder. One in every 500 people will have HCM. Hypertrophic cardiomyopathy is also a major cause of sudden cardiac death (SCD) in young people (i.e., younger than 30 years) and is the most common cause of SCD in young athletes, accounting for 36% of deaths. The annual frequency of HCM-related SCD is 0.5% to 1% in adults. Almost 50% of HCM-related deaths happen during or just after the person has done some type of physical activity. Sudden cardiac death is often the only indication of HCM presence. Ninety percent of HCM-related deaths in athletes occur in males. This is potentially due to the higher frequency of participation at a higher intensity in male athletics; however, a true understanding of this gender bias has not been fully elucidated. As is seen with DCM, there are different types of HCM. Extensive genetic heterogeneity is common. Heterogeneity refers to the fact that a disease's etiology can result from different conditions or contributing factors. The majority of idiotic forms of HCM are genetic (Ackerman et al., 2011).

Genetic Basis of HCM

Hypertrophic cardiomyopathy is usually inherited through an autosomal dominant inheritance pattern. Thus far, 21 genes have been associated with HCM. Sarcomere protein gene mutations cause most forms of HCM, with 80% of cases being associated with MYH7, MYBPC3,

TNNT2, and TNNI3 mutations. As was discussed with DCM, sarcomere genes involve muscle formation and function. With regard to HCM, the genetic mutations cause force generation malfunctions. As is common in most cardiogenetic disorders, incomplete penetrance and variable gene expressivity are common with HCM; 50% to 60% of patients with a high index of clinical suspicion for HCM will have a mutation in at least one out of nine sarcomeric genes. MYH7 mutations are considered to be the most severe phenotype of sarcomere protein mutation–related HCM. De novo MYH7 mutations have also been noted in patients who have HCM but have no family history of the disease. This type of mutation causes early onset of HCM and is often associated with early decompensation requiring transplantation. MYBPC3 is considered a milder form of sarcomere protein gene mutation and results in later onset of HCM, usually around the age of 50-60 years. TNNT2 mutation has a high incidence of SCD. An insertion/deletion polymorphism of the gene responsible for encoding ACE is also associated with HCM. The deletion/deletion genotype of ACE is associated with more marked LV hypertrophy and may be associated with higher rates of SCD (Masry & Breall, 2008).

Genetic Testing

Genetic testing for the aforementioned gene mutations/deletions is available for people who are being considered for HCM diagnosis.

Current detection rate is 40% for isolated cases and 66% for cases with a family history of HCM/SCD. Genetic testing should be accompanied by genetic counseling by both a genetic counselor as well as a cardiologist who specializes in cardiogenetics. Specifically, discussion of HCM pathophysiology, symptoms, prohibition of sports participation, SCD, and possible need for invasive intervention should be included.

HCM Screening and Diagnosis

Hypertrophic cardiomyopathy screening has become prevalent in young athletes (see **Table 21-2**). Healthcare providers have been taught that 80% of diagnoses lie in the history and physical. In the case of HCM, however, physical exam and medical history are ineffective because only 3% of cases are caught. Electrocardiogram detection of left ventricular hypertrophy (LVH) is common. Seventy percent of asymptomatic HCM is diagnosed by using ECG. This test, however, cannot describe the type of hypertrophic abnormality. Echocardiogram detects 80% or more HCM cases and is used to specifically diagnose HCM. Upon recognition of LVH in ECG readings, most clinicians will do further studies to investigate the cause of LVH. Most patients will have echocardiographic studies as well as cardiac magnetic resonance imaging (MRI) to detect myocardial fibrosis or degree of LVH.

Table 21-2   Athlete's Heart Versus HCM

	Athlete's Heart	HCM
Septum thickness	Less than 15 mm	Greater than 15 mm
Symmetry	Yes (for septum and LV wall)	No (septum much thicker)
Family history	None	Possibly
Deconditioning	Reduction within 3 months	None

Source: Data from Maron, B., & Zipes, D. (2005). Introduction: Eligibility recommendations for competitive athletes with cardiovascular abnormalities—General considerations. *Journal of the American College of Cardiology, 45*(8), 1318–1321.

Treatment

Because of HCM pathophysiology, dehydration must be avoided at all costs. Because of the tachycardia and dehydration associated with sports, young patients with HCM are precluded from participating in sports activities. Beta blockade agents are used to reduce myocardial oxygen demand as well as maintain a lower heart rate. For those who do not tolerate beta blockade therapy, calcium channel therapy is an acceptable alternative as long as the patient has preserved LV function. For those patients who continue to have symptoms despite optimization of medical management, there are more invasive management alternatives.

Alcohol septal ablation (ASA) therapy can be provided by interventional cardiologists. This procedure was introduced in 1994 to reduce the need for invasive myectomy. Procedure qualification must occur prior to ASA therapy. Patients had to demonstrate limited functional capacity secondary to exertional dyspnea and chest pain classified as either NYHA III or IV. Septal hypertrophy of 18 mm or more and resisting or provocable LV gradient of 50 mmHg or more was also required. Now, these restrictions have been relaxed. In a systematic review of almost 3,000 patients undergoing ASA (Alam, Dokainish, & Lakkis, 2006), the mean NYHA Class was noted to be 2.9 and only 51% to 53% were on beta blocker or calcium channel therapy. One restriction of this therapy that has not been modified is for the patient to have no evidence of hemodynamically significant coronary artery disease (CAD).

The procedure is performed by introducing a catheter-based injection of absolute alcohol into the septal perforator to induce a controlled infarction of the hypertrophied septum. This helps abolish the dynamic outflow obstruction. Gradient reduction has been shown to correlate with significant clinical improvement in patient symptoms as well as assist with LV remodeling. The most common complication of ASA has been conduction issues, where up to 10% of patients undergoing this procedure have had complete heart block refractory to medication, thereby requiring permanent pacemaker insertion. Myocardial infarction is a less common complication but has been seen in up to 3.5% of patients undergoing ASA (Masry & Breall, 2008). Another consideration of ASA is that this procedure induces myocardial tissue necrosis, thereby leaving a scar. This scar can result in an arrhythmogenic substrate that predisposes some patients to lethal re-entrant ventricular tachycardias. Up to 32% of patients undergoing ASA redevelop hypertrophic septal tissue that requires myectomy (Maron, 2007).

Surgical myectomy is a surgical procedure for HCM when other treatments have not worked. This procedure is still considered the gold standard of care for symptomatic obstructive HCM. In this procedure, a rectangular, 3–4 cm myectomy trough is created by a cardiac surgeon from just below the aortic valve to the site of mitral–septal contact and intraventricular obstruction. As a result, the redundant tissue causing LV outflow tract obstruction is surgically removed. This allows for improved hemodynamics and LV remodeling.

Complications of myectomy include the usual post-cardiac surgery complications, including infection, atrial arrhythmias, and bleeding. Specifically, because the atrioventricular conduction system can be affected, high-degree conduction blocks may occur. This necessitates permanent pacemaker insertion. Approximately 6% of patients who undergo myectomy have regrowth of obstructive tissue requiring another myectomy surgery (Maron, 2007). Rarely (less than 2% of cases), heart transplantation is needed for HCM.

FAMILIAL HYPERCHOLESTEROLEMIA

Familial hypercholesterolemia (FH) is characterized by raised serum low density lipoprotein (LDL) cholesterol levels, which result in excess cholesterol in tissues. This leads to acceleration of atherosclerosis and increased risk for premature CHD. Because of the often markedly elevated LDL levels, deposition of LDL-derived cholesterol, called xanthomas, can be found in tendons and the skin.

Genetics

Mutations in the low density lipoprotein receptor (LDLR) gene have been found to be the primary cause of FH. Low density lipoprotein receptor mutation databases currently list more than 800 different mutations. Apolipoprotein B (apoB) mutations have been noted, but these are rare. Most cases have been identified in those with European ancestry. Mutations in apoB tend to have incomplete penetrance, thereby resulting in a milder form of FH than that seen in LDLR mutations.

The most common inheritance pattern for FH is autosomal dominant. Autosomal recessive FH is extremely rare and involves LDLRAP1 mutation. Patients with this type of mutation often have a milder form of FH. Autosomal recessive FH is most commonly seen in patients with consanguinity being notable in their family pedigree.

Two types of autosomal dominant FH exist: homozygous and heterozygous. Heterozygous FH is milder than homozygous FH. There may be up to a twofold elevation in cholesterol (350–550 mg/dL). Coronary artery disease develops after age 30. Homozygous FH is rare, with only one in 1 million people being affected. Severe hypercholesterolemia (650–1,000 mg/dL) is commonly seen. Coronary artery disease develops in childhood and frequently causes MI-related deaths.

In the LDL receptor gene, the short arm of chromosome 19 is affected. There are five classes of mutations, with each class having subdivisions. Class 1 includes null alleles, which means that there is a failure to produce an immunoprecitable protein. Class 2 is the most common mutation. In this subdivision, there are defective transport alleles.

Class 3 includes binding defective alleles. Class 4 is the rarest form, with internalization-defection alleles. This entails proteins that are encoded reaching the cell surface and binding LDL normally; however, they fail to cluster in coated pits and thereby do not internalize bound LDL. Class 5 includes recycling defective alleles. Patients with heterozygous FH have one normal allele and one mutant allele at the LDL receptor locus. This means that cells are able to bind and take up LDL at approximately half the normal rate. Those with homozygous FH have two mutant alleles. This causes total or near-total inability to bind or take up LDL. Some inherit two identical alleles. Some have two different mutant alleles.

PCSK9 mutations are associated with a particularly severe clinical phenotype. These patients seem to respond well to statins (Repas & Tanner, 2014).

Screening

Approximately 85% of patients with FH have not been diagnosed and are not on appropriate lipid-lowering therapy (Repas & Tanner, 2014). Familial hypercholesterolemia begins at the age of 3 in patients with a family history. Cholesterol levels are checked frequently. Cardiac catheterization to ascertain presence of early CHD is done at earlier ages than in the general population. Those patients with homozygous FH will often be placed under cardiac catheterization in early childhood.

Management

Statin therapy is initiated at an early age (usually around age 15–18) in those with heterozygous FH. Most will likely need escalating doses of statins as they age. Lomitapide (Juxtapid®) is a new medication that has been specifically designed for FH. Those patients with homozygous FH are under constant surveillance. Frequent cardiac catheterizations are common, with the first being in early childhood at times.

Percutaneous coronary intervention and coronary artery bypass grafting are often required, even in children. Medications to combat hypercholesterolemia are ineffective in patients with homozygous FH; frank discussion regarding stringent heart-healthy lifestyle is paramount in this patient population.

Because of the higher incidence of development of ischemic cardiomyopathy, heart failure is common in patients with homozygous FH. Cardiac transplantation is typically not explored in this population because of the high likelihood for CAD development in the transplanted organ. Moreover, tacrolimus, an anti-rejection medication, has a propensity to cause early development of CAD. In some cases, heart transplantation can be explored if concomitant liver transplant is also performed. With liver transplantation, the hope is that the new organ will assist in LDL uptake improvement, thereby decreasing the risk for early CAD development (Repas & Tanner, 2014).

AORTOPATHIES

Aortopathy refers to any disease or malfunction of the aorta. There are five main aortopathic conditions that have clinical focus: Marfan syndrome (MFS), Loeys–Dietz syndrome (LDS), Ehlers–Danlos syndrome (EDS—Types I/II, IV, and VI), idiopathic thoracic aneurysm/dissection, and coarctation of the aorta. Note that three of the five are syndromes, which means that multiple body systems are affected by the disease process. Marfan syndrome, LDS, EDS, and coarctation of the aorta all have genetic components. This chapter focuses on the first three syndromes without discussion of coarctation of the aorta because of its usual repair in pediatric settings.

Marfan Syndrome (MFS)

The gene responsible for MFS was not discovered until 1991. Dr. Francesco Ramirez discovered the occurrence of misfolding of the protein fibrillin-1 (FBN1). There are no currently documented gender, geographical, or ethnic biases associated with MFS. Fifteen to thirty percent of MFS cases occur secondary to a de novo genetic mutation—not inheritance from a parent. Therefore, sole reliance on pedigree/family history can cause missed MFS diagnosis in some patients. See **Table 21-3**.

MFS Genetics

Glycoprotein is an essential part of elastic fiber formation in connective tissue. The gene responsible for this is located on Chromosome 15 q21.1. Fibrillin has an essential role in glycoprotein production. There are believed to be three types of fibrillin. Fibrillin-1 is a major component of microfibrils that form a sheath surrounding elastin, a component of all connective tissue. Fibrillin-1 has a direct role in connective tissue formation and maintenance. Fibrillin-1 also has direct relationship with transforming growth factor beta (TGF-β). Misregulated TGF-β has injurious effects on vascular smooth muscle development and the integrity of the extracellular matrix. Because of both the FBN1 and TGF-β errors, the characteristic features of MFS are manifested. Marfan syndrome has notable excess TGF-β in the lungs, aorta, and heart valves. Fibrillin-2 plays a major role in joint and musculoskeletal formation. Fibrillin-2 malfunctions are seen in Beals syndrome, also known as congenital contractural arachnodactyly. Marfan syndrome has an autosomal dominant inheritance pattern. Therefore, there is a 50% chance of passing a copy of the Marfan FBN1 gene to offspring (Boileau, Jondeau, Mizuquchi, & Matsumoto, 2005).

MFS Key Cardiac Characteristics

Cardiovascular compromise is common in MFS. Many patients will have sluggish peripheral circulation, resulting in cold feet,

Table 21-3 Marfan Syndrome Diagnostic Criteria	

Skeletal System

Major Criteria	Presence of at least four of the following manifestations:
	• Pectus carinatum
	• Pectus excavatum requiring surgery
	• Reduced upper to lower segment ratio or arm span to height ratio greater than 1.05
	• Wrist and thumb signs
	• Scoliosis of > 20 degrees
	• Reduced extension at the elbows (< 170 degrees)
	• Medial displacement of the medial malleolus causing pes planus
	• Protrusio acetabuli of any degree (on x-ray)
Minor Criteria	Pectus excavatum of moderate severity
	Joint hypermobility
	Highly arched palate with crowding of teeth
	Facial appearance (dolichocephaly, malar hypoplasia, enophthalmos, retrognathia, down-slanting palpebral fissures)

Ocular System

Major Criterion	Ectopic lentis
Minor Criteria	Abnormally flat cornea (measured by keratometry)
	Increased axial length of globe (ultrasound)
	Hypoplastic iris/ciliary muscle causing decreased miosis

Cardiovascular System

Major Criteria	Dilatation of the ascending aorta with or without aortic regurgitation
	Dissection of the ascending aorta
Minor Criteria	Mitral valve prolapse
	Mitral valve prolapse with/without mitral valve regurgitation
	Dilatation of the main pulmonary artery, in the absence of valvular or peripheral pulmonary stenosis before the age of 40
	Calcification of the mitral annulus before the age of 40
	Dilatation and/or dissection of the abdominal aorta or descending thoracic aorta before age 50

Pulmonary System

Minor Criteria	Spontaneous pneumothorax
	Apical blebs (on chest x-ray)

Skin/Integumentary

Minor Criteria	Stretch marks not associated with weight changes, stress, and/or pregnancy
	Recurrent or incisional hernia

Dura

Major criterion	Lumbosacral dural ectasia by CT or MRI

Table 21-3   Marfan Syndrome Diagnostic Criteria *(Continued)*

Family/Genetic History

Major Criteria	Having a parent, child, or sibling who meets these diagnostic criteria independently
	Presence of a mutation in FBN1 known to cause MFS
	Presence of a haplotype around FBN1, inherited by descent, known to be associated with unequivocally diagnosed MFS in the family

CT, computed tomography; FBN1, fibrillin-1; MFS, Marfan syndrome; MRI, magnetic resonance imaging.

Source: Data from De Paepe, A., Devereux, R., Dietz, H., Hennekam, R., & Pyeritz, R. (1996). Revised diagnostic criteria for the Marfan syndrome. *American Journal of Medical Genetics, 62*(4), 417–426; and Rand-Hendriksen, S., Lundby, R., Tjeldhorn, L., Andersen, K., Offstad, J., Ove Semb, S., Smith, J. Paus, B. & Geiran, O. (2015). Prevalence data on all Ghent features in a cross-sectional study of 87 adults with proven Marfan syndrome. *European Journal of Human Genetics, 17*, 1222-1230.

hands, or both. Mitral valve prolapse is seen in approximately 28% to 45% of patients with MFS. Aortic valve formation and function have also been noted to be problematic in MFS. Many patients will have aortic valvular prolapse, resulting in aortic insufficiency. The most worrisome cardiovascular concern in MFS is the high propensity of aortic aneurysms and dissections. The most vulnerable parts of the aorta for MFS patients are the aortic root and ascending aorta. Descending thoracic aorta aneurysms are also common. Less commonly, aneurysms of the iliac and renal arteries are noted (less than 1% of cases). Pulmonary complications of MFS include spontaneous pneumothoraces, sleep apnea, and obstructive lung disease (Habashi et al., 2006).

Dysautonomia is also seen in MFS. Rather than affecting the central nervous system, dysautonomia affects the autonomic nervous system (ANS). There are four associative symptoms of dysautonomia seen in MFS:

1) *Postural orthostatic tachycardia syndrome (orthostatic intolerance)*: This is associated with tachycardia when patients move from a supine to sitting/standing position. Heart rate increase can be well over 50% higher than that of normal orthostatic heart rate changes.

2) *Vasovagal syndrome*: ANS response to overstimulation of the vagus nerve resulting in nausea, vomiting, syncope, diaphoresis, and neurally mediated hypotension.

3) *Neurocardiogenic syndrome*: Similar to vasovagal syndrome, except syncope is usually worse and there can be associated seizures.

4) *Mitral valve prolapse dysautonomia*: Atypical chest pain, dyspnea on exertion, palpitations, and hypotension associated with ANS dysfunction. Supraventricular tachycardia has also been noted when there is increased parasympathetic tone (Hayek, Gring, & Griffin, 2005).

MFS Screening/Testing

Genetic testing should be considered for anyone with a 50% risk of MFS development. Given that many characteristics of MFS are also seen in other aortopathies, genetic testing is more widely suggested for patients who have an unclear aortopathic etiology. Echocardiogram should be performed to evaluate for aortic root and valvular issues, especially mitral valve prolapse and aortic insufficiency. Computed tomography (CT) scans of the chest are routinely ordered to obtain definitive aortic measurements. If the clinician desires to obtain only aortic dimensions, a CT scan without contrast will suffice. However, if there is a possibility of aortic dissection, a CT scan with contrast will be required. For patients with confirmed MFS or aortopathy, serial CT scans are performed. Frequency of CT scans will vary but range from every 6–12 months. Close monitoring of the aortic root and ascending aorta is performed. Growth of either the aortic area by more than 0.5 cm in 6 months or aortic root diameter larger than 5 cm is usually deemed appropriate (Gott et al., 1999).

MFS Treatment

Aortic dimension surveillance should be deemed as treatment. As previously discussed, patients with MFS have excess TGF-β. Angiotensin II receptor blockers have been known to decrease TGF-β levels. Data suggest that there was aortic aneurysm stabilization and mild reduction in aortic size (Habashi et al., 2006; Pyeritz, 2008).

For those who require surgery, ascending aortic and aortic root replacement with a Dacron graft occurs. Postoperative complications may include pneumothoraces and more pronounced dysautonomia. Prognosis for patients with MFS has dramatically improved since prophylactic monitoring and therapies have been employed (Habashi et al., 2006).

Loeys–Dietz Syndrome (LDS)

Loeys–Dietz syndrome is a newly recognized connective tissue disorder with associated aortopathy. This syndrome has an autosomal dominant inheritance pattern. Mutations in transforming growth factor beta-receptor 1 (TGFBR1: LDS Type 1) and transforming growth factor beta-receptor 2 (TGFR2: LDS Type 2) genes have been reported as the genetic causes of LDS. As was noted in MFS, these receptors play a major role in vascular stability. Among the first notable characteristics of LDS was aortic aneurysm; SMAD 3

(LDS Type 3) and TGFB2 (LDS Type 4) gene mutations have also been reported. Mutations in all of these genes show similarly altered TGF-β; therefore, they impart similar cardiovascular, craniofacial, skin, and skeletal features (MacCarrick et al., 2014).

Clinical Presentation

Patients with LDS all seem to have a much higher risk for arterial tortuosity and aneurysm than patients with MFS or EDS. Rapid progression of aortic aneurysms is a distinct feature of LDS. This is especially notable in patients with Type 1 or 2 LDS. These patients are known to have aortic rupture at young ages and at a smaller dimension than those with other aortopathies. Aortic dissection has been reported in patients as young as 3 months to 3 years. Mean age of death of patients with LDS has been reported as 26.1 years, with aortic dissection and cerebral hemorrhage as the major causes of death.

Bicuspid aortic valve (BAV), atrial septal defect, or patent ductus arteriosus is frequently seen in Type 1 or 2 LDS. Mitral valve prolapse can be seen in all types of LDS, with mild to severe mitral valve disease being reported. Twenty-four percent of patients with Type 3 LDS have been noted to have chronic AF and LVH. Left ventricular hypertrophy associated with LDS has been reported as mostly concentric in the absence of aortic stenosis or hypertension and ranges from mild to moderate. Type 1 LDS has associated decreased systolic function, heart failure, and arrhythmias. Arterial tortuosity can be generalized; most typically, neck vessels have been noted to have a higher degree of tortuosity. Type B (descending thoracic aorta) dissections have been reported in minimally or non-dilated aortas (3.7–4.2 cm) in Types 1, 2, and 3 LDS. There have also been reports of rapid expansion of aneurysm within dissections within a few days. Aneurysms and dissections of other major arteries have also been reported (MacCarrick et al., 2014).

LDS Genetic Testing/Screening

Because of its relatively new status as a diagnosis, routine genetic testing is still being developed. Aortopathy panels readily include the four associated LDS genes, which increases the likelihood of appropriate diagnosis. Patients with LDS should have echocardiograms at least every 6 months (MacCarrick et al., 2014).

LDS Management

Because of the aggressive and rapidly progressive aortic aneurysms associated with LDS, valve-sparing aortic root replacement is advised. In MFS, aortic root dimensions of 5 cm or greater are deemed the appropriate measurement necessitating surgery. However, experts advise LDS patients to undergo surgery when aortic root dimensions reach 4 cm. Valve-sparing surgery is more widely done to avoid the need for anticoagulation, given these patients often have higher incidence of bleeding problems. Postoperative echocardiograms should be done at 3- to 6-month intervals for 1 year after surgery and every 6 months thereafter because of the report of coronary button aneurysm after valve-sparing aortic root replacement. Patients with known aortic dissections should be monitored every 2–3 months with surveillance CT scans. Because of the higher incidence of arterial tortuosity, especially in the neck, ultrasound-guided catheter placement needed for post-surgical management should be performed. As is seen with MFS, angiotensin receptor blocker therapy has been shown to be effective in aortic stabilization as well as hypertension management (MacCarrick et al., 2014).

Ehlers–Danlos Syndrome (EDS)

Unlike MFS, EDS has been shown to have multiple inheritance patterns, including autosomal dominant, autosomal recessive, and X-linked. Many patients with EDS will have crossover symptoms that appear in multiple syndromes; therefore, diagnosis is often missed or misdiagnosis occurs.

Types of EDS

There are currently six major types of EDS. Type 4 has cardiac implications and is the most clinically worrisome because it affects vascular collagen/connective tissue. Type 4 EDS has an autosomal dominant inheritance pattern. Of those with Type 4 EDS, 25% develop significant health problems, including heart failure, by the age of 20. More than 80% develop life-threatening complications by age 40. Because of the COL3A1 genetic mutation, vascular connective tissue is extremely vulnerable; these patients often have spontaneous blood vessel and organ rupture (Rombaut et al., 2011).

Genetics

Type 4 EDS is associated with COL3A1 gene mutations (Rombaut et al., 2011).

Clinical Presentation

Vascular problems seen in EDS are often as severe, if not more severe, than those seen in MFS. All blood vessels, not just the aorta, are fragile and have a tendency toward aneurysm. Arterial rupture has been seen with Type 4 EDS. Mitral valve prolapse is also seen in Type 4 EDS and is often associated with endocarditis. Finally, these patients often have platelet aggregation failure and have a tendency to bleed (Rombaut et al., 2011).

EDS Screening/Testing

Ehlers–Danlos syndrome is often a diagnosis of exclusion because of its associated crossover and often vague symptoms. Genetic testing and counseling should be performed only by those associated with a strong background in this type of disorder.

EDS Management

Ehlers–Danlos syndrome has no cure. Palliative treatment is the primary cornerstone of management. Even if genetic testing does not provide definitive diagnosis of Type 4 EDS, close monitoring of these patients' cardiovascular systems should be done. Those patients with valvular malfunction or aortic aneurysm may require surgery. Unlike those with MFS, prognosis does not necessarily improve with aortic replacement. These patients may still have spontaneous rupture of other organs. These patients also have been seen to have high incidence of bleeding and profound hematoma development after arterial and venous catheter placement. As a result, these patients require careful line insertion by qualified personnel (Rombaut et al., 2011).

BICUSPID AORTIC VALVE DISEASE

Normal aortic valves are tricuspid. Bicuspid aortic valve disease is the most common congenital cardiac abnormality, with an estimated worldwide prevalence of 1% to 2%. These estimates may be much lower than actual cases due to lack of routine echocardiogram screening of the general population (Ward, 2000). Bicuspid aortic valve disease is almost three times more common in males than females. There do not seem to be ethnic biases for BAV (Ercan, Ekici, Atalay, & Nacar, 2005).

Pathogenesis

Embryologically, the definitive fetal cardiac structure is developed by 8 weeks' gestation. The semilunar valves form the division between the truncus arteriosus and create two separate channels that form the aortic and pulmonary trunks. The channels are created by the fusion of two truncal ridges across the lumen. Small swellings appear on the inferior margins of each truncal ridge, forming the

basis for adult valve leaflets. A third channel is created in each channel occurring opposite the first, which will form the third leaflet. In the normal aortic valve, the left and right leaflets of the adult valve are formed from the respective swellings, while the posterior leaflet is formed from an off branch of the aortic trunk. The exact pathophysiology of the formation of BAV is not fully understood. It is thought to have a genetic component, especially given the association of BAV with other congenital abnormalities such as coarctation of the aorta. Three types of BAV are described in literature:

1) *Type 1*: Two commissures of the BAV are located in an anteroposterior direction giving left and right cusps
2) *Type 2*: Commissures located on the right and left sides of the annulus leading to anterior posterior cusps
3) *Type 3*: Fusion of the left and non-coronary cusps (most rare: seen in less than 1%)

A raphe, a seam that forms the line of union between symmetric parts, is present on the right and anterior cusps, respectively. This makes the valve appear tricuspid on echocardiography. The site of cusp fusion can have prognostic effects of BAV. Type 1 BAV has been associated with a higher incidence of stenosis; Type 2 valves have complications at younger ages, with most having aortic insufficiency (Roberts, 1992).

Coronary anatomy may also be abnormal. The posterior descending artery (PDA) supplies the inferior wall of the left ventricle and inferior part of the septum. The coronary artery that supplies the PDA determines coronary dominance. Approximately 70% of people have right coronary artery dominant circulation, meaning that the PDA originates from the right coronary artery. Twenty percent have codominance, meaning both the right coronary artery and circumflex artery feed the PDA. Ten percent are left coronary dominant, meaning that the circumflex alone supplies the PDA (Pelter, Al-Zaiti, & Carey, 2014).

Most patients with BAV disease have a left dominant coronary circulation. This left coronary can arise from the pulmonary artery. The left main coronary artery can also be up to 50% shorter than in normal patients in up to 90% of cases. This is an extremely important consideration in any aortic valve surgery. The most common non-valvular abnormality associated with BAV is thoracic aortic dilatation. This is thought to be due to alteration in aortic flow but is also due to cellular structural abnormalities including decreased fibrillin, which causes smooth muscle cell detachment and cellular death. Approximately 5% of patients with BAV disease will have aortic dissection, while at least one-third will have a serious complication because of aortic dilation. Coarctation of the aorta is also seen in 20% to 85% of cases. Presence of aortic coarctation and a poor result from aortic valve repair can lead to more rapid failure of the valve or aortic dissection. Conditions seen in association with BAV include labile hypertension, mitral regurgitation, and kidney/liver cysts (which give rise to concern that there could be an association between BAV and polycystic kidney disease).

BAV Genetics

Heritability of BAV has now been widely supported. Gene mutations in NOTCH1 have been noted in BAV. NOTCH1 is a transmembrane receptor that has a role in organ development. Other genetic mutations possibly tied to BAV are currently under investigation. Currently, chromosomes 18q, 5q, and 13q have been identified as possible genetic causes for BAV.

Screening

Although the 2% incidence of BAV may be higher than currently reported, there have been no guidelines suggesting BAV screening in the general population. Rather, screening for BAV in patients with first-degree relatives known to have BAV has been recommended by the American College of Cardiology (ACC) and the AHA. Screening includes echocardiography to screen for evidence of BAV and aortic root dilatation. If there is echocardiographic evidence of BAV and aortic root dilation, further investigation for aortopathy is recommended by obtaining a CT of the chest to obtain precise aortic root and ascending aortic measurements.

BAV Diagnosis

Type 1 BAV is the most common type. In these patients, presentation is typically from ages 40–60 years. In this population, aortic stenosis is most commonly seen. However, mixed aortic stenosis and aortic insufficiency is not uncommon. In Type 2 BAV, presentation usually is seen between the ages of 20 and 30. These patients tend to present with mild to severe aortic insufficiency and ascending aortic aneurysms. Physical examination will usually be limited to auscultation with most patients having a systolic ejection murmur associated with aortic stenosis that is best heard at the apex. An ECG will usually be normal; however, if there is moderate to severe aortic stenosis, associative LVH may be noted. The mainstay of BAV diagnosis is echocardiography (both transthoracic and transesophageal). With adequate images, there is a 92% sensitivity and a 96% specificity for definitive BAV diagnosis. Parasternal short axis views allow for the best and direct visualization of aortic valve cusps. In this view, the normal triangular opening shape is lost. The commonly described "fish mouth"-like appearance can be noted. This appearance is similar to that of the mitral valve. This "fish mouth" appearance is especially pronounced in systole. In diastole, the raphe can appear similar to a commissure of the third cusp, which can result in inaccurate diagnosis of tricuspid aortic valve rather than

BAV. Echocardiography cannot fully quantify the extent of any aortopathy; therefore, cardiac MRI and CT are used to assist with better diagnosis.

BAV Treatment

The only curative treatment for BAV is surgical replacement of the aortic valve. Medical therapy is used to alleviate symptoms and to slow progression of aortic valve disease and aortopathies. Joint guidelines from ACC/AHA suggest beta blockers as a first-line therapy in patients with BAV (Mordi & Tzemos, 2012). Angiotensin receptor blocker therapy may have a role, but there is lack of supporting evidence of efficacy. Surgical management is dependent on the patient. Valvular replacement is usually not deemed as practical because patients outgrow the prosthetic valve. The 2005 AHA/ACC guidelines suggest combined replacement of the ascending aorta if it is greater than 4.5 cm in diameter. Estimated 15-year freedom from complications was 86% in patients with an aortic diameter less than 4 cm, dropping down to 81% in those with 4–4.4 cm, and 43% in patients with an ascending aortic diameter 4.5 cm or greater. New techniques of repair such as transcatheter aortic valve implantation have been reported.

PHARMACOGENOMICS

As has been demonstrated in this chapter, cardiogenetics can play a huge role in disease development. Similarly, ICU nurses may be faced with challenges related to pharmacogenomics. Pharmacogenomics refers to the study of genetic/genomic differences in *multiple* genes' influence on variability in drug response (e.g., efficacy, toxicity). Pharmacogenetics refers to the study of how genetic differences in a *single* gene influence variability in drug response (e.g., efficacy, toxicity). Components of both pharmacogenomics and pharmacogenetics include drug targets and transporters, drug-metabolizing enzymes, pharmacodynamics, and pharmacokinetics. All of these factors play roles in the variability seen in drug efficacy and toxicity.

Other factors that contribute to drug distribution and action variability include age, gender, ethnicity/race, concomitant drug administration, concomitant diseases, psychosocial factors, and socioeconomic factors. When considering the clinical relevance of this emerging field, two questions should come to mind: 1) Can we predict who will derive an optimal response? and 2) Can we predict who will have toxicity? As these questions have been the cornerstone of research, evidence has supported that patient genotype determines optimal drug therapy approach; however, pathogen genotype can also determine optimal drug approach.

Drug Metabolism Pharmacogenetics

Drug metabolism considerations are considered pharmacogenetics rather than genomics because of their monogenic nature. This means that a single gene is the focus of the character difference. Drug metabolism mutations have a phenotype-to-genotype approach, meaning that the characteristics presented in the clinical setting are considered prior to exploring genetic mutations/cause. Drug metabolism can occur in several organs; the liver frequently has the greatest metabolic capacity and is the major site for drug metabolism. Chemical modifications to drugs occur so they can eventually be eliminated. These chemical reactions usually increase water solubility to promote elimination. In the case of genetic mutations, these chemical reactions may be halted, sped up, or altered in some manner. In the liver, the drug-metabolizing enzyme cytochrome P450 is well known. This enzyme has subunits that often have genetic mutations that cause significant clinical consequence.

Warfarin

The widely known drug warfarin (Coumadin®) has a narrow range between efficacy and toxicity. Warfarin metabolism and subsequent inactivation are mediated by CYP2C. There are two known variants: CYP2C9*2 and CYP2C9*3. These variants result in a protein with decreased function or nearly abolished function, respectively. With mutation of CYP2C9, there is up to three times higher risk of serious or life-threatening bleeding episodes in patients requiring warfarin therapy. Greater than 90% of deleterious CYP2C9 mutations are found in Caucasians. Clinical sensitivity for other ethnicities is currently still being investigated. Vitamin K epoxide reductase (VKOR) is the site of action for warfarin.

Vitamin K, the antidote for warfarin, regulates clotting in humans. The associated gene, VKORC1, has a common promoter variant that reduces the expression of the gene. This, therefore, lowers the amount of VKOR and leads to warfarin sensitivity and the need for markedly high doses of warfarin to reach therapeutic levels. The combination of the two CYP2C9 (*2 and *3) variants with the VKORC1 promoter mutations is estimated to account for 40% to 63% of therapeutic warfarin doing variability. Genetic testing is available; caution should be used when ordering. Mutations other than those previously described will not be detected. Mutations in other genes and nongenetic factors that may affect drug metabolism (e.g., drug–drug interactions) are not detected. Genetic variant detection does not replace the need for therapeutic drug monitoring or other appropriate clinical monitoring.

CYP2C19 Mutations

CYP2C19 protein regulation is controlled by the CYP2C19 gene. This protein, like CYP2C9, produces an enzyme that controls drug metabolism for several antidepressants (e.g., tricyclics, selective serotonin reuptake inhibitors), anti-epileptics (diazepam [Valium®], phenytoin [Dilantin®], phenobarbital [Luminal®]), proton pump inhibitors (omeprazole [Prilosec®], lansoprazole [Prevacid®], pantoprazole [Protonix®]), clopidogrel (Plavix®), beta blockers (propranolol, Inderal®), nonsteroidal anti-inflammatory drugs (indomethacin [Indocin®]), and warfarin. Three to five percent of Caucasians and 15% to 20% of Asians with CYP2C19 mutations are deemed "poor metabolizers" with no CYP2C19 function. In the case of clopidogrel, this could lead to considerable risk, including MI, stroke, and death. As a result, in 2010, the U.S. Food and Drug Administration put a black box warning on clopidogrel for healthcare providers and patients to be aware that CYP2C19 poor metabolizers, representing up to 14% of patients, are at high risk for treatment failure and that genetic testing for a CYP2C19 mutation is available. A Roche AmpliChip® CYP450 test is used to identify CYP2C19 and CYP2D6 mutations. Pharmacies have begun routine testing for this mutation when new clopidogrel prescriptions are received. Other CYP mutations, such as in CYP2D2, exist that may affect drug metabolism, including commonly used analgesic agents used in the ICU.

CARDIOGENETIC NURSING CONSIDERATIONS

Intensive care unit nurses employed at academic or tertiary centers, or both, will most likely provide care for patients with a genetic foundation for their disease process. Insomuch, these nurses should familiarize themselves with common cardiogenetic disorders that may be seen in patients routinely cared for. For those nurses who practice in smaller community hospitals, this does not mean that they will be excluded from seeing patients with cardiogenetic disorders. Given that many patients present without prior symptoms, this is especially true.

Careful review of pathophysiology is paramount. For example, when caring for a patient who has undergone surgical myectomy for HCM, the nurse must be aware that the left ventricle will require time to recover from the HCM-associated stiffness and high pressure gradient. As such, the patient will most likely be volume dependent for several hours in the postoperative phase. Therefore, early diuresis with diuretics should be avoided. Further, given postoperative patients have autodiuresis, extra volume may be required to maintain adequate filling pressures. Tachycardia should be avoided. This can usually be controlled by volume

resuscitation; pharmacologic intervention may also be required. Conversely, patients who undergo cardiac surgery and have DCM will require early diuresis because of their higher risk for CHF.

Patients with familial aortopathic disease will also have connective tissue problems. Many patients with MFS have spontaneous pneumothoraces; close observation after chest tube removal is required. Increased intrathoracic pressure created with vomiting can increase the risk for pneumothoraces; early use of anti-emetics should be employed.

SUMMARY

Understanding the importance of history taking of the patient with a focus on family health is crucial to the identification of genetic predisposition to cardiovascular disorders associated with hereditary.

CASE STUDY

On his first visit, a 55-year-old male presents with shortness of breath, fatigue, 1+ pitting edema in the lower extremities, and chest pain. His symptoms seem to have come on in a short period of time. Dilated cardiomyopathy is the differential diagnosis.

Critical Thinking Questions

1. What should be included in the history for this patient?
2. What are the cardiogenetic red flags to watch for during the interview process?
3. What are the screening guidelines for the first-degree relatives of patients with DCM?

Answers to Critical Thinking Questions

1. The 2009 HFSA guidelines recommend a careful family history for three generations or more for all patients with cardiomyopathy. Family history and pedigree analysis for unexplained heart failure before age 60 or sudden cardiac death in the absence of ischemic disease should be assessed for family members.

2. When completing family histories, there are cardiogenetic red flags to watch for during the interview process. These include:

   • "Heart attack" in a person younger than 50 years old (could be cardiomyopathy, aortic dissection, or arrhythmias)

- Two or more closely related family members on the same side of the family with the same or related condition (e.g., heart disease, arrhythmia, stroke)
- Unexplained sudden death (could be indicative of MI, cardiomyopathy, arrhythmia, aortic dissection)
- Individual who has been diagnosed with a specific type of hereditary disease (e.g., HCM, MFS)
- Coronary heart disease at an early age (males younger than 55, women younger than 65)
- Two or more family members with congenital heart defects/disease
- Family history of symptoms and procedures suspicious for hereditary arrhythmia syndrome: syncope, seizures, multiple family members with pacemaker/ICD, sudden death, sudden infant death syndrome

3. The 2009 HFSA genetic evaluation of cardiomyopathy guidelines recommend the following screening for first-degree relatives of patients with DCM. This screening should include: history (with special focus on heart failure symptoms, arrhythmias, presyncope, syncope), physical examination (special attention to cardiac/skeleton muscle systems), ECG, echocardiogram, and serum CK-MM. Even though initial screening may not reveal any problems, asymptomatic patients should be re-screened at 3- to 5-year intervals beginning in childhood or at any time symptoms begin to appear. Repeat clinical screening at 1 year is suggested in first-degree relatives with any abnormal clinical screening tests (Hershberger et al., 2009).

SELF-ASSESSMENT QUESTIONS

1. Pedigrees (also known as genograms) are schematic renderings of family history and should include _____ generation(s) of both paternal and maternal family history.
   a. One
   b. Two
   c. Three
   d. Four

2. With regard to cardiogenetics, females with the Duchene muscular dystrophy gene mutation should be evaluated for which disorder?
   a. Hypertrophic cardiomyopathy
   b. Arrhythmogenic right ventricular cardiomyopathy
   c. Dilated cardiomyopathy
   d. Left ventricular non-compaction cardiomyopathy

3. The 2009 HFSA genetic evaluation of cardiomyopathy guideline recommends screening for first-degree relatives of patients with DCM. If a first-degree relative has an abnormal clinical screening test, he or she should be reevaluated within which of the following time periods:
   a. 3 months
   b. 6 months
   c. 9 months
   d. 12 months

4. Most inherited cardiovascular diseases have a(n) _____ pattern.
   a. Autosomal dominant
   b. Autosomal recessive
   c. Y-linked inheritance
   d. X-linked inheritance

5. The "G" of the MOGE(S) classification stands for which of the following?
   a. Glycogen storage diseases
   b. Level of generation

c. Gradient pressures

d. Nature of genetic transmission

6. Which of the following is the most common cause of sudden cardiac death in young athletes?

   a. Hypertrophic cardiomyopathy

   b. Arrhythmogenic right ventricular cardiomyopathy

   c. Dilated cardiomyopathy

   d. Left ventricular non-compaction cardiomyopathy

7. Tendon manifestation of deposition of LDL-derived cholesterol is most often recognized in which tendon?

   a. Patellar

   b. Achilles

   c. Trapezoid

   d. Calcaneofibular

8. Diagnosis of Marfan syndrome may be misleading if relying totally on pedigree/family history because some patients have:

   a. a de novo genetic mutation.

   b. poor penetrance levels.

c. an autosomal dominant gene mutation.

d. glycogen storage diseases.

9. An easily usable screening test to determine joint flexibility for MFS diagnosis is the:

   a. Romberg test.

   b. Rhine Test.

   c. Steinberg's sign.

   d. Ghent nosology.

10. A distinct feature of Loeys-Dietz Syndrome is:

    a. severe muscle weakness.

    b. outflow obstruction.

    c. keloid formation.

    d. aortic aneurysms.

Answers to Self-Assessment Questions

1. b	6. a
2. c	7. b
3. d	8. a
4. a	9. c
5. d	10. d

Clinical Inquiry Box

Question: Are psychological well-being and health-related quality of life impacted by a family cardiac screening?

Reference: McGorrian, C., McShane, C., McQuade, C., Keelan, T., O'Neill, J., Galvin, J., . . . Codd, M. (2013). Family-based associations in measures of psychological distress and quality of life in a cardiac screening clinic for inheritable cardiac diseases: A cross-sectional study. *BMC Medical Genetics*, *14*, 1.

Objective: To determine the anxiety and depression burden associated with family-based cardiac screening, to examine whether these traits cluster within families, and to examine the associations between higher levels of anxiety and depression states in this population.

Method: Prospective survey of patients attending a cardiac screening clinic over 1 year. Two health measurement tools were used.

Results: Depression scores increased with age ($p < 0.0001$), indicating increasing prevalence of depressive symptoms, and the physical quality of life decreased with age ($p = 0.01$), indicating worsening physical health. Out of the 316 subjects, 62 had scores indicating risk of anxiety and depression, but the subjects did not have significantly higher depression or anxiety scores.

Conclusion: The approach of using a family screening clinic whereby the entire family comes in to be screened and then receives results together may be the best approach for genetic screening and counseling.

REFERENCES

Ackerman, M., Priori, S., Willems, S., Berul, C., Brugada, C., Brugada, R., . . . Zipes, D. P. (2011). HRSA/EHRA expert consensus statement on the state of genetic testing for the channelopathies and cardiomyopathies. *Heart Rhythm, 8*(8), 1308-1318.

Alam, M., Dokainish, H., & Lakkis, N. (2006). Alcohol septal ablation for hypertrophic obstructive cardiomyopathy: A systematic review of published studies. *Journal of Interventional Cardiology, 19*(4), 319-327.

Boileau, C., Jondeau, G., Mizuquchi, T., & Matsumoto, N. (2005). Molecular genetics of Marfan syndrome. *Current Opinion in Cardiology, 20*(3), 194-200.

Dahm, R. (2008). Discovering DNA: Friedrich Miescher and the early years of nucleic acid research. *Human Genetics, 122*(6), 565-581.

Elliott, P. (2003). Classification of cardiomyopathies: Evolution or revolution? *Journal of the American College of Cardiology, 62*(22), 2073-2074.

Ercan, T., Ekici, F., Atalay, S., & Nacar, N. (2005). The prevalence of bicuspid aortic valve in newborns by echocardiographic screening. *American Heart Journal, 150*(3), 513-515.

Gott, V., Greene, P., Alejo, D., Cameron, D., Naftel, D., Miller, D. C., . . . Pyeritz, R. E. (1999). Replacement of the aortic root in patients with Marfan's syndrome. *New England Journal of Medicine, 340*(12), 1307-1313.

Habashi, J., Judge, D., Holm, T., Cohn, R., Loeys, B., Cooper, T., . . . Diets, H. C. (2006). Losartan, an AT1 antagonist, prevents aortic aneurysm in a mouse model of Marfan syndrome. *Science, 312*(5770), 117-121.

Harmon, K. (2010). *Genome sequencing for the rest of us.* Retrieved from http://www.scientificamerican.com/article/personal-genome-sequencing/

Hayek, E., Gring, C., & Griffin, B. (2005). Mitral valve prolapse. *Lancet, 365*(9458), 507-518.

Hershberger, R., Lindenfeld, J., Mestroni, L., Seidman, C., Taylor, M., & Towbin, J. (2009). Genetic evaluation of cardiomyopathy—A Heart Failure Society of America practice guideline. *Journal of Cardiac Failure, 15*(2), 83-89.

MacCarrick, G., Black, J., Bowdin, S., El-Hamamsy, I., Frischmeyer-Guerrerio, P., Guerrerio, A., . . .

Dietz, H. C., III. (2014). Loeys-Dietz syndrome: A primer for diagnosis and management. *Genetics in Medicine, 16,* 576-587. Retrieved from http://www.nature.com/gim/journal/vaop/ncurrent/full/gim201411a.html

Maron, B. J. (2006). Contemporary definitions and classification of the cardiomyopathies. *Circulation, 113,* 1807-1816.

Maron, B. J. (2007). Surgical myectomy remains the primary treatment option for severely symptomatic patients with obstructive hypertrophic cardiomyopathy. *Circulation, 119*(20), 196-206.

Maron, B. J., & Zipes, D. P. (2005). Introduction: Eligibility recommendations for competitive athletes with cardiovascular abnormalities—General considerations. *Journal of the American College of Cardiology, 45*(8), 1318.

Masry, H., & Breall, J. A. (2008). Alcohol septal ablation for hypertrophic obstructive cardiomyopathy. *Current Cardiology Reviews, 4*(3), 193-197.

Mestroni, L., Rocco, C., Gregori, D., Sinagra, G., Di Lenarda, A., Miocic, S., . . . Camerini, D. (1999). Familial dilated cardiomyopathy: Evidence for genetic and phenotypic heterogeneity. *Journal of the American College of Cardiology, 34*(1), 181.

Mordi, I., & Tzemos, N. (2012). Bicuspid aortic valve disease: A comprehensive review. *Cardiology Research and Practice, 2012.* Retrieved from http://www.ncbi.nlm.nih.gov/pmc/articles/PMC3368178/

Newton, G. (2004). *Discovering DNA fingerprinting.* Retrieved from http://genome.wellcome.ac.uk/doc_wtd020877.html

Olson, T., Michels, V., Ballew, J., Reyna, S., Karst, M., Herron, K., . . . Anderson, J. L. (2005). Sodium channel mutations and susceptibility to heart failure and atrial fibrillation. *Journal of the American Medical Association, 293*(4), 447-453.

Pelter, M., Al-Zaiti, S., & Carey, M. (2014). Coronary artery dominance. *American Journal of Critical Care, 20*(5), 401-402.

Pyeritz, R. (2008). A small molecule for a large disease. *New England Journal of Medicine, 358*(26), 2829-2831.

Rand-Hendriksen, S., Lundby, R., Tjeldhorn, L., Andersen, K., Offstad, J., Ove Semb, S., Smith, J. Paus, B. & Geiran, O. (2015). Prevalence data on all Ghent features in a cross-sectional study of 87 adults with proven Marfan syndrome. *European Journal of Human Genetics, 17,* 1222–1230.

Repas, T., & Tanner, J. (2014). Preventing early cardiovascular death in patients with familial hypercholesterolemia. *Journal of the American Osteopathic Association, 114*(2), 99–108.

Roberts, W. (1992). Morphologic aspects of cardiac valve dysfunction. *American Heart Journal, 123*(6), 1610–1632.

Rombaut, L., Malfait, F., De Wandele, L., Cools, A., Thijs, Y., De Paepe, A., . . . Calders, P. (2011). Medication, surgery, and physiotherapy among patients with the hypermobility type of Ehlers-Danlos syndrome. *Archives of Physical Medicine and Rehabilitation, 92*(7), 1106–1112.

Ward, C. (2000). Clinical significance of the bicuspid aortic valve. *Heart, 83*(1), 81–85.

WEB RESOURCES

Aortopathy genetic testing: This document provides an overview of common genes associated with the different types of aortopathies as well as testing provided: http://ltd.aruplab.com/Tests/Pdf/100

Ehlers-Danlos National Foundation: This website has excellent information and support resources for patients with EDS as well as for healthcare providers: http://ednf.org

Warfarin genetic testing and overall dosing: http://warfarindosing.org/Source/Home.aspx

Glossary

ACORN CorCap™ cardiac support device: A polyester mesh fabric that is wrapped snugly around the ventricles. It provides passive support to the ventricles, which should reduce wall stress and prevent further remodeling.

Afterload: The resistance against which the left ventricle must pump to move blood forward. The pressure of the arterial systemic circulation produces afterload. Smooth muscle tone in the arterioles can increase the resistance to blood flow and increase afterload. Medications can alter the amount of resistance that arteriolar smooth muscle generates.

Alcohol septal ablation (ASA): A procedure performed in the catheterization lab to remove hypertrophied heart muscle. It entails injection of 100% alcohol into one of the branches of the coronary artery that leads to the enlarged septum and the hypertrophied myocardium; it is left in place for a few minutes. This results in immediate cell death to that area. The end result is improved blood flow as the hypertrophied myocardium is no longer obstructing blood flow.

Allograft: The transfer of an organ from one person to another. The donor is not a twin but is of the same species.

Allograft coronary artery disease (ACAD): Development of coronary artery disease in heart transplant patients. It can be described based on the degree of stenosis of the affected vessel(s). This disease is often associated with graft failure.

Alveolar-arterial oxygen gradient (A-a gradient): A method of measuring intrapulmonary shunt. The calculation is the difference between the concentration of alveolar oxygen entering the alveoli and the concentration of oxygen diffused into the arterial blood.

Ankle-brachial index: An assessment used to evaluate arterial blood flow to the lower extremities. Results of this calculation are used to rate the degree of peripheral artery disease and to determine if the saphenous vein is suitable for use during cardiac surgery.

Annuloplasty: Surgical repair of an ineffectual heart valve.

Aortic regurgitation: Incomplete closure of the aortic valve leaflets, resulting in a backflow of blood. There is a reflux of blood from the aorta into the left ventricle (LV) during diastole because the valve leaflets fail to close completely and remain tightly closed during diastole. Acute aortic regurgitation imposes a large volume load on the LV, which a normal heart cannot accommodate. The sudden increase in end-diastolic volume (preload) will result in increased left ventricular end-diastolic pressure and decreased cardiac output. Aortic regurgitation is identified by the presence of an early diastolic murmur that can be heard at the second and third intercostal spaces at the right sternal border and the second and fourth intercostal spaces at the left sternal border. The murmur of aortic regurgitation usually decreases in intensity and disappears before S1.

Aortic stenosis: Narrowing or constriction of the aortic valve that creates a pressure gradient. The aortic valve does not open completely, which creates a left ventricular outflow tract obstruction and increases both the workload and afterload of the left ventricle. The calcification of aortic stenosis is regarded as a proliferative and inflammatory process, similar to atherosclerosis.

Aortopathy: Any disease or malfunction of the aorta. There are five main aortopathic conditions that have clinical focus: Marfan syndrome, Loeys-Dietz syndrome, Ehlers-Danlos syndrome (Types I/II, IV, and VI), idiopathic thoracic aneurysm/dissection, and coarctation of the aorta.

Arterial pulse contour continuous cardiac output monitoring: A method that estimates cardiac output by use of pulse contour analysis; it is an indirect method based on analysis of the arterial pressure pulsation waveform. The key underlying concept is that the contour of the arterial pressure waveform is proportional to stroke volume. The arterial pressure waveform is used to calculate cardiac output, stroke volume variance, intrathoracic volumes, and extravascular lung water. These data may predict response to fluid therapy.

Assisted aortic end-diastolic pressure: The pressure in the aorta at the end of diastole when counterpulsation has assisted the cardiac cycle. It is usually lower than the unassisted end-diastolic pressure.

Assisted systole: The systolic aortic pressure when counterpulsation has assisted the cardiac cycle. It is usually lower than the unassisted systole due to the action of balloon deflation.

Atrial cuff technique (bicaval technique): A method used during heart transplantation in which the donated heart is attached to the recipient's atrial "cuffs."

Atrial septal defect (ASD): An opening between the right and left atria. Oxygenated blood leaves the left atrium and returns to the right atrium through this opening rather than continuing forward to deliver oxygen to cells, organs, muscles, and tissues throughout the body.

Balloon valvotomy/valvuloplasty: Use of a balloon to stretch open a narrowed heart valve or to break adhesions in a scarred valve.

Beating heart surgery: *See* **off-pump coronary artery bypass**.

Bicaval technique: A method used during heart transplantation in which the anastomoses are made in the superior and inferior vena cavae.

Biologic valves: Valves that are constructed from bovine, porcine, and human cardiac tissue.

Biventricular assist device (BiVAD): A type of mechanical support for the heart. It is used when both the right and left ventricles are failing. Blood is drained from each ventricle through cannulae to centrifugal pumps, which provide circulatory support in severely decompensated heart failure patients until a heart transplant can be performed. A BiVAD is typically used when a left ventricular assist device does not provide sufficient circulatory support.

Bridge to recovery: Use of a mechanical circulatory device (ventricular assist device [VAD]) to support circulation in patients with heart failure. If myocyte damage is not permanent, myocardial cells may regain their ability to function. The VAD supports the patient until heart function improves and is adequate without mechanical support.

Bridge to transplantation: Use of a mechanical circulatory device (ventricular assist device) to support circulation in patients with severe heart failure until a donor heart becomes available and a transplant can be performed.

Cardiac allograft vasculopathy: *See* **coronary artery vasculopathy**.

Cardiac catheterization: An invasive diagnostic test whereby a catheter is inserted and advanced into the heart chambers or coronary arteries. It reveals information about the blood pressure of the heart and the heart's ability to pump, blood flow in the heart chambers, presence and degree of narrowing of the coronary arteries, and valve function.

Cardiac output (CO): A measure of the amount of blood that is ejected by the heart each minute. It is affected by the individual's preload, afterload, and contractility.

Cardiogenetics: The specialized focus on genetics related to the cardiovascular system within humans.

Cardiomyopathies: A heterogeneous group of diseases of the myocardium associated with mechanical or electrical dysfunction, or both, that usually (but not invariably) exhibit inappropriate ventricular hypertrophy or dilatation and are due to a variety of causes that are frequently genetic. There are two categories of cardiomyopathies: primary and secondary. (*See* **primary cardiomyopathy** and **secondary cardiomyopathy**.)

Cardioplegia: A method of intentionally arresting the heart's motion with infusion of a solution to facilitate performance of cardiac surgery. The solution contains potassium (to decrease myocardial oxygen consumption and the rate of anaerobic metabolism while the heart is ischemic), magnesium (to decrease myocardial oxygen consumption), calcium (to decrease the chance of reperfusion injury), procaine (vasodilator and antiarrhythmic; may decrease dysrhythmias following aortic cross-clamping), bicarbonate (to counter the metabolic acidosis that occurs secondary to

anaerobic metabolism while the heart is in arrest), hypothermia (decreases myocardial oxygen consumption and increases the heart's tolerance to ischemia), mannitol (to decrease edema related to hypothermia and ischemia, and may minimize reperfusion injury), dextrose (to counter edema due to hypothermia and ischemia, and for continued energy production), amino acids (for energy production, may minimize reperfusion injury, and has a role as a scavenger for oxygen free radicals), and oxygenated blood (to optimize the heart's metabolic environment and minimize reperfusion injury). The patient's circulation is diverted to a heart–lung machine that takes over the function of these two organs. The heart is isolated from the body with cross-clamping of the aorta. A cold cardioplegic solution is then instilled to decrease myocardial oxygen consumption and increase the heart's tolerance to ischemia, thereby preventing heart damage during the procedure.

Cardiopulmonary bypass (CPB): The temporary rerouting of blood from the right atrium to the aorta via an oxygenator (bypass machine), thereby bypassing the heart and lungs during the surgical procedure.

Carotid bruit: A sound associated with turbulent blood flow that may indicate arterial stenosis.

Central venous oxygen saturation (ScvO$_2$): A method used to determine how much oxygen the tissues are extracting. It entails analysis of a blood sample from a central venous catheter.

Cold ischemia time: The time from cross-clamping of the donor heart, with subsequent excision and immersion of the heart in iced saline, to removal of the cross-clamp after the donor heart's implantation into the recipient.

Commissurotomy: A procedure that opens commissures (the contact area for the valve leaflets), which have developed scarring and do not open to allow blood to flow.

Contractility: The rate and ability of the myocardial muscle to shorten itself, or the amount of strength evidenced by the myocardium when it ejects blood. It is influenced by heart rate, neural factors, and certain metabolic states.

Coronary artery bypass grafting (CABG): *See* **surgical revascularization**.

Coronary artery vasculopathy (CAV): A type of stenosis caused by plaque in the coronary arteries. The lesions contain inflammatory cells (including T cells). Coronary artery vasculopathy is a major cause of long-term morbidity and mortality in heart transplant patients who survive past the first year. Innate and adaptive immune responses result in development of vascular lesions.

Cox Maze III procedure: A modification of a procedure that interrupts the reentrant pathways required for atrial fibrillation using surgical incisions. The Cox Maze III procedure remains the standard surgical therapy for atrial fibrillation. It entails a number of incisions being made on the right and left atria. "Maze" refers to the pattern of incisions made in the atrium. The incisions cause scarring, which does not conduct electricity, stops irregular electrical activity, and eradicates atrial fibrillation. The scarring also prevents future irregular electrical signals from developing.

Cox Maze IV procedure: A procedure that uses radiofrequency ablation to eradicate atrial fibrillation.

Deep sternal wound infection: Infection of the sternum and underlying structures.

Destination therapy: Use of a ventricular assist device in patients with severe heart failure who are not candidates for or have declined heart transplant.

Diastolic augmentation: The increase in pressure in the aorta above the balloon catheter that results with balloon inflation during diastole. This phenomenon increases perfusion in the coronary arteries and myocardial oxygen supply.

Dicrotic notch: When referring to an intra-aortic balloon pump or intra-arterial pressure monitoring, an area on the downstroke of the arterial waveform that results from the slight pressure increase created by closure of the aortic valve.

Dilated cardiomyopathy (DCM): One of the main causative factors for congestive heart failure. Dilated cardiomyopathy is characterized by dilatation and systolic dysfunction of one or both ventricles, with specific detriment to left ventricular function.

Dor procedure: Also known as endoventricular circular patch plasty repair. A procedure whereby the left ventricle is reconstructed using a purse-string suture to isolate nonfunctional segments of myocardium (rather than excising them) and a circular patch to control the shape of the ventricle. The Dor procedure is usually performed concomitantly with a coronary artery bypass graft.

Drug-eluting stent (DES): A metal tube or "scaffold" inserted into a coronary artery following dilation of the vessel with a balloon (balloon angioplasty). The tube is coated with a drug to prevent reblockage (restenosis) of the vessel.

Dynamic cardiomyoplasty (DCMP): An innovative technique whereby the latissimus dorsi muscle is wrapped around the heart. An implanted stimulator is then used to stimulate the muscle to contract in synchrony with ventricular contraction. Due to the borderline clinical improvement associated with this technique, DCMP is rarely used in the United States, though it remains in use in other areas.

Dynamic response test: *See* **square wave test**.

Ejection fraction (EF): The percentage of blood volume of the left ventricle that is ejected with each contraction. A normal ejection fraction is approximately 65–70%.

Electrical bioimpedance: A noninvasive method to determine cardiac output. Using this technology, cardiac output is identified by changes in impedance that take place as blood is ejected from the left ventricle into the aorta and is calculated from changes in thoracic impedance. Change in thoracic blood volume during the cardiac cycle can be used to calculate cardiac output.

Endoaneurysmorrhaphy: A procedure that involves excising an aneurysm and reapproximating the wall edges using a Dacron patch to control the shape and size of the ventricle. It is used to treat ventricular tachycardia. Although this approach attempts to restore more normal ventricular geography, data indicate that it does not improve left ventricular function.

Endoscopic atraumatic coronary artery bypass grafting (EndoACAB): A combination of two methods to perform off-pump coronary artery bypass grafting. The internal thoracic artery is harvested using an endoscopic approach, and the anastomosis is performed with direct visualization through a small thoracotomy incision.

Endovascular/"keyhole" procedure: A type of minimally invasive procedure. It entails use of a small (5-mm or 3-mm) endoscope to access the heart through the intercostal space. The 5-mm scope makes it easy to maneuver between ribs, increasing visibility, and has been used to close a patent ductus arteriosus, thereby eliminating the need for a thoracotomy. The digital camera and processing make pictures from the 5-mm scope better than the pictures provided by the traditional surgical 10-mm scope. The 3-mm scopes are designed to feel and work like standard instruments used by cardiac surgeons.

Endoventricular circular patch plasty repair: *See* **Dor procedure**.

Ethanol septal ablation: A procedure for relieving outflow obstruction symptoms that is accomplished by infusing ethanol into the first septal branch of the left anterior descending coronary artery via an angioplasty catheter. This technique reduces outflow tract obstruction, increases exercise capacity, and improves symptoms.

Ex-Maze procedure: A cutting-edge technique for the Maze procedure. It is performed endoscopically on the outside of a beating heart. The ablation device uses unipolar radiofrequency energy with vacuum-maintained contact and suction-controlled saline perfusion to ensure uniform energy transmission and transmural lesion development. Because the procedure is performed on a beating heart, atrial function can be monitored during treatment. Patients can convert to normal sinus rhythm during the procedure or within 6 weeks. The Ex-Maze procedure is less invasive and does not require cardiopulmonary bypass. It is safer, associated with less postoperative pain, and has fewer complications.

Extracorporeal membrane oxygenation (ECMO): Use of a machine that can provide oxygen to the blood while it is circulating outside of the body. Blood is removed from the body via a catheter, pumped through a machine to be oxygenated by an artificial lung, and returned to the body through another catheter. The heart and lungs are bypassed, providing both hemodynamic and respiratory support. Blood oxygenation is a distinct advantage with this technique.

Fast flush: *See* **square wave test**.

Geometric mitral reconstruction (GMR): A procedure in which an annuloplasty ring is used to restore a more normal mitral valve anatomy that has achieved favorable outcomes. Geometric mitral reconstruction has consistently resulted in significant improvements in ejection fraction. It is indicated for patients with cardiomyopathy and mitral regurgitation.

Graft closure: Failure of the harvested vein (graft) to maintain patency, usually due to platelet aggregation. Antithrombotic therapy is initiated to prevent this complication of coronary artery bypass surgery.

Heterotopic method: A heart transplantation technique utilizing end-to-end anastomoses of the donor to the superior vena cava, pulmonary artery, and aorta. The donor heart is placed "piggyback" to the recipient heart. This method may be used in patients with severe pulmonary hypertension or if there is a mismatch between the donor and recipient heart size. It is rarely used.

Hypertrophic cardiomyopathy (HCM): A condition in which the myocardium becomes abnormally thick or hypertrophied. The thickened myocardium makes it more difficult for the heart to pump blood. It is a common genetic cardiovascular disease characterized by abnormal myocytes leading to hypertrophy without dilatation and preserved systolic function. Hypertrophy is most severe in the ventricular septum. It is asymmetrical and usually occurs at the level of the left ventricular outflow tract, leading to subaortic stenosis or asymmetrical HCM. In addition, abnormal systolic anterior motion of the mitral valve contributes to the outflow obstruction.

Hypothermia: A decrease in internal (core) body temperature below normal values. Often, a temperature less than 95 °F (35 °C) is considered hypothermia.

Infective endocarditis: A condition that occurs when bacteria attach to and destroy the surface of a valve leaflet or chordae. If a valve is damaged, immune cells, platelets, and fibrin migrate to the site to initiate healing of the valve. If bacteria become trapped under layers of these cells, "clumps" of tissue (called vegetations) can develop on the valves and within the heart muscle (endocarditis). Vegetations may break off and become emboli.

Internal thoracic artery (ITA): An artery in the chest located adjacent to the left anterior descending coronary artery. There is one ITA on either side of the sternum. This artery is resistant to cholesterol buildup (atherosclerosis), which makes it a good choice for use as a graft in coronary artery bypass surgical procedures.

International Society for Heart & Lung Transplantation (ISHLT) grading system: The standardized cardiac biopsy system that is used to grade acute heart rejection.

Intra-aortic balloon pump (IABP): A mechanical device that is used to improve cardiac function on a temporary basis. It increases blood flow, oxygen delivery to the heart, and cardiac output, and decreases the amount of work the heart must do to eject blood through a process called counterpulsation.

Intrapulmonary shunt (IPS): The percentage of cardiac output that does not participate in gas exchange. This portion of blood passes through the lungs but is not exposed to ventilated alveoli, so gas exchange does not take place and the blood leaves the lungs desaturated.

Keyhole procedures: *See* **endovascular/ "keyhole" procedures**.

Left-to-right shunting: Diversion of blood from the left heart to the right heart, rather than forward into the systemic circulation. Oxygenated blood from the arterial circulation mixes with deoxygenated blood from the venous system. Chronic left-to-right shunting may cause right ventricular failure, tricuspid regurgitation, atrial arrhythmias, paradoxical embolization, and cerebral abscesses.

Left ventricular assist device (LVAD): A type of mechanical support for the left ventricle. Blood is drained from the apex of the left ventricle to a pump via an inflow cannula. It is returned to the body via an outflow cannula, which is attached to the aorta. The pump is housed in the pre-peritoneal space of the abdomen, near the stomach. A percutaneous driveline that is tunneled across the pre-peritoneal space to the left side of the body carries an electrical cable and air vent to the electrical controller outside the patient's body.

Lower and Shumway method: A method used during heart transplantation in which the donor heart is anastomosed to the left atrium, right atrium, pulmonary artery, and aorta.

Maze procedure: *See* **Cox Maze III procedure**.

Mean arterial pressure (MAP): The driving force for peripheral blood flow and the preferred pressure to be evaluated in unstable patients. It is measured electronically by first integrating the area under the arterial pressure waveform and then dividing by the duration of the cardiac cycle.

Mechanical assist device: A device used to support cardiac function over the short or long term. Mechanical circulatory support has three primary functions: bridge to transplantation, bridge to recovery, and destination therapy. Short-term, temporary devices are often used as bridge to recovery in the setting of acute cardiogenic shock or cardiopulmonary arrest. Under these circumstances, circulatory assistance provides immediate hemodynamic support, restoring blood flow to vital organs while decompressing the heart, avoiding pulmonary edema, and minimizing cardiac workload to maximize the patient's chances of recovery.

Mediastinitis: Inflammation of the mediastinum; an uncommon but severe complication following cardiac surgery. Its incidence is reportedly higher in patients who have undergone grafting with bilateral internal thoracic arteries.

Minimally invasive cardiac surgery (MICS): An approach to coronary artery bypass grafting surgery that entails use of a laparoscopic procedure to perform cardiac surgery. Minimally invasive cardiac surgery has also been defined as cardiac surgery without the use of cardiopulmonary bypass or sternotomy; rather, smaller incisions are made. This term also refers to various procedures used to bypass blocked coronary arteries.

Minimally invasive direct coronary artery bypass (MIDCAB): An approach to traditional coronary artery bypass grafting (CABG). Differences between the two approaches are threefold. First, the incision size is much smaller for MIDCAB; several 3- to 5-inch incisions are made between the ribs as compared to a 10- to 12-inch median sternotomy incision in conventional CABG procedures. Second, because MIDCAB is a beating heart procedure, no cardioplegia is instilled to stop the heart. Third, because MIDCAB is a beating heart surgery and no cardioplegia is instilled, cardiopulmonary bypass is not required for MIDCAB procedures. These procedures are performed on patients with one or two blockages to the right coronary artery, left anterior descending coronary artery, or its branches on the front of the heart.

Minimally invasive direct view: Techniques that were developed to repair or replace the mitral valve and repair or replace the aortic valve. The main benefit of minimally invasive direct view valve surgery is the avoidance of a median sternotomy. An 8-cm incision is made and cartilage is removed to allow for direct visualization of the valves.

Minute ventilation: The volume of gas exchange (inhaled and exhaled) in 1 minute. It is measured by multiplying respiratory rate and tidal volume.

Mitral regurgitation: Incomplete closure of the mitral valve leaflets, resulting in a backflow of blood into the left atrium during ventricular systole.

Mitral stenosis: Narrowing or constriction of the mitral valve that creates a pressure gradient. The narrowing creates resistance to the forward flow of blood into the left ventricle during diastole.

Mitral valve annuloplasty ring: A three-dimensional ring that improves mitral valve function and left ventricular shape.

Myocardial revascularization: Restoration of blood supply to the myocardium. It may be accomplished by either percutaneous intervention or surgery.

Myectomy: A procedure that involves excision of a section of subaortic septal muscle approximately 3–7 cm long and 3–12 g in weight, with or without mitral valve replacement. Left ventricular myectomy is recommended for patients with drug-refractory symptomatic outflow obstruction (peak gradient > 50 mmHg under resting conditions and/or gradient > 50 mmHg measured). Surgery may also be considered in symptomatic patients with documented outflow obstruction under physiologic exercise but with absent or very mild resting obstruction. One additional subset of patients may benefit from left ventricular myectomy: young, asymptomatic patients with documented severe outflow tract obstruction (gradient 75–100 mmHg).

Myxoma: A benign cardiac tumor. It causes obstruction of blood flow, which leads to the clinical presentation of heart failure; signs of central nervous system embolization; and constitutional symptoms such as fever, weight loss, fatigue, weakness, arthralgia, myalgia, or any combination of these. Tumor resection is the only effective treatment.

Negative inspiratory pressure: Also referred to as negative inspiratory force. The amount of negative pressure that the patient generates during a forced inspiration when working against an obstruction to flow. It is a reflection of a patient's ability to take a deep breath and generate a cough that is strong enough to clear secretions.

Nitric oxide (NO): A product that is released by endothelial cells. It produces vasodilation and increased vascular permeability.

Obesity: Obesity is defined based on body mass index (BMI). Obesity is defined as a BMI > 30 kg/m^2. Obese class I corresponds with a BMI of 30–34.99 kg/m^2, class II is a BMI of 35–39.99 kg/m^2, and class III is a BMI ≥ 40 kg/m^2.

Obesity hypoventilation syndrome (OHS): A condition in which a person with obesity has a CO_2 level greater than 45 mmHg while awake.

Off-pump coronary artery bypass (OPCAB): Also known as a beating heart procedure. This type of minimally invasive cardiac surgery entails a median sternotomy or thoracotomy incision; no bypass machine is required. The surgeon sews the grafts onto the beating heart using specialized instruments to stabilize the myocardial tissue. Off-pump coronary artery bypass may be performed on patients needing four or five vessels repaired, as compared with minimally invasive direct coronary artery bypass, where only one or two vessels can be repaired. With OPCAB, an artery or vein from the lower extremities is used to make the bypass.

Orthotopic heart transplant: A heart transplant approach that entails replacing the recipient heart with the donor heart.

Overdamped waveform: A situation in which a pressure waveform is sluggish and has an exaggerated or falsely widened and blunt tracing. It will cause the patient's systolic pressure to be recorded as falsely low and the diastolic pressure to be recorded as falsely high.

Oxygen consumption: The amount of oxygen used by the body's tissues.

Oxygen delivery: The amount of oxygen that is carried to the body's tissues each minute.

PaO$_2$/FiO$_2$ ratio: An index of oxygenation. A PaO$_2$/FiO$_2$ ratio of less than 200 is associated with a significant intrapulmonary shunt.

Papillary fibroelastoma: A benign cardiac tumor that occurs on the heart valves and may cause obstruction or central nervous system embolization.

Paroxysmal nocturnal dyspnea (PND): A feeling of shortness of breath that awakens the patient. It is usually relieved when the patient assumes an upright position.

Partial left ventriculectomy: A procedure to restore the proper mass-to-diameter ratio for the left ventricle. In this procedure, a section of the left ventricular wall from the apex to the mitral annulus is removed, and the edges are reapproximated. Improvements in signs of heart failure and ejection fraction have been achieved with this technique. Because other surgical procedures have achieved results superior to those produced with the partial left ventriculectomy, this procedure is no longer in use in most of North America; however, it is still used in other areas where cardiac transplantation is less readily available.

Percutaneous mitral balloon valvotomy (PBMV): *See* **commissurotomy**. This technique has very successfully reduced left atrial gradient, increased mitral valve area, and improved symptoms of mitral stenosis.

Percutaneous transluminal coronary angioplasty (PTCA): A technique that uses an arterial catheter and various mechanical means to increase the diameter of diseased coronary arteries, thereby improving blood flow.

Pericardiectomy: Surgical removal of part of the membrane that surrounds the heart (pericardium). It is usually performed to treat inflammation and prevent collection of fluid in the pericardial sac (between the pericardium and heart), which can cause hemodynamic compromise from poor cardiac filling and emptying.

Pharmacogenetics: The study of how genetic differences in a single gene influence variability in drug response (e.g., efficacy, toxicity). Components of both pharmacogenomics and pharmacogenetics include drug targets and transporters, drug-metabolizing enzymes, pharmacodynamics, and pharmacokinetics.

Pharmacogenomics: The study of how genes affect the person's response to drugs.

Phlebostatic axis: An anatomic landmark located at the fourth intercostal space, midpoint of the anterior–posterior diameter. Leveling at the phlebostatic axis is performed to eradicate the effects of hydrostatic forces on the hemodynamic pressures.

Phrenic nerve injury: A complication following cardiac surgery with cardiopulmonary bypass. The extent of injury can range from neuropathy to paralysis of the diaphragm. It is often reported to be attributed to the use of hypothermia, application of ice slush around the heart, and harvesting of the internal thoracic artery that occur during surgery.

Postcardiotomy cardiogenic shock: Heart failure that develops as a result of heart surgery or a heart attack.

Preload: The pressure found in the left ventricle at the end of diastole. It is sometimes referred to as left ventricular end-diastolic pressure. Right-sided preload is the pressure found in the right atrium at the end of diastole.

Primary cardiomyopathy: The heart is predominantly the main organ affected. Primary cardiomyopathies are then subdivided into those that are genetic, mixed (predominantly nongenetic or less commonly genetic), or acquired. The most commonly known cardiomyopathies include dilated cardiomyopathy, hypertrophic cardiomyopathy (HCM), left ventricular non-compaction cardiomyopathy (LVNCC), arrhythmogenic right ventricular cardiomyopathy (ARVC), and restrictive cardiomyopathy. Hypertrophic cardiomyopathy, LVNCC, and ARVC are classified as genetic cardiomyopathies.

Prosthetic valves (mechanical valves): Valves that are manufactured from manmade materials such as metal alloys, pyrolytic carbon, and Dacron. Mechanical prosthetic valves are more durable and last longer than biologic valves.

Pulmonary hypertension: High blood pressure in the arteries that supply the lungs and right side of the heart. It develops when these vessels become constricted or obstructed, which slows blood flow. The result is an increase in pressure in the pulmonary arteries, making it more difficult for the right ventricle to eject blood to the pulmonary arteries.

Pulmonary stenosis: Narrowing or constriction of the pulmonic valve that creates a pressure gradient.

Pulse oximetry: A noninvasive method of monitoring the percentage of hemoglobin that is saturated with oxygen.

Pulse pressure variation (PPV): An alternative, less invasive method of evaluating cardiac output. It may be used as a means for determining the patient's ability to respond to fluid. Pulse pressure variation is the difference between the maximum and minimum values of the arterial pulse pressure during one mechanical breath divided by the mean of the two values. In the evaluation of the Frank-Starling curve, an increase in preload causes a decrease in PPV; decreasing preload causes an increase in PPV and contractility.

Pulsus alternans: An exaggeration of the normal variation in the pulse during the inspiratory phase of respiration, in which the pulse becomes weaker as the person inhales and stronger as the person exhales. It is an indicator of the presence of severe ventricular systolic failure and decreased myocardial contractility.

Right-to-left shunting: The flow of blood from the right to left side of the heart, usually through an opening between the two atria or ventricles. Great vessels in the chest may be affected as well. Right-to-left shunting can be attributed to a patent foramen ovale, especially with conditions that increase right atrial pressure (e.g., tricuspid stenosis). An example is a patient with an atrial septal defect. The affected patient may have periods of cyanosis.

Right ventricular assist device (RVAD): A type of mechanical support for the right ventricle. Blood is drained through a pump from the right ventricle to the pulmonary artery.

Robot-assisted coronary artery bypass (RACAB): A cutting-edge surgical technique. Unaccommodating places is what robot-assisted surgery is about; the human surgeon is not optimized for tiny spaces. In RACAB, the surgical robot consists of a collection of wristed tools called manipulators, which receive digital instructions from an interfaced computer. The surgeon, who is seated at a computer console with a three-dimensional display, acts as the "driver" of the computer. The surgeon initiates the digital instructions by controlling the hand grips. By using the hand grips, the surgeon's hand movements at the console are then duplicated in the robot, with software filtering out physiologic hand tremors.

Saphenous vein: A vein in the patient's leg that runs near the leg's surface. It is used as a graft for coronary artery bypass procedures. There are actually two saphenous veins in the leg—the great (large) and small veins. When harvested for bypass procedures, long incisions are usually made. Almost directly upon harvest, the surface of the saphenous vein becomes vulnerable to platelet aggregation because of the loss of the vascular endothelium. For this reason, patients require anti-thrombotic therapy to prevent graft closure.

Secondary cardiomyopathy: Involves another organ besides the heart.

Square wave test: Also referred to as a fast flush or dynamic response test; a test that is performed to ensure that the waveforms that appear on the monitoring screen accurately reflect pressures. It is accomplished by pulling and releasing the "pigtail" or squeezing the button of the flush device so that the flow through the tubing increases (from 3 mL/hr obtained with a pressure bag inflated to 300 mmHg). The sudden rise in pressure in the system generates a square wave on the monitor oscilloscope.

Stabilizer: A device used in minimally invasive cardiac surgery that provides a direct view of the operating field, dampens the movement of the epicardium, and permits the surgeon to maintain a nontraumatic grip on the beating heart. The device helps the surgeon isolate the diseased vessel and stabilizes the localized region of epicardium for anastomosis.

Steroid pulse: Administration of large doses of steroids over a short period of time to treat heart transplant rejection.

Stroke volume: The amount of blood ejected by the left ventricle with each contraction. Stroke volume is affected by the amount of blood in the ventricle and by the force of contraction of the ventricle. It can also be affected if the aortic valve restricts flow out of the left ventricle.

Stroke volume variation (SVV): An alternative, less invasive method of evaluating cardiac output. It may be used as a means for determining the patient's ability to respond to fluid. Stroke volume variation occurs due to changes in intrathoracic pressure during spontaneous breathing. It produces data on changes in preload that occur with mechanical ventilation. Stroke volume variation is the difference between the maximum and minimum stroke volume during one mechanical breath relative to the mean stroke volume.

Subendocardial resection (SER): A procedure that involves surgical removal of scar tissue, portions of an aneurysm, or other sites of abnormal electrograms. It is used to treat ventricular tachycardia.

Superficial sternal wound infection: An infection involving only the skin and subcutaneous fat. It is characterized by drainage from the wound and local inflammation while the underlying sternum remains stable.

Surgical anterior ventricular endocardial restoration (SAVER): A procedure that is a modification of the original Dor procedure. It is associated with a significant reduction of left ventricular volume and a significant increase in ejection fraction as well as significant reductions in hospitalizations for heart failure.

Surgical revascularization: Also known as coronary artery bypass grafting (CABG). Use of arterial or venous vessels to create a new pathway for blood to reach the coronary arteries, thereby "bypassing" a stenosis.

Sympathomimetics: Agents that activate adrenergic receptors by direct receptor binding, promotion of norepinephrine (NE) release, blockade of NE reuptake, and inhibition of NE inactivation.

Systolic pressure variation (SPV): An alternative, less invasive method of evaluating cardiac output. It may be used as a means for determining the patient's ability to respond to fluid. SPV is the difference between the maximum and minimum systolic blood pressure during one mechanical breath.

Tidal volume: The amount of air inhaled during a normal breath (versus a forced inhalation).

Total artificial heart (TAH): A treatment alternative for patients with biventricular failure who are hospitalized candidates for heart transplant. A TAH replaces the function of both ventricles and the four heart valves. It is implanted in the patient's chest and attached to the atria. Tubes from the ventricles continue from the patient's chest to a power-generating console. The TAH can deliver cardiac output at a rate as high as 9.5 L/min. It reportedly augments renal and hepatic blood flow and improves survival of heart transplant patients with preoperative biventricular failure.

Totally endoscopic coronary artery bypass (TECAB): A method of performing off-pump coronary artery bypass grafting. It entails using endoscopy, as opposed to the minimally invasive direct coronary artery bypass approach, which uses small thoracotomy incisions.

Transmyocardial laser revascularization (TMR): A procedure whereby transmyocardial channels are created from the epicardium into the ventricle via a laser. The channels then allow blood from the ventricle to reach the myocardium directly.

Transplantation: The surgical removal of a diseased heart and replacement with a healthy donor heart.

Transplant vasculopathy: Accelerated coronary artery disease in the transplanted heart.

Tricuspid regurgitation: Incomplete closure of the tricuspid valve leaflets, resulting in a backflow of blood.

Tricuspid stenosis: Narrowing or constriction of the tricuspid valve, which creates a pressure gradient.

Tricuspid valve: The heart valve that is located between the right atrium and ventricle, near the atrioventricular node, right coronary artery, and coronary sinus. Its function is to maintain forward flow of blood. The tricuspid valve has an annular ring and three leaflets connected via chordae tendineae to papillary muscles that are integrated with the right ventricle.

Unassisted aortic end-diastolic pressure: The pressure in the aorta at the end of diastole when counterpulsation via the balloon pump has not assisted that cardiac cycle.

Unassisted systole: The systolic aortic pressure when counterpulsation has not assisted the cycle.

Underdamped waveform: A situation in which a pressure waveform has an overresponse, revealed visually as an exaggerated, narrow, and artificially peaked tracing. In this case, the waveform overestimates the patient's systolic pressure and underestimates the diastolic pressure.

Valvuloplasty: A procedure that entails insertion of a balloon to stretch or enlarge the valve opening.

Venous oxygenation saturation (SvO_2): A method used to determine how much oxygen the tissues are extracting. Venous oxygen sat-

uration reveals the association between oxygen delivery (the amount of oxygen that is carried to the tissues each minute) and oxygen consumption (the amount of oxygen used by the tissues).

Ventricular assist device (VAD): A device used for longer term mechanical circulatory support. This implanted mechanical pump is used in patients with end-stage heart disease. Ventricular assist devices assist a weakened heart by pumping blood throughout the body.

Ventricular reconstruction: Techniques that are based on the principle that the ventricular wall tension is proportional to the left ventricular radius and pressure and inversely proportional to the wall thickness (Law of Laplace). By changing the size and shape of the ventricle, these techniques seek to reduce wall tension and improve left ventricular function. Specifically, surgical reconstruction techniques remove or isolate dysfunctional myocardium, reduce the diameter of the ventricle, and attempt to restore a more elliptical ventricular shape. Additional goals are to relieve ischemia by revascularization, if possible, and to further reduce ventricular size and volume via mitral valve repair.

Ventricular septal defect (VSD): An opening in the wall (septum) between the right and left ventricles. The result of this opening is the return of oxygenated blood in the left ventricle to the right ventricle, rather than the blood continuing forward into the systemic circulation to deliver oxygen to the cells, organs, muscles, and tissues. A VSD also results in an increase in ventricular workload because greater volumes of blood are being circulated; this effect ultimately leads to heart failure.

Vital capacity: The amount of air that can be exhaled forcibly following a full inspiration.

Zero balance: A process of establishing atmospheric pressure as zero to obtain accurate hemodynamic values.

Index

B

N

S